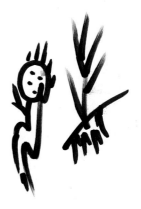

E-Z ECG Rhythm Interpretation

Henry B. Geiter, Jr., RN, CCRN

F. A. DAVIS COMPANY • Philadelphia

F. A. Davis Company
1915 Arch Street
Philadelphia, PA 19103
www.fadavis.com

Printed in the United States of America

Last digit indicates print number: 10 9 8 7 6 5 4 3 2 1

Acquisitions Editor: Lisa B. Deitch
Developmental Editor: Anne-Adele Wight
Project Editor: Ilysa H. Richman
Art and Design Manager: Carolyn O'Brien

As new scientific information becomes available through basic and clinical research, recommended treatments and drug therapies undergo changes. The author(s) and publisher have done everything possible to make this book accurate, up to date, and in accord with accepted standards at the time of publication. The author(s), editors, and publisher are not responsible for errors or omissions or for consequences from application of the book, and make no warranty, expressed or implied, in regard to the contents of the book. Any practice described in this book should be applied by the reader in accordance with professional standards of care used in regard to the unique circumstances that may apply in each situation. The reader is advised always to check product information (package inserts) for changes and new information regarding dose and contraindications before administering any drug. Caution is especially urged when using new or infrequently ordered drugs.

ISBN 0-8036-1043-2 978-0-8036-1043-9

Library of Congress Cataloging-in-Publication Data
Geiter, Henry B.
     E-Z ECG rhythm interpretation / by Henry B. Geiter, Jr.
        p. ; cm.
     Includes bibliographical references and index.
     ISBN-13: 978-0-8036-1043-9
     ISBN-10: 0-8036-1043-2
     1. Electrocardiography—Interpretation. 2. Heart—Diseases—Diagnosis.
     I. Title.
     [DNLM: 1. Electrocardiography. 2. Heart Diseases—diagnosis.
     WG 140 G313e 2006]
     RC683.5.E5G45 2006
     616.1'207547—dc22
                                        2005026200

PREFACE

So, you want to learn how to interpret ECGs. It may surprise you to learn that you already know some of the core concepts. Do you know what a superhighway is? Do you know how a tollbooth works? Have you watched a teacher quickly silence a rowdy classroom? Have you ever seen a boxing match or watched a football game? If you answered "yes" to any of these questions, then you're already on your way to interpreting ECGs.

I believe the best way to learn something new is to relate it to something common, some everyday thing that you already understand. Some people call this "learning by analogy"; I call it using what you know to learn something new. You see, the difference between prior knowledge and new knowledge can be as simple as a difference in descriptive language. The concepts of ECG interpretation aren't radically different from things you already know; we just describe them using a new set of words and a new set of rules. Instead of screaming children, we talk about ventricular fibrillation; instead of a tollbooth, we see the atrioventricular node; where you watch a boxing match, we observe AV node block; where you see superhighways, we see bundle branches. This book uses ordinary, familiar ideas to help you understand the heart and soul of ECG interpretation.

Learning ECG terminology is comparable to learning a foreign language. Imagine traveling to France, Italy, or Japan. The first time you visit, you won't be too familiar with the language. You may try to learn some French, Italian, or Japanese before your trip, but when you try to use your limited knowledge, you'll make all kinds of mistakes. You run into the same difficulties when you first try to speak ECG language. But after you've used this book for a while, you'll learn vocabulary, grammar, and exceptions to the rules. If you go on to study ECG in more depth, you'll soon be speaking like a native.

This book teaches you the basics: words and sentence construction. When you study the language of a country you plan to visit, you learn important questions like "Where am I?" or "Where is the bathroom?" You'll be able to understand a lot of what you hear—maybe not word for word, but you'll get the general idea. In ECG language, you'll learn to identify rhythms. Once you can do that, you're ready to visit ECG country (float to the telemetry or step-down unit or work as a monitor tech). When you visit this new country, you may not understand everything you hear, but you'll understand enough to ask intelligent questions and answer simple ones. You'll still be a tourist, but you won't sound so much like one. The words you know will become familiar and comfortable; meanwhile, new words and sentence structures will begin to sound comprehensible, if not completely clear yet. For many of you, this is as far as you need or want to go in learning ECG language. For those who want to go farther, more complex material abounds.

If you study ECG interpretation in greater depth, you will learn more complex sentence structure, more vocabulary, and some exceptions to the rules you learned in the first book (think of "*i* before *e* except after *c*"). You'll speak ECG as if you'd been doing it all of your life, although natives will be able to tell that you're really a well-educated tourist. (Yes, I know there are no true natives of ECG, but let's pretend.) You will be able to ask more complex questions, like "How do I get to the grocery store at 3rd and Elm?" and the more complex answers will make sense. In ECG language, you will learn treatments, new rules, exceptions to rules, and secrets of rhythm interpretation. In practical terms, you can emigrate to ECG land (become a staff nurse on the telemetry or step-down unit) and hold your own while you become even more comfortable with the language. Conversation will get more interesting: you'll exchange ideas with tourists, émigrés, and, yes, natives.

If you explore ECG interpretation as far as you can go, the subtle nuances of the language—the slang, idioms, and euphemisms—will become your own. You will finally become a native speaker. Tourists and émigrés will depend on you to help them learn the language, and you'll answer all their questions or at least know where to direct them for the answers. They'll turn to you as the resource person, the wise provider of answers, and the mentor for the next generation of tourists.

Preface

This book is structured for your benefit. I've devoted it to the basics so you can focus on mastering what you need to know before you can move on to the next level. Many ECG books—"everything to everybody" books—cram too much information between their covers; in fact, this type is prevalent in bookstores. As a result, the inexperienced reader often has to decide what's important to learn and what isn't.

Think about your grammar school career, starting with kindergarten. In every beginning course, whether language, mathematics, or science, you most likely used one book. When you completed that first course and that first book, the next course moved you on to a new, slightly more advanced book, and the next course, to one still more advanced.

Or think of undergraduate nursing education. When I was in nursing school, learning how to take a blood pressure in the first semester, I had a book that showed me the steps in case I forgot them. Lots of practice helped me learn my new skill on both a mental and a physical level. The next semester—in a different course, using a different book—I learned about conditions that can cause high or low blood pressure. I put this knowledge into clinical practice during the next several weeks, connecting actual patients with what I knew about blood pressure and other health issues. The following semester—using a third book and building on the previous two semesters—I learned about how the medications used to treat high or low blood pressure worked. At that point, with this minimal amount of knowledge, I was able to work in the hospital environment, where I continued to learn from other books, my clinical experiences, and my coworkers. I've brought the same concept to ECG interpretation: it's a new language, which you must acquire in easy steps and use every day to set it in your mind.

This book will teach you the basics of interpreting ECG rhythms and will prepare you for taking the next step toward fluency. Stick around, and together we'll build your language skills slowly but logically. If you go far enough in your studies, you can step off a plane in ECG land with the exact degree of fluency you want.

ACKNOWLEDGMENTS

Writing a book, especially a complex, technical book such as this one, is a daunting task. It took years to hone my original manuscript into the simple text you see today. There are a number of people who deserve credit for this book. The first is my Publisher (Saint) Lisa (Biello) Deitch. She took a chance on me and my unique way of explaining this complex material. Her ebullient personality was a major factor in my persevering through this long, arduous task. Her patience qualifies her as a saint, at least to me!

Many of my coworkers at the variety of Pinellas County medical institutions in which I have worked in my 15-year career provided me with some of the great strips that appear in this book. They also helped me refine my explanations and analogies by asking for my assistance in interpreting ECG strips and then sitting through my several explanations. We discovered together what worked best, and I thank them for asking and listening. Some who consistently provided me with "good" strips and listened to more than their fair share of explanations are Sherri Wenzel, Aurelia Miller, and Matt Handwerk.

There are a few people who went above and beyond, providing encouragement when I thought I would never finish the book. To Dr. Pyhel, a patient cardiologist; to David Deering, Krissy Sfarra, and Tina Lemiere, three nursing students who are currently working as ECG and Patient Care techs and who bring me many ECGs to see if I can use them; to Debbie Vass, my ever-optimistic boss; and to Cathy Massaro, a social worker with special skills, I offer my appreciation for their constant support and their belief in my ability to accomplish this almost overwhelming task.

Creativity is not something that comes easily to me; it flourishes best when I am surrounded by creativity. To that end, I must thank people whom I've never met but who provided a creative environment for my writing and fostered the development of the analogies found in this book; they were whispering in my ears every time I sat down to write. Elton John, Billy Joel, Helen Reddy, Tori Amos, Queen, James Taylor, David Bowie, and Dr. Hook are just a few of the artists whose musical creativity allowed me to achieve a state of mind in which I became more creative, more at ease, and more self-confident than I could have been without them. They each have a signed, dedicated copy of this book should they be interested.

Of course, any list of acknowledgements would be incomplete without mentioning my mother, Mary Cushman. Besides allowing me to survive my childhood, a test of tolerance if there ever was one, she instilled a desire to do more than just know, more than just understand, but to learn deeply and fully; so fully that the knowledge seeps out my pores. She is a smart lady, but she would rarely give me an answer to a question. She would question me and help me figure out the answer, or we would sometimes look up the answer together and discuss the topic. "What do you think?" was her mantra. She was a firm believer in the adage, "Give a man a fish and he eats for a day, teach a man to fish and he eats for a lifetime." My belly is full, I will never want for fish, and this book will, I hope, help others to learn to fish for themselves, too.

Finally, but most importantly, I must thank my family: my wife Lynn and my three children, Ryan, Kim, and Hope. The hour after hour I sat at my desk banging out manuscript on the keyboard, scanning the more than 1000 strips that went into developing this book, and reviewing editorial changes and artwork not only boggled the mind but diverted my time and attention from them. (Also, they put up with the deluge of ECG strips that inundated the house—well over 4000 in all.) They gave me the time to accomplish this dream of writing an ECG book.

Denise Thornby, RN, MS, CNAA
Director, Education & Professional Development
Virginia Commonwealth University Health System
Richmond, Virginia

Eleanor Elston, RN, BTech, MCE
Educational Consultant
Vancouver Health Authority and Elston Learning and Leading Solutions
Victoria, British Columbia
Canada

Jennifer Whitley, RN, MSN, CNOR
Instructor
Huntsville Hospital
Huntsville, Alabama

Barb Durham, RN, BSN, CNRN, CCRN
Critical Care Educator, Staff Development
Salinas Valley Memorial Healthcare System
Salinas, California

Samantha Venable, RN, MS, FNP
Professor
Saddleback College
Mission Viejo, California

Lori Baker, RN, CNCC (C), CCCN(C), Dip. B. Admin.
Surgical Nurse Educator (LGH)
Lions Gate Hospital and The Justice Institute of B.C.
North Vancouver, British Columbia
Canada

Susan Moore, PhD, RN
Professor Nursing
New Hampshire Community Technical College
Manchester, New Hampshire

Faith Addiss, BSN, RN
Instructor/Principal
Bryant & Stratton College
Buffalo, New York

Consultants

Catherine Richmond, MSN
Professor of Nursing
State University of New York, Alfred State College
Alfred, New York

Rita Tomasewski, RN, MSN, ARNP, CCRN
Cardiovascular Clinical Nurse Specialist
St. Francis Health Center
Topeka, Kansas

Contents

Contents

Contents

SECTION

1

Learning the Basics

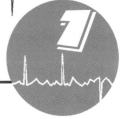

A Hearty Tour

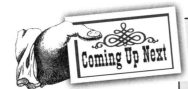

Coming Up Next

○ Where is the heart located?

○ How big is the normal heart?

○ What protects the heart?

○ What is the path that blood takes through the heart?

○ What is the purpose of the valves in the heart?

○ How does the heart get the blood it needs?

○ What is cardiac output and how can it be changed?

An Elegant Design

The heart is a powerful, complex, beautifully designed organ. In fact, the heart is a muscle. It's placed a little off center, just left of the middle of the chest, and tilts slightly down and to the left. In front of it is a large, wide, flat bone called the *sternum.* This bone is connected to the ribs on both sides and protects the heart from physical injury. The sternum in front, the spine in back, and the ribs on both sides form a cage that can absorb shock from trauma or stop objects from penetrating the chest wall and puncturing the heart (Fig. 1–1).

The size of a person's heart is as individual as the person. It depends on characteristics such as stature, physical condition, age, and sex. In the average adult, the heart is a little larger than a 3- by 5-inch index card. A good rule of thumb is that the heart is generally a little larger than the person's closed hand. As with all muscles, the well-conditioned heart weighs more because the muscle is larger.

HOW IT WORKS

To put it simply, the heart is a pump, just like the pump in your fish tank or pool. Similarly, there are two basic components to understand—the mechanical aspect, or how the pump does its job, and the electrical aspect, or what drives the pump. This chapter is dedicated to the basics of the mechanical aspects, while the rest of the book is devoted to the electrical aspects.

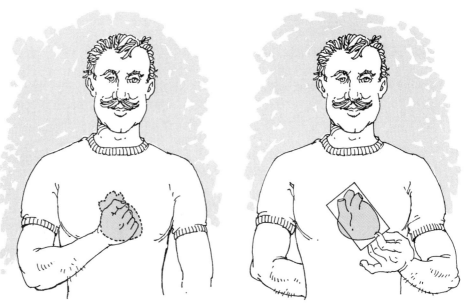

Estimate of normal heart size.

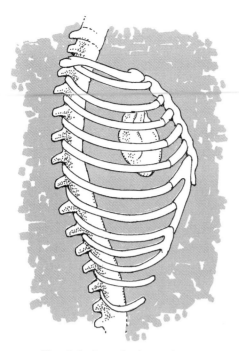

Fig. 1-1 Protection for your heart.

The heart is divided neatly into a right side and a left side (Fig. 1–2). The right side receives blood returning from the body. This blood is full of waste products, mostly carbon dioxide, and is depleted of oxygen by the tissues of the body. The blood is pumped into the blood vessels in the lung; there the red blood cells dispose of the carbon dioxide and pick up a fresh supply of oxygen.

Meanwhile, the left side of the heart receives the oxygen-rich blood from the blood vessels in the lungs and proceeds to pump the blood to all parts of the body. This blood then gives up some of its oxygen to all the various cells, allowing them to function, takes the waste products from the cells, and returns to the right side of the heart.

This sounds like a simple process: from the right side of the heart to the lungs, from the left side of the heart to the body, and back to the right side of the heart. Usually this happens more than a billion times in our lives without difficulty. However, it really is a complicated event and must be well coordinated to take place efficiently.

HOW IT'S PUT TOGETHER

In addition to having a right side and a left side, the heart contains four *chambers,* two on either side (Fig. 1–3). The upper chambers are called *atria,* which means "corridors" in Latin. Each *atrium* (the singular form of "atria") is a collection chamber for the blood when it returns to the heart, whether it returns from the body on the right or from the lungs on the left. The lower chambers, called *ventricles* (*ventricle* means "little belly"), receive the blood from the atria. Their job is to pump the blood out of the heart. The right ventricle pumps blood to the lungs, and the left ventricle pumps it to the rest of the body (Table 1–1).

The Value of Valves

To maintain an orderly flow of blood in only one direction—forward—we need something to help control the backward flow. Since the right atrium and right ventricle are connected, what stops the blood from going back into the right atrium when the right ventricle contracts? Well, think

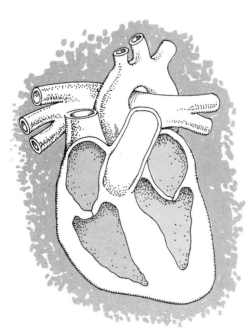

Fig. 1-2 Learning to distinguish left from right.

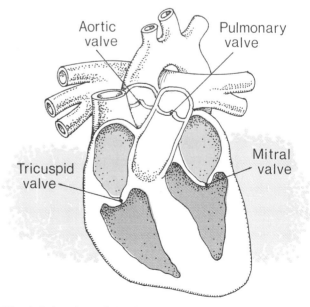

Aortic valve

Pulmonary valve

Tricuspid valve

Mitral valve

Fig. 1-3 Learning to distinguish top from bottom and to identify the heart's four valves.

3

Table 1–1 Where does the blood go now?

Heart Chamber	Receives Blood from	Sends Blood to
Right atrium	Entire body	Right ventricle
Right ventricle	Right atrium	Blood vessels in lungs
Left atrium	Blood vessels in the lungs	Left ventricle
Left ventricle	Left atrium	Entire body

about the plumbing in your home. What stops it from traveling all the way back to the utility company when you turn off the water? You guessed it—valves.

The heart contains four valves, all designed to allow flow in only one direction—forward. When blood flows back-ward, it's because the valves are not doing their job. Back-ward flow can decrease the heart's efficiency, even to the point of death.

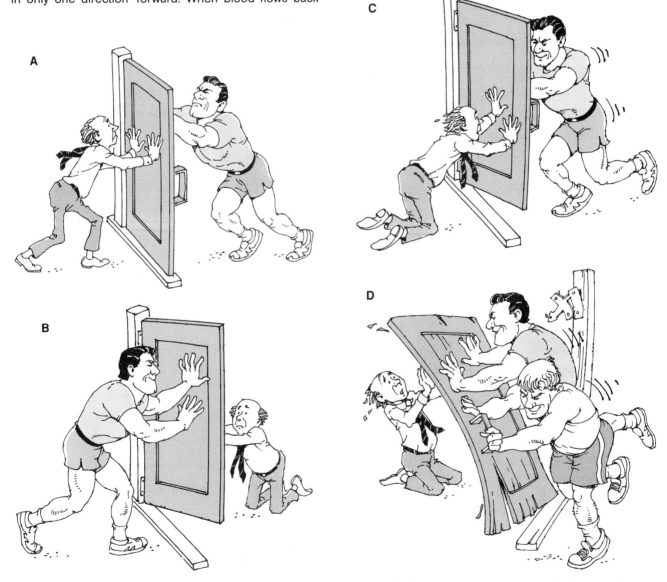

A, A normal valve should not open in the wrong direction just because a larger force is used. B, If the larger force pushes the valve in the correct direction, the valve opens. C, If the valve is open and a larger force pushes back against it, the valve will close. D, If the valve receives too much pressure, it will fail and allow flow in the wrong direction.

GO WITH THE FLOW

The right atrium receives blood from the body through the *superior vena cava* (SVC) and the *inferior vena cava* (IVC). The right atrium is located higher in the chest cavity than the right ventricle. Therefore, left to its own devices, the blood would simply fall through the bottom of the atrium and into the right ventricle, just as the sand in an hourglass falls from the upper chamber to the lower chamber. This would present a problem if we stood on our heads.

Luckily, it doesn't work that way. The blood stays in place because of the *tricuspid* (three-leafed) valve, located between the right atrium and right ventricle. Its three cusps, or leaves, come together and form a seal to stop blood from flowing back into the right atrium once the ventricle is full and begins to contract.

The pressure in the right ventricle approaches zero as the ventricle begins to relax after contraction. Meanwhile, a small amount of pressure remains in the right atrium from the blood that's been forced back into the heart. When the pressure in the right ventricle becomes less than the pressure in the right atrium, the tricuspid valve opens. Then the right atrium begins to contract fully and forces a large portion of the remaining blood, under pres-

sure, into the right ventricle. The right ventricle stretches to accommodate this pressurized blood rushing in. This stretch in the right ventricle is vital to maximizing the output of the heart.

CONTENTS UNDER PRESSURE

No Place to Go Just like a stretched rubber band, the stretched ventricle is constantly trying to relieve pressure by returning to its normal shape and dimensions. When the force stretching the rubber band is released, the band snaps back to its normal shape with a lot of force— if you've ever snapped yourself with a rubber band, you can attest to this. The right ventricle tries to snap back by pushing the blood back into the right atrium. However, the pressure in the atrium is now less than the pressure in the right ventricle, so the normal tricuspid valve snaps shut.

An Exit Valve There's another valve that lets the blood out of the right ventricle. This valve leads to the blood vessels that enter the lung tissue. These blood vessels are called the *pulmonary arteries,* and the valve that leads from the right ventricle to the pulmonary arteries is called the *pulmonic valve.* It takes more pressure to open the pulmonic

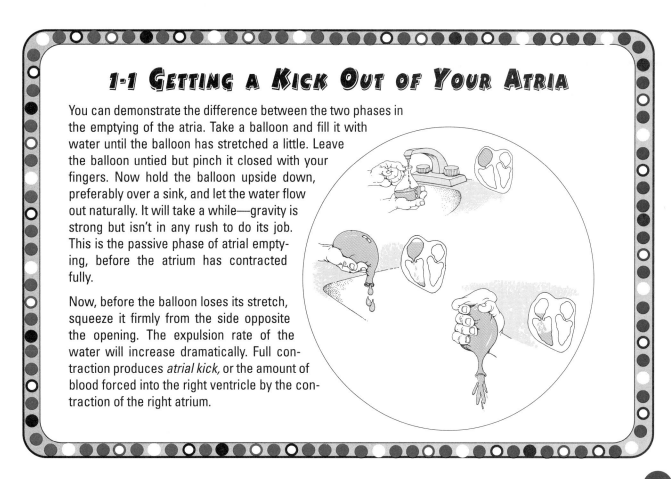

1-1 GETTING A KICK OUT OF YOUR ATRIA

You can demonstrate the difference between the two phases in the emptying of the atria. Take a balloon and fill it with water until the balloon has stretched a little. Leave the balloon untied but pinch it closed with your fingers. Now hold the balloon upside down, preferably over a sink, and let the water flow out naturally. It will take a while—gravity is strong but isn't in any rush to do its job. This is the passive phase of atrial emptying, before the atrium has contracted fully.

Now, before the balloon loses its stretch, squeeze it firmly from the side opposite the opening. The expulsion rate of the water will increase dramatically. Full contraction produces *atrial kick,* or the amount of blood forced into the right ventricle by the contraction of the right atrium.

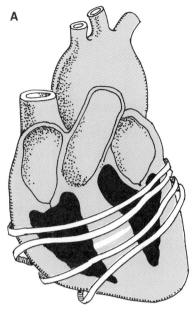 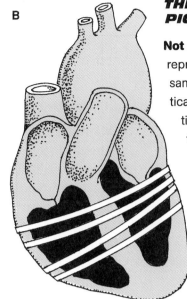

A, The ventricles behave like rubber bands; when the muscles are relaxed, there is no tension. B, As with a rubber band, stretching the muscles increases tension.

THE OTHER HALF OF THE PICTURE

Not a Moment's Rest Remember, all this action represents only the right side of the heart. At the same time, the left side is putting on a nearly identical show featuring valves, pressure, and contraction. To blow your mind even more, remember that this coordinated sequence of events normally happens 60 to 100 times a minute, every day of every year of our lives—without any rest!

The left side of the heart works much the same way as the right side. Although the chambers and valves have different names, you'll find that you're already familiar with the process.

Moving the Blood After the blood travels through the lungs and performs the necessary exchange of gases, the pulmonary veins bring it back to the heart. These veins empty directly into the left atrium. As with the right atrium, no valve is needed to admit blood into the left atrium.

The valve separating the left atrium from the left ventricle is called the *mitral,* or *bicuspid* (two-leafed) *valve.* The mitral valve has only two leaves, not three, to seal the opening between the chambers. As in the right side of the heart, the blood first empties passively from the left atrium into the left ventricle. Next, the left atrium contracts, ejecting the blood under pressure into the left ventricle, as the left ventricle relaxes. The left ventricle then stretches to accommodate the large volume of blood entering. This stretch is essential to maximizing the amount of newly oxygenated blood pumped out to the body. When the pressure in the left ventricle is greater than the pressure in the left atrium, the mitral valve closes.

Ejecting the Blood The exit valve in the left ventricle leads to the largest artery in the body—the *aorta.* Therefore, the valve connecting the left ventricle to the aorta is called the *aortic valve.* When the left ventricle begins to contract, the pressure inside it increases because the blood is being squeezed and has nowhere to go. Then, when the pressure in the left ventricle exceeds the pressure in the aorta, the aortic valve springs open and the blood in the left ventricle is forced upward into the aorta and out to the rest of the body.

However, before all the blood in the left ventricle is ejected, the pressure in the aorta increases drastically because of all the newly received blood. Eventually the aortic pressure becomes greater than the pressure in the

valve than the modest stretch in the right ventricle can provide, so the blood in the right ventricle is trapped. Then the filled ventricle begins to contract. This increased pressure also pushes on the tricuspid valve. However, the tricuspid is sealed shut, and its design prevents it from allowing backward, or retrograde, flow.

When the pressure in the right ventricle exceeds the pressure in the pulmonary arteries, the pulmonic valve is finally forced open, just as in our earlier door examples. The blood in the right ventricle has only one place to go—into the hole created by the opening of the pulmonic valve. Because the pressure generated by the right ventricle is much greater than the pressure in the pulmonary arteries, most of the blood in the right ventricle is ejected into the pulmonary arteries. It then travels through the blood vessels in the lung tissue to collect oxygen and dispose of carbon dioxide. As the blood moves into the pulmonary arteries, the pressure there increases until it exceeds the pressure in the right ventricle. At that point the pulmonic valve slams shut (Table 1–2).

Table 1–2 What are the valves doing now?

Chamber Contracting	Tricuspid Valve	Pulmonic Valve
Right atrium	Open	Closed
Right ventricle	Closed	Open

1-2 STRETCH BEFORE YOU EXERCISE

Take your balloon and empty out all the water. Now blow it up just a little bit so it takes on its natural shape without any stretch in the rubber. Let the balloon go and watch it make a beeline for the floor or tabletop. Recapture the balloon and blow it up a little more this time, enough to give it some stretch, and then let go. The balloon will probably travel a short distance before falling to the floor. That's because the stretch has increased the air pressure in the balloon and thus the force with which the air is ejected.

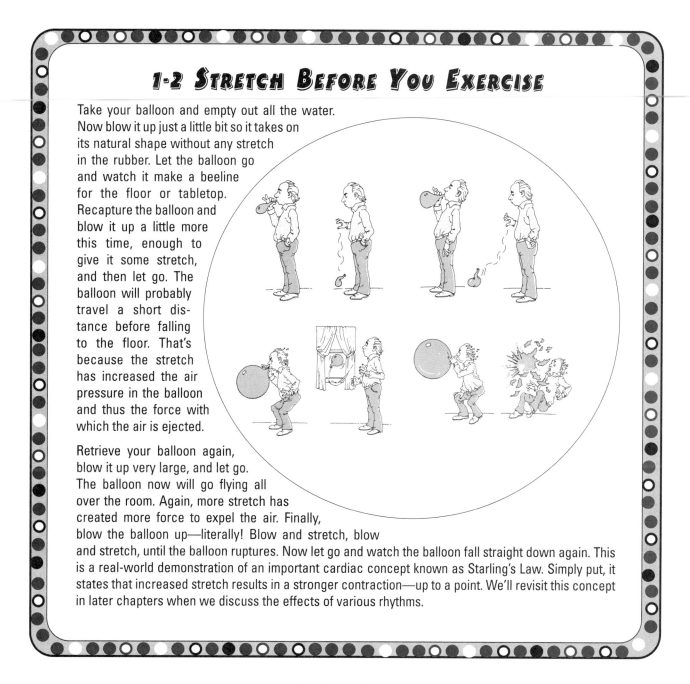

Retrieve your balloon again, blow it up very large, and let go. The balloon now will go flying all over the room. Again, more stretch has created more force to expel the air. Finally, blow the balloon up—literally! Blow and stretch, blow and stretch, until the balloon ruptures. Now let go and watch the balloon fall straight down again. This is a real-world demonstration of an important cardiac concept known as Starling's Law. Simply put, it states that increased stretch results in a stronger contraction—up to a point. We'll revisit this concept in later chapters when we discuss the effects of various rhythms.

left ventricle. With nothing to keep it open, the aortic valve slams shut. The ejected blood now circulates through the body, eventually returning to the right atrium, where the process begins all over again (Table 1–3).

Telling Left from Right Many people have difficulty remembering which valves are on which side. Table 1–4 shows you a simple way to remember which valves go where. It relates the first letters of the valves to the sides of the heart. Each valve is located on the side of the heart that goes in the same half of the alphabet. So the aortic (A) and mitral (M) valves are on the left (L); the pulmonic (P) and tricuspid (T) valves are on the right (R).

Table 1–3 What's the left side doing?

Chamber Contracting	Mitral Valve	Aortic Valve
Left atrium	Open	Closed
Left ventricle	Closed	Open

Table 1–4 Location of heart valves

Left	Right
Aortic valve	**P**ulmonic valve
Mitral valve	**T**ricuspid valve

The Heart Needs Its Wheaties™ Too

BREAKFAST IS SERVED

This valve stuff is all well and good, but where does the heart get the energy to do all that work? Remember, the heart is a muscle. Because it needs oxygen to do its work, it also needs a way to get rid of carbon dioxide, the toxic waste product of metabolism. Most people think wrongly that the heart exchanges these two gases with the blood as it passes through the various chambers. But if that were true, the right side of the heart would be at a distinct disadvantage. The blood coursing through the right atrium and right ventricle is already filled with carbon dioxide and depleted of oxygen; after all, that's why the blood is returning. Well, then, how *does* the heart get its revitalized blood?

The blood is delivered to the heart tissue, or *myocardium* (heart muscle), through a pair of openings at the base of the aorta called the *coronary arteries.* When the oxygenated blood is ejected from the left ventricle, it goes into the aorta, increasing the pressure there. Like all pressurized blood, it looks for a way to decrease the pressure. It can't return to the heart through the aortic valve, which is closed now. Instead, aortic stretch and increased aortic pressure force the blood back toward the heart, where it fills the coronary arteries at the base of the aorta (Fig. 1–4).

WHERE TO NEXT?

Many Delivery Routes There are two main branches off the base of the aorta, the *right coronary artery* (RCA) and the *left main coronary artery* (LM). The left main coronary artery travels a very short distance before splitting into the *left anterior descending artery* (LAD), which travels down the front of the heart, and the *left circumflex* (LCx), often known as the "circ," which wraps around the left side and down the back of the heart. These vessels branch off further into smaller and smaller vessels that eventually feed every cell in the heart. Each of these three primary coronary arteries—the RCA, LAD, and LCx—is responsible for delivering blood to a specific portion of the heart tissue. They can overlap somewhat in the areas they supply; however, most areas are fed by only one artery. Chapter 19 discusses what areas of the heart are usually supplied by which coronary arteries.

Death by Starvation When one of these vessels becomes completely blocked, or occluded, blood may not reach a certain portion of the myocardium and the patient will experience a "heart attack," or *myocardial infarction* (MI), if blood flow is not restored quickly. Infarction results in

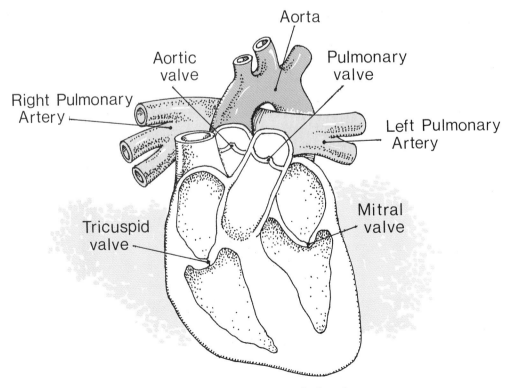

Fig. 1–4 How the heart gets what it needs.

tissue death, or *necrosis,* from lack of blood flow. The part of the heart that dies depends on which vessel is occluded; the severity of the infarction depends on how much of the vessel is blocked and for how long. The topics of MIs and the coronary arteries will be more fully developed in Chapter 19.

HANDLING THE WORKLOAD

We need to cover another important concept: *cardiac output,* or how much blood the heart pumps out into the body in 1 minute. The amount of blood that the heart ejects in one beat is called *stroke volume* (SV) and is normally about 60–80 mL at rest. Stroke volume depends on many factors, including activity level, physical condition, and prior heart disease.

Let's pretend for a moment that all heartbeats are identical and that every heartbeat pumps out the same amount of blood. Then, if we know the heart rate, we can compute cardiac output very simply: CO = HR × SV. That is, cardiac output (CO) equals the number of heartbeats in 1 minute (HR) times the amount ejected by each heartbeat (SV).

For example, if Mr. XYZ has a stroke volume of 80 mL and his heart rate is 80 bpm, his cardiac output would be 80 × 80 mL, or 6400 mL, or 6.4 L per minute. When discussing cardiac output, we usually omit "per minute"

because that's already part of the definition of cardiac output. Therefore, we say that this patient's cardiac output is 6.4 L. The normal range of cardiac output is 5 to 8 L.

If Mr. XYZ increases his physical activity or some part of his body demands more oxygen, his heart must increase its output. It can accomplish this in two ways. Because the heart is a pumping system, you can either speed it up so it pumps more often per minute or you can make it more efficient so it ejects more each time it pumps. In other words, you can increase either the heart rate or the stroke volume. If Mr. XYZ kept his stroke volume at 80 mL but increased his heart rate to 100 bpm, his new cardiac output would be 80 × 100 mL, or 8000 mL, or 8 L. If he kept his heart rate at 80 bpm but increased his stroke volume to 100 mL, his new cardiac output would be the same but for different reasons.

In reality, the body is constantly adjusting the speed and efficiency of the pump we call the heart. Stroke volume can vary by small amounts from beat to beat, and heart rate can change slightly from minute to minute. The many reasons for this include stress, fear, illness, disease, and activity, healthy or otherwise.

The heart is an amazing muscular pump that we take for granted—until something goes wrong. More about that later; now it's time to recap.

1-3 PICKING UP ROCKS

Say you need to move a large pile of rocks from point A to point B. You start out moving one rock every minute, so your output is 60 rocks per hour. But your boss says you're going too slowly and need to speed up. What do you do? Well, instead of picking up one rock every minute, you could pick the rocks up faster, say, one every 30 seconds. That would raise your output to 120 rocks per hour. However, this increase will cost you. You'll need more energy to work at a faster pace because your muscles are working twice as often per minute.

What if, instead of picking up one rock every minute, you pick up two rocks at a time and do that once every minute? Your rock output is still 120 rocks per hour, but you're only using your muscles once per minute. However, now they're working twice as hard as when they carried only one rock at a time. So your muscles are working about as hard as when you picked up one rock twice per minute.

Either way, your muscles must work harder to increase your rock output. Either way, they'll need more energy and more oxygen. Because the heart is also a muscle, it makes little energy difference whether you increase cardiac output by increasing stroke volume or heart rate. The heart works harder either way and needs more oxygen to perform properly.

Test Yourself

1. The heart has _____ chambers.

2. The two upper chambers are called _____.

3. The two lower chambers are called _____.

4. A change in _____ is the primary reason that valves open and close.

5. You can increase cardiac output by increasing _____ or _____.

6. The heart receives its blood supply from the _____ that start at the base of the _____.

7. The large, flat bone in front of the heart is the _____.

8. The _____ valve separates the left atrium from the left ventricle, and the _____ valve separates the right atrium from the right ventricle.

9. Starling's Law states that increased _____ results in increased strength of _____ —up to a point.

10. When the right ventricle is contracting, the _____ valve is open and the _____ valve is closed.

11. Label the parts of the heart in the picture below:

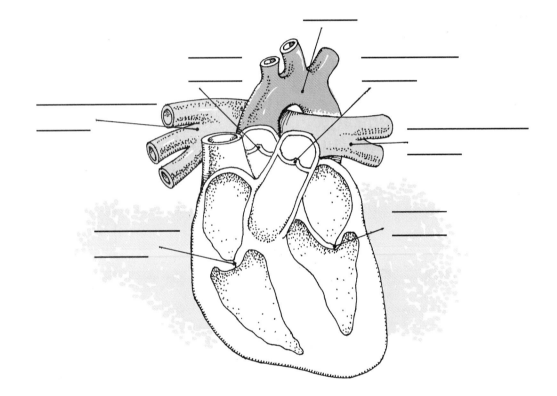

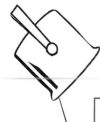

Now You Know

The heart is located slightly off center in the middle of the chest behind the sternum.

A "normal" heart is a little bigger than an index card, or a little larger than the person's closed hand.

The heart is protected by a cage formed by the sternum, ribs, and spine.

The blood travels from the body to the right atrium, through the tricuspid valve into the right ventricle, and then through the pulmonic valve into the pulmonary arteries. Then it travels into the left atrium, through the mitral valve into the left ventricle, and through the aortic valve into the aorta and out to the body.

Valves make sure the blood travels in only one direction.

The three primary coronary arteries (LAD, LCx, and RCA) supply blood to the heart.

Cardiac output is the amount of blood the heart pumps out in 1 minute and can be changed by altering heart rate, stroke volume, or both.

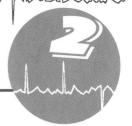

(Dis)Charge It!

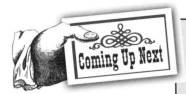

Coming Up Next

○ What are depolarization and repolarization?

○ What makes the heartbeat start?

○ What is the difference between an intra-atrial pathway and an internodal pathway?

○ What are some of the most important ions in the heart conduction system?

○ How do we know that the electrical signal is actually following the correct pathway in the heart?

○ What is a pacemaker cell?

Start the Pump

WHO RUNS THE SHOW?

The heart, as we discovered in Chapter 1, is a pump driven by electrical signals. However, the heart doesn't come with a cord. We can't plug it into an outlet like the pumps in our pools or fish tanks. So where do the electrical signals that drive the heart pump come from?

All cardiac muscle cells are capable of initiating a signal, but certain groups of cells are given the responsibility of running the show. These cells are called *pacemaker cells* because they can set the pace of the heart rhythm. Pacemaker cells generate an electrical signal that gets sent in turn to every other cell in the heart. They can generate this signal without any external force or stimulation, a unique ability among cardiac cells known as *automaticity*. Automaticity is the ability of a cell to generate a spontaneous signal automatically, without any prompting from outside itself.

CELLULAR BATTERIES

Looking at the Positive and Negative These pacemaker cells of the heart are filled with ions—atoms and molecules that have a positive or negative charge, just like the ends of a battery. The more important ones for our discussion here are potassium (K^+) and sodium (Na^+), each of which has a single positive charge, and calcium (Ca^{2+}), which has a double-positive charge. There are many negative ions, such as bicarbonate (HCO_3^-) and chloride (Cl^-), each of which has a single negative charge, but they aren't important for our understanding at this level.

The most important cell feature is the membrane. The cell membrane is designed to allow certain chemicals through specialized gates called *channels*. In pacemaker cells, these channels selectively allow or prevent movement of chemicals, especially sodium, potassium, and calcium ions (Fig. 2–1).

A Negative Balance The cardiac pacemaker cell is said to be *polarized* in its resting state. A polarized cell has a charge, or an imbalance of positive and negative ions. Cardiac cells have a negative charge because they contain more negative ions than positive ions. The charge of the resting cardiac cell is normally around −90 mV (Fig. 2–2).

Different types of positive ions occur in greater or lesser numbers inside and outside the polarized cell. Inside it, potassium ions far outnumber sodium ions, while the reverse is true outside the cell.

Polarity is maintained by the cell membrane. Without its control, positive ions would rush in and negative ions would rush out to try to balance the charge. The cell membrane prevents this from happening until the pacemaker gives it the go-ahead.

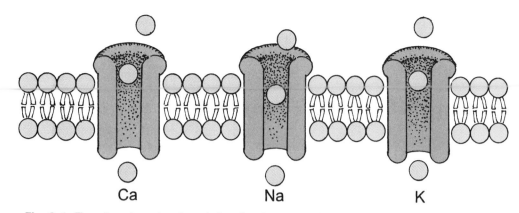

Fig. 2–1 The cell membrane has channels that allow the passage of sodium, potassium, calcium, and other ions.

Keep It Going
COORDINATED SIGNALS

A Positive Change: Phase 0 When the pacemaker's internal clock calls time, the pacemaker cells begin to depolarize, or to try to eliminate the negative charge inside the cell. The pacemaker cells do this slightly differently than all the other cardiac cells. They allow Ca^{2+} to slowly leak into the cell to raise the charge inside to 0 mV. We will not cover pacemaker cells in depth, but understand that they depolarize automatically and slightly differently than the rest of the cardiac electrical system.

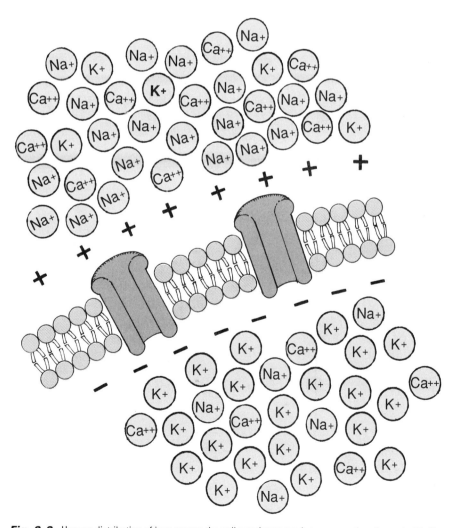

Fig. 2–2 Uneven distribution of ions across the cell membrane produces a negative charge inside the cell compared with the outside of the cell.

The other cells in the heart depolarize by opening specialized channels on the cell membrane called sodium channels. These allow sodium ions to enter the cell.

There are two types of sodium channels: slow and fast. The slow sodium channels are active initially, but the inflow of sodium ions is partially balanced by positive potassium ions leaving the cell. As the number of positive sodium ions increases, so does the charge inside the cell. When the charge in the cell reaches approximately −65 mV, the fast sodium channels open and the sodium inflow overcomes the potassium outflow. The goal is to reach 0 mV, or a neutral (nonpolarized) state. However, the massive influx of positive ions causes the charge to overshoot the mark until it reaches +30 mV. At this point, the sodium channels close. This process is called "phase 0."

This massive shift of positive ions inside the cell also lowers the charge outside the cell so that it becomes more negative. This in turn triggers the adjacent cells to begin depolarizing themselves. Another specialized set of cells gets involved here. These cells are referred to collectively as the *conduction system*. The role of the conduction system is to transmit the change in the electrical charge, the depolarization, from the pacemaker cells to the individual cardiac muscle cells. The muscle cells then depolarize and (we hope) cause the cardiac cell to contract. All cardiac muscle cells are able to transmit the depolarization signal, but the conduction system is specially designed to deliver the signal in a coordinated manner. It's important that all the cardiac cells contract in a particular order; this specialized conduction system ensures that they do. Different cardiac cells depolarize in slightly different ways, but this gives us a better understanding of the complexity of the process and the basic mechanisms involved.

Potassium Shipment: Phase 1 Remember phase 0, the process that ends when the sodium channels close? After

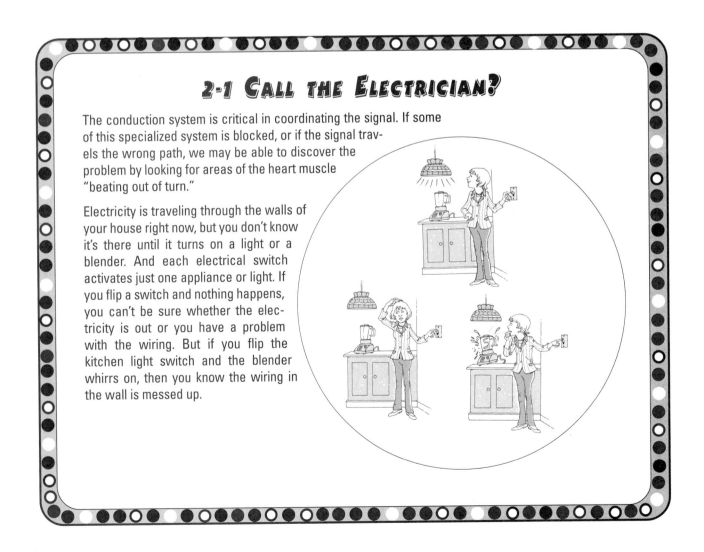

2-1 CALL THE ELECTRICIAN?

The conduction system is critical in coordinating the signal. If some of this specialized system is blocked, or if the signal travels the wrong path, we may be able to discover the problem by looking for areas of the heart muscle "beating out of turn."

Electricity is traveling through the walls of your house right now, but you don't know it's there until it turns on a light or a blender. And each electrical switch activates just one appliance or light. If you flip a switch and nothing happens, you can't be sure whether the electricity is out or you have a problem with the wiring. But if you flip the kitchen light switch and the blender whirrs on, then you know the wiring in the wall is messed up.

2-2 ELECTRICAL HEART WRITING

The machine that measures the depolarization signal is called an *electrocardiograph* (*electro*—electrical; *cardio*—heart; *graph*—writing). The electrocardiograph, or ECG machine, picks up the signal delivered by depolarizing cardiac cells. Normally the conduction system uses only a small number of cells, so its signal is too faint to be recorded by our external ECG machine.

The term ECG is an Americanized version of the real term, EKG. You see, most of the original development in the field of electrocardiography came from Germany and the Netherlands. In these countries, the hard "K" sound in electrocardiography, is represented by a "K", not a "C", thus the term EKG.

But the machine records activity when large areas of the heart are depolarizing at the same time. That's how we map the pathway of the depolarization signal—not by the actual path but by the timing of the results. Therefore, the ECG machine doesn't directly measure the transmission of the signal through the heart but tells us which area of the heart is depolarized and (hopefully) contracting.

phase 0 is complete and the cell is depolarized, it must quickly return to its normal state—polarized, with a larger negative charge inside the cell. This return to polarity begins in phase 1.

After the influx of positive sodium ions, the cell tries to repolarize, or get back to the highly negative charge of its resting state, to prepare for the next depolarization. First, the cell sends out potassium, another positive ion. This lowers the charge inside the cell, but the charge must become even lower to get back to the resting state of −90 mV.

Getting Enough Calcium: Phase 2 During phase 2, potassium outflow increases and calcium begins to flow into the cell in smaller amounts than before. Calcium is vital in proper heart function. This ion is responsible for making the cell contract, and no amount of potassium and sodium movement can act in its place. In fact, all muscle cells, not just cardiac cells, require calcium to contract properly.

In this phase, the potassium ions flow out of the cell much faster than the calcium ions flow in. Remember, though, that calcium has double the positive charge of potassium; therefore, the charge inside the cell drops by only an insignificant amount.

Redistributing the Goods: Phase 3 During phase 3, the calcium channels close, while the potassium and sodium are redistributed across the cell membrane until they reach the same concentration as before the depolarization took place. Most of the change in charge occurs during this phase.

A Spontaneous Act: Phase 4 Finally, phase 4 occurs. In pacemaker cells, the charge inside the cell increases slowly until the cell can depolarize spontaneously. Non-pacemaker cells normally wait for the next wave of depolarization to give them their cue, at which point we see a rapid change in charge. As we'll learn, phases 0 through 4 behave differently in different types of cells.

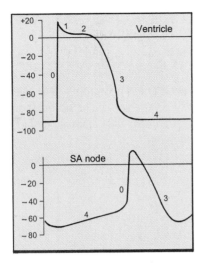

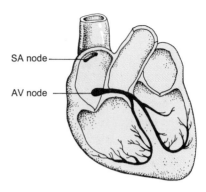

Fig. 2–4 The conduction system is vital to the contraction of the heart.

Fig. 2–3 The standard action potential curve for the sinus node and ventricular tissue. The sinus node depolarizes slowly and continuously, in contrast to the sudden depolarization in the ●ntricular tissue.

A LOOK BACK AT THE ACTION

This whole process is called an *action potential* and can be represented as a graph (Fig. 2–3). If you learn visually, you might feel more comfortable with the graph than with the previous detailed description of the action potential.

Do you really need all this information about depolarization and repolarization? Yes. Later we'll learn how to use this knowledge to help us choose drugs that alter the rhythm of a patient's heart!

Now that we understand how pacemaker cells work and how the action potential is transmitted from cell to cell, it's time to discuss the specialized conduction path that's designed to carry this signal.

A CLOSER LOOK AT THE CONDUCTION SYSTEM

Let's examine the conduction system in greater detail. Two main groups of tissue transmit the signal to large areas of the heart. The first, the *sinoatrial node,* is located high up in the right atrium. It's also called the sinus node, or SA node. This small area of tissue is the preferred pacemaker location for normal hearts. Signals are generated here and transmitted to all the cells of the heart. The sinus node will reappear in Chapter 9, where we introduce rhythms, and in Chapter 10, where we focus on sinus rhythms.

The other important cluster of cells in the conduction system is called the *atrioventricular node,* or AV node. Its job is to process the signals received from the sinus node, coordinate them, and transmit them to the ventricles. Each of these two areas of cells is vitally important in normal

transmission. Any disruption in their function can cause serious trouble, even death (Fig. 2–4).

Each area of cells capable of "running" the heart has a characteristic action potential. In normally functioning sinus node cells, a gentle increase in charge begins as soon as the cell returns to its normal state. Cells in the atria, AV node, and ventricles have a longer phase 4. That allows these cells to take over the heart rhythm if the sinus node fails. In fact, they're trying to depolarize all the time, and the sinus node just beats them to it. Figure 2–5 shows the general shape and timing of the depolarization-repolarization cycle in each type of cell.

A High Sign From the Sinus Node The sinus node, being the preferred pacemaker, normally depolarizes first. Because it's only a small group of cells, its signal is not

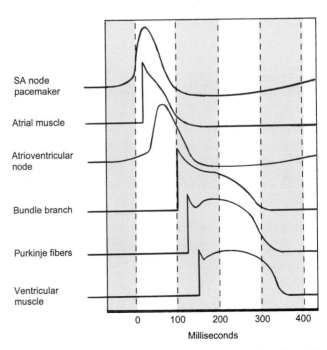

Fig. 2–5 The action potential curve for different types of cardiac cell.

recorded on the ECG tracing. After the cells in the sinus node depolarize, they must transmit their signal in many directions at the same time. We'll discuss each location individually.

The right and left atria must depolarize at approximately the same time for maximum efficiency. Here's where the *intra-atrial pathway* comes in. This group of cells allows the signal to travel within the atria, much as an *intra*state highway lets cars travel from one part of the state to another. The intra-atrial tissue allows such speedy travel within the atria that, although the right atrium is closer to the sinus node, the left atrium can receive the signal at nearly the same time and can contract along with the right atrium.

Although we have a right and a left atrium, we talk about only one intra-atrial pathway. That's because the right atrium is in direct contact with the sinus node and doesn't need to have the signal delivered anywhere.

Bachmann's bundles are a group of independent pathways. Because they transport the signal down to the atrioventricular node, they are called *internodal pathways*. As *inter*state highways allow travel from one state to another state, the internodal pathways allow the signal to travel quickly from one node (the sinus node) to a different node (the AV node). This is vitally important in maintaining the maximum efficiency of the heart pump.

A Slow Wink From the AV Node The atrioventricular node receives the signal before the atria have finished depolarizing and contracting, but it doesn't send out the signal immediately. The signal travels slowly through the AV node toward a group of cells formed into a large bundle of tissue called the *bundle of His*. The bundle of His then transmits the signal to two different smaller bundles of tissue—the left and right bundle branches.

The left bundle branch divides into two major pieces, which then divide further into smaller and smaller tracts until they're no longer bundles but individual fibers. These fibers are called *terminal Purkinje fibers* (Fig. 2–6). The

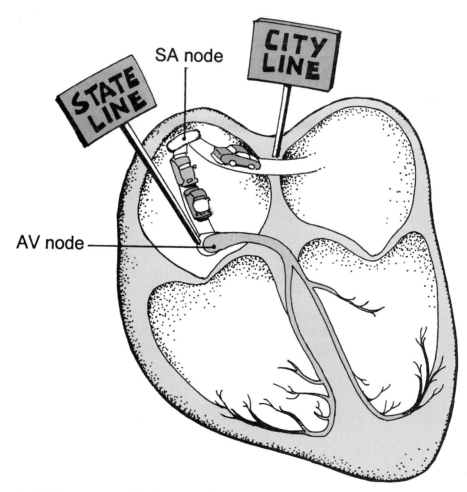

*Intra*state highways connect cities in one state. *Intra*-atrial pathways connect parts of one type of chamber—the atria. *Inter*state highways connect two different states. *Inter*nodal pathways connect two different nodes.

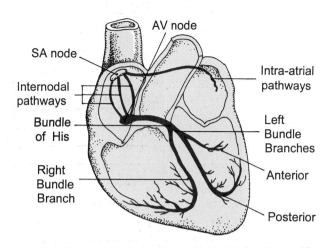

Fig. 2–6 The intra-atrial, internodal, and His Purkinje (bundle branch) systems.

same thing happens with the right bundle branch, although it doesn't break into two main branches. This process is explained in detail in Chapter 7.

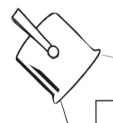

As we've seen, when large numbers of muscle cells depolarize in unison, they make a big enough splash for the ECG machine to pick up. The heart's fast conduction system doesn't generate a strong signal directly. But if these small cell clusters didn't work the way they were supposed to, the machine wouldn't detect any signal at all.

Test Yourself

1. The _____ controls the depolarization of the cardiac cell.

2. The _____ is a group of cells that is the heart's preferred pacemaker.

3. _____ is the positive ion responsible for actually causing the muscle cell to contract.

4. The cell membrane has a normal resting charge of about _____.

5. _____ atrial pathways transmit the signal from the sinus node to the AV node.

6. _____ atrial pathways transmit the signal from the sinus node to the left atrium.

7. The _____ normally holds on to the signal for a brief period of time before sending it on.

NOW YOU KNOW

The cardiac cells are normally in a polarized state, with different electrical charges inside and outside the cell.

Depolarization occurs when the movement of charged particles across the cell membrane changes the electrical charge both inside and outside the cell.

Repolarization occurs when the cell membrane returns to its original polarized state.

Usually the sinus node initiates the signal to cause the heart to contract; however, all cardiac muscle tissue can generate the signal under certain circumstances.

An intra-atrial pathway delivers the sinus node signal to the left atrium, while the internodal pathways deliver the signal from the sinus node to the atrioventricular node.

Sodium (Na^+), potassium (K^+), and calcium (Ca^{2+}) are very important in cardiac conduction and contraction.

The only way to know if the signal is traveling the correct pathway through the heart is to observe the order of cardiac muscle cell contractions on the ECG strip.

A pacemaker cell is one that can depolarize itself, with no outside stimulation, to trigger (we hope) a contraction of the heart.

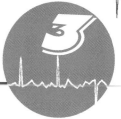

THE ECG CANVAS

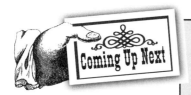

○ How do the lines get on the paper?

○ How fast does the ECG paper run?

○ What is a small box and what does it represent?

○ What is a large box and what does it represent?

○ What are the special markings on the top and bottom of the strips for?

○ What are three methods for estimating heart rate and when should each be used?

○ How do you determine whether a rhythm is regular or irregular?

○ What other information can be on the ECG strip and why does it matter?

○ What should we do with the computer's interpretation?

Doing the Background Work

All artwork needs a canvas on which to be displayed, and what could possibly be more beautiful and artistic than the rhythmic, life-giving contractions of the heart? So, to properly display this work of art, we need a canvas that will do it justice.

No, I haven't lost my mind—it's still in the jar right next to me—although I may be getting a little carried away. But choosing the right background can mean the difference between seeing something and missing it. If you paint a white polar bear on a white canvas, we'll have trouble appreciating the details; if you chose a black background, the contrast will let us appreciate the bear's finer points.

KEEPING IT SIMPLE

The background of an ECG tracing should be simple enough not to intrude on the tracing itself. At the same time, it should help you see the details and make the measurements you need to interpret the faint signals the heart is sending to the surface of the chest wall.

The universal background is simply a grid, or an approximation of a grid. Altering the background isn't usually an option. Each ECG machine has a predetermined background, although some models allow you to choose between two or more backgrounds (Fig. 3–1A–C).

GRID OR BLANK SLATE?

The backgrounds fall into two different categories: *preprinted* and *print as you go*. With preprinted paper, the background grid is already on the paper, and the ECG tracings are drawn over that. The advantage of this method is that the background grid can be of a different color than the ECG tracing (see Fig. 3–1A). This enhances the contrast between background and tracing and allows for easier interpretation.

The print-as-you-go method draws both the tracing and the background on the paper at the same time. This can lower the cost of the paper, but the method has a disadvantage. The background is the same color as the tracing, and interpretation can suffer (see Fig. 3–1B–C). To minimize this disadvantage, some of the lines may be left out and replaced by dots where the lines would normally intersect. That way you still have a grid, but the lines of the ECG tracings are less likely to get confused with the lines of the background grid.

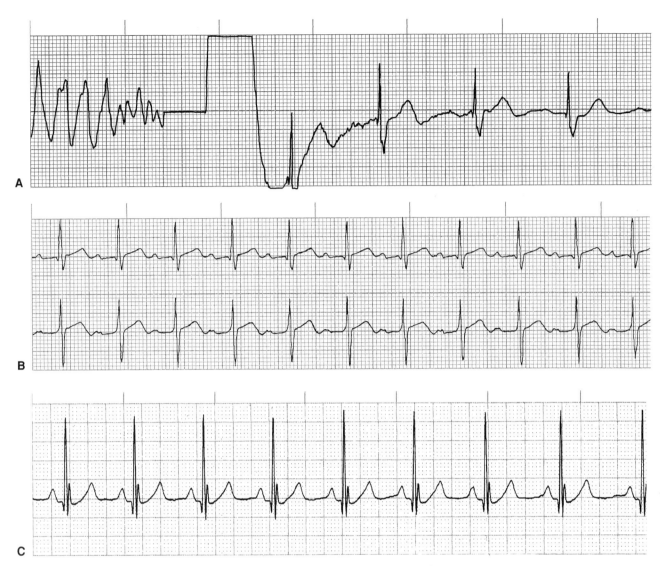

Fig. 3–1A–C Various ECG strip backgrounds.

The Tracing Takes Shape
DRAW IT OR BURN IT?

Now that you've decided on a background, you have another choice to make. There are two ways to get the tracings onto the paper. One way is to draw the tracing with ink; the other is to burn it onto special heat-sensitive paper. The ink method has the advantage of permanency because the ink takes a long time to fade.

The burning method lacks permanency by its very nature. A rapidly moving, high-temperature stylus leaves a black mark wherever its hot tip passes close enough to the paper, while the rest of the paper remains white. Unfortunately, the paper can't distinguish between the heat of the stylus and heat from other sources, such as the sun, a bright light, or even warm machinery. So, even

after the tracing is recorded, the paper will still react to any sufficient heat, which can ruin the tracing.

MARKING TIME

Basic Boxes The lines on ECG paper are always spaced at specific intervals. This allows precise and consistent measurement of the ECG waveform characteristics (Fig. 3–2). It's crucial to remember that the intervals between the markings don't represent distance. Left-to-right markings represent time, while vertical markings represent voltage, or the energy of each signal. If you look at Figure 3–2, you will notice that not all the markings are identical—some lines are darker than others. In fact, if you look carefully you'll see a repeating pattern: four fine lines followed by a heavier line, in both the vertical and horizontal dimensions. This pattern of

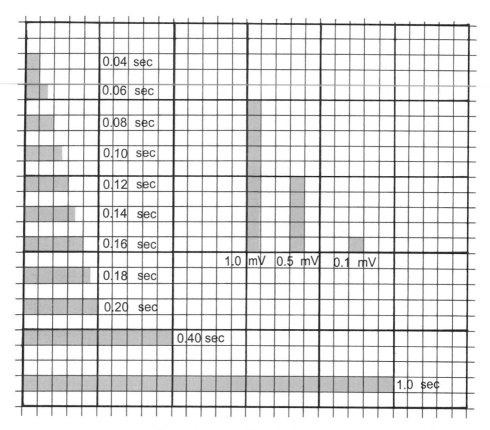

Fig. 3–2 Boxes and their standard values.

small boxes and *large boxes* will prove helpful in measuring our ECG strip.

The small boxes represent 0.04 seconds horizontally and 0.1 mV (millivolts) vertically in standard mode when the paper moves at 25 mm per second. At different speeds, of course, the values assigned to the horizontal boxes changes, but it is extremely rare to use any speed other than 25 mm per second. These are indeed tiny measurements. Just to give you some perspective, 1 second uses 25 horizontal small boxes. The energy of

one 9-volt battery would take up 90,000 vertical small boxes!

Boxes Within Boxes Look at Figure 3–2 again. You'll notice that every pair of heavy lines contains five small boxes, again in both horizontal and vertical dimensions. These heavy lines define the large boxes. Each large box represents 0.20 seconds (5 small boxes × 0.04 sec per small box) horizontally, or 0.5 mV vertically. The box system will come in handy later, when we start measuring intervals and calculating heart rates.

3-1 SPECIAL MARKINGS

Almost all ECG tracings have some additional markings that indicate larger intervals at a quick glance. These markings vary dramatically with the brand of equipment. For example, in Figure 3–1A, one-second intervals are shown by red lines enclosing five large boxes and extending past the top of the grid (5 large boxes × 0.20 sec per large box). Red lines extending past the bottom of the grid represent six-second intervals. However, in Figure 3–1B, we find triangles at the bottom of the strip at three-second intervals. Figure 3–1C shows small horizontal lines, also at three-second intervals. As you can see, knowing the markings on the strips you use is vital to quick interpretation of the results.

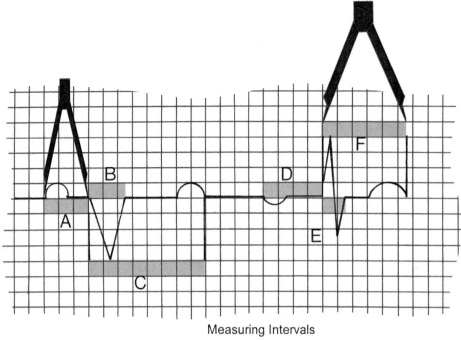

Measuring Intervals

A- 0.12 sec B- 0.10 sec C- 0.32 sec

D- 0.16 sec E- 0.06 sec F- 0.22 sec

Fig. 3–3A–F Practice measuring intervals on a standard ECG strip. A, 0.12 sec. B, 0.10 sec. C, 0.32 sec. D, 0.16 sec. E, 0.06 sec. F, 0.22 sec.

In measuring ECG intervals, it's customary to measure certain characteristics down to the nearest half of one small box. This represents 0.02 seconds (0.04 sec÷2). This is indeed a tiny fraction of a second. Because of limitations on human eyesight and the accuracy of the ECG tracing, we shouldn't go any further without using the 12-lead ECG, in which precision can reach 0.001 seconds.

Now for some practice. On the strip in Figure 3–3A–F, measure the intervals indicated in each part of the figure. The first 3 small boxes is 3 × 0.04 sec, or 0.12 sec; check your measurements against the answers provided.

Speed Reading

Now that you understand basic time measurement using the box system, you can put that information to good use. One of the key features of any ECG tracing is the heart rate. Knowing the heart rate is mandatory to naming the rhythm, as well as to understanding its implications for the patient. There are three ways to measure heart rate, all of which depend on your understanding the time measurement system we just covered. Before we get into measuring heart rate, however, we need to talk about regular and irregular rhythms.

PICKING UP THE BEAT

Imagine listening to your favorite song, the one you really get into. What happens while you're listening to it? Well, if you're like me, you start snapping your fingers, tapping your toes, or bobbing your head to the music. Most music has a regular beat to it; you snap your fingers at a set interval. If you snap your fingers once, snap them again a second later, and continue to snap them every second, that's a regular beat, or *rhythm*.

Imagine yourself beating a drum, striking it once and then striking it again one second later. Is that a regular beat? You can't tell because you haven't hit the drum

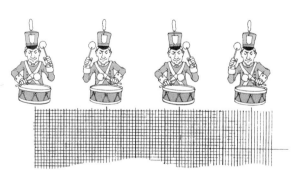

The drumbeat of the ECG rhythm.

3-2 RUNNING LAPS

Imagine that you're driving a car around an oval race track at a constant speed. You ask a friend to time you for one lap. He can start the stopwatch when you pass the starting line and stop it when you pass the starting line again. However, if he's far away from the starting line, he can just as easily start the stopwatch when you turn at a specific point, then stop it when you come to that point again. Or else he can start the stopwatch when you pass any specific point and stop it when you pass that point again. The key is to start and stop the measurement when you're at exactly the same place; this will measure the time you took to do one lap.

often enough. You won't be able to determine whether you have a regular beat until you've hit that drum several times at one-second intervals.

TALKING ABOUT COMPLEX THINGS

The heart beats in a cyclical rhythm: the blood enters the atria, and then flows into the ventricles and out of the heart. Eventually this same blood will return to the heart to repeat the cycle. The electrical signals of the heart, which we interpret as ECG rhythm strips, also tend to be cyclical; curves with the same shape and lines of the same size repeat throughout the strip. This cyclical feature allows us to measure the heart rate.

In the following chapters we'll learn to name the different curves and lines of the ECG, but for now that doesn't matter. What's important is to recognize when two things look the same. In the next few sections we will use the straight lines on the ECG rhythm strip as a reference point for our measurements. This part of the ECG strip is known as the *QRS complex*. We can choose any part of the QRS complex to start our measurement

as long as we use the same point of the next QRS to end on.

KEEPING COUNT

At Regular Intervals A heart rhythm is considered regular if the QRS complexes are approximately equidistant from each other (remember, distance means time on the ECG strip). We can determine regularity by counting the number of small boxes between the same point on two consecutive QRS complexes, or simply by measuring the physical distance between them. This is best done with ECG calipers. Place one tip of the calipers on any point of a QRS complex. Then stretch the second tip to the *identical* point on the following QRS complex, with the first tip still in its original position (Fig. 3–4). This distance, or time, is known as the *R to R interval;* we'll revisit that concept several times in later chapters.

Now that you know the distance between two consecutive QRS complexes, you need to determine whether the distance, or time, between every two QRS complexes is the same or whether it varies.

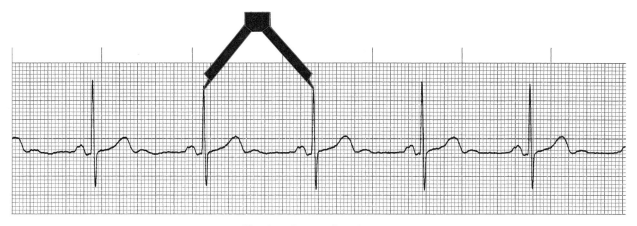

Fig. 3–4 Proper caliper placement.

3-3 A Little Wiggle Room

In measuring heart rate we allow a bit of leeway. Heart rate is never static, but makes constant small adjustments to meet the body's continually changing needs. If the time between the different QRS complexes varies by only one or two small boxes, the rhythm is still usually considered regular. We'll get into the details of regularity when we discuss the various regular and irregular rhythms in Chapter 8.

Pick up the first tip of your calipers, being careful not to change the distance between the two tips (see Fig. 3–4). Now spin your calipers so that the first tip moves to the next QRS complex. If the rhythm is regular, the second tip should fall within one or two small boxes of the same point on the next QRS. Continue moving the calipers from one set of QRS complexes to the next for the entire length of the strip.

When the Pattern Varies If the distance between even one QRS pair varies significantly from the distance between another pair, the rhythm is considered irregular. The strip in Figure 3–5 shows an irregular rhythm. You can see that the distance between the fourth and fifth QRS complexes is much smaller than the distance between the third and fourth ones. Just by looking at the strip in Figure 3–5, you can see that the QRS complexes aren't evenly spaced. But in Figure 3–4, even without measuring the R to R interval, you can guess that the spacing is pretty even. Your visual inspection skills will develop as you hone your interpretation skills. However, it's still a good idea to actually measure the intervals, as appearances can be deceiving.

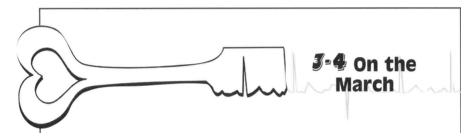

3-4 On the March

When the calipers fall on each consecutive QRS, we often say that the rhythm "marches out." This is easy to understand when you imagine the caliper points as the heels of soldiers "marching" from QRS to QRS as in Figure 3–4. When the QRS complexes come at irregular intervals throughout the strip, the rhythm "does not march out."

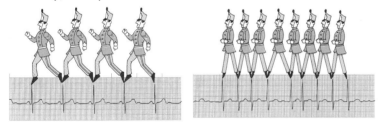

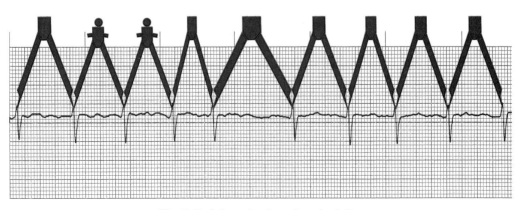

Fig. 3–5 Calipers showing an irregular rhythm.

Estimating Heart Rate

We can estimate heart rate in three basic ways. They all give approximate results because they're usually based on a six-second rhythm strip, not a full minute. Therefore small differences are insignificant, and we've even come to expect them.

QUICK ESTIMATE: THE SIX-SECOND METHOD

The first method of calculating heart rate is the easiest and can be used on any rhythm strip, whether the rhythm is regular or irregular. It's called the *six-second method,* and the process is simple and painless. Just count the number of QRS complexes in a six-second length of strip and multiply by 10 (for you non–math majors out there, just put a zero after the number). This is where the extra time markings on the strip come in handy. If you look at Figure 3–4, you'll notice markings on the strip at one-second intervals. All you have to do is count the number of QRS complexes in six of those one-second intervals. Figure 3–4 shows five QRS complexes in a six-second interval, and therefore the estimated heart rate is 50 bpm.

The six-second method is generally used to assess heart rate quickly in an emergency, or to assess the accuracy of the ECG machine in calculating heart rate. It's the least precise technique and can be off by 10 bpm or more. This amount is usually not important in practice and has minimum impact on treatment. However, actual interpretation of the strip demands a more precise measurement. Also, this method can result in different values depending on which six-second interval you choose.

If the rhythm is irregular, the estimate can be less accurate, but still close enough to help us out. With an irregular rhythm, any given six-second period will represent the overall rhythm well enough to give us the general heart rate. The rhythm in Figure 3–5 is irregular, but the strip has the same three-second markings as in Figure 3–4. Here we find nine QRS complexes in a six-second period, and therefore the estimated heart rate is 90 bpm.

Calculate the heart rate on the three strips in Figure 3–6A–C and compare your answers with the answers listed.

A LARGE-BOX ESTIMATE

The next method is called the *large-box method* and only works with regular rhythms. To understand the large-box method you must refer back to the measurement section earlier in this chapter headed "Marking Time." Remember that each large box represents 0.20 seconds. Therefore five large boxes represent 1 second. If there are 60 seconds in 1 minute and five large boxes in each second, then there are 300 large boxes (60×5) in 1 minute.

Now, to estimate the heart rate, all we have to do is determine the number of large boxes between any two consecutive QRS complexes. In Figure 3–7, first verify that the rhythm is regular. Then measure the distance between two consecutive QRS complexes. Using your calipers, place one tip on the first QRS and the second tip on the same point in the next QRS. Now, *carefully,* lift your calipers and move them so the first tip is directly on any heavy line. Now count the number of large boxes between the tips of the calipers. The second tip will rarely fall directly on a heavy line, so you must frequently round to the nearest box. In Figure 3–7, the measurements are done for you. You can count about three large boxes between the second and third QRS complexes.

Remember, this strip represents a regular rhythm. If you were drumming this rhythm, you'd strike your drum at about every third large box. How many groups of four large boxes are there in 1 minute? Well, this is easily computed. All you need to do is divide the number of large boxes in your measurement into 300 (the number of large boxes in 1 minute) and get about 100 bpm.

If you look at Figure 3–8, you'll find the heart rates for various numbers of large boxes. Commit the numbers in Figure 3–8 to memory, in order: 300, 150, 100, 75, 60, 50. Then, when you want a quick estimate of heart rate on a regular strip, just count off the large boxes using this list of numbers, and voilà, you'll have the heart rate by the large-box method.

Now try this method on the three strips in Figure 3–9A–C, and compare your answers with those provided.

SMALL-BOX PRECISION

If you try to measure the dimensions of a room with a foot-long stick of wood, you will get a pretty good estimate to the nearest foot. However, if you want more a more precise measurement, you can get a new measuring device or simply mark the wood with a finer measurement, such as inches. Then you can use the original measurement, but with more precision. In the case of an ECG strip you can use the same caliper measurement, but instead of counting the large boxes, simply count the small boxes.

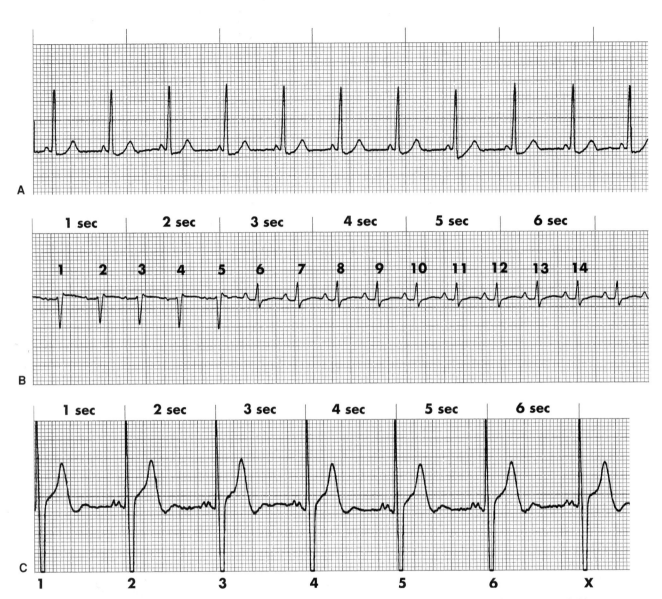

Fig. 3–6A–C Measurement using the six-second method. A, A heart rate of 100 bpm. B, A heart rate of 140 bpm. C, A heart rate of 50 bpm.

If there are 300 large boxes in 1 minute and five small boxes in each large box, then there must be 1500 small boxes in 1 minute. Count them if you must, but trust me, there really are 1500. Remember that earlier section, "Marking Time"? Small boxes measure a shorter time interval than large boxes, 0.04 seconds for a small box, 0.20 seconds for a large box. Obviously, a minute contains many more small boxes than large boxes; this is the key to the precision we're looking for.

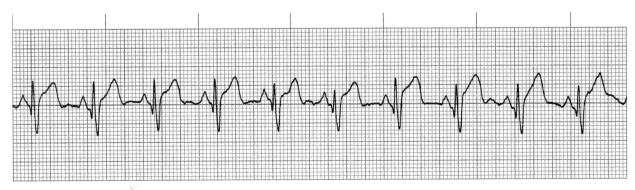

Fig. 3–7 The R-to-R interval can be calculated from any point on one QRS complex to the identical point on the next QRS. Usually the R-wave, the measuring point of the R-to-R interval, is the most easily identifiable point on the QRS complex.

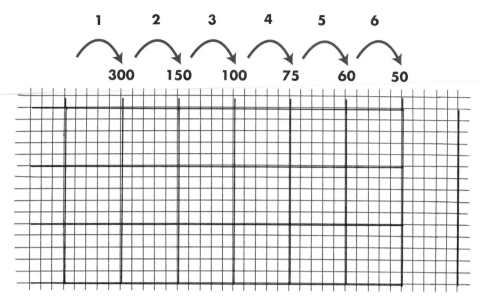

Fig. 3–8 The large-box method. The number of large boxes between two consecutive QRS complexes can be used to estimate the heart rate in regular rhythms.

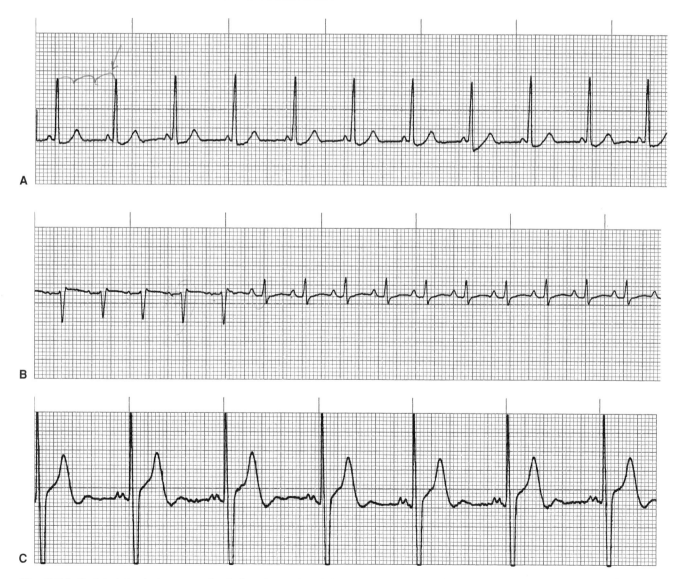

Fig. 3–9A–C Calculating the heart rate using the large-box method. A, Approximately three large boxes; the heart rate is 100 bpm. B, Almost two large boxes; the heart rate is about 150 bpm. C, Approximately five large boxes; the heart rate is about 60 bpm.

Returning to Figure 3–7, measure the same R to R interval you measured before. But now, instead of counting the large boxes, count the small boxes. You should get a number somewhere near 17. What do you do with it? As in the large-box method, you divide it into the number of similar (in this case small) boxes in 1 minute. Therefore the heart rate is 1500 ÷ 17, or about 88 bpm.

"Hey," some of you are saying, "this is too much math!" True, there is some math involved. However, if you look in the back of the book, you'll find a removable heart rate table that's already done the math for you. If you look up 17 small boxes on this table, you'll find a heart rate of 88, which our calculation has just confirmed.

Now look at the three strips below, and measure the heart rate using the small-box method. Compare the accuracy of the various methods in Figure 3–10.

The Small-box Method and Irregular Rhythms Some frequently occurring rhythms are highly irregular, and people often ask why they can't use the large- or the small-box method to measure them. Refer back to Figure 3–5, the strip that we determined was irregular. Count the number of small boxes between the first two QRS complexes. Then count the number of small boxes between the fifth and sixth QRSs. As you can see, the difference is dramatic. The first measurement is 19 small boxes, which the heart rate table translates into 79 bpm. In contrast, the measurement

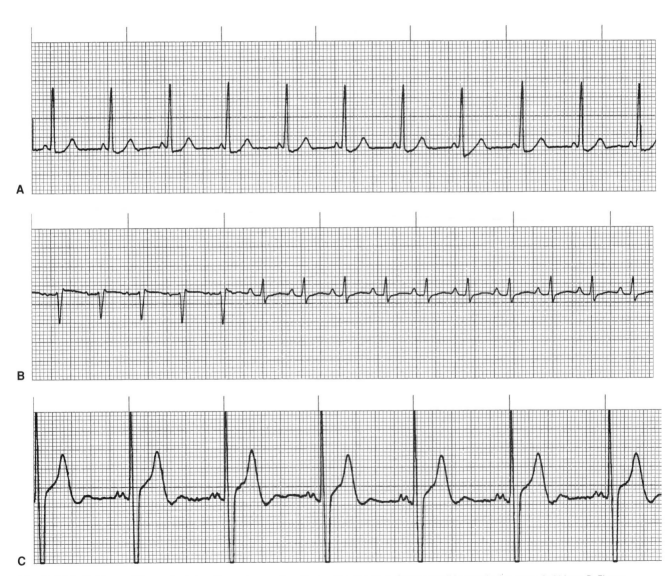

Fig. 3–10A–C The small-box method gives the most accurate estimate of heart rate. A, Sixteen small boxes; the heart rate is 94 bpm. B, Eleven small boxes; the heart rate is 136 bpm. C, Approximately 26 small boxes; the heart rate is 58 bpm.

between the fifth and sixth complexes is 27 small boxes, which translates into 56 bpm. These two heart rates will result in dramatically different rhythm strip interpretations.

The small-box method can help us understand the *range* of heart rates in an irregular strip. The six-second method will give the average heart rate over 6 seconds, but the small-box method will give us the highest and lowest heart rates over the same period. In the small-box method, the key is to find the extremes. First, measure the distance between the two closest consecutive QRS complexes; next, measure the distance between the two farthest from each other. The closest pair will give us the maximum heart rate, while the most widely spaced pair will give us the minimum heart rate.

To practice measuring range on an ECG strip, refer back to Figure 3–5. Measure the number of small boxes between the fourth and fifth QRS complexes. This represents the maximum heart rate because these two consecutive QRS complexes are the closest together. We can easily determine that the heart rate is 115 bpm. Now measure the number of small boxes between the fifth and sixth QRS complexes. There are 27 small boxes, which, according to the table in the back of the book, translate into a heart rate of 56.

Now, on the following three irregular rhythm strips (Fig. 3–11A–C), measure the average heart rate using the six-second method, and then determine the highest and lowest heart rates using the small-box method.

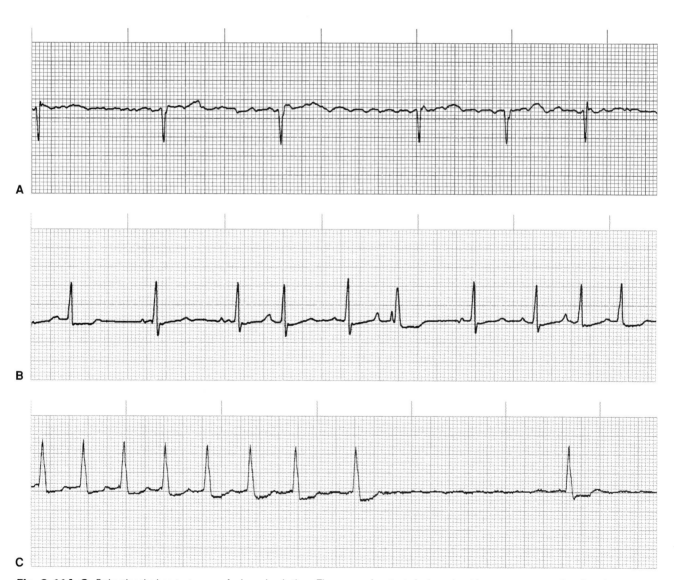

Fig. 3–11A–C Estimating the heart rate range for irregular rhythms. The average heart rate for irregular strips may not accurately reflect the range within a rhythm. A, A range of 42 bpm to 71 bpm, with an average of 60 bpm. B, A range of 68 bpm to 150 bpm, with an average of 110 bpm. C, A range of 26 to 136 bpm, with an average of 90 bpm.

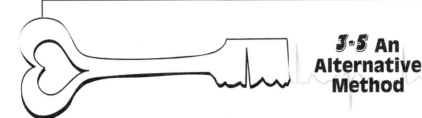

3-5 An Alternative Method

Calipers are not always readily accessible when we need to measure heart rate. But there is another way: with a piece of paper and a sharp pencil. To use this method, you place the flat edge of a piece of paper at one point of a QRS complex, then make a pencil mark on the paper at the same point of the following QRS complex. Then you lift the paper up and move the edge of it to a dark line to make the measurement—just as if the paper were calipers.

One benefit of this method is that, unlike the caliper method, there's no chance that you'll alter the measurement when you move the paper.

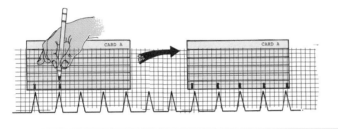

Thinking Outside the Box

The ECG rhythm strip tells us a lot more than just the heart rate. Some of this information is mandatory and should be written in if it's missing. If you review real strips, you'll notice that some strips contain writing in addition to the ECG tracing. This information can be as simple as the patient's name, or the lead from which the tracing was obtained.

The amount and type of information depend on the environment in which the tracing was recorded. For instance, patients in the intensive care unit have designated ECG monitors all to themselves. They frequently have automatic blood pressure monitors connected as well. Therefore, a strip obtained in the ICU environment can show the patient's name, heart rate, blood pressure, and more. But in the emergency room, when a patient is brought in and connected to a portable ECG monitor, the only available information may be the heart rate

and the lead designation. Emergency personnel may not know the patient's name, and the patient usually isn't connected to an automatic blood pressure monitor, at least initially.

Other information that's important to record is the gain. Gain compares the height of the ECG tracing with the standard, where 10 small boxes equal 1.0 mV. This value lets us know whether the tracing is larger or smaller, and by how much. Gain is usually indicated on the strip as "X" followed by a number, which ranges from X1/4 (one quarter of the standard height) to X4 (four times the standard height) (see Fig. 3–6). Although this information usually isn't vital for basic interpretation, it can help in some cases, as we'll see later. Since it may be on the strip, you should know what it means even if you don't need it for that particular case.

As I mentioned earlier, the patient's name and the lead designation must appear on every strip in the patient's

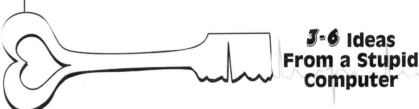

3-6 Ideas From a Stupid Computer

Some ECG machines actually attempt to interpret the rhythm for you. I stress the word "attempt" because the computer is often wrong. When the computer identifies an abnormal rhythm, it may automatically print out a strip showing the offending rhythm. Pay attention to these strips; look at them carefully before dismissing the computer as stupid. Even if the rhythm isn't dangerous, you need to know the computer's idea of a bad rhythm so you can correct it.

When the computer detects an abnormal rhythm, it frequently prints the word "ALARM" or a synonym on the strip, along with its interpretation of the rhythm. When you print out a routine strip for interpretation (which the computer doesn't do automatically), the strip will read "DELAY" or "AUTO," indicating that you requested the printout.

record. The date and time of each recording must be included. Also, it's important to list any additional information, such as chest pain or nausea. Any signs or symptoms associated with unusual rhythm strips should also be documented because they may assist in diagno-sis. This information protects you and the patient from confusion and misdiagnosis. So be careful when you tear your strips to fit them into the patient's chart. Make sure you don't remove this vital information, and if you find that you have, write it in yourself.

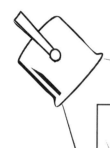

Now You Know

The ECG strip can be generated by burning the information onto special paper or tracing it with ink.

The ECG machine normally moves the paper at 25 mm per second.

Time is measured using the horizontal boxes.

Voltage is measured using the vertical boxes.

One vertical small box equals 0.1 mV.

One horizontal small box equals 0.04 seconds.

One horizontal large box equals 0.20 seconds.

Five horizontal large boxes equal 1.0 second.

The additional lines on the strip are reference points to quickly identify longer intervals.

A rhythm is considered regular if consecutive QRS complexes occur at a defined interval, or within a couple of small boxes.

There are three methods for measuring heart rate:

    The six-second method, used for regular or irregular rhythms

    The large-box method, used only for regular rhythms

    The small-box method, used for regular rhythms, or to determine range of heart rate for irregular rhythms

The patient's name, date, time, lead, gain, and any associated signs and symptoms should be recorded on each strip to aid in diagnosis and protect the interpreter.

Any computer-generated interpretation should be used only as a guide and not substituted for an analysis of the strip.

Test Yourself

1. One small box equals _____ seconds horizontally and _____ mV vertically.

2. One large box equals _____ small boxes.

3. One large box represents _____ seconds horizontally.

4. There are _____ small boxes and _____ large boxes in 1 minute.

5. There are _____ small boxes and _____ large boxes in 1 second.

6. Why can't the small-box method of calculating heart rate give you an accurate heart rate for an irregular rhythm?

7. Which method of calculating heart rate is the most accurate for a regular rhythm?

8. Why are there extra markings for time on the ECG strip?

9. What additional information should always be on a rhythm strip?

10. Circle the lead designation and the computer's calculated heart rate, and fill in the appropriate information, for the following ten strips:

   A. Is the rhythm regular or irregular?
   B. Use the six-second method to determine the heart rate.
   C. Use the large-box method to determine the heart rate.
   D. Use the small-box method to determine the heart rate.

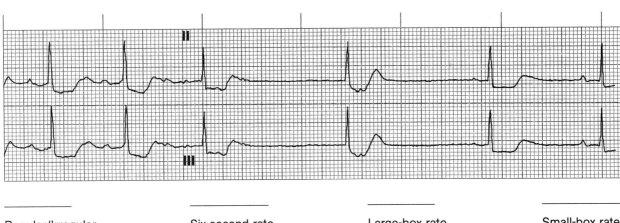

_____   _____   _____   _____
Regular/Irregular   Six-second rate   Large-box rate   Small-box rate

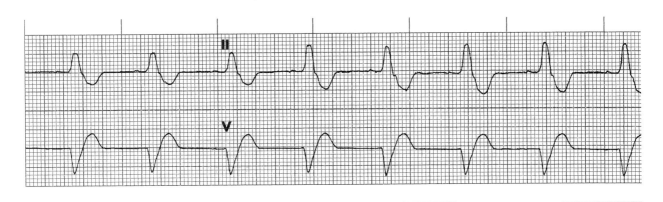

_____   _____   _____   _____
Regular/Irregular   Six-second rate   Large-box rate   Small-box rate

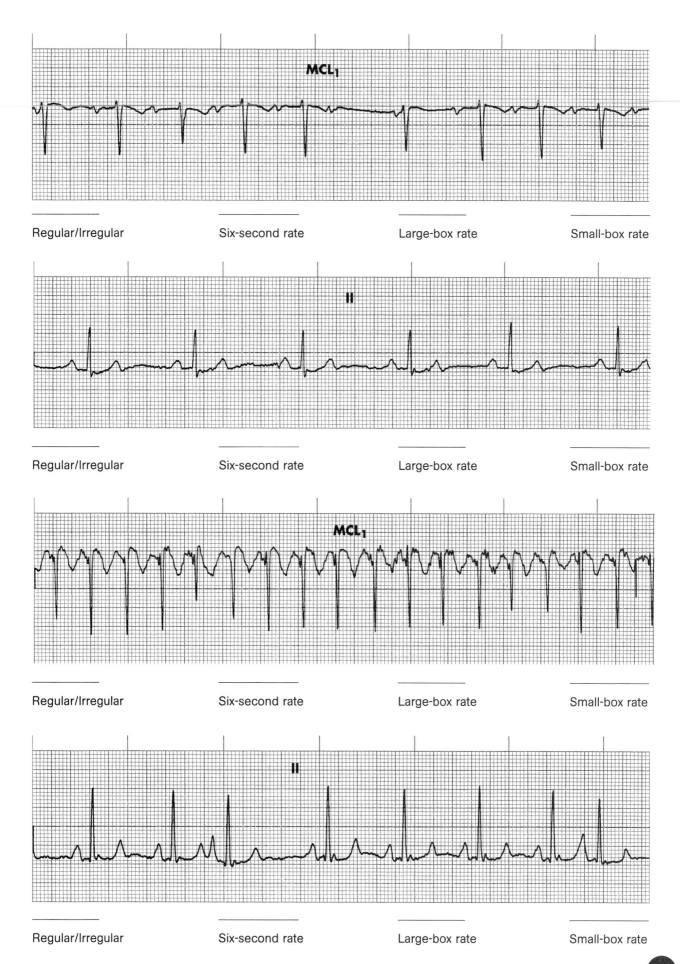

MCL₁

Regular/Irregular   Six-second rate   Large-box rate   Small-box rate

II

Regular/Irregular   Six-second rate   Large-box rate   Small-box rate

MCL₁

Regular/Irregular   Six-second rate   Large-box rate   Small-box rate

II

Regular/Irregular   Six-second rate   Large-box rate   Small-box rate

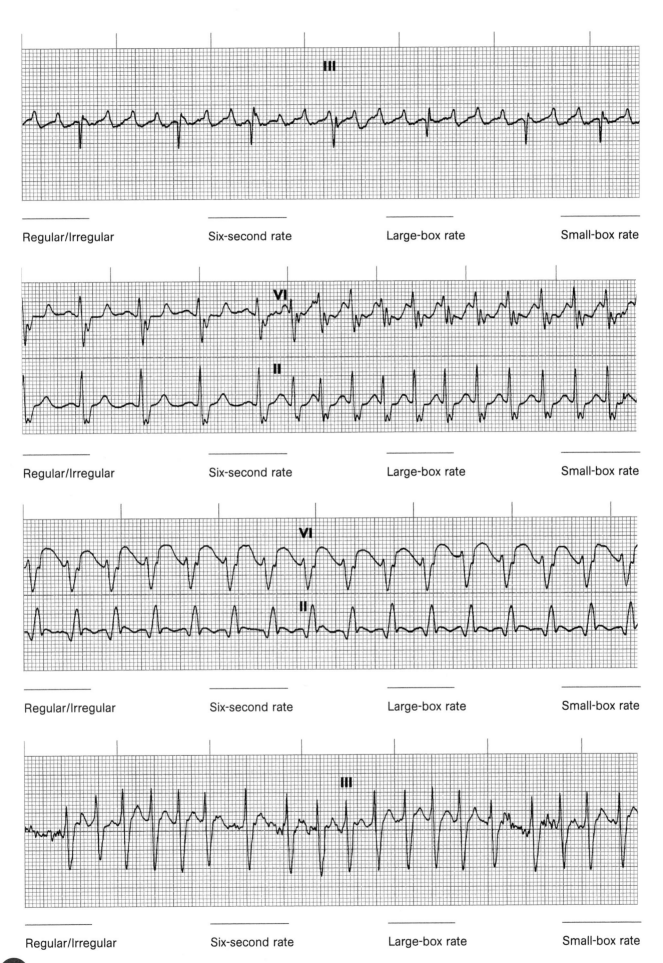

Regular/Irregular   Six-second rate   Large-box rate   Small-box rate

Regular/Irregular   Six-second rate   Large-box rate   Small-box rate

Regular/Irregular   Six-second rate   Large-box rate   Small-box rate

Regular/Irregular   Six-second rate   Large-box rate   Small-box rate

LOCATION, LOCATION, LOCATION

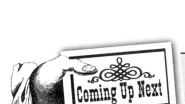
Coming Up Next

- ○ What is a vector?
- ○ How do vectors relate to the ECG tracing?
- ○ What are the basic features of an ECG patch?
- ○ What things can interfere with the electrical signal reaching the ECG patch?
- ○ How do we correct the problems caused by interference?
- ○ Where are the standard locations for the ECG patches?
- ○ What are limb leads? What are precordial leads?
- ○ What is the difference between unipolar and bipolar leads?

Lines of Force

We've learned that the heart generates electrical signals. These signals cause the heart to contract, and to do so (we hope) in a coordinated fashion. We've learned that these signals form an identifiable pattern when written on paper with special markings. What we don't know is how the electrical signals get from the patient to the paper. That's what we'll cover in this section. But before we get there, we need to look at an important concept: vectors.

Electrical forces inside the heart are traveling in all different directions. Because all these forces are vectors, we can represent each one as an arrow. The problem is, we can't measure and trace the thousands of individual vectors in the heart, and even if we could, the result would be a mess to interpret. Our solution is to measure just a few vectors, representing the average of the thousands of vectors moving through the heart, and then to trace those few.

You can find higher mathematics courses devoted to vectors; in fact, you can learn to average any number of

4-1 HOW HARD CAN YOU PULL?

A *vector* is simply a force, or energy, exerted in a general direction. Let's say you need to drag a large, heavy object, such as a grand piano. If you tie a rope to the piano and pull, you create a vector. The vector has two components: the force and the direction of your pull. We can represent the vector as an arrow, with the tail at the place where the piano starts moving, the tip pointing the same way you're pulling, and the thickness indicating how hard you're pulling. (You also create a vector if you push the piano. Any force, whether electrical or physical, generated in any way, creates a vector.)

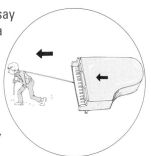

them. However, you don't need higher math to understand the concept of averaging vectors; you see it in action every day.

In Search of an Arrow
OBEYING THE LAW OF AVERAGES

The electrical conduction signal in the heart is like all those different ropes pulling on the piano. The signal is being sent in all directions at the same time. Therefore, we have a large number of vectors, all with different intensities and directions. But what we actually measure is the *average* force and direction of the signal.

We measure this average vector by measuring the difference in the electrical signals at two points. For this we attach electrodes to different areas of the body. Each electrode measures all the electrical forces moving both toward it and away from it. Therefore, just as our piano responds to the average of several physical forces, our electrodes measure the average of all the electrical forces. This average is what appears as the ECG tracing.

To make an ECG tracing, then, we need to know the direction and intensity of the average signal as it travels through the heart. Now we need some way to transmit the signal to the ECG machine. The skin is the closest we can get to the heart without exposing the patient to injury or infection. Therefore, we connect the electrodes to the patient's skin using patches.

LEARNING PATCHWORK

From Torture to Technology To measure the heart's faint signals through the skin, we need to capture them somehow. The original technique used needles that actually pierced the outer layer of dead skin cells and penetrated into the living dermis and subcutaneous areas. This hurt, especially if the patient moved. Later we advanced to gauze dipped in a dilute saline solution and then applied to the patient.

Today we use adhesive patches made of a better electrical conductor, frequently silver chloride (AgCl). The patch has an area of sticky adhesive surrounding a small gelatinous disk of the conductor, usually about 1 cm in diameter. The sticky area is connected to a small metal disk with a snap that sticks out at the top of the patch. This snap is where the cables from the ECG monitor are connected. The electrical signal is transmitted from the skin to the gel, to the metal disk, to the snap, to the ECG cable, and finally to the monitoring equipment.

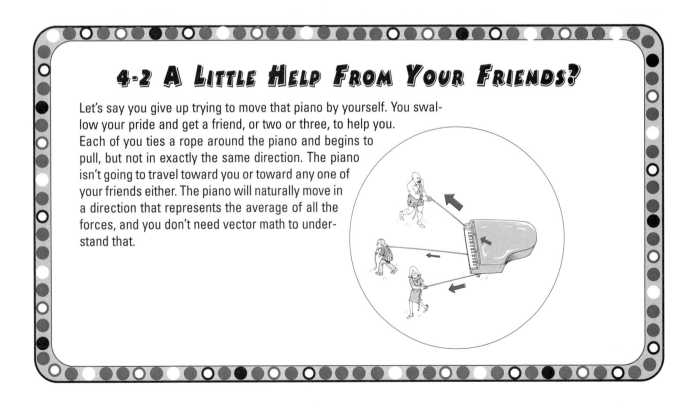

4-2 A Little Help From Your Friends?

Let's say you give up trying to move that piano by yourself. You swallow your pride and get a friend, or two or three, to help you. Each of you ties a rope around the piano and begins to pull, but not in exactly the same direction. The piano isn't going to travel toward you or toward any one of your friends either. The piano will naturally move in a direction that represents the average of all the forces, and you don't need vector math to understand that.

Can You Make It Stick? These high-tech patches present a few problems that the old-fashioned needles didn't. First, the surface layer of skin is made completely of dead cells, which don't conduct electricity as well as live skin cells. The dead cells can be abraded off gently with a fine grade of sandpaper, but you must take care not to damage the underlying tissue or cause bleeding. Newer patches are more efficient, and so abrading the skin has become less popular, but it can still improve signal reception in some cases.

Oil and sweat are often present on the skin surface. Both these substances inhibit signal conduction. A quick cleansing with an alcohol swab or soap and water will usually remove them.

Hair can interfere with patches by reducing the amount of skin surface that touches the patch. Usually it's sufficient to clip the hairs as close to the skin surface as possible. If the hair is particularly dense, you may have to shave the area. Again, it's important to preserve skin integrity. A patch over broken skin can cause poor conduction, significant irritation and itching, and even infection.

The location chosen for the patch must be as flat as possible. The patch is flexible enough to keep contact with a slightly irregular surface, but a flatter surface is always better.

Finally, try to keep patches away from places where large bones come near the skin surface. Bones are not good conductors and can diminish the signal traveling through them.

WHERE, OH WHERE, DO THE PATCHES GO?

Now you can't just start sticking ECG patches all over a patient and connecting wires. If you did, you'd get an ECG tracing—your patches would pick up the heart's signal—but the tracing wouldn't give you any useful information. Also, my placement would probably vary from yours, so we wouldn't be able to compare tracings if we needed to look for changes. To get a correct interpretation, you need to put the patches in designated locations, shown in Figure 4–1. These locations have been chosen for the specific information they provide. These locations are for a 12-lead ECG. We will discuss them to understand all possible leads, but we will vary the placement for continuous monitoring for convenience and patient comfort.

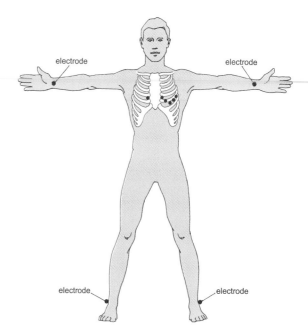

Fig. 4–1   The proper locations of the 10 electrodes used for a 12-lead ECG.

We don't really care about the signal if it's measured at just one point. We do care how the signal travels through the heart; therefore, we need at least two points to measure it from.

Lead and the Signal Will Follow

Two patches placed at a distance from each other are called a *lead*. Think back to the discussion of polarity in Chapter 2. Well, each lead has poles also, a positive and a negative pole—just like a magnet. Each of these poles is a patch with an electrode. The signal is measured as it travels between the two poles. The placement of the positive electrode usually tells us which part of the heart is being monitored. We'll visit this point again at the end of the chapter and explore it more deeply later in the book.

If the ECG tracing moves up, or is *positively deflected,* the signal is traveling toward the positive electrode and away from the negative one. Conversely, if the ECG tracing moves down, or is *negatively deflected,* then it's moving toward the negative electrode and away from the positive one.

The leads that monitor the vertical plane are called *limb leads* because they use the patches located near the patient's arms and legs. These leads are I, II, III, aVR, aVF, and aVL. The leads that monitor the horizontal plane are called *chest leads* because they use the patches located

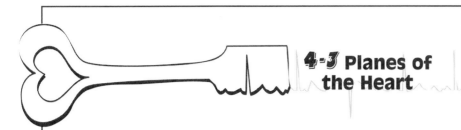

4-3 Planes of the Heart

For the purposes of this book, the heart can be divided into two distinct planes: the vertical and the horizontal (Fig. 4–2). The vertical plane cuts through the heart from top to bottom, and the horizontal cuts through the heart from back to front. To get a complete picture of the heart's electrical conduction, we must measure in both planes. The vertical plane measures the top-to-bottom movement of the signal; the horizontal plane measures its back-to-front movement.

cal plane, measuring the signal as it travels from top to bottom or from side to side. Each consists of two actual, distinct patches, one labeled "negative" (−) and the other "positive" (+), like the poles of a battery. These leads usually give the best views for identifying the individual parts of the ECG tracing, which we'll discuss in Chapter 5.

The bipolar leads are leads I, II, and III (Fig. 4–3A–C). Bipolar leads actually use three electrodes—the positive, negative, and ground

on the patient's chest wall. They're also called *precordial leads,* from the combining forms meaning "in front of" and "heart." These leads are V₁, V₂, V₃, V₄, V₅, and V₆. Each lead monitors a specific area of the heart. Later in the book we'll pay more attention to the functions of the different leads.

We go further than just distinguishing between chest and limb leads. Some leads use only one electrode to capture the electrical signal; others use two.

electrodes—to generate a tracing. The ground electrode helps to eliminate the noncardiac electrical signals, such as those from the nerves, skin, and muscles. So, even though three patches are used, the tracing measures the difference between two electrodes, using a third electrode to help eliminate information we don't need. These leads can also be generated by using the two paddles of a defibrillator monitor.

BIPOLAR LEADS

Bipolar leads are the type used most frequently for monitoring patients. These leads monitor the heart in the verti-

UNIPOLAR LEADS

The other type of lead is unipolar. Instead of using two electrodes, unipolar leads use only one.

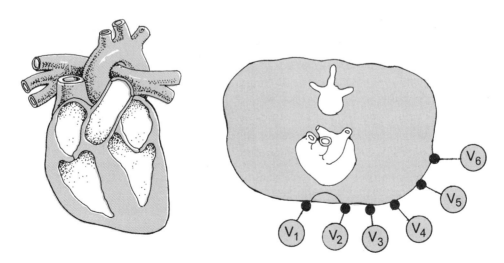

Fig. 4–2 The limb leads view the signal as it travels through the vertical plane (pink). The precordial, or chest, leads view the signal as it travels through the horizontal plane (blue).

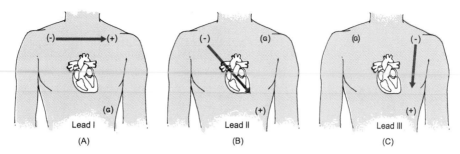

Fig. 4–3A–C In a system that uses three electrodes, leads I, II, and III can be obtained by placing the electrodes as shown. A, Lead I uses RA as negative, LA as positive, and LL as ground. B, Lead II uses RA as negative, LL as positive, and LA as ground. C, Lead III uses LA as negative, LL as positive, and RA as ground.

I know, you're asking, "How can a lead be unipolar?" The other location, instead of being an actual electrode, is an imaginary point that represents the center of the heart. Calculated from the placement of several other patches, it represents both the second electrode and the ground electrode found in bipolar leads. Therefore, unipolar leads really do have the two points they should have, but only one of them is an actual electrode. Unipolar leads can be monitored only if there are other electrodes attached to the patient.

The unipolar leads are leads aVR, aVL, aVF, V_1, V_2, V_3, V_4, V_5, and V_6 (Fig. 4–4A–B).

A LOT OF LEADS TO FOLLOW

Together there are 12 possible leads, three bipolar and nine unipolar, that make up the standard 12-lead ECG. However, in most cases the bedside monitoring equipment can't track all 12 leads continuously. More commonly, it monitors between one and seven leads at once.

Some monitors display the tracings from more than one lead at a time. If a patient is in intensive care, the bedside monitor may display two or more leads while the central monitor displays only one. In cardiac telemetry units, which don't have bedside-monitoring capabilities, patients are in more stable condition, so it's usually

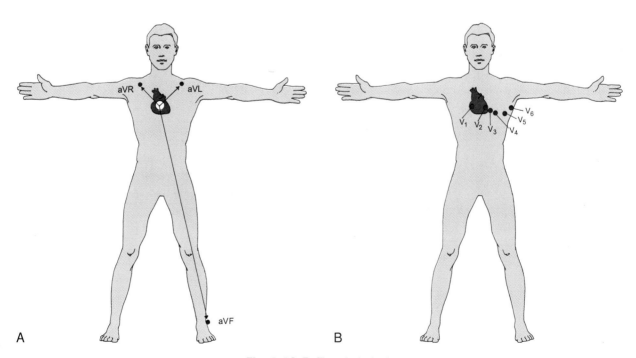

Fig. 4–4A–B The unipolar leads.

considered sufficient to display one lead on the central monitor.

Electrode Placement and Leads

Electrode placement has been standardized to make it easier and quicker. The wires that connect to individual electrodes are frequently coded with specific colors (Table 4–1). Sometimes only the ends of the wires are colored, so you have to keep your eye out. (Note: These color designations are for the United States; other countries use different ones.)

All ECG monitoring devices label the wires with the letter designation, the color, or both. Not all monitoring equipment has five wires; some systems have only three. But, however many wires are present, their placement will always follow the listings in Table 4–1.

LEADS I, II, AND III

Leads I, II, and III are bipolar limb leads that can be generated by using only three electrodes. Systems that work this way always use electrodes RA, LA, and LL in the standard position (see Table 4–1). By changing what each electrode represents, we can alter the tracing we get. Looking at Table 4–2, we can see that if RA is the negative pole, LA is the positive pole, and RL is the ground, we get lead I. If RA is negative, LA ground, and LL positive, we get lead II. Finally, if RA is ground, LA negative, and LL positive, we get lead III. The computer inside the ECG monitoring equipment switches the roles of the electrodes automatically. All we have to do is change settings, from lead I to lead II, for instance.

Table 4–2 Placement of ECG bipolar limb leads

Lead I	Lead II	Lead III
RA negative	RA negative	LA negative
LA positive	LL positive	LL positive
RL ground	LA ground	RA ground

LEADS aVR, aVL, AND aVF

Leads aVR, aVL, and aVF are unipolar limb leads. Like leads I, II, and III, they're generated from electrodes RA, LA, and LL. Usually a fourth electrode, RL, is used along with them. Because these leads are unipolar, they use only one actual electrode and average the signal from all the electrodes attached to the patient. The fourth electrode, RL, allows a more accurate calculation of the second (imaginary) electrode signal, which represents the center of the heart.

These leads are known as *augmented leads*. Because they're generated differently, they produce a much smaller ECG tracing than any of the other leads. Therefore, the computer amplifies their signal to make the tracing size consistent with that of the tracings from all the other leads.

You may be wondering why we designate these leads the way we do. Well, the uppercase "V" stands for "vector"; the lowercase "a" stands for "augmented." The final letter tells you which electrode is positive: "R" for RA, "L" for LA, and "F" for LL ("F" stands for "foot" to help differentiate it from aVL). We read aVR as *augmented vector right*, aVL as *augmented vector left*, and aVF as *augmented vector foot*.

Table 4–1 ECG Electrode designations and wire colors

Location	Letter Designation	Wire Color
Right arm	RA	White
Left arm	LA	Black
Right leg	RL	Green
Left leg	LL	Red
Chest	V	Brown

Table 4–3 Placement of ECG chest leads

Lead	Electrode Placement
V_1	Fourth intercostal space at right sternal border
V_2	Fourth intercostal space at left sternal border
V_3	Midpoint of a straight line connecting V_2 and V_4
V_4	Fifth intercostal space on midclavicular line
V_5	Fifth intercostal space anterior axillary line
V_6	Fifth intercostal space midaxillary line

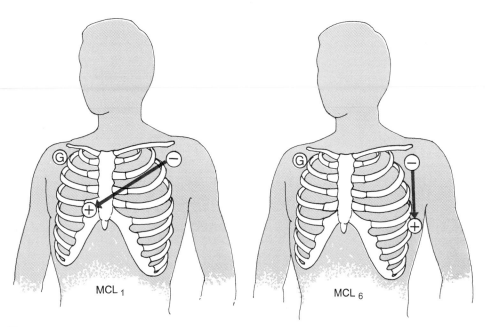

MCL ₁   MCL ₆

Fig. 4–5 For modified chest leads (designated by MCL$_x$), place the white-wire (usually labeled RA) electrode in the same position as the equivalent V lead you want to monitor (i.e., place the white wire [RA] at the fifth intercostal space, midaxillary line, to monitor MCL$_6$).

LEADS V₁ THROUGH V₆

Leads V_1 through V_6 are unipolar chest leads. We can generate any one of these leads using only five electrodes: RA, LA, RL, LL, and the chest lead. We don't use all six V leads unless we're working with a 12-lead ECG tracing.

The placement of the V electrode (connected to a brown cable in a five-wire system) determines which chest lead we're monitoring. Placement is critical. The leads and the placement of the electrodes are listed in Table 4–3.

MODIFIED CHEST LEADS

In a system that only uses three wires, it is sometimes necessary to approximate the chest leads. In this case, we refer to *modified chest leads* (MCL$_x$, where "x" indicates which of the six chest leads is being approximated). This involves moving wires and electrodes (Fig. 4–5). The ground electrode, which is connected to the red wire, is placed on the right shoulder area, not on the left leg, where it usually goes. The negative lead is placed on the left shoulder area and is connected to the white wire (RA wire). The

remaining electrode is placed at the correct location for the chest lead that you want to approximate. This electrode is connected to the black wire.

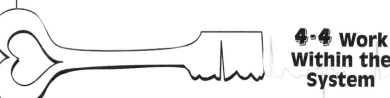

4-4 Work Within the System

Suppose you want to monitor a chest lead in a three-wire system lead. MCL should be selected on the monitor if the system allows it. Some systems do; others force you to choose another lead, let's say lead I, II, or III, to record the tracing, and then you have to label the strip by hand as MCL. With this kind of system, select lead I and record your tracing. Be sure to cross out the lead designation and write the correct MCL designation in its place. The most common modified chest leads to be monitored are MCL$_1$ and MCL$_6$.

I Spy with My Little Lead

Why do we have 12 potential leads when we have only one heart? The answer is that each lead views the heart from a slightly different perspective; we'll develop this concept as we move through the book. For right now, remember this: the placement of the positive electrode with respect to the heart usually indicates which part of the heart is being monitored. For instance, lead V_6 monitors the side of the heart, or the lateral wall; leads V_3 and V_4 monitor the front of the left ventricle; and leads II and III monitor the bottom of the heart, or the inferior wall. This knowledge becomes critical when we're deciding which leads to monitor for a particular condition.

Also, remember that if the signal travels toward a positive electrode in a lead, then the tracing will be positive, and if it travels towards the negative electrode (or away from the positive electrode), the tracing will be negative.

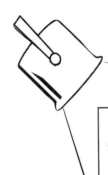

Now You Know

A vector is simply a force applied in a specific direction.

The ECG tracing is a graphical representation of the average vector at a given time.

ECG patches have a conductive gel (usually silver chloride), a sticky applicator, and a metal snap on which to attach the ECG wire.

It's important for the conductive gel to make good contact. Interference with proper conduction can come from dry or irritated skin, excessive or thick hair, large bones, dead skin cells, and lotion or sweat.

We can gently abrade the skin, clean it with soap and water or alcohol, clip or carefully shave the hair, or change the lead position as a last resort.

The white patch goes on the right shoulder area and the black lead on the left shoulder area. The green wire goes on the right side of the upper abdomen, the red wire goes on the left side of the upper abdomen, and the brown wire attachment depends on which V lead we wish to monitor.

Limb leads are I, II, III, aVR, aVL, and aVF and are formed using the four patches RA, RL, LA, and LL, located near the arms and legs. Chest leads, also called precordial leads, consist of leads V1–V6 and use the patches that are placed on the anterior and lateral chest wall.

Bipolar leads measure the difference between two actual ECG patch locations to make the ECG tracing. Unipolar leads use one actual ECG patch and average the signal received by several other patches to approximate the second patch location as the center of the heart.

Test Yourself

1. A vector can be represented by an _____.

2. The ECG tracing represents the _____ of all the electrical vectors in the heart.

3. Name four impediments that can interfere with the electrical signal: _____.

4. Silver chloride (AgCL) is used as an electrical _____ in many ECG patches.

5. Which leads are limb leads? _____
Which leads are precordial leads?

_____

Which leads are unipolar? _____
Which are bipolar? _____

6. Bipolar leads use two _____ electrodes. Unipolar leads use one _____ lead and one _____ electrode, which is an average of the remaining electrodes.

7. Match the electrode with its proper location:

A. White

B. Black

C. Red

D. Green

E. V_1 (MCL$_1$)

F. V_2 (MCL$_2$)

G. V_3 (MCL$_3$)

H. V_4 (MCL$_4$)

I. V_5 (MCL$_5$)

J. V_6 (MCL$_6$)

a. Fourth intercostal space left sternal border

b. Fifth intercostal space midaxillary line

c. Right arm (shoulder area)

d. Left arm (shoulder area)

e. Fifth intercostal space midclavicular line

f. Fourth intercostal space right sternal border

g. Fifth intercostal space anterior axillary line

h. Left leg or midclavicular line on abdomen

i. Right leg or midclavicular line on abdomen

j. Midway between V_2 and V_4

SECTION

2

Getting More Technical

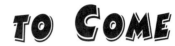

THE SHAPE OF THINGS

TO COME

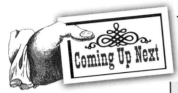

○ What do the parts of the PQRSTU tracing look like?

○ What are waves, intervals, complexes, and segments?

○ Can more than one of each letter appear in a single complex?

○ Do the letters always occur in the PQRSTU order?

Telling Dogs From Wolves

PATTERN RECOGNITION

Do you know what a car looks like? How about a dog? Can you instantly recognize your best friend in a crowded room? If you can answer yes to these three questions, you can learn to recognize the lines and curves that make up the ECG rhythm strip.

Whether or not you realize it, when you look at a person or an object for the first time, your brain identifies key features and remembers them. Then it uses them to recognize what you've seen the next time you see it. These key features are vital to quick recognition. If I had never seen a dog and I asked you to describe it, what would you do say? It's not easy, is it? One way would be to give specific features and then show me several pictures as examples. Then I'd have a pretty good idea. However, I'd get an even better idea if I tried to pick out the dogs in a pack of similar animals, such as wolves. That way you could tell me if I was right or wrong and explain why.

That's how most of this book will be organized. First I'll list the specific features of a particular rhythm, and then I'll show some perfect examples of that rhythm. I'll also give you several examples of the rhythms to

practice on, with the correct answers at the end of the book. But you must learn how all the parts of a perfect ECG tracing fit together before you can study the various rhythms. This chapter will teach you how to identify the different parts of the ECG tracing; the next two chapters will tell you which parts of the heart they correspond to.

START AT THE BOTTOM

The most easily identified portion of the ECG tracing is the *baseline*. This is the straight, flat line that connects all the curves, waves, and complexes. We also call it the *isoelectric line* ("iso-" means "same") because no electrical activity from the heart is being picked up. All waves and complexes are measured from this line. In other words, a wave begins when the tracing leaves the baseline and ends when it returns there.

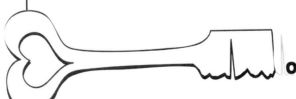

5-1 Process of Elimination

There is another way to identify the baseline: if you identify all the other portions of the tracing, the baseline is whatever's left over. Ideally this line is perfectly flat. However, in real strips it may have occasional bumps or may drift slightly upward or downward.

The Perfect Wave

SURFING THE ALPHABET

A *wave* is a rounded curve or a straight line that leaves the baseline and returns to it. The ECG waveform is a group of waves that record the electrical signal as it depolarizes the heart muscle cells. It's important to identify the pieces of the ECG tracings correctly because the measurements of each individual wave can affect the rhythm strip interpretation.

To describe the waveform in detail, we break it down into parts that are easily recognizable and that correspond to various parts of the heart. Each part of the waveform is designated by one or more of the letters P, Q, R, S, T, and U. The different parts of the waveform frequently occur in alphabetical order, although some parts may be absent and some may appear more than once in the same waveform. It's important to understand what part of the heart, and therefore what part of the depolarization-repolarization cycle, the letters are associated with. This chapter will give you a basis on which to begin interpreting different heart rhythms. Once you understand each rhythm, you'll be able to learn its possible complications and their consequences to the patient.

Figure 5–1 is the prototype of the normal ECG waveform. It contains all the letters, and everything is perfect and easy to identify. Don't get used to it, though. You'll almost never encounter a perfect ECG strip in a real patient; there aren't even many perfect strips in this book. However, learning to read ECG strips is like learning a language. First you must learn the letters and words and how they're supposed to go together. Only then can you go on to learn the dialects and slang terms of your new language.

TALL, STRAIGHT LINES

After the baseline, the easiest feature to recognize is the QRS complex. The QRS complex is a set of straight lines, usually the tallest part of the tracing. This portion is usually the most prominent and, as we'll find out later, the most important feature of the ECG strip. The QRS is the only part of the tracing to have a three-letter designation. That's because it can actually have three distinct pieces. Its shape doesn't necessarily change the rhythm interpretation but may affect other ECG phenomena.

The first piece of the QRS complex is the Q-wave. The Q-wave is defined as the first downward, or negative, deflection of the QRS *before* any upward deflection. So, if the first QRS deflection is upward, there is no Q-wave. Even without a Q-wave, the entire complex is still called a QRS complex.

The R-wave is defined as any upward, or positive, deflection of the QRS complex above the baseline. If the first deflection is positive, that's the R-wave. If the first deflection is negative and the second positive, you have both a Q-wave and an R-wave (Fig. 5–2A–B). Sometimes you'll find only a single positive deflection; that's an R-wave by itself (Fig. 5–2C).

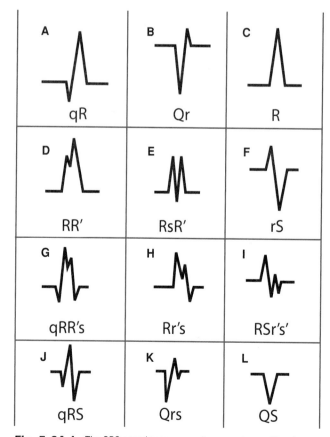

Fig. 5–2A–L The QRS complex can come in many shapes. The shape indicates only what path the electrical signal took through the ventricles.

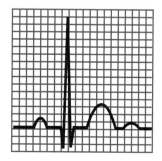

Fig. 5–1 The ECG tracing prototype.

The S-wave is defined as any negative deflection after the R-wave. That is, if you see a positive deflection and then a negative deflection, you're looking at an R-wave followed by an S-wave. See Figure 5–2F–K for examples of QRS complexes with S-waves. Some shapes are normal in some leads and abnormal in others. For example, a tall R-wave is normal in lead II, but the same waveform is always abnormal in leads aVR and V$_1$.

If there are no positive deflections at all, only negative deflections, this part of the tracing is labeled a QS complex. This departure from the rules is simply convention. Figure 5–2I shows an example of a QS complex.

There can be more than one R-wave (Fig. 5–2D–H) and more than one S-wave (Fig 5–2I), but there's never more than one Q-wave. This is because the Q-wave is defined as the *first* negative deflection. If the QRS complex has more than one R- or S-wave, the second one is designated with a prime (') symbol to differentiate it from the other wave of the same type. See Figure 5–2D–I for some examples.

Identify the QRS complexes and their individual waves on the following four strips (Fig. 5–3). The first one is done for you.

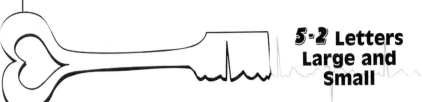

5-2 Letters Large and Small

As if naming the QRS complex weren't intricate enough, the sizes of individual waves are indicated by uppercase and lowercase letters. As the examples in Figure 5–2 show you, lowercase letters indicate that the corresponding wave is small; uppercase letters are used for larger waves. Small q-waves may be benign, but large Q-waves usually indicate heart attacks. If there are two R-waves, the larger usually gets an uppercase R and the smaller a lowercase r, in addition to the prime (') notation applied to the second wave. This convention helps to describe more phenomena that you'll probably encounter in a more advanced course.

Fortunately, we can identify a rhythm without this thought-provoking exercise. But because the configuration of the QRS complex can vary so widely, it's important to be as specific as possible when identifying it in an ECG strip. When we begin measuring the QRS later, we will know where to start and stop measuring.

A GENTLE CURVE

The tall, straight lines calm down after the QRS complex. Then comes the T-wave. The T-wave always follows the QRS. If you have a QRS complex, you *must* have a T-wave; you can't have one without the other. You always find the T-wave after the QRS, never before it.

The T-wave is usually small and rounded. Its distance from the QRS complex can vary—sometimes it's closer, sometimes it's farther away. Although T-waves are almost always rounded, they can be nearly flat in some leads. If you're unable to identify the T-wave in one lead, check another lead.

Identify the T-waves on the four strips in Figure 5–4 and notice how they vary. The first one is done for you.

A GENTLER CURVE

The final piece of the ECG tracing is the U-wave. When you can find it, it always follows the T-wave and is usually much smaller and rounded. Its presence is very uncommon, and its significance is still debated. Some conditions can cause it to appear larger. Although it normally can be present in slower rhythms and may indicate an electrolyte imbalance, its presence doesn't affect the interpretation of the rhythm. We need to recognize the U-wave so we can distinguish it from the next wave of the perfect ECG—the P-wave.

IN THE BEGINNING WAS THE P-WAVE

The P-wave is rounded, much smaller than the QRS complex, and usually smaller than the T-wave. It usually occurs before the QRS and can appear inverted (negative deflection) or upright (positive deflection). On rare occasions it follows the QRS, but I'll explain those circumstances when we discuss the associated rhythms. For the purposes of this chapter, the P-wave always appears before the QRS.

Some rhythms have more than one P-wave for every QRS complex. But the T-wave, and the U-wave if it's present, never appear more than once in relation to any QRS complex.

Identify the P-wave or P-waves on the following four strips (Fig. 5–5A–D). The first one is done for you.

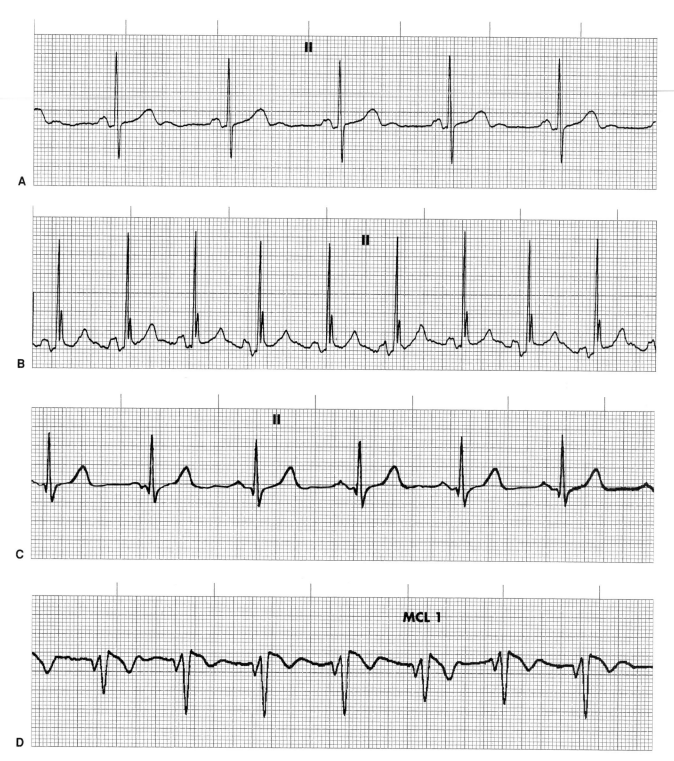

Fig. 5-3A-D Identify the QRS complexes on these strips.

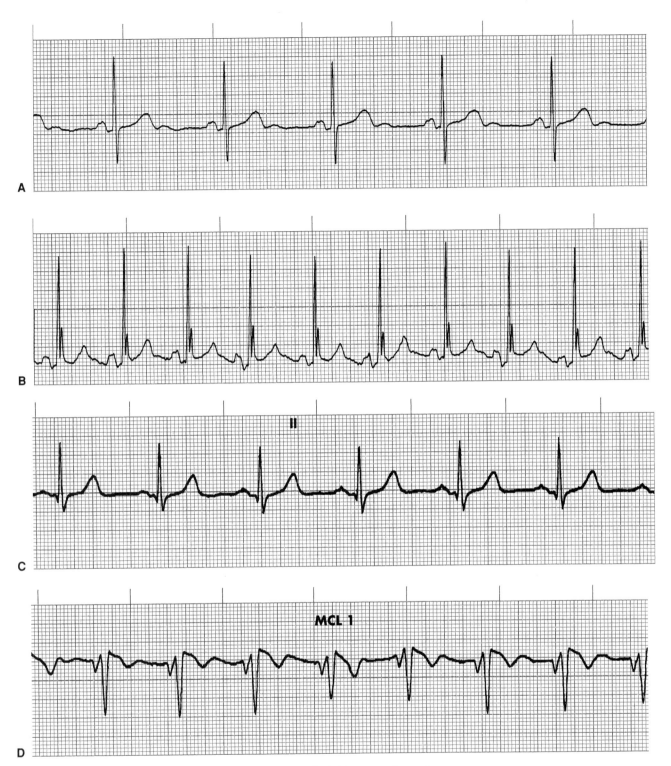

Fig. 5–4A–D Identify the T-waves on these strips.

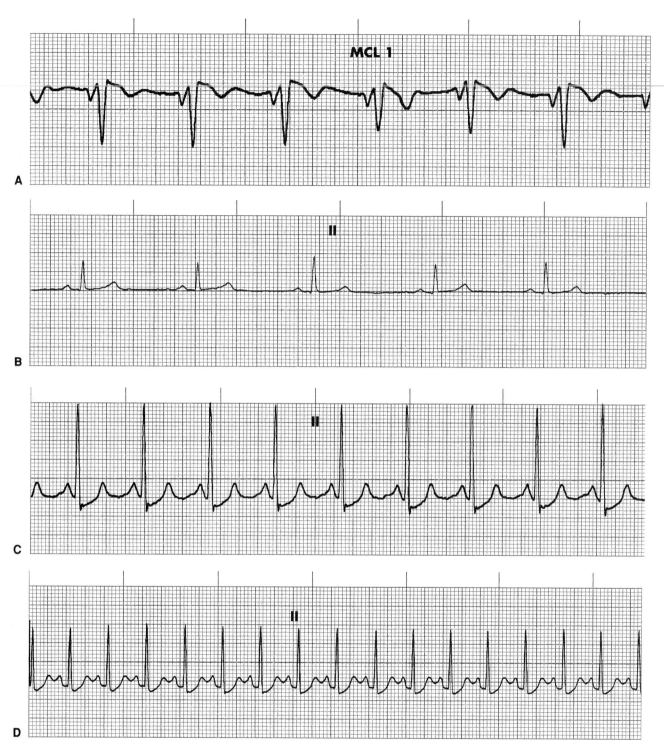

Fig. 5–5A–D Identify the P-waves on these strips.

Waves, Complexes, Segments, and Intervals

A COUPLE YOU'VE MET

You already know a good deal about waves. As we've seen, a wave can be rounded or straight, provided it leaves the baseline and returns there. Examples include the P-, T-, Q-, and U-waves.

You also know something about complexes. A *complex* is a group of waves; for example, the QRS complex can consist of a Q-wave, R-waves, and S-waves or variation combinations of these.

A COUPLE YOU HAVEN'T MET

A *segment* is a piece of the baseline that connects two waves. Examples include the PR segment, which connects the end of the P-wave to the beginning of the QRS complex. Technically this should be called a PQ segment. However, it's more common for the Q-wave to be missing than to be present, so the R-wave becomes the first portion of the QRS complex. Another example is the ST segment, which connects the end of the QRS (frequently an S-wave) to the beginning of the T-wave. We'll revisit the ST segment when we discuss myocardial infarctions. There's also a TP segment, which connects the end of the T-wave to the beginning of the P-wave if no U-wave is present. See Figure 5–6 for examples of the PR, ST, and TP segments.

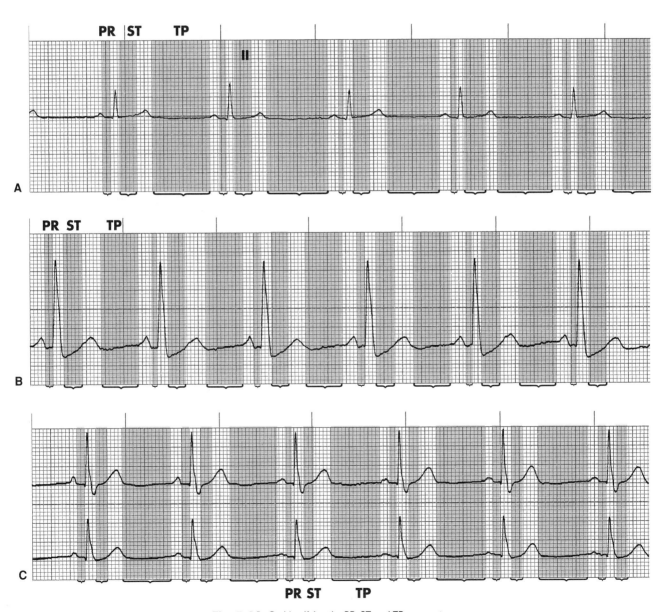

Fig. 5–6A–C Identifying the PR, ST, and TP segments.

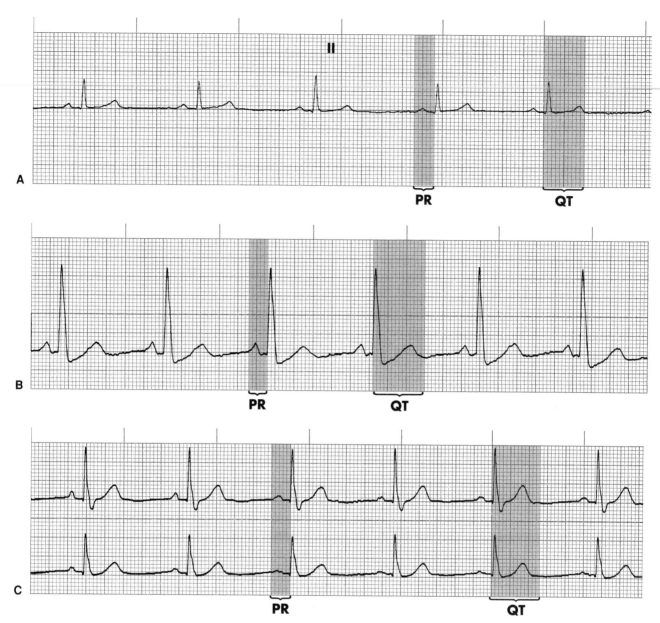

Fig. 5-7A-C Identifying the PR and QT intervals.

Intervals are the most inclusive elements of the ECG tracing. An *interval* contains at least one wave and one segment. Examples include the PR interval, which contains the entire P-wave and the PR segment, and the QT interval, which contains the entire QRS complex and the ST segment as well as the T-wave. See Figure 5-7 for examples of these intervals.

Identify the PR segment, PR interval, and ST segment in the four strips shown in Figure 5-8.

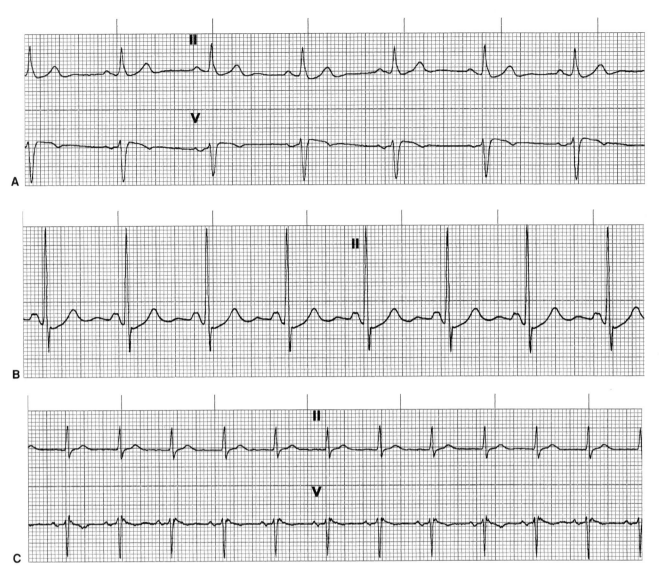

Fig. 5–8A–C Identify the PR segment, PR interval, and ST segment in these strips.

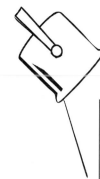

Now You Know

Two waves are connected by a segment.

The P-wave usually comes before the QRS complex. There may be more than one P-wave or none at all.

Complexes consist of at least one wave and frequently more than one.

Intervals begin at the beginning of one wave and end before the next wave.

Without exception, the T-wave always comes after the QRS complex.

The U-wave is usually not present. If it does appear, it occurs after the T-wave and is small and rounded.

If there is a QRS complex, there must be one and only one T-wave.

QRS complexes frequently don't have all three waves (the Q-, R-, and S-waves) and can have more than one R- or S-wave.

Test Yourself

1. Label and measure all the parts of the ECG tracing in the following 10 strips:

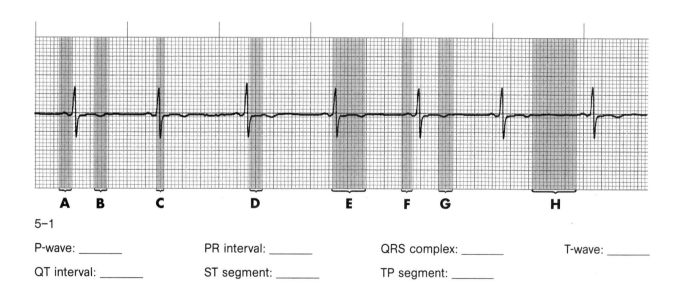

5–1

P-wave: _____   PR interval: _____   QRS complex: _____   T-wave: _____

QT interval: _____   ST segment: _____   TP segment: _____

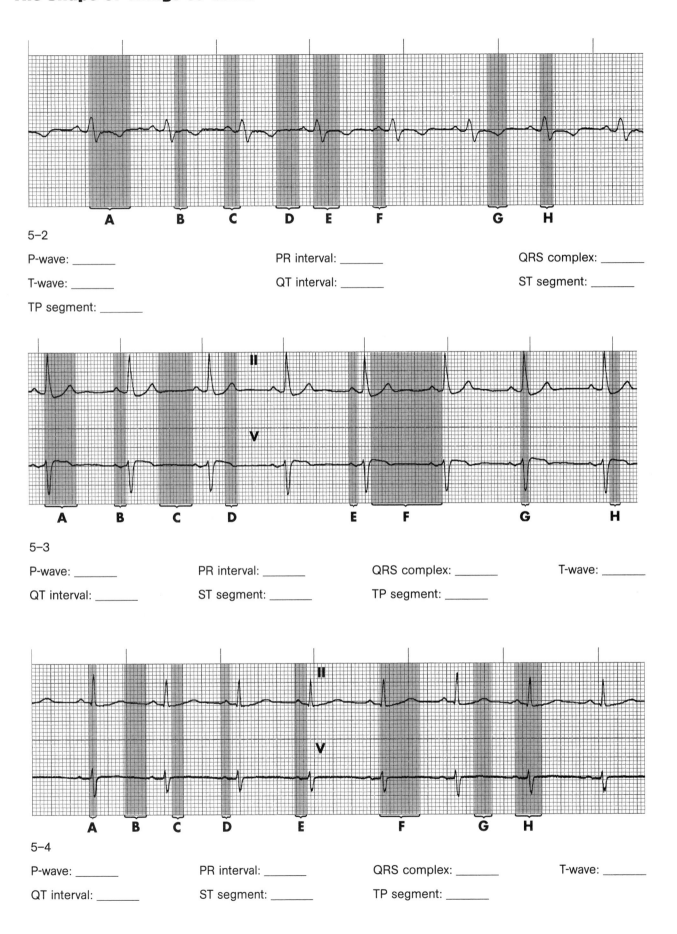

5–2

P-wave: _____   PR interval: _____   QRS complex: _____

T-wave: _____   QT interval: _____   ST segment: _____

TP segment: _____

5–3

P-wave: _____   PR interval: _____   QRS complex: _____   T-wave: _____

QT interval: _____   ST segment: _____   TP segment: _____

5–4

P-wave: _____   PR interval: _____   QRS complex: _____   T-wave: _____

QT interval: _____   ST segment: _____   TP segment: _____

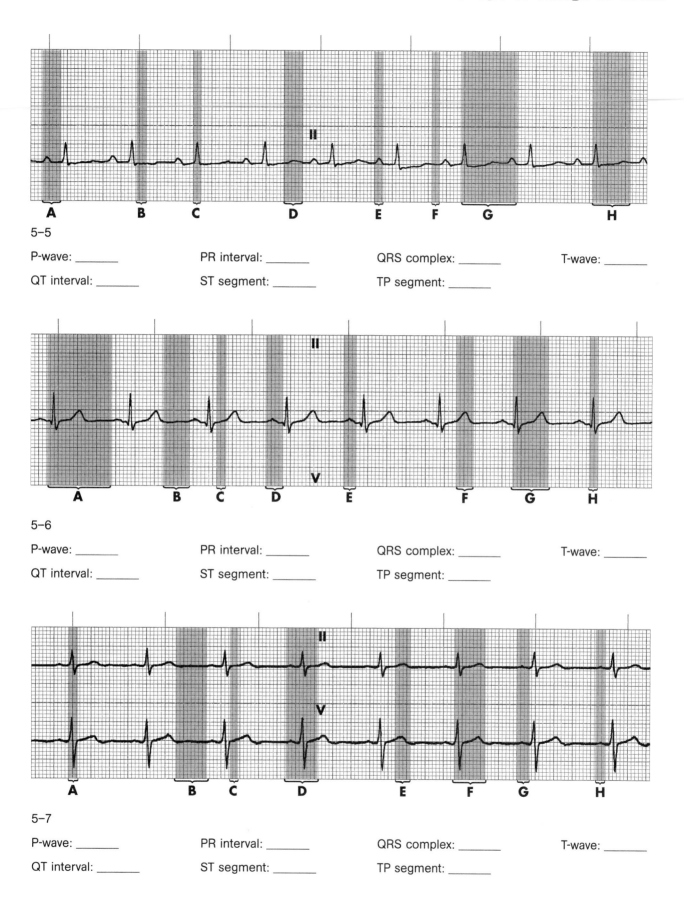

5–5

P-wave: _____   PR interval: _____   QRS complex: _____   T-wave: _____

QT interval: _____   ST segment: _____   TP segment: _____

5–6

P-wave: _____   PR interval: _____   QRS complex: _____   T-wave: _____

QT interval: _____   ST segment: _____   TP segment: _____

5–7

P-wave: _____   PR interval: _____   QRS complex: _____   T-wave: _____

QT interval: _____   ST segment: _____   TP segment: _____

The Shape of Things to Come

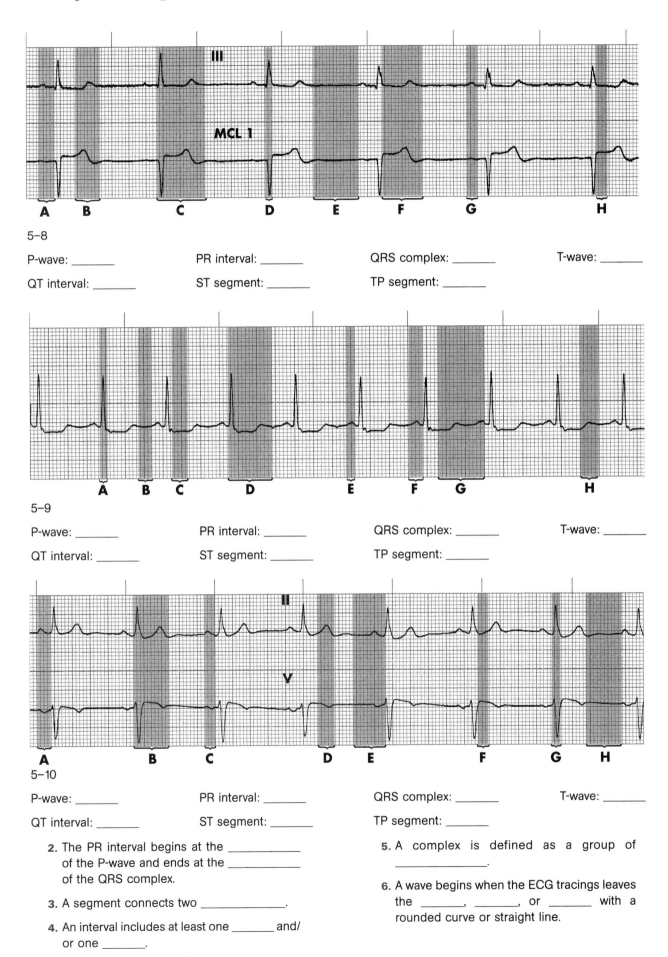

5–8

P-wave: _____   PR interval: _____   QRS complex: _____   T-wave: _____

QT interval: _____   ST segment: _____   TP segment: _____

5–9

P-wave: _____   PR interval: _____   QRS complex: _____   T-wave: _____

QT interval: _____   ST segment: _____   TP segment: _____

5–10

P-wave: _____   PR interval: _____   QRS complex: _____   T-wave: _____

QT interval: _____   ST segment: _____   TP segment: _____

2. The PR interval begins at the _____ of the P-wave and ends at the _____ of the QRS complex.

3. A segment connects two _____.

4. An interval includes at least one _____ and/ or one _____.

5. A complex is defined as a group of _____.

6. A wave begins when the ECG tracings leaves the _____, _____, or _____ with a rounded curve or straight line.

Cars and Carts: From P-Wave to QRS Complex

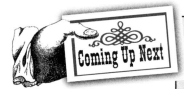

Coming Up Next

- ○ What is the shape of a normal P-wave?
- ○ Where do P-waves occur in relation to the QRS complex?
- ○ Do all QRS complexes have one and only one P-wave?
- ○ Do all rhythms have a P-wave?
- ○ What is the PR interval and what does it represent?
- ○ How do you measure the PR interval?
- ○ Are all PR intervals on a given strip always the same?
- ○ What is the normal range for PR intervals?
- ○ What happens if the PR interval is too short or too long?

How to Tie a Shoelace

Have you ever tried to teach a child how to tie a shoelace? If you're like me, when you try to do it slowly, you often mess it up. And when you're in a hurry, you mess up again. However, you can tie that shoelace perfectly every time if you do it at the "right" speed—the speed you're accustomed to. The heart is no different. The signal has a certain route to follow and a certain order and speed in which to follow it.

We already know how to measure the heart rate using the methods taught in Chapter 3. Now we'll learn how to make the other measurements we need for rhythm interpretation.

Remember the discussion of the conduction system in Chapter 2? As you recall, we can check on the status of the conduction system by figuring out which areas of the heart depolarize in what order. Part of doing that is to determine whether the signal is traveling through the heart at the right speed. Why does it matter how fast the signal travels? Well, think about it. If the signal travels through any area too quickly, that part may not be coordinated with the rest. Conversely, if the signal travels too slowly, the heart may not produce an effective contraction.

First Comes the P-Wave

The P-wave represents the depolarization of both the left and right atria. We don't normally single it out in basic rhythm interpretation, but you need to be able to identify it. The P-wave usually appears as a small, rounded wave on the ECG strip. It may be upright, inverted, or biphasic (partly upright and partly inverted, or "notched"). P-waves are normally less than 0.12 seconds, or three small boxes. Figure 6–1 shows examples of these three different P-wave types.

The height of the normal P-wave is less than 2.5 small boxes. Larger waves can indicate that more tissue is being depolarized, which suggests an enlargement of one or both atria. Again, this detail isn't important in basic rhythm interpretation.

WHERE ARE THE P-WAVES?

Some rhythms have no P-waves at all, and for them this chapter becomes moot. Other rhythms have more than one P-wave for every QRS complex. We'll learn more about these rhythms in later chapters.

To complicate matters, P-waves don't always occur before the QRS complex; sometimes they occur during or

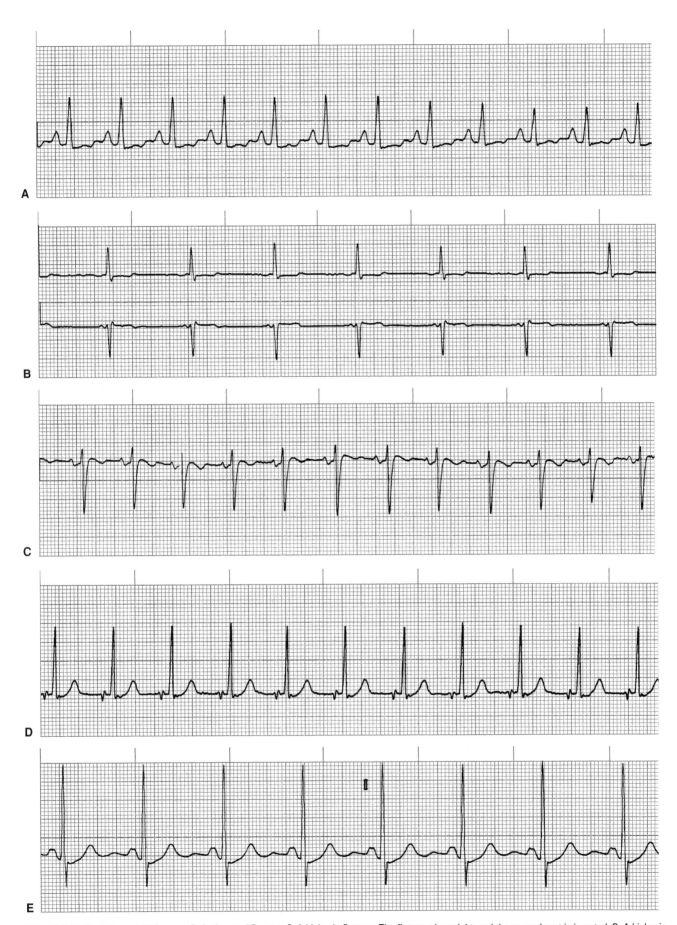

Fig. 6–1A–E A, An upright P-wave. B, An inverted P-wave. C, A biphasic P-wave. The first part is upright, and the second part is inverted. D, A biphasic P-wave. The first part is inverted, and the second part is upright. E, A notched P-wave.

6-2 WHICH BRAND OF TISSUES?

Many people confuse arrhythmias and dysrhythmias, but they're two different entities. An arrhythmia is a loss or an irregularity of rhythm. That's a lot more specific than a dysrhythmia. So an arrhythmia is a type of dysrhythmia, but not all dysrhythmias are arrhythmias.

What's your favorite brand of facial tissue, if you have one? That particular brand is an arrhythmia; generic, any-old-kind tissues are dysrhythmias.

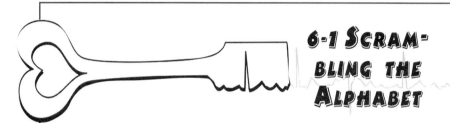

6-1 SCRAMBLING THE ALPHABET

Dysrhythmias are rhythms with something wrong. Dysrhythmias may be regular or irregular. Sometimes the problem is the number of waves, the heart rate, or the order of the waves. So don't be fooled by the PQRSTU designation; waves don't necessarily occur in that order.

even after it. In such cases, it's important to identify the P-wave, but we can't measure the PR interval because it has no meaning in those situations.

THE P-WAVE AND QRS CONNECT

After the P-wave, there is the PR segment—a short, flat line. Flat lines indicate no measurable electrical activity in the heart. Does the signal actually stop as it travels through the heart? Let's think about it. As you know, the baseline, or isoelectric line, connects one PQRSTU complex to the next. Because it represents no measurable electrical activity, the baseline is flat. But that flat line doesn't mean there's nothing going on! It just means that the electrical activity occurring in the heart can't be measured from outside the body.

In a sense, the signal does stop in the AV node, but just briefly and for a good reason. A programmed delay in the signal maximizes the efficiency of the heart's contractions. This delay occurs as the signal travels through the AV node and helps to coordinate the atrial and ventricular contractions so they can work together.

The AV Node Tollbooth

WELL-TIMED SIGNALS

Located at the base of the atria, the AV node acts like a tollbooth. By spacing out the communication of signals from the atria to the ventricles, it makes sure that too many signals aren't communicated at once. The intervals of time between signals let the atria contract and empty as much of their contents as possible into the ventricles. Think back to Chapter 1: more blood means more stretch in the ventricles, which means stronger contractions, which ultimately increase cardiac output.

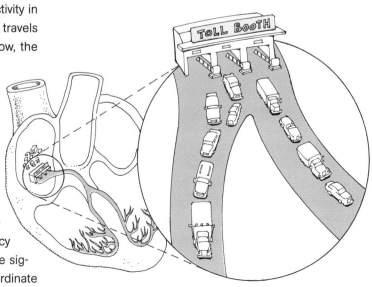

As the signal reaches the AV node, the atria are still contracting. What would happen if the much stronger ventricles opposed them by contracting at the same time? A lot of blood would get forced back into, or be blocked from leaving the atria. If the signal weren't delayed by the AV node, it would be transmitted directly to the bundle branch system, and the amount of blood transferred from the atria to the ventricles could be compromised severely. Less blood transferred to the ventricles means a lower cardiac output.

Instead, when the signal reaches the AV node, its brief delay gives the atria time to empty more effectively. Ventricular filling is maximized, and so is cardiac output. That's how the AV node tollbooth works—by delaying the transmission of signals from atria to ventricles.

This brief delay, usually about 0.10 seconds, is responsible for atrial kick. As we discussed earlier, atrial kick can represent a large percentage of cardiac output.

KEEP THEM COMING

However, as with all good things, more delay is not necessarily better. The atria contract for only a short time and then relax as they prepare to contract again during the next cycle. After the atrial contraction is over, the pressure in the atria decreases rapidly.

Then, if the ventricles aren't contracting, the pressurized blood there can begin to flow backward into the atria. The blood in the ventricles is now under more pressure than that in the atria. Blood always flows from high pressure to low pressure, never the other way. So, if the delay at the AV node is too short, the atria don't get a chance to empty completely. If the delay is too long, the blood may back up when the atria relax.

WAIT YOUR TURN

A highway tollbooth limits the number of cars that can get onto the highway in a given amount of time. This protective mechanism prevents catastrophic accidents and miles-long traffic jams. Another function of the AV node tollbooth is to limit the ventricular rate. In some rhythms, the atria can send 250 signals or more per minute. If all of these signals got through and the ventricles contracted in response to each one, the result would prove as catastrophic as any of those traffic accidents. The ventricles need time to fill, and rates this high can markedly decrease stroke volume. In some cases the decrease is

worse than that caused by a loss of atrial kick. The end result is a dangerously low cardiac output.

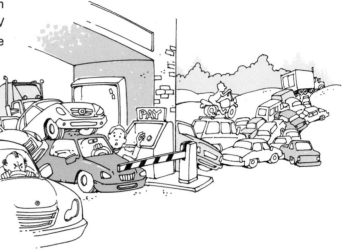

Like all cardiac cells, the AV node must repolarize before it can accept and transmit another signal. However, the speed of the approaching signal, in part, determines how long it takes the AV node to get ready for the next one.

PAST THE TOLLBOOTH

After the signal travels through the AV node, it enters the bundle of His and then is dispersed to the bundle branches, which we met in Chapter 2. Because the bundle branches are part of the conduction system, the signal doesn't show up on the ECG tracing. So how do we know that the bundle of His and the bundle branches have depolarized? We look at the PR interval.

If the AV node conduction is defective, the PR interval will change; we'll learn how in the section called "Renegade P-Waves." However, if the conduction problem is in the bundle branches, it will show up in the QRS complex. We'll explore the QRS more deeply in Chapters 7 and 15.

Variations on a P-Wave

NORMAL P-WAVES

Normal P-waves travel from the sinus node to the AV node. If you look at the various leads presented in Chapter 4, you'll see that this path is best viewed in lead II, where the signal travels the same path as the vector. The ECG will show a large positive deflection, giving a positive (upright) P-wave in lead II. An upright P-wave in lead II usually originates in the sinus node and is considered normal.

6-3 HOW MANY GREEN LIGHTS?

The faster the atrial signals arrive, the faster the AV node can accept them. If that sounds strange, imagine a superhighway with several tollbooths. If you drive on that highway at midnight, you'll find just a couple of tollbooths open. But try driving through at rush hour. As the number of cars begins to increase, more tollbooths open, allowing more cars to go through at one time. The tollbooth system has become more efficient.

When you think about it, this mechanism does make sense in the heart. If the heart rate needs to increase because of a stimulus such as trauma, fear, blood loss, or dehydration, the AV node can repolarize faster. Therefore, more signals can be transmitted through the AV node in a given time, producing a higher ventricular rate.

In other leads, "normal" P-waves can vary in shape; this is why lead II is often monitored to identify P-waves.

RENEGADE P-WAVES

Normally, of course, P-waves occur just before the QRS complex. But don't always expect them to fall into line the way they're supposed to. P-waves come in all shapes and sizes. Not only that—they can also occur anywhere in the PQRSTU complex. It's important, but not always easy, to be able to distinguish renegade P-waves from other types, such as T-waves and U-waves.

Putting the Cart Before the Horse Suppose you find a P-wave occurring after the QRS complex. This P-wave has caused an atrial contraction after the ventricles have already contracted. Such lack of synchronization can diminish cardiac output significantly. In this case, we can't measure the PR interval because it doesn't mean anything. Remember, the PR interval defines the amount of

time from the beginning of atrial depolarization to the beginning of ventricular depolarization. If the P-wave comes after the QRS, it obviously isn't causing the QRS; that leaves us no PR interval to measure.

Figure 6–2 shows a tracing in which the P-wave distorts the T-wave. Notice that the T-wave shape changes in the fourth beat. That little notch is the P-wave.

Putting the Horse in the Cart The P-wave can also occur inside the QRS complex. We'll explore the reasons further on in this book. However, the impact on the PR interval should be obvious—once again, there isn't any PR interval. If the atria depolarize during the QRS, again the cause-and-effect relationship is lost, and the PR interval means nothing.

P-waves buried in the QRS complex are almost always hard to identify, but later we'll discuss techniques to help pinpoint them. Figure 6–3 shows an example of P-waves occurring in the QRS complex.

A Cart Without a Horse In certain rhythms, some more common than others, the P-wave is missing entirely. Always be careful when determining an absence of P-waves. As you've discovered, P-waves can hide in either the QRS

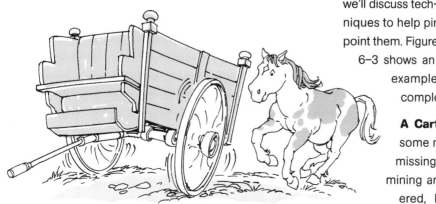

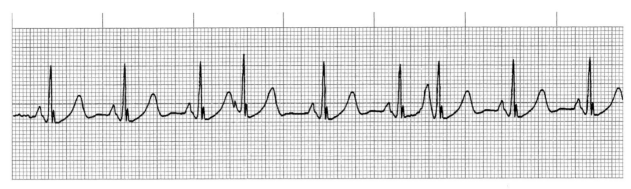

Fig. 6–2 P-wave occurring after the QRS complex. The T-wave after the third beat is slightly different from the rest of the T-waves on the strip; the small distortion is a P-wave. Also, the T-wave after the sixth beat is more pointed than the other T-waves, again because of a P-wave.

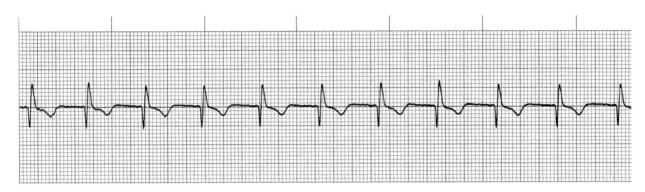

Fig. 6–3 The P-waves in this ECG strip occur at the same time as the QRS complex and are therefore not visible.

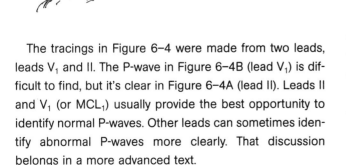

complex or the T-wave and can come before, during, or after the QRS. Look carefully for the P-wave and consider checking multiple leads.

The tracings in Figure 6–4 were made from two leads, leads V₁ and II. The P-wave in Figure 6–4B (lead V₁) is difficult to find, but it's clear in Figure 6–4A (lead II). Leads II and V₁ (or MCL₁) usually provide the best opportunity to identify normal P-waves. Other leads can sometimes identify abnormal P-waves more clearly. That discussion belongs in a more advanced text.

The basic rule is, until you become comfortable identifying P-waves, look carefully and look everywhere. Because they can try to hide, look where you don't expect to find them.

Appearances can be deceiving. If a P-wave occurs before a QRS complex, it didn't necessarily cause the QRS complex. It's important to measure the PR interval throughout the strip so you can thoroughly assess the cause-and-effect relationship. See the next section, "One Cart, Many Horses," for more of this discussion.

One Cart, Many Horses If many horses are pulling one cart, they have to work as a team. Because P-waves are independent of each other, they never work together, so it's not good to have more than one P-wave for any QRS complex. Multiple P-waves mean multiple atrial contractions for every ventricular contraction—not very efficient! They can also make it hard to identify the PR interval—which P-wave is actually causing the QRS? You may think it's the one directly before the QRS, but that isn't always the case.

Any P-wave that comes before the QRS complex can depolarize the ventricles; it doesn't have to be the closest

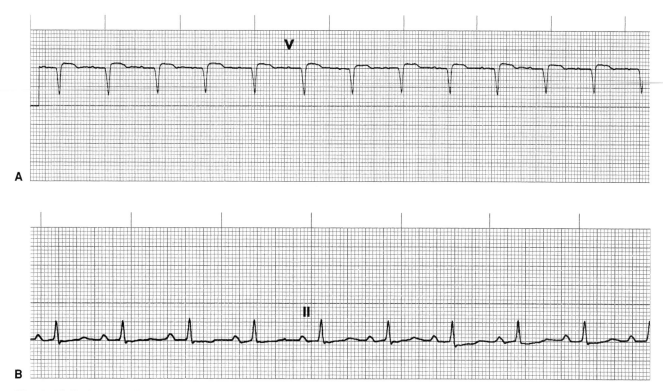

Fig. 6–4A–B A, Lead V₁. If you look carefully, you can identify the P-waves. B, Lead II. The P-waves are much easier to identify in this tracing.

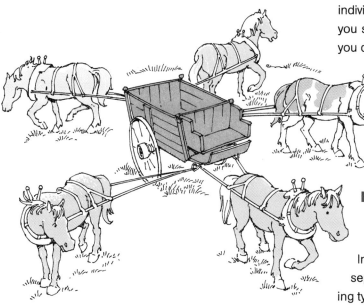

individual rhythms in which they occur. For the time being, you simply need to know that these variations exist. Once you do, you can find examples of P-waves in all their different shapes, sizes, and locations, which in turn will help you understand the PR interval and the relationship of P-waves to the QRS complex. When you can identify P-waves and measure PR intervals, rhythm interpretation will become easier and more accurate.

Measuring the PR Interval

WAVE PLUS SEGMENT

In normal conduction, a short period of time usually separates the P-wave and the QRS complex. The tracing typically shows a flat line called the PR segment, which we met in Chapter 5. As you remember, the PR segment connects the end of the P-wave to the beginning of the QRS complex. When you look at the PR segment, you're seeing how long the signal took to travel through the AV node, the bundle of His, and the bundle branches before any ventricular muscle cells depolarized.

The PR interval, therefore, is the combination of the P-wave and the PR segment. (If you remember from Chapter 5, an interval contains at least one segment and one wave.)

one. In certain rhythms, it's impossible to determine the PR interval (Fig. 6–5). However, some rhythms do make it clear which P-wave is causing the QRS, even if each QRS complex has more than one P-wave (Fig. 6–6); with this information, we can find our PR interval.

Becoming a Horse Expert We'll explore all of these situations—no P-waves, extra P-waves, P-waves during or after the QRS complex, and more—when we examine the

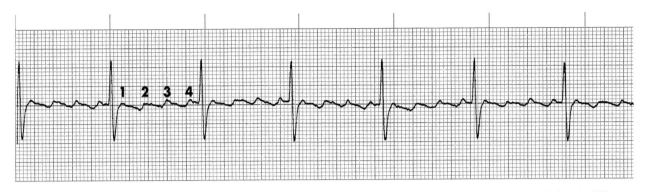

Fig. 6–5 Here there are four P-waves (labeled 1–4) for every QRS complex. Testing demonstrated that P-wave 4, immediately before the QRS complex, did not cause the QRS; in fact, P-wave 3 did. The PR interval is not measurable because, with four P-waves, there are four possible points from which to start measuring.

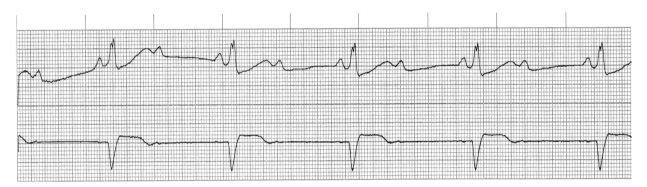

Fig. 6–6 Here there are two P-waves (labeled 1 and 2) before every QRS complex. Because only one P-wave is close to each QRS, it is easy to identify the P-wave (2) that caused the QRS. In this rhythm, the PR interval is measurable.

CHECK AND CHECK AGAIN

To measure the PR interval, place one point of your calipers at the beginning of the P-wave and the other at the beginning of the QRS complex as shown in Figure 6–7. Be careful to not include any portion of the QRS because the PR interval ends where the QRS begins. If you look closely at Figure 6–7, you'll see that the PR interval doesn't include the small Q-wave at the beginning of the QRS. Normally the PR interval measures between 0.12 and 0.20 seconds inclusive, but PR intervals up to 0.40 seconds or even longer are possible if the AV node is dysfunctional.

Now try measuring a few on your own.

Because the PR interval can vary in some rhythms, you should check all the PR intervals on a tracing and make sure that they're the same. Your confidence will increase with lots of practice, but until then, check and double check.

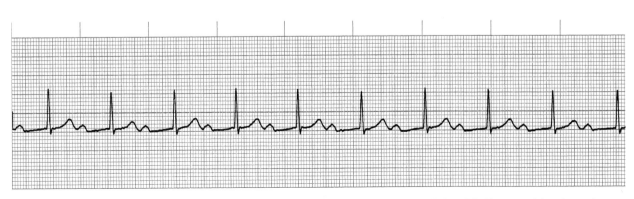

Fig. 6–7 Proper caliper placement for measuring the PR interval. Place one caliper point at the beginning of the P-wave and the other at the beginning of the QRS complex. Then, without changing the distance between points, place the first point on a dark line.

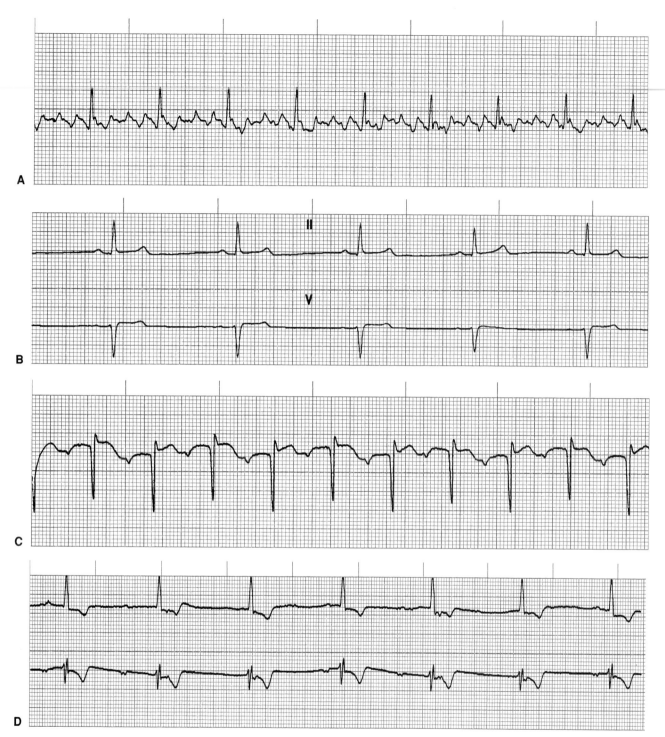

Fig. 6–8A–D   A, The PR interval is not measurable. B, The PR interval is 0.18 seconds. C, The PR interval is 0.26 seconds. D, The PR interval is variable.

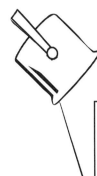

Now You Know

A "normal" P-wave can be upright, inverted, or biphasic depending on which lead is monitored. P-waves can also be notched, but this is abnormal.

P-waves normally occur just before the QRS complex but may also occur during or after the QRS in some rhythms.

Some QRS complexes can have more than one P-wave, and some have no P-waves at all.

The PR interval represents the amount of time the signal takes to travel through the atria, AV node, bundle of His, and bundle branches; its length shows how much time the ventricles have to fill before contracting.

The PR interval is measured from the beginning of the P-wave to the beginning of the QRS complex.

Occasionally the PR interval can vary from beat to beat; therefore, all PR intervals must be measured.

The PR interval is normally from 0.12 to 0.20 seconds inclusive, but it can be much longer with AV node dysfunction.

Improper ventricular filling, caused by poor coordination between atrial and ventricular contractions, can lead to loss of cardiac output.

Test Yourself

1. If the PR interval is too short, what effect does that have on the cardiac output?

2. The PR interval is made up of the ____ and the PR _____.

3. When does the P-wave occur in relation to the QRS complex?

4. A rhythm can have one, no, or many _____ for each QRS complex.

5. All PR intervals must be carefully examined because PR intervals can ___ throughout a tracing.

6. In the following 10 rhythm strips, identify all the P-waves and measure the PR interval if that is appropriate:

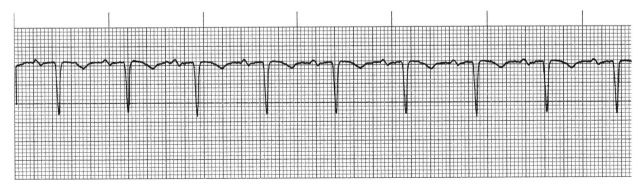

6–1

PR interval = _____

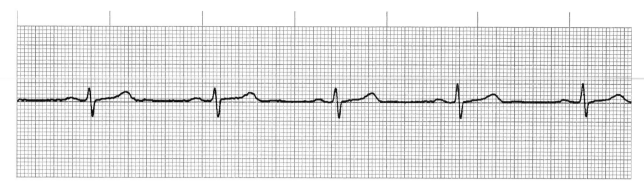

6–2

PR interval = _____

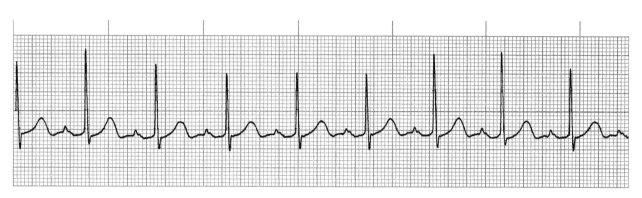

6–3

PR interval = _____

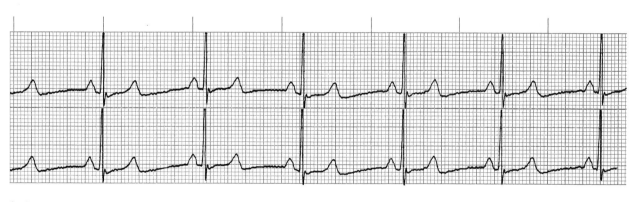

6–4

PR interval = _____

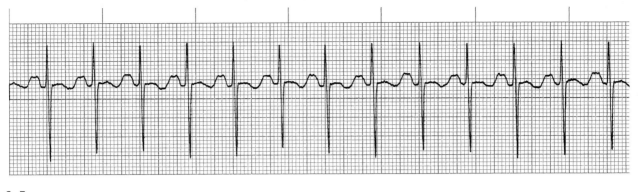

6–5

PR interval = _____

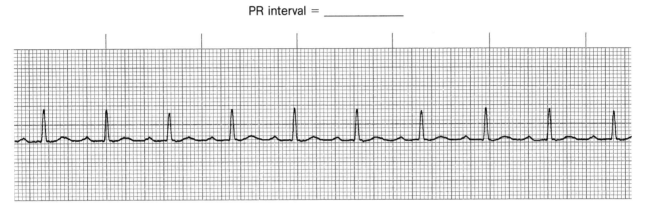

6–6

PR interval = _____

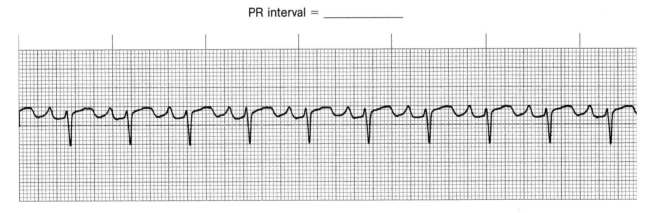

6–7

PR interval = _____

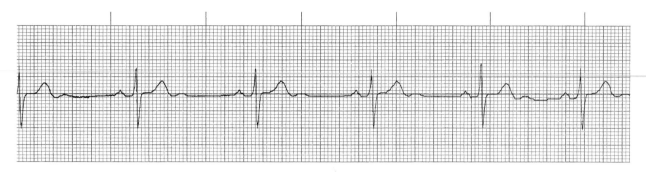

6–8

PR interval = _____

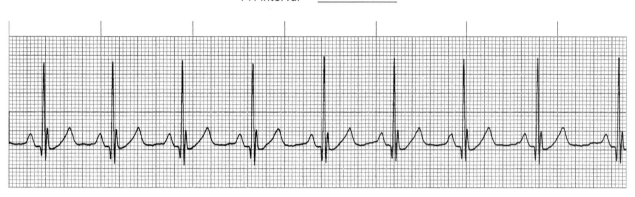

6–9

PR interval = _____

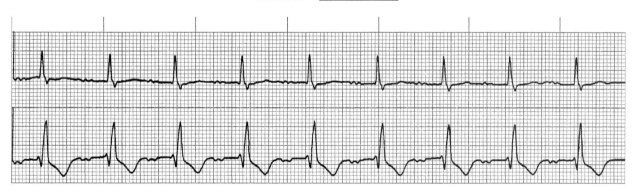

6–10

PR interval = _____

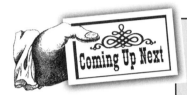

THE INTRAVENTRICULAR SUPERHIGHWAY

Coming Up Next

- ○ What are bundle branches, and what is their role?
- ○ How do we know which part of the ECG is the QRS complex?
- ○ What is the J-point and what does it represent?
- ○ Where does the QRS complex begin and how do we know where it ends?
- ○ What is the normal range of values for the QRS complex?
- ○ Why are some QRS complexes upright and some inverted?
- ○ How can we make measuring the QRS complex easier?

Traveling the Bundle Branch Routes

A FAST RIDE THROUGH THE VENTRICLES

Well, so far we have covered the electrical conduction system of the heart through the atrioventricular (AV) node. Now that we've made it through the tollbooth of the AV node, it's time to jump on the "Intraventricular Superhighways."

These highways are a special set of thoroughbred thoroughfares. Extremely fast conductors, they are often referred to as the "fast path through the ventricles." Even faster than the expressways through the atria, they transport the signals that emerge from the AV node toll booth to all parts of the ventricles. This is not an insignificant feat, as we will soon see.

These intraventricular highways are called the *bundle branches*, and are simply groups of long Purkinje fibers.

The bundle branches are superefficient in their role as transmitters. They carry a signal too faint to be recorded from outside the body. Remember that any signal recorded by an external ECG monitor must travel through many layers. It must go through the heart muscle, the fat

cushion surrounding the heart, the pericardial fluid, the other tissue in the chest cavity (lungs, thymus gland), the chest muscles, the ribs, the subcutaneous fat, and finally the skin. The signal transmitted by the bundle branches is not strong enough to travel through all that insulation, and therefore the ECG records no electrical activity (the tracing stays at the isoelectric line, or baseline).

WHAT'S HAPPENING ON THE STRIP?

Let's review the ECG rhythm strip and identify the part of it that we are dealing with now. Remember, the P-wave is caused by depolarization of, and conduction through, the atria after the sinus node depolarizes. The PR segment is the delay following transmission through the atria, and represents the signal traveling through the AV node and the bundle branches to the terminal Purkinje fibers. Therefore, the process of elimination tells you that the QRS complex is the depolarization of all parts of the ventricles (Fig. 7–1a–c). Many people, even experienced critical care

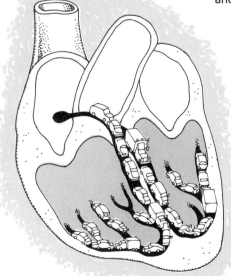

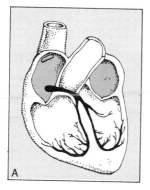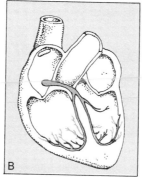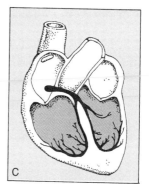

Fig. 7–1A–C Correlating the ECG tracing with the electrical conduction through the heart. A, The P-wave reflects conduction through and depolarization of the atrial tissue. B, The PR segment reflects conduction through and depolarization of the AV node and conduction through the bundle branches. C, The QRS complex reflects conduction through and depolarization of the ventricular tissue.

nurses, incorrectly believe that the transmission of the signal through the bundle branches is part of the QRS, not the PR segment.

THE INTRAVENTRICULAR ROAD MAP

You can take two main bundle branch routes after you emerge from the AV node tollbooth. Initially, after leaving the AV node tollbooth, the two bundle branches are fused into one mega-superhighway, called the *Bundle of His*. Shortly thereafter, this mega-superhighway separates into two distinct highways, or bundle branches. The first branch transmits the signal to the right ventricle and therefore is called the *right bundle branch*. A short distance further down, the left bundle branch breaks again into two separate highways. These two highways direct the signal to the left ventricle. However, they serve very distinct areas. One serves the front of the left ventricle and the other the back. They are called the *left anterior fascicle* and *left posterior fascicle*, respectively. There is also a septal branch, but that is not important for our purposes at this level.

The signals to both ventricles travel down these multilane highways and exit to smaller and smaller roads until they terminate at the Purkinje fibers, where the signal (we hope) causes ventricular contraction (see Fig. 7–2). The signals must be transmitted quickly and evenly; otherwise the contraction will be poorly coordinated and therefore less effective.

You may ask why we need three paths, the right bundle branch and the two left fascicles, to feed only two ventricles. As we will learn later, you need only *one* working path to conduct the signal to *both* ventricles, but the human body has survived as well as it has because of redundancy. (For example, we have two lungs and two kidneys, although we could survive comfortably with just one of each).

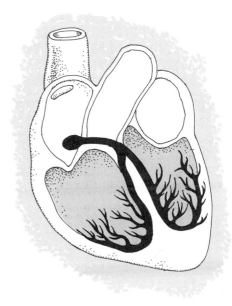

Fig. 7–2 The bundle branches are the fast path through the ventricles. They coordinate delivery of the signal from the AV node to all parts of the ventricles.

We've already said that bundle branch depolarization is included in the PR interval. However, the bundle branches and their divisions also determine how the signal is distributed, and whether the left and right ventricles receive the signal simultaneously or in succession. By doing so, they ultimately determine the shape and size of the QRS in the various leads. This concept will be further developed in later chapters.

Tracking the QRS Complex

HEIGHT AND STRAIGHT LINES

Now that we understand how the highways work, let's see how their jobs translate into the ECG tracing. Remember that the amplitude, or height, of the tracing gives us a

7-1 YOUR FRIENDLY UTILITY COMPANY

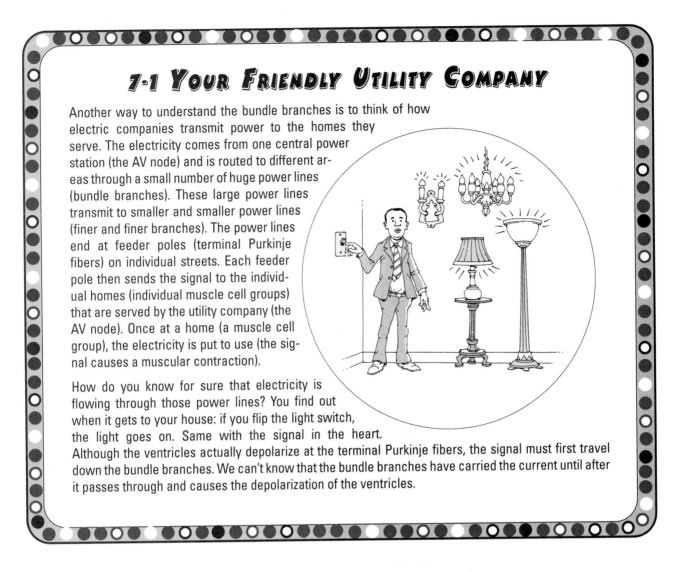

Another way to understand the bundle branches is to think of how electric companies transmit power to the homes they serve. The electricity comes from one central power station (the AV node) and is routed to different areas through a small number of huge power lines (bundle branches). These large power lines transmit to smaller and smaller power lines (finer and finer branches). The power lines end at feeder poles (terminal Purkinje fibers) on individual streets. Each feeder pole then sends the signal to the individual homes (individual muscle cell groups) that are served by the utility company (the AV node). Once at a home (a muscle cell group), the electricity is put to use (the signal causes a muscular contraction).

How do you know for sure that electricity is flowing through those power lines? You find out when it gets to your house: if you flip the light switch, the light goes on. Same with the signal in the heart. Although the ventricles actually depolarize at the terminal Purkinje fibers, the signal must first travel down the bundle branches. We can't know that the bundle branches have carried the current until after it passes through and causes the depolarization of the ventricles.

general idea of the power of the signal *approaching* the lead we are viewing (refer back to Chapter 4, "Location, Location, Location," for a review of the leads). Because the ventricles are significantly larger than the atria, the tracings from the signals traveling through the ventricles will most likely be larger than the tracings from the signals traveling through the atria. Therefore the tallest waves are usually the QRS waves, or QRS complexes, which we met in Chapter 5. This knowledge helps us to differentiate the QRS complex from the P-wave and the T-wave.

Another distinguishing characteristic of the QRS complex is straight lines. In almost all ECG tracings, the P-wave, T-wave, and U-wave (when present) are always small, rounded curves. The QRS complex, as we've seen, is large and usually consists of straight or nearly straight lines. Note the different ECG strips, and the labels identifying the various waves, in Figure 7–3.

The amount of tissue (and thus the total signal strength) partly determines the amplitude of the QRS complex. The

direction of the signal also affects it. A signal coming straight at the lead will appear taller than a signal that is moving obliquely toward the lead. Just as a flashlight shone right at you will appear very bright, the same flashlight shone slightly to your right would appear less bright (see Fig. 7–5).

THE EFFECT OF PERSPECTIVE

A question will probably come up when you go out into the real world and begin applying your interpretation skills to non-textbook strips. However people may phrase it, the basic question is the same: "Why are some people's QRS complexes upside down while others are not? Why don't they all look the same, or at least all go in the same direction?"

In addition to heart shape, location, and condition (all of which will be covered in future chapters), the answer also has to do with perspective. Remember Chapter 4, where we discussed the way different leads take pictures of the heart's electrical system from different viewpoints? That's the

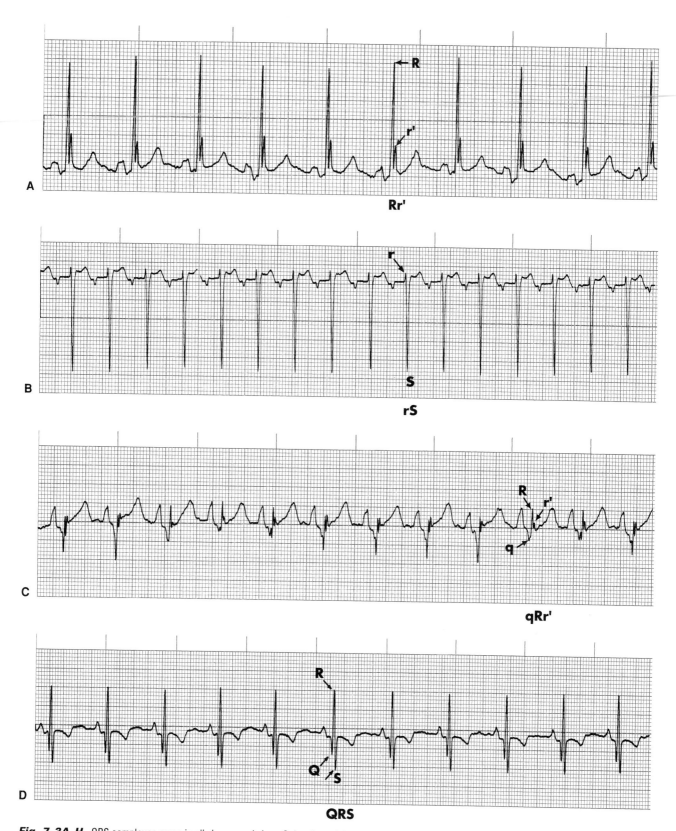

Fig. 7-3A-H QRS complexes come in all shapes and sizes. Only a few of the possibilities are shown here. The differently shaped QRS complex shapes simply indicate the path the signal traveled through the ventricles.

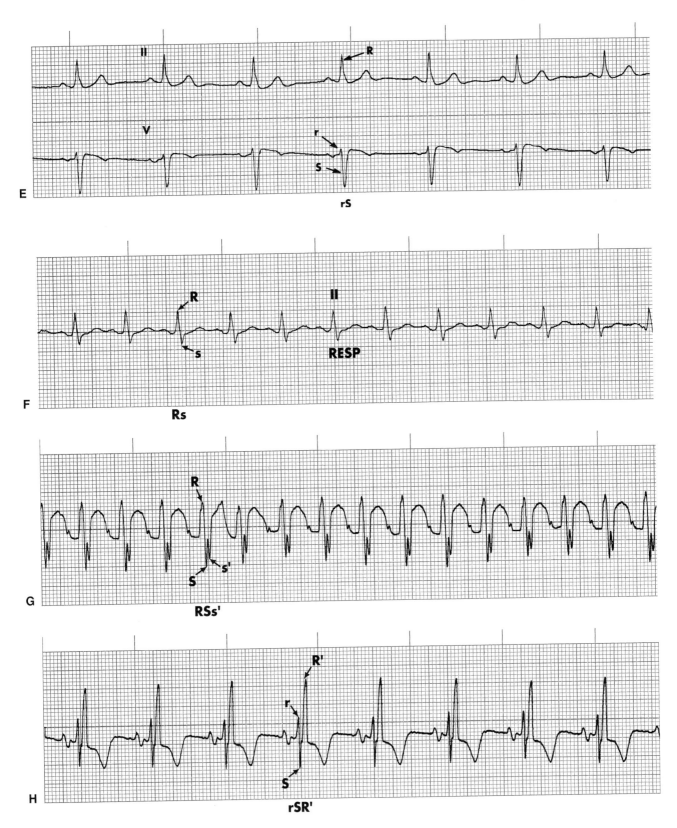

Fig. 7–3A–H (Continued)

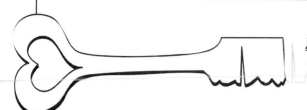

7-2 Two For the Price of One

There are actually *two* QRS complexes in every ECG tracing, although only one is normally seen. Wait a minute, you say. How come we're talking about one if there are really two?

Let's look at what happens before you get your P-wave in a knot. The AV node sends the signal to the right and both left bundle branches simultaneously. Therefore all three branches receive and transmit the signal together, causing the right and left ventricles to depolarize at the same time. The depolarization of each ventricle creates a separate QRS complex. Because they occur simultaneously, the two complexes combine to form a single complex bigger than that created by either ventricle alone. The ventricles then contract together, causing a heartbeat. (Remember, ventricular depolarization causes the ECG tracing; ventricular contraction is a separate event.) The QRS complex does not last longer than either of its components because they've occurred simultaneously (Fig. 7–4). The QRS is normally less than 0.12 seconds in duration.

Remember the vector discussion in Chapter 4, and the example of several people pulling different ways? Depolarization of the ventricles produces two vectors in different directions. Because the vectors occur simultaneously, they produce a single vector in a third direction. We see only this combined vector on the ECG. The vector concept will reappear in our discussion of what happens when the ventricles *don't* contract together.

lead we are viewing. Just like the train whistle, the amplitude of the QRS wave drops when the signal moves away, falling below the baseline.

The shape of the QRS complex also depends on perspective. A lead that views the left ventricle from the bottom, such as Lead II, will show a tall, upright shape in a normal ECG. "Why?" you ask. The large mass of the left ventricle sends a large signal toward the lead. If you reversed the lead patches for Lead II, the QRS complex would still be large. However, the signal would then be moving away from the positive lead, and the QRS complex would be large and would point *down*. In the next few chapters we will learn more about the many possible shapes of the QRS complex, and exactly why those shapes are the way they are. (Experiment with lead placement at your facility to see how it changes the QRS complex shape.)

answer to the question. When the signal through the ventricles travels toward the lead we are viewing, the QRS wave is above the baseline. When the signal travels away from the lead, we see the QRS wave from below the baseline. In some leads, upright QRS complexes are the norm; in other leads, they can indicate a problem. The leads that normally have upright QRS complexes are I, II, aVf, V3, V4, V5, and V6. Those that are normally inverted are aVr, V1, and V2.

To understand more easily, think of a passing train. When a train blows its whistle from far away as it comes toward you, the pitch of the sound is high. If the whistle continues to blow at the same pitch, the sound gets lower as the train moves away from you. The amplitude of the QRS wave is also high when the signal travels from above the baseline toward the

NOT THE SAME OLD LINE: HOW QRS SHAPES VARY

Although the QRS complex can appear in many forms, most QRS complexes share certain characteristics. First, as we saw earlier, they consist mostly of straight lines. The QRS complex begins with the first movement of a straight line away from the baseline, after the P-wave. Whether that line moves up or down doesn't matter at this point; however, it's important that the line be relatively straight. The QRS ends when the straight lines return to the baseline. If all QRS complexes behaved this way, you wouldn't need a whole book to learn ECG interpretation. Unfortunately, not all QRS complexes return to baseline when they end. The numerous reasons will be explored further in later chapters.

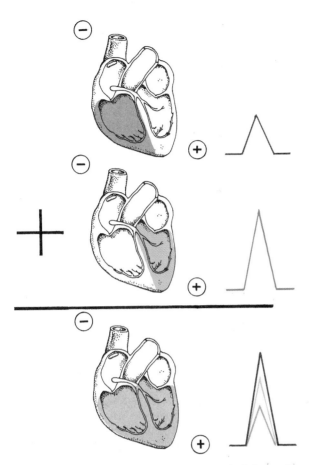

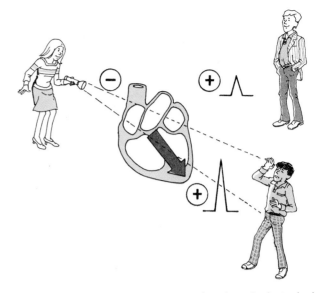

Fig. 7–5 If the signal travels directly toward an electrode, the tracing is larger than if the signal travels slightly to the side of the electrode.

Fig. 7–4 The ventricles normally depolarize independently, but nearly simultaneously. The QRS complex represents the sum of both depolarizations.

You don't need several patients to demonstrate the different forms of the QRS complex. The same patient can have differently shaped QRS complexes in different leads, as shown in Figure 7–6. When more than one QRS complex shape occurs in the same lead, we have a different situation. We will discuss this situation in the next several chapters.

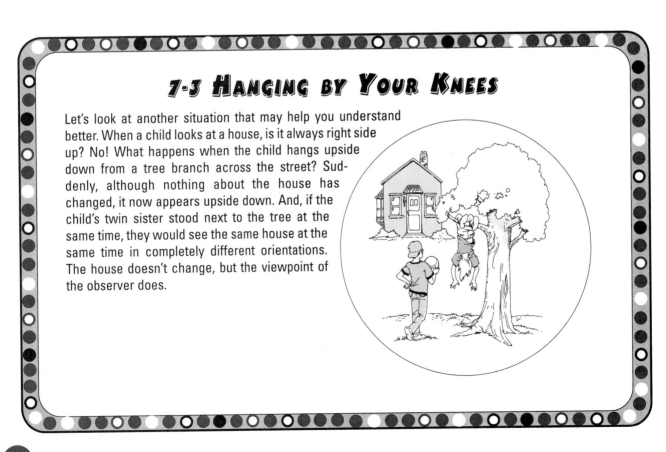

7-3 HANGING BY YOUR KNEES

Let's look at another situation that may help you understand better. When a child looks at a house, is it always right side up? No! What happens when the child hangs upside down from a tree branch across the street? Suddenly, although nothing about the house has changed, it now appears upside down. And, if the child's twin sister stood next to the tree at the same time, they would see the same house at the same time in completely different orientations. The house doesn't change, but the viewpoint of the observer does.

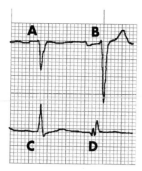

Fig. 7–6a–d QRS complexes taken from the same patient at the same time, but with different leads. The difference in their shapes reflects the direction of the signal and the perspective of the different leads.

As you can see on the ECG strips in Figure 7–7, sometimes the QRS complex can be difficult to identify.

A DIFFERENT ENDING: IDENTIFYING THE J-POINT

Return to baseline is not the only signal that a QRS complex has ended. Another indication is that the straight line starts to bend or curve. Identifying the end of the QRS this way is more difficult and requires a little more effort. For several examples of this concept see Figures 7–8 and 7–9.

The point where the QRS begins to curve from the straight and narrow is called the J-point. You may well be asking where that letter came from: "I thought we were dealing with the PQRSTU part of the alphabet?!" Yes, that's true, but the J-point was named for its appearance. Look at a capital J—how would you describe it? In ECG terms, the letter J is a straight line that ends in a curve, or bend. Well, that's what happens to the QRS complex. The QRS, as we know, is a series of connected straight lines. When these straight lines suddenly end in a curve, the result looks like a J (Fig. 7–10). (So, I think we should forgive the person who chose the name "J-point" because it actually makes sense.)

The J-point is not always easy to identify. That is one of many reasons why it's important to monitor patients using more than one lead. Because different leads display different QRS complex shapes, in certain leads the J-point is more readily identified, and in some the QRS complex may even return to baseline. So, if you can't find the J-point in one lead, switch to another. You may ask if this is cheating. The answer is a resounding "No!" Why is that?

Although our perspective changes in different leads, the length of each segment of our ECG tracing doesn't change. Each segment length tells us how long it took that wave to move through a certain area. That length of time does not change within one QRS complex.

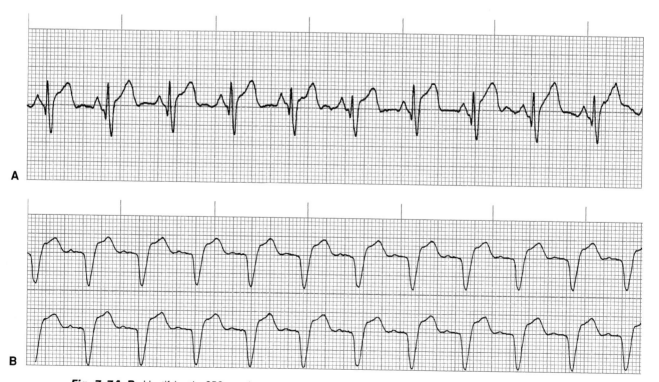

Fig. 7–7A–B Identifying the QRS complexes can present a challenge, especially for a novice in ECG interpretation.

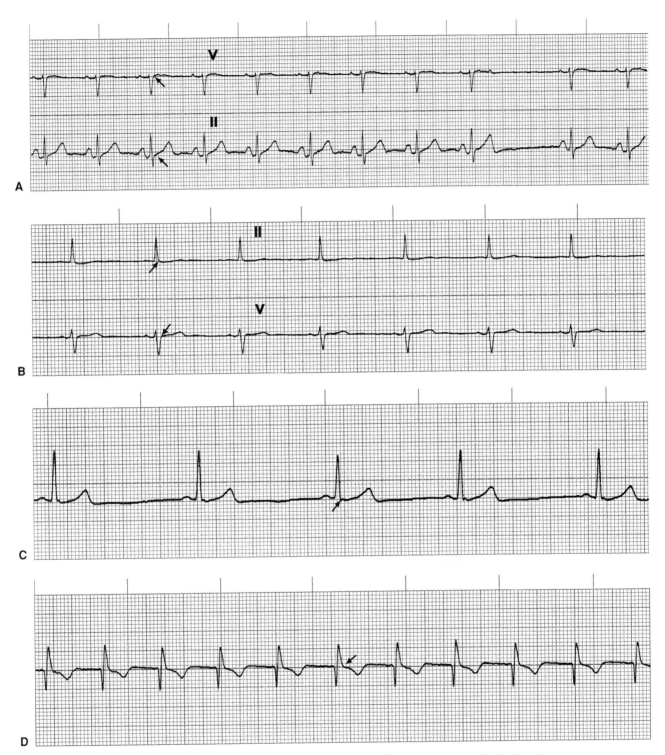

Fig. 7–8A–D When the QRS complex simply returns to baseline, identifying the beginning and end of it can be easy.

Measuring Tools and Techniques

Now that we've learned to identify the beginning and end of the QRS complex, we can learn to measure it. Just as we measured the PR interval and heart rate in previous chapters, so must we measure the QRS interval. Deviations from the normal ranges of measurement give us clues to interpreting rhythms, and to diagnosing and treating patients in our care.

It's important to choose the leads that make our job the easiest, especially during the learning process. Many factors will influence our choice of which lead to monitor. We

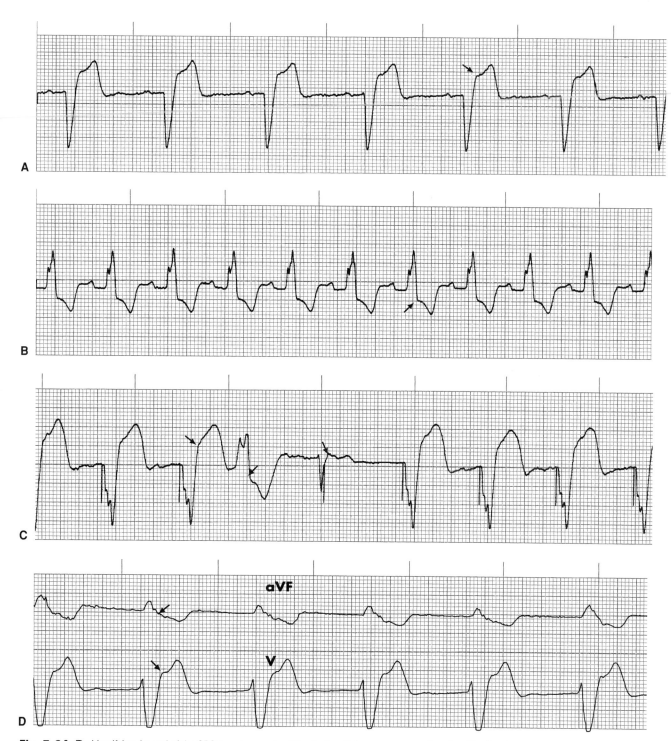

Fig. 7–9A–D Identifying the end of the QRS complex can be difficult when it does not return to baseline. The line changes subtly from straight to curved at the end of these QRSs.

need to consider what's wrong with the patient, what parts of the ECG tracings we need to see, and why we are monitoring the patient at all. Although we may choose to monitor certain leads for specific reasons, we can take our interval measurements from any lead.

The following pages give you many QRS complexes to practice measuring. The ones at the bottom of this page

are done for you, including the correct placement of your calipers on the tracing and on the paper to measure the interval (Fig. 7–11). The QRS complexes on the following page are for your practice. In all cases, the correct measurements are listed for comparison.

In the first QRS complex, place one tip of your calipers on the first arrow and, without moving it, stretch the

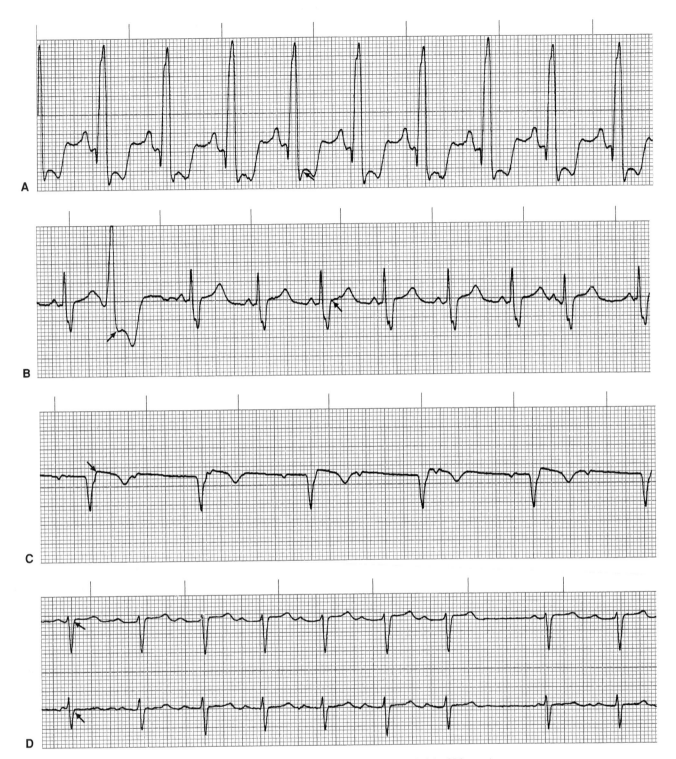

Fig. 7–10A–D Here the J-point is used to identify the end of the QRS complex.

second tip to the point of the second arrow. Gently lift your calipers off the page and place them so that the left tip touches a heavy line. Because heavy lines are easier to identify, it's customary to use them when measuring heart rate, PR interval, and QT interval (discussed later in this book). Be careful not to squeeze the calipers inadvertently, as this will change your measurement. If you are unsure

whether you moved the calipers, simply place the points back on the QRS complex to verify that they haven't moved.

Now note the number of small boxes between the left and right tips. This is your QRS measurement and is recorded as part of your documentation of the strip. In the

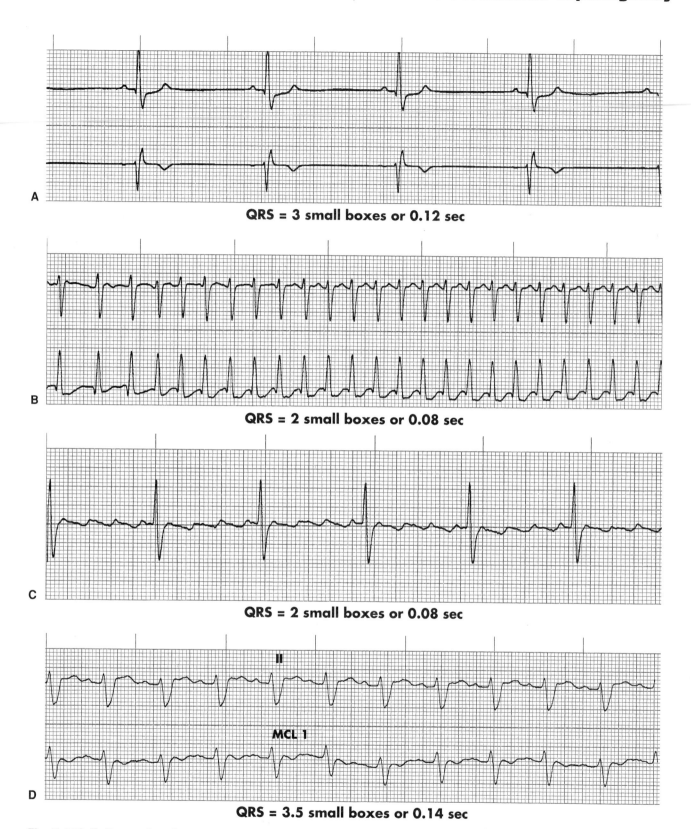

QRS = 3 small boxes or 0.12 sec

QRS = 2 small boxes or 0.08 sec

QRS = 2 small boxes or 0.08 sec

QRS = 3.5 small boxes or 0.14 sec

Fig. 7–11A–D Proper caliper placement for measurement of the QRS complex. A, QRS is 0.12 sec. B, QRS is 0.06 sec. C, QRS is 0.08 sec. D, QRS is 0.16 sec.

first practice strip, the QRS measures 0.08 seconds, or exactly two small boxes (remember, each small box is 0.04 seconds; for a review see Chapter 3). Be forewarned, reading the number of small boxes can be tricky. Also, we count small boxes to the nearest half box. Valid measurements are 0.02 (unlikely), 0.04, 0.06, 0.08, or 0.10 seconds. We will discuss in another chapter what happens if the QRS is 0.12 seconds or more.

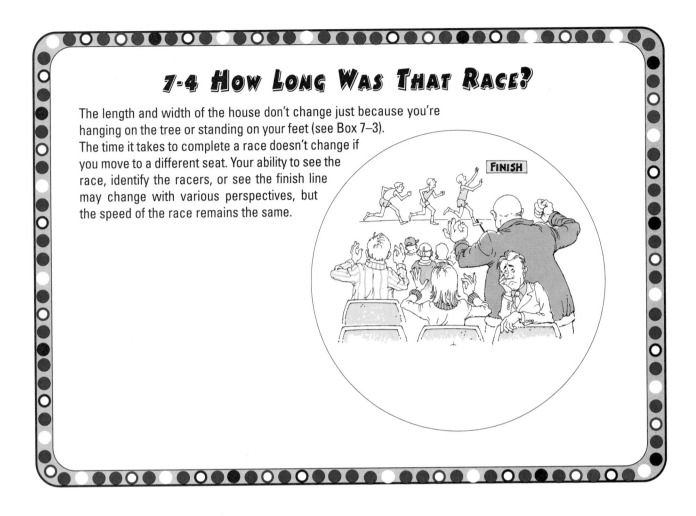

7-4 How Long Was That Race?

The length and width of the house don't change just because you're hanging on the tree or standing on your feet (see Box 7–3). The time it takes to complete a race doesn't change if you move to a different seat. Your ability to see the race, identify the racers, or see the finish line may change with various perspectives, but the speed of the race remains the same.

FINISH

Practice identifying and measuring the QRS complexes in these eight strips.

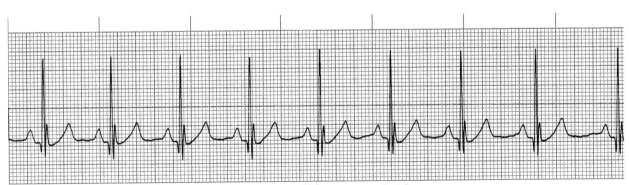

QRS = 2.5 small boxes or 0.10 sec

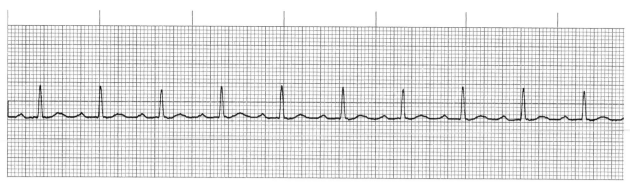

QRS = 1 small box or 0.04 sec

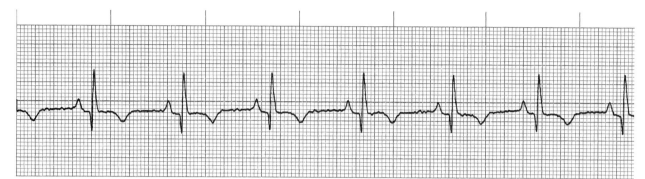

QRS = 0.08 sec

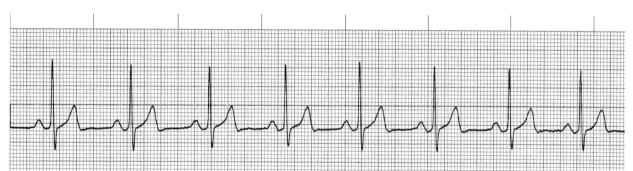

QRS = 0.08 sec

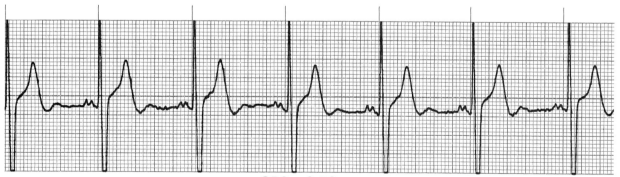

QRS = 0.12 sec

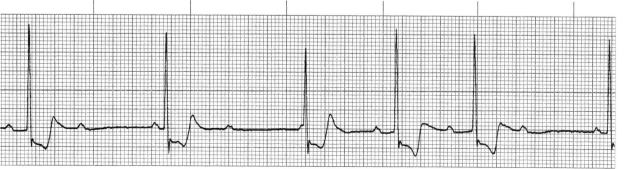

QRS = 0.06 sec

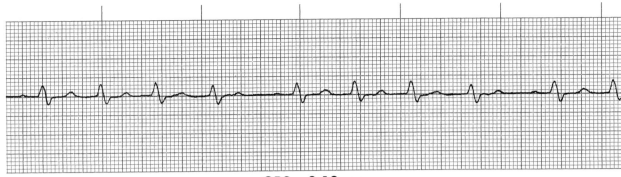

QRS = 0.12 sec

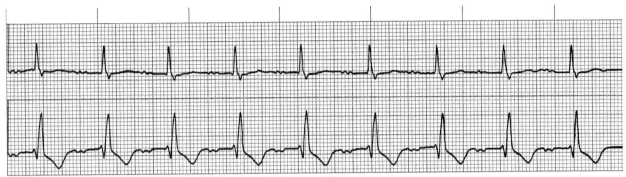

QRS = 0.12 sec

From this and previous chapters, we've learned about the PR interval, heart rate, and QRS interval. This information tells us a great deal about the heart. In fact, this is all the measuring necessary to identify most rhythm strips! We are well on our way, but now it's time for a brief review.

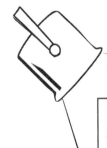

Now You Know

The left and right bundle branches are bundles of Purkinje fibers and are responsible for transmitting the signal from the AV node to both ventricles in a coordinated manner.

The QRS complexes are composed of straight or nearly straight lines and start with the first movement above or below the isoelectric line after the P-wave.

The J-point is the point where the straight lines of the QRS complex start to bend or curve and, along with a return to baseline, designates the end of the QRS.

The normal range of QRS complexes is 0.04 to 0.10 seconds.

QRS complexes are primarily upright in leads I, II, aVf, V3, V4, V5,V6 and primarily inverted in leads aVr, V1, V2. Their orientation depends on whether the signal is traveling toward or away from the lead we are looking at.

All intervals, PR or QRS, are the same no matter what lead they are measured from; therefore we can chose the lead that makes measurement the easiest.

Test Yourself

1. The QRS complex represents the signal travelling through the _____ and depolarizing the ventricles.

2. There are _____ main bundle branches.

3. The _____ _____ bundle branch, or _____ ___, sends the signal to the **front,** or anterior portion of the left ventricle.

4. The _____ _____ bundle branch, or ___ ___, sends the signal to the **back,** or _____, of the left ventricle.

5. The normal length of the QRS complex is between _____ and _____ seconds.

6. Most QRS complexes consist of _____ _____, unlike the P-wave and T-wave.

7. The J-point is the point where the QRS complex begins to ___ or ___.

8. The J-point marks the _____ of the QRS complex.

9. Measure the QRS complex width in the following 10 strips:

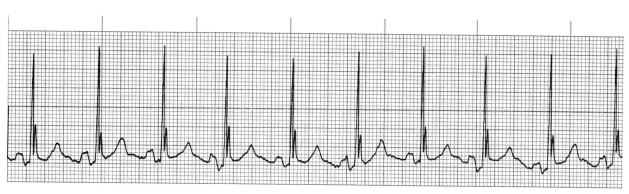

7–9

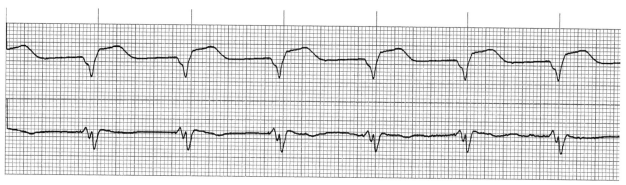

7–10

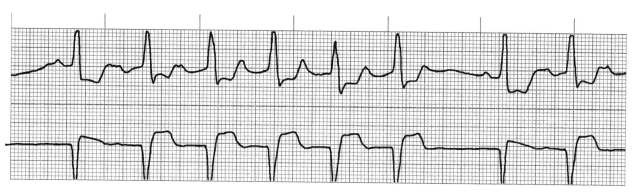

7–11

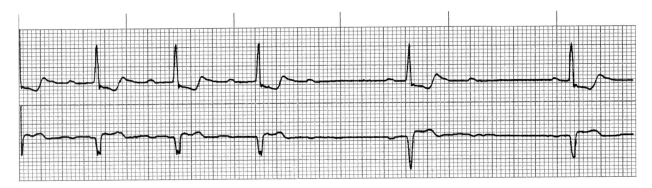

7-12

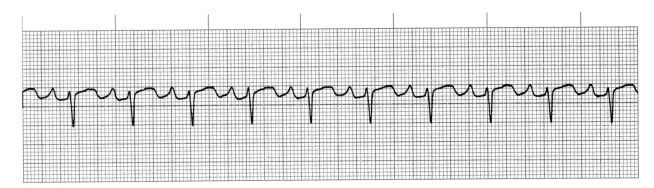

7-13

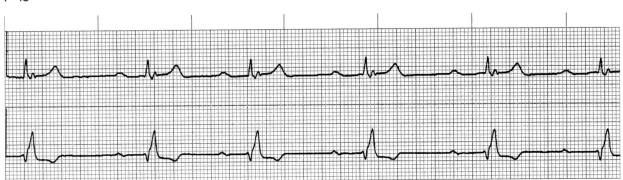

7-14

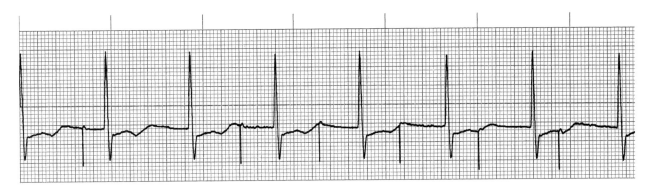

7-15

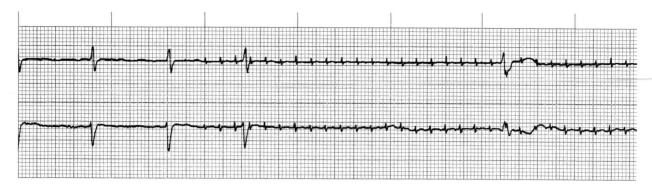

7–16

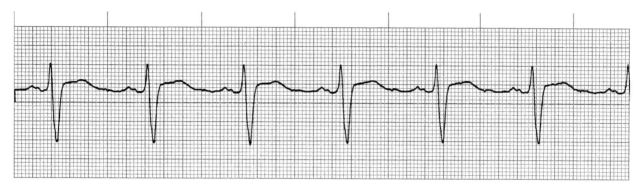

7–17

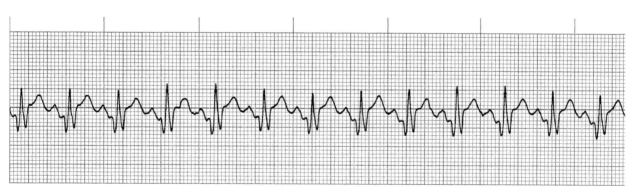

7–18

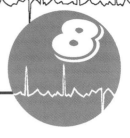

THE LANGUAGE OF ECG

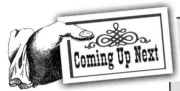

Coming Up Next

○ What are the four areas of the heart that can initiate a rhythm?

○ What terms are used to describe the heart rate?

○ Why can't you have a premature sinus contraction?

○ What is the difference between a premature and an escape beat and why do we care?

○ What do *bigeminal* and *trigeminal* mean?

○ What are modifiers?

Starting With the Basics

Whenever you learn a new language, you start by learning certain basic words and some rules by which you can combine those words into intelligent phrases. The language of ECG is no different. In this chapter, we're going to learn the basic terms of "ECGese," what they mean, and the rules for combining them.

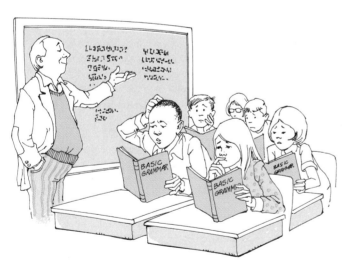

WHERE DOES THE RHYTHM BEGIN?

The most important part of interpreting any rhythm is to know its point of origin. If you look at the chapter titles for Section III of this book, you'll see four basic divisions, which correspond to the four main areas of the heart. They are "Sinus," "Atrial," "Junctional," and "Ventricular." When you describe a rhythm or part of a rhythm, one of these terms must be present in some form. Which part of the heart the rhythm, or individual beat, comes from is vitally important. You must know where it begins before you can anticipate its effect on the patient and determine the treatment needed, if any.

The term *sinus* refers only to rhythms that begin in the sinus node. Although this statement sounds deceptively simple, we will see shortly that it can't be taken for granted.

The term *atrium* comes from the Greek word meaning "corridor." This word aptly describes the function of the atria (plural of "atrium")—the blood travels through them from the blood vessels to the pumping chambers, the ventricles. The term *atrial* describes any rhythm that arises in either atrium and does not come from the sinus node. It also refers to individual beats that interrupt another type of rhythm.

Junctional, or *nodal*, refers to signals that arise in the *atrioventricular node*. The term *junctional* usually refers to rhythms and individual beats, whereas the term *atrioventricular* (AV) is reserved for describing conduction problems within the AV node itself.

The term *ventricle* comes from a Latin word meaning "little belly." That's what the ventricles really are: little

Table 8-1 Normal (intrinsic) rates for various tissues of the heart

Sinus Node (bpm)	Atrial Tissue (bpm)	Junctional Node (bpm)	Ventricular Tissue (bpm)
60–100	60–100	40–60	20–40

bellies for holding and ejecting blood. The term *ventricular* refers to any rhythm that originates in the ventricles.

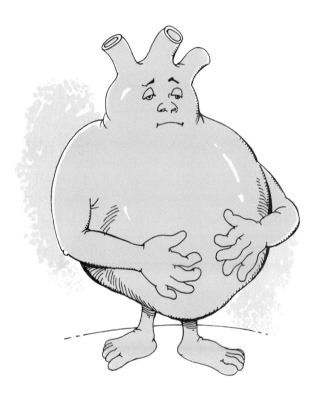

All of these Greek and Latin terms may seem like just so much esoteric nonsense. However, when you combine them with the rest of the information in this chapter, you'll be able to name a significant portion of all the basic rhythms discussed in this book.

HOW FAST DOES IT GO?

Now that we know where our rhythm originates, we must also know how fast it is. This is the second major piece of the interpretation puzzle, and it's vital to knowing how we should expect our patient to look and whether emergency interventions are needed.

If you've ever taken a medical terminology course, you will recall some of the word forms I'm about to use to describe the speed of rhythms. *Brady-* describes an abnormally slow rhythm. *Idio-* denotes a normal, or *intrinsic,* rhythm. An *accelerated* rhythm is somewhat faster than normal. And *tachy-* describes an abnormally fast rhythm.

Ranging Far and Wide: What's Normal? A normal ventricular rhythm is called *idioventricular;* we'll discuss this term a little further on. Otherwise, you can follow general rules to arrive easily at the correct term, but some of those rules depend on your knowing where the rhythm originates. For example, a normal speed for the sinus node is too fast for a normal junctional rhythm. Each area of the heart that can initiate a signal has its own normal range. Those ranges are listed in Table 8–1, and it's vitally important that you memorize them. You need them to determine the origin of your rhythm and to arrive at its correct name.

Life in the Slow Lane Table 8-2 provides general information on how to name a rhythm, given its origin and rate. As we've seen, the term *bradycardia* describes a slower-than-normal rhythm. The rate depends on what's normal, or intrinsic, for the tissue of origin. The bradycardia cutoff point for rhythms originating in the sinus node is higher than the bradycardia cutoff for rhythms originating in the junctional tissue because the normal rate for the sinus node is faster than the normal rate for junctional tissue. For example, a heart rate of 50 bpm originating in the sinus node is considered *sinus bradycardia.* However, the same rate originating in the junctional tissue is termed *junctional rhythm,* not "junctional bradycardia," because 50 is within the normal range for the junctional tissue. You'll notice that *tachycardia* always describes a rhythm faster than 100 regardless of where it originates.

If a patient's sinus node is normal and the heart rate is less than 100 bpm, the sinus node will override the atrial tissue's attempt to control the rhythm and will take over the work of determining the rhythm. Therefore, atrial rhythms below 100 are unusual and frequently are hard to identify from one- or two-lead rhythm strips.

Atrial rhythms below 100 bpm are called *ectopic,* which comes from the Greek word meaning "displaced." The rhythm is being generated from a point in the atrium other than the sinus node. This other point now acts as the primary pacemaker even though it's firing at a rate normally reserved for the sinus node. Ectopic rhythms don't usually cause much trouble, but they do indicate that the sinus

Table 8–2 Converting heart rates and origins to rhythm names

Rhythm Type	Sinus Node (bpm)	Atrial Tissue (bpm)	Junctional Node (bpm)	Ventricular Tissue (bpm)
Bradycardia	<60 Sinus bradycardia	<60 Ectopic atrial bradycardia	<40 Junctional bradycardia	<20 Ventricular (agonal) bradycardia
Normal rhythm	60–100 Sinus rhythm	60–100 Ectopic atrial rhythm	40–60 Junctional rhythm	20–40 Idioventricular rhythm
Accelerated rhythm	NA	NA	60–100 Accelerated junctional rhythm	40–100 Accelerated idioventricular rhythm
Tachycardia	>100 Sinus tachycardia	>100 Atrial tachycardia	>100 Junctional tachycardia	>100 Ventricular tachycardia

node is diseased and unable to consistently fulfill its royal duties as king of the heart rhythms.

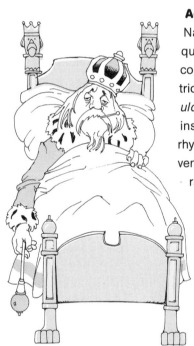

Agonizing Slowness

Naming rhythms is a quirky business. Most confusing are the ventricular rhythms. *Ventricular bradycardia,* for instance, describes a rhythm originating in the ventricles and having a rate of less than 20 bpm. Although the term is technically correct, a patient with a heart rate below 20 is in serious trouble. In reality, ventricular bradycardia usually occurs just before the heart stops, when the heart is making its last effort to fight but may be too sick to recover. Therefore, this rhythm is more commonly called "agonal." Does that sound like a word that you hear in everyday usage? Yes, "agony." Both words come from the same root, meaning "death" or "severe pain," a good description of what's going on inside the heart.

How Fast Is Too Fast? When the rhythm originates in the ventricles and produces a heart rate of 20 to 40 bpm, the prefix *idio-* is added to the term *ventricular,* making the rhythm *idioventricular.* The prefix *idio-* is Greek and simply means "own," or "individual." This may seem redundant, and I agree it is, but that's the accepted naming method. The same prefix applies when the rate is 40 to 100 for a rhythm originating in the ventricles, only the term is preceded by the word "accelerated." *Accelerated* means the same as it does in everyday language—faster than normal. It describes a rhythm faster than the rate at which the originating tissue usually fires and applies only to junctional and ventricular tissue, for example, *accelerated idioventricular rhythm.* Because the usual rates for junctional and ventricular tissue are too slow to meet the body's needs, accelerated rhythms are generally good. Therefore, if the heart tissue is in pretty good shape and the body does its job right, junctional and ventricular rhythms will normally accelerate to meet the body's demands.

However, things change once the rate increases to over 100 bpm. Now we're dealing with tachycardia. Heart rates greater than 100 normally are not necessary to meet the resting demands of the body. If they exceed 100, there's usually something else going on to drive the heart rate that high. The body's needs aren't being handled well enough by the rhythm at normal heart rates, so the body tries to increase blood flow by increasing heart rate. (Remember, CO = HR × SV.) Regardless of where the rhythm originates, we need to be able to express that it's a cause for concern; therefore, we identify rhythms greater than 100 as tachycardias.

So now, if you're given both the origin and the heart rate for a basic ECG rhythm, you can name the rhythm. In later chapters, you will learn the clues that help you determine the point of origin, and you've already learned how to calculate heart rates.

A Little Less Basic

If that were all the knowledge necessary for naming heart rhythms, you wouldn't need an entire book. Frequently, however, a rhythm strip contains elements besides the basic rhythm.

A COUPLE OF CRANKY CUSTOMERS

Sick or Just Greedy? The next two terms we'll discuss are *premature* and *escape beats*. *Premature* describes a beat that comes before the next beat is expected. Premature beats occur because the small area of tissue that generates them needs more than it's getting from the heart. The tissue is trying to increase the heart rate, usually to get more blood flow because it needs more oxygen. The tissue is described as *irritable,* which, as you can imagine, is not normally a good thing. The problem is that the tissue generating the beats is going against the crowd: it's the only area not happy with the way the heart is functioning. You could almost call it greedy, although "sick" would be a more accurate description.

Premature beats can originate from the atrial, junctional, or ventricular tissue. Like other beats, they are named according to their point of origin.

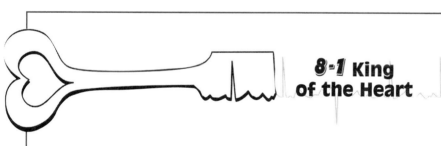

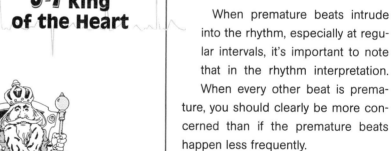

8-1 King of the Heart

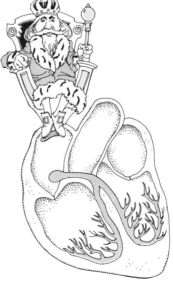

You'll notice the conspicuous absence of the sinus node from any discussion of premature beats. Because the sinus node is the preferred pacemaker for the heart, it can originate a beat at any time and at any rate, so the beat is never considered premature. The sinus node is the king of the heart. Even if it makes whimsical decisions about when to generate a beat, it's still the king, and we wouldn't think of questioning it by terming its beat premature.

Where Did That Beat Go? *Escape beats,* the opposite of premature beats, take place after the next beat should have occurred. Something happens to the pacemaker generating the signal so that it fails to generate a beat when it should. Again the tissue becomes irritated because of insufficient blood flow, but this time it isn't greedy, it has simply been abandoned.

The escape beat, when it finally comes, provides an "escape from death". If the pacemaker controlling the heart stops functioning and no other area sends out a signal, the heart rate will be zero and the patient will surely die. Escape beats can originate in the same locations as premature beats. Occasionally they can take over a rhythm that has failed; the escape beats are then termed an *escape rhythm*.

Never Seen Alone Premature and escape beats and rhythms appear in association with the basic or underlying rhythm, never by themselves. Therefore, you must have a named rhythm in addition to a premature or escape beat. Examples include sinus rhythm with a premature atrial beat or accelerated junctional rhythm with a ventricular escape beat. When you name an escape rhythm, you must name both rhythms in order of appearance. An example would be sinus rhythm with an accelerated junctional escape rhythm.

When premature beats intrude into the rhythm, especially at regular intervals, it's important to note that in the rhythm interpretation. When every other beat is premature, you should clearly be more concerned than if the premature beats happen less frequently.

MEET THE TWINS

Now for some more terminology. Some terms describing premature beats are based on the Latin suffix -*geminy,* which means "twin" or "twinning," just like the zodiac sign of Gemini. The term is used generally to describe a group of beats that occurs in a repeating pattern or cycle.

The prefixes describing premature beats come from Latin and indicate

8-2 Waiting for a Friend

The difference between the premature beat and the escape beat can be better understood if you imagine a regular excursion with your best friend. Suppose you and your friend always go for a walk every Saturday at three o'clock. This event, which happens at evenly spaced intervals, is like a regular heartbeat.

Now suppose that this Saturday you arrive very early. You get impatient and start the walk at two o'clock but don't call to let your friend know. A premature beat is like that. On the other hand, if you wait until four o'clock and then leave because your friend never shows up, that's like an escape beat. Either way you do the same thing, but you wait too long in one case and not long enough in the other.

the total number of beats in the repeating group. You're familiar with some of the most commonly used ones: *bi-*, meaning "two" as in "bicycle," and *tri-,* meaning "three" as in "tripod." *Bigeminy* describes a group of two beats, one normal beat and one premature beat, while *trigeminy* describes a group of three, two normal beats and one premature beat. Theoretically the term can stretch all the way up to dodecageminy, a group of 12 beats, but the reality goes only as far as *quadrigeminy,* a group of four beats (three normal and one premature). The cutoff comes here because the total number of premature beats in a minute decreases to tolerable levels when it exceeds quadrigeminy.

Remember, the *-geminy* terms describe the total number of beats in the repeating group, not the number of normal beats or premature beats. This is a common mistake and one you should take care to avoid.

ARRIVING TOO SOON

A Single Visitor Premature beats are called *ectopic beats* because, as we discussed before with atrial rhythms, the location generating the beat has been displaced from the sinus node to the location of the premature beat. The location of the premature beat is called a *focus,* which simply means "point." Occasionally, however, premature beats come from multiple locations, or *foci* (plural of "focus"). Premature beats that come from one location are termed *unifocal*—coming from the same point every time. Those that come from more than one location are termed *multifocal*—coming from more than one point—and are more serious than unifocal beats. The reason is simple: if only one part of the heart is irritated,

that's bad, but it's much worse if more than one part is irritated.

When a Crowd Shows Up Moving from bad to worse, we find couplets and triplets. *Couplets* are two consecutive premature beats of the same type. For example, two consecutive premature ventricular beats make up a ventricular couplet. Two consecutive premature atrial complexes make up an atrial couplet. However, one premature ventricular beat followed by one premature atrial beat is not a couplet. *Triplets* are three consecutive premature beats of the same type. The triplet phenomenon used to be called a "salvo"; although that term is outdated, you may hear it bandied about now and then, especially by old timers such as myself. Nowadays triplets are usually referred to as a *short run* of the offending premature beat, as in sinus rhythm with a short run of premature ventricular beats. The three beats may also be described as a *second rhythm,* as in sinus rhythm with a three-beat run of ventricular tachycardia, as long as the original rhythm takes over again.

As you may already have gathered, there are several ways to refer to premature beats. For example, premature beats from the ventricles can be called premature ventricular beats (PVBs), premature ventricular contractions or complexes (PVCs), ventricular premature beats (VPBs), or ventricular premature contractions or complexes (VPCs). Simply substitute "atrial" or "junctional" for "ventricular," and you get the terms describing premature beats from other foci. I'm sure that even more ways to describe premature beats exist, but whichever one you choose, most people will understand what you're talking about. My personal preference is for "premature ventricular complexes" because of my previous training, not for any other significant reason.

NOT QUITE USUAL

Finally, we have terms called *modifiers.* Modifiers describe something unusual about rhythm. They usually refer to blocks, such as bundle branch block or first-degree AV block, which we will cover later in the book. Modifiers are usually appended to a rhythm descriptor—for example, sinus rhythm with a bundle branch block.

We'll discuss the details of determining modifiers as they arise throughout the book. For now you need to know only that they exist and that they don't alter the basic description but simply provide more detail about the rhythm being described.

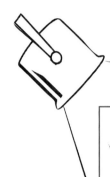

NOW YOU KNOW

The four areas that can initiate a rhythm are the sinus node, the atria, the junctional or atrioventricular node, and the ventricles.

Brady- describes an abnormally slow rhythm. *Idio-* denotes a normal, or *intrinsic,* rhythm. An *accelerated* rhythm is somewhat faster than normal. And *tachy-* describes an abnormally fast rhythm, always above 100 bpm.

Heart rate is termed *bradycardia, accelerated, tachycardia,* and *normal* or *intrinsic,* denoted by *idio-.*

The sinus node is king of the heart, and whenever it wants to produce a beat, that's just fine.

A premature beat occurs before the next expected beat; an escape beat occurs after the next expected beat should have occurred.

Bigeminal and *trigeminal* describe the relationship between normal and abnormal beats. *Bigeminal* describes one normal and one abnormal beat in a repeating pattern; *trigeminal* describes two normal beats and one abnormal beat in a repeating pattern.

Modifiers are used to describe additional features of the ECG tracing that are independent of the rhythm itself.

Test Yourself

1. An ECG tracing originating in the sinus node with a heart rate of 52 bpm would be described as _____.

2. An ECG tracing originating in the sinus node with a heart rate of 89 bpm, with two consecutive premature ventricular complexes, would be described as _____ with a _____.

3. Accelerated junctional rhythm could have a heart rate from _____ to _____ bpm.

4. Any rhythm with a heart rate above 100 bpm is considered a _____.

5. A rhythm that has a heart rate of 56 bpm, originates in the junctional tissue, and has two beats followed by a premature ventricular complex (PVC) in a repeating cycle would be called _____ with _____.

6. Junctional tachycardia originates in the _____ and has a heart rate of at least _____ bpm.

7. When a rhythm has premature atrial complexes (PACs) that come from different locations, the PACs are considered _____.

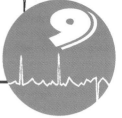

RHYTHM RULES

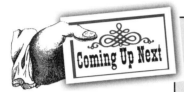
Coming Up Next

○ What are the key areas to evaluate when you interpret a cardiac rhythm?

○ Is a rhythm either regular or irregular?

○ What are the five steps to identifying a rhythm?

○ Why is evaluating the PR interval important?

○ Can a rhythm have more than one P-wave per QRS complex?

How Many Questions?

When trying to interpret any rhythm strip, we focus on certain features. This chapter will discuss these features and why each one is important. You must answer anywhere from 5 to 12 questions to interpret a cardiac rhythm; it depends on what book you read. However many questions you end up with, they can be easily grouped into five general areas.

How Regular Is Regular?

Whether a rhythm is regular is not as simple a question as it seems. You learned in Chapter 3 that a rhythm is considered regular if the distance between any two consecutive QRS complexes varies by three small boxes or less. So identifying a regular rhythm is easy (Figs. 9-1, 9-2). However, identifying an irregular rhythm is a lot more complicated. Not all irregular rhythms are created equal.

REGULARLY IRREGULAR

A rhythm can be *regularly irregular* (Figs. 9-3, 9-4). This means that although the rhythm doesn't march out like a regular rhythm, it still has a pattern. For instance, it may slow down, speed up, and slow down again, repeating the sequence over and over. To identify a rhythm as regularly irregular, you should usually be able to recognize a pattern and predict what will happen next, although you may not be able to anticipate the exact timing of each individual QRS complex.

IRREGULARLY IRREGULAR

The next type of irregular rhythm is *irregularly irregular* (Fig. 9-5). This rhythm has no pattern to its irregularity and no periods of regularity. You can't predict when the next beat should occur or identify any pattern to the rhythm at all.

9-1 SLEEPING IN ON WEEKENDS

Think about getting up in the morning. (Yes, you have to think about it!) If you get up every day at 6 AM no matter what, that's a regular pattern. But if you get up Monday through Friday for work at 6 AM and sleep in until noon on the weekends, your pattern is regularly irregular. The pattern is identifiable–a stretch of 5 early rising days, followed by 2 days when you get to sleep in. Your wake-up time changes, but predictably; therefore, the pattern is regularly irregular.

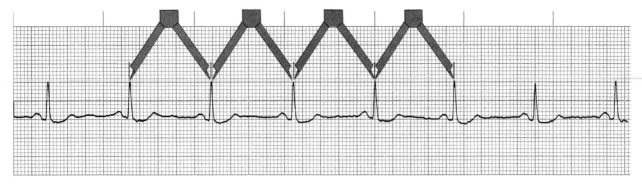

Fig. 9–1 This rhythm is regular because the QRS complexes are equally spaced. The P-waves are also regular.

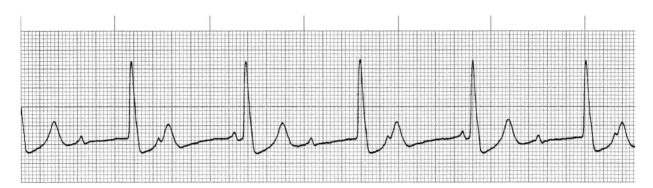

Fig. 9–2 The QRSs and the P-waves are regular in this strip, but note that they seem unrelated to each other.

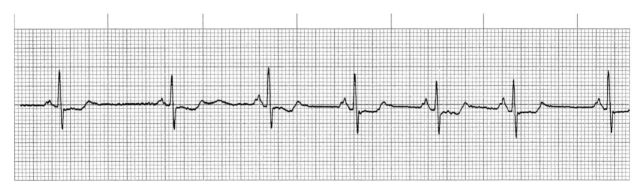

Fig. 9–3 The QRSs and the P-waves first grow closer together and then move farther apart. This pattern repeats, and therefore the rhythm is regularly irregular.

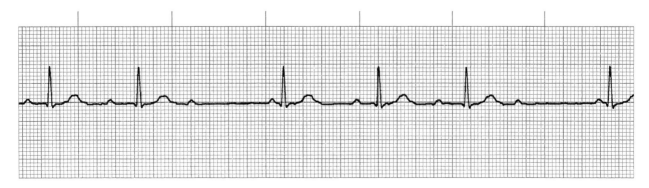

Fig. 9–4 The QRSs in this rhythm look regular at first glance. On closer inspection, they grow farther apart incrementally, then suddenly move very far apart. This rhythm is regularly irregular, but for a different reason than in Fig. 9–3.

9-2 SLEEPING IN ANYTIME

Let's say you have trouble sleeping. You may get up early one day, sleep in the next, and not sleep at all the following night. You don't know when you'll get up on any given morning or whether you'll sleep at all on any given night. This is irregularly irregular.

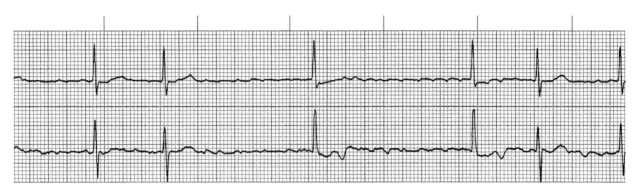

Fig. 9–5 The QRSs in this rhythm seem randomly spaced. First they are close, then farther apart, then closer, then farther apart, and then still farther apart. There is no identifiable pattern to the rhythm, which could even be called an arrhythmia.

"REGULAR EXCEPT"

Some rhythm strips are what I call *"regular except"* (Figs. 9–6, 9–7). Those rhythms fit the definition of regularity, except for a portion or portions that throw them off. These portions can occur once or recur over and over. They can happen randomly or in a repeating pattern. The important thing to remember is that the rhythm would be regular without the irregular portions.

In short, when answering the question of regularity, we have more choices than just "yes" and "no." We have regular, regularly irregular, irregularly irregular, and "regular except." The characteristics of each are listed in Table 9–1.

Fast, Slow, or Just Right?

Back in Chapter 3 you learned how to calculate the heart rate. If the rhythm is regular, you should use the small-box method. If it's irregular, you should use the small-box method to determine the range of heart rates and the 6-second method to determine the average rate.

In Chapter 8 we reviewed the basic reasons why heart rate is important in naming a rhythm. Remember, each area of the heart has its own intrinsic rate, and if we know where the rhythm originates, the heart rate will tell us whether this tissue is going faster or slower than it's programmed to.

9-3 SLEEPING IN WHEN YOU'RE SICK

How does a "regular except" rhythm fit into our sleep analogy? Imagine that you get up at 6 AM 7 days a week *except* when you're sick. You may get sick every payday, on the first of every month, or just randomly. The key is that if I eliminate your sick days, I can predict with certainty what time you'll get up in the morning. If I include your sick days, however, I can't predict your wake-up time accurately.

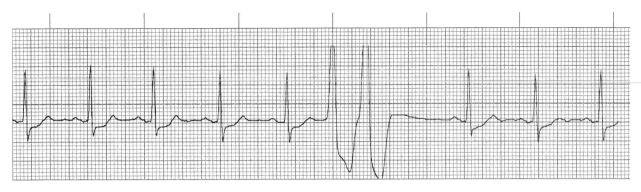

Fig. 9–6 The first six QRSs are evenly spaced, and then suddenly then next two beats disrupt the regularity. The remaining beats are again evenly spaced. The disruption makes this rhythm "regular except."

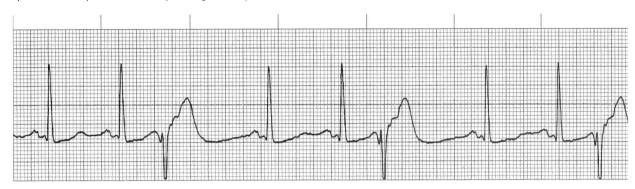

Fig. 9–7 The consecutive, upright QRSs are all separated by the same distance. However, every third beat disrupts the regularity, making this "regular except."

P or Not P?

KNOW WHAT TO ASK

The next area we need to investigate is the P-wave. It's important to search carefully for P-waves in all rhythms. This step helps you determine where the rhythm is starting from.

Table 9–1 Types of regular and irregular rhythms

Characteristic	Description
Regular	Distance between consecutive QRS complexes differs by less than three small boxes.
Regularly irregular	Distance between consecutive QRS complexes varies by more than three small boxes, but with a repeating pattern.
Irregularly irregular	Distance between consecutive QRS complexes varies by more than three small boxes, with no recognizable pattern.
"Regular except"	Distance between consecutive QRS complexes varies by less than three small boxes, except for specific portions that leave a regular rhythm when removed.

Finding the P-wave requires you to answer several questions. First and foremost, is there is a P-wave or isn't there? That question can be tough to answer. A poor rhythm strip with interference, or the wrong lead, can make it difficult if not impossible to identify the P-wave. P-waves can be shy wallflowers; frail and small, they can sometimes easily blend into the background. If it isn't buried or hidden, the P-wave may turn up where you least expect it.

Now you've identified all the P-waves on the strip. Next question: are they all the same shape (Fig. 9–8)? This step is important. If the P-waves have different shapes, they either originated in different places or followed different paths. This study of the shape of ECG waveforms is known as *morphology* and helps us to find the starting point of the rhythm.

Next, how many P-waves can you find for every QRS complex? To determine this, simply look at the segment before each QRS and identify the P-waves. In most cases you'll find one P-wave for every QRS. Occasionally, however, you may find QRS complexes without P-waves or QRSs with two or more P-waves (see Figs. 9–2 and 9–4). Although a QRS may have more than one P-wave, only one P-wave gets through the AV node and causes the ventricles to

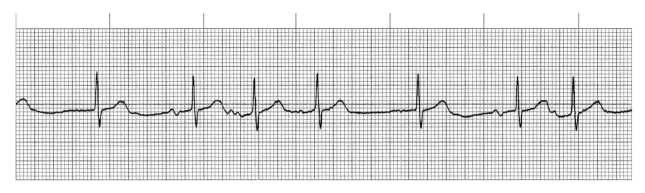

Fig. 9–8 Each of the first four P-waves has a different shape (morphology). The differing shapes tell us that the P-waves started at different points in the heart.

depolarize. This is important to remember. If you need a refresher, look again at the section of Chapter 6 called "Renegade P-Waves"–remember the carts and horses?

Last question: are the P-waves regular? Many people think that a regular rhythm means regular P-waves and that an irregular rhythm means irregular P-waves. Not necessarily.

ALLOW FOR EXCEPTIONS

Although the P-waves usually determine whether a rhythm is regular or not, we find some rhythms in which this doesn't apply. For an example, look again at Figure 9–4; you'll see that, although the P-waves march out, the QRS complexes are irregular. Although such outlaw rhythms are uncommon, they do turn up, so be careful to check both the P-waves and the QRSs for regularity. We'll run into these unusual rhythms again later in the book.

When analyzing P-waves you must determine three things. First, do they all have the same shape, and if not, how many different shapes do they have? Second, are the P-waves regular according to the definitions we discussed earlier in this chapter? Finally, how many P-waves occur before each QRS complex? This last answer has to be "none," "one," or "more than one."

How Far From P to R?

The next step is to evaluate the PR interval. The purpose of this step is to check the AV node function. Many books simply tell you to measure the PR interval, but I think this method is incomplete. You should evaluate *each* PR interval and make sure they're all the same or that they differ by no more than half a small box. If that's the case, simply record the measurement.

If you look back at Figure 9–2, you'll see that all the PR intervals are different. If they vary, simply note that in your

analysis. If they're missing altogether (because there are no P-waves), make a note of that.

To sum up, our three choices for interpreting the PR interval are as follows: a single number, "variable," and "not measurable."

How Complex Is Your QRS?

You already know the next step from Chapter 7: you need to measure the QRS complex. Also, as with the P-waves, you must compare the QRSs and make sure they all have the same shape. It's important to make a note of any difference. Remember, if the shape of the QRSs vary, they either originated in different locations or followed different paths; determining which one will help you understand how the bundle branches are functioning.

When analyzing the QRS complex, you must note its duration and whether it's normal or too long. Also, you must make sure that all QRSs have the same morphology; if they don't, note those with abnormal shapes.

If the QRS complexes are all the same shape, then the T-waves should all be the same shape also. If the T-waves are different, but the QRS complexes the same, then be on the look out for P-waves buried in the T-waves.

What Was All That Again?

STEP 1: DETERMINE REGULARITY

Is the rhythm regular, regularly irregular, irregularly irregular, or "regular except"?

STEP 2: CALCULATE HEART RATE

Are the atrial and ventricular rates different? If so, calculate both.

STEP 3: EVALUATE THE P-WAVES

Are there P-waves?

What is the P-wave morphology (are all P-waves the same shape)?

Is there one P-wave per QRS complex? If not, how many are there?

STEP 4: EVALUATE THE PR INTERVAL

If all PR intervals are the same, note the measurement.

If the PR intervals are different, note that the interval is "variable."

If there are no P-waves, note that the interval is "not measurable."

STEP 5: EVALUATE THE QRS COMPLEX

Are there QRS complexes?

What is the QRS morphology (are they all the same shape)?

If the QRS complexes are the same, are the T-waves all the same?

Why All the Questions?

Do you question the need for all these questions? Well, you'll need them because you'll come up with a different set of answers for each type of rhythm. For example, you'll get one set of answers for sinus rhythm. In sinus arrhythmia, you'll get the same answers except for the regularity question. In sinus bradycardia, the answers are all identical except for the heart rate question.

In theory, if you memorize each set of answers to the questions, you'll know all the rhythms discussed in this book. However, a better approach is to learn the reasons behind the answers for each rhythm. That way, when you decide to continue your education in ECG interpretation, you won't have to memorize anything. Adjust your questions a little and you'll be all set.

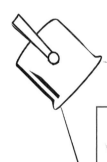

NOW YOU KNOW

To identify a rhythm, you must

  (1) Determine regularity,

  (2) Calculate the heart rate,

  (3) Evaluate the P-waves,

  (4) Evaluate the PR interval,

  (5) Evaluate the QRS complexes and T-waves.

A rhythm can be regular, regularly irregular, irregularly irregular, or "regular except."

If the QRS complexes are irregular, the P-waves may still be regular.

Evaluating P-waves helps to determine where the rhythm originates.

Evaluating the PR interval helps to determine how the AV node is functioning.

Rhythm Rules

Test Yourself

1. In a regular rhythm, the distance between consecutive QRS complexes varies by less than _____ small boxes.

2. In an irregularly irregular rhythm, there is no _____ to the occurrence of the QRS complexes.

3. In a _____ rhythm, one or more complexes disturb an otherwise regular rhythm.

4. Identifying P-wave morphology can help determine where the rhythm _____.

5. PR interval measurements can be a fixed number, _____ or ___ _____.

6. Answer the questions in the five areas for the following five strips:

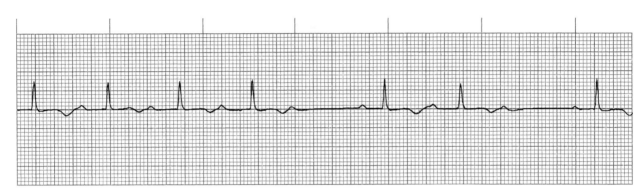

9–1

Regularity: _____   Heart rate: _____   PR interval: _____

P-waves: _____   QRS complex: _____

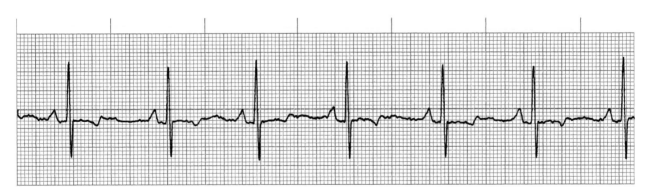

9–2

Regularity: _____   Heart rate: _____   PR interval: _____

P-waves: _____   QRS complex: _____

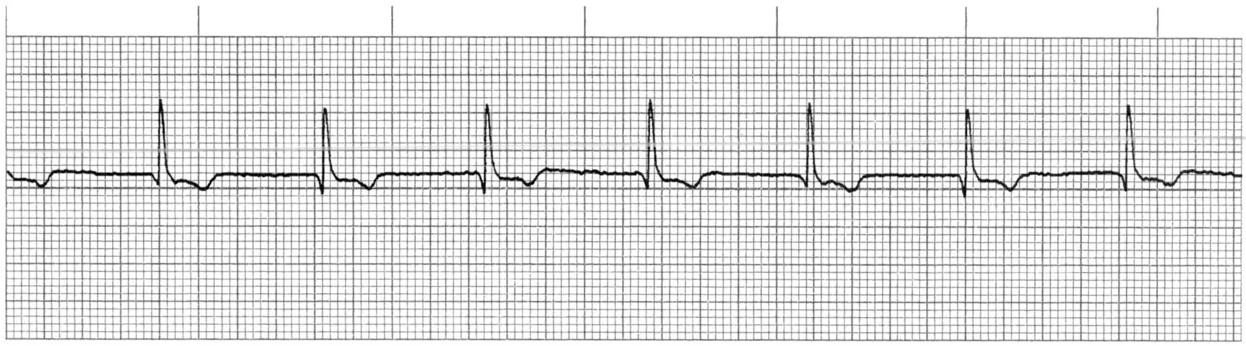

9–3

Regularity: _____   Heart rate: _____   PR interval: _____

P-waves: _____   QRS complex: _____

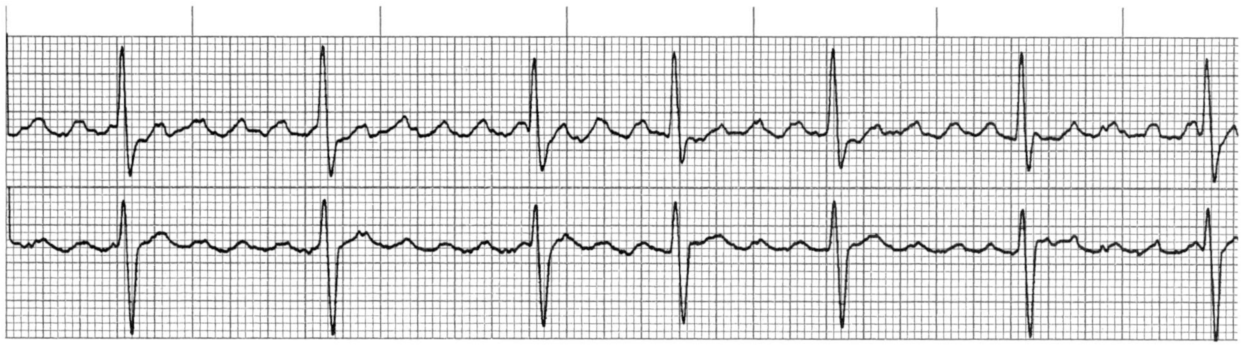

9–4

Regularity: _____   Heart rate: _____   PR interval: _____

P-waves: _____   QRS complex: _____

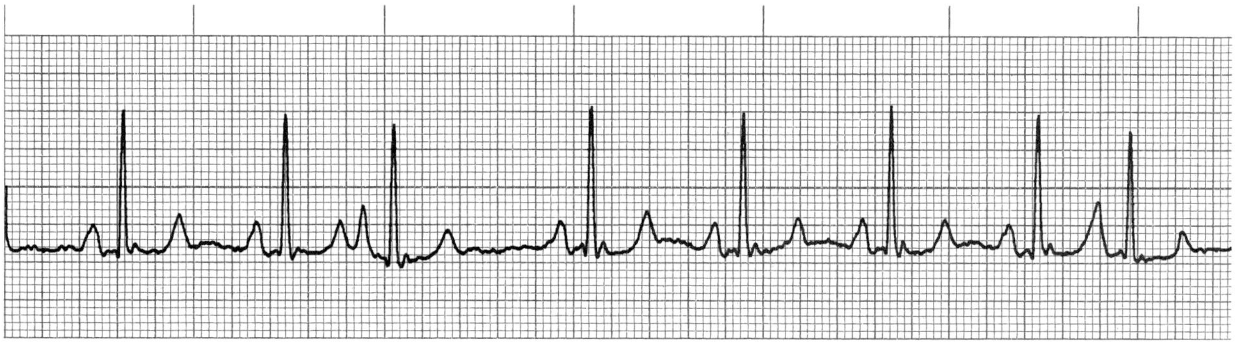

9–5

Regularity: _____   Heart rate: _____   PR interval: _____

P-waves: _____   QRS complex: _____

Interpretation: _____

SECTION

Moving to the Rhythm

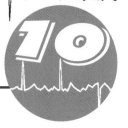

SINUS RHYTHMS

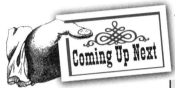

Coming Up Next

○ What are the criteria for sinus rhythms?

○ How do the types of sinus rhythms differ from each other?

○ Are all sinus rhythms regular?

○ Is normal sinus rhythm always "normal"?

○ What is the preferred treatment for most cases of sinus tachycardia?

○ What is the maximum heart rate for sinus tachycardia?

○ What is the difference between sinus arrest and sinus exit block?

One Who Sets the Pace

The *sinoatrial node,* also called the *sinus node* or SA node, is the preferred pacemaker of the healthy heart. The whole electrical conduction system of the heart is designed around it.

Sinus rhythm is frequently called *normal sinus rhythm.* This can be a misnomer. Highly conditioned athletes can have a resting heart rate between 30 and 40 bpm, which is less than the usual range for sinus rhythm. An athlete's heart rate can be that low because he or she has an extremely efficient heart. The stroke volume with each contraction is very large, so the heart doesn't need to beat as frequently. A heart rate of 96, within the normal range for most people, would be nearly three times normal for our athlete. It would mean that the heart's efficiency had declined dramatically and that the athlete was in trouble.

Normality is highly individual—what is normal for you is not normal for me. I recommend that we stick with *sinus rhythm,* or *regular sinus rhythm,* and not concern ourselves with normality until we assess the patient's condition.

Recognizing Sinus Rhythms

CAPABLE AND SUFFICIENT LEADERSHIP

In Chapter 8 we referred to the sinus node as king of the heart rhythms. In case you like a more democratic system,

let's say that the heart is set up like the government of our country and the sinus node is the executive branch. Under normal circumstances, the sinus node rules the heart. All the other parts of the heart follow its lead as long as that leadership is capable and sufficient.

All rhythms are named for their point of origin in the heart. Sinus rhythms originate in the sinus node, and all sinus rhythms share certain characteristics. If we apply the five rhythm interpretation questions from Chapter 9, we can discuss the different answers that different sinus rhythms provide.

CHARACTERISTICS OF A SINUS BEAT

All sinus rhythms have one P-wave per QRS complex, and all sinus P-waves viewed in the same lead have the same characteristic shape (Fig. 10–1). That's because they all originate from the same point in the heart, the sinus node, and follow the same path through the atria.

The PR interval is normal. That's because the signal travels through the atria as we'd expect, then to the AV node, where it encounters the usual delay, and finally through the bundle branches. The signal uses all the normal pathways, so the time it takes to travel should fall into the usual range.

Because the QRS complex depends on normal conduction through the bundle branches, we can expect it to be normal as well. The different rhythms initiated in the sinus node vary only in rate and regularity.

10-1 It's Up to the Drummer

Pretend you're the drummer in a rock band. What are you doing—besides venting your frustrations—when you bang on that drum?

Think back to the section of Chapter 3 called "Picking Up the Beat." In a band, the drummer sets the pace, establishing the rhythm for everybody. If the drummer starts to beat the drum faster, the whole band will play and sing faster to keep up. The band can play without a drummer, but the result may not be well coordinated and the music won't sound too good.

Now think of the band as your heart and the drummer as its pacemaker. If the heart's pacemaker speeds up or slows down, so does the heart rate.

Sinus Discharge Can Be a Good Thing

In sinus rhythm (Figs. 10–2 and 10–3; Table 10–1), the signals start with the depolarization of the sinus node. The sinus node discharges regularly at a rate of 60 to 99 bpm. The P-waves are upright in leads I, II, III, V_5 and V_6, as well as in others, and should be inverted in lead aVR, and we always find one and only one for every QRS complex. The PR interval is within the normal range, as we've seen, and all the QRS complexes are normal in shape, size, and duration.

Sinus Tachycardia

WHEN SINUS DISCHARGE IS TOO MUCH

The sinus node normally discharges in the range of 60 to 99 times per minute. However, many things can cause it

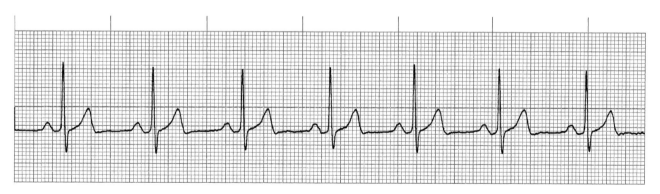

Fig. 10–1 Sinus rhythm. All of the P-waves on this strip are identical: upright and rounded.

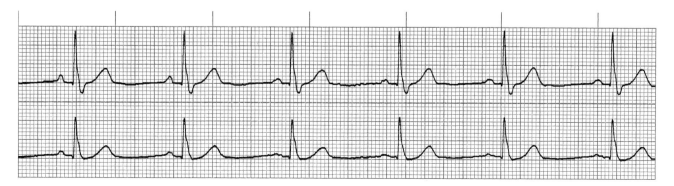

Fig. 10–2 Sinus rhythm in leads II and III. All of the P-waves are identical in each lead, but the P-waves in lead II are slightly different from those in lead III.

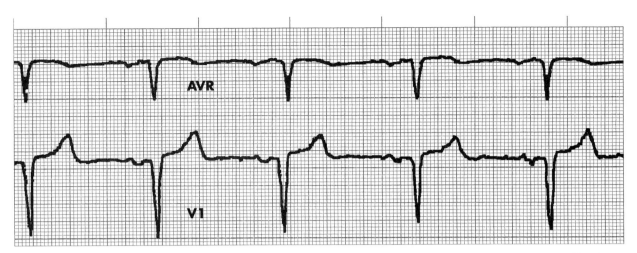

Fig. 10–3 Sinus rhythm in leads aVR and V₁. All of the P-waves in each lead are identical but different from those in the other lead. Also, the P-waves in lead aVR are negative, a normal finding in this lead.

Table 10–1 Criteria for sinus rhythm

Regularity	Always regular
Heart Rate	60–99 bpm
P-Wave	1 per QRS, all the same shape
PR Interval	0.12–0.20 seconds (three to five small boxes)
QRS Complex	All the same shape, <0.12 seconds (three small boxes)

to depolarize faster. When the rate of sinus node discharge exceeds the normal range of 60 to 99 bpm, the rhythm is called *sinus tachycardia* (Figs. 10–4 and 10–5). Although the rhythm still originates in the sinus node, it has become a tachycardia because the rate is 100 or more. Table 10–2 shows the heart rate in bold type to distinguish it from normal sinus rhythm.

Sinus tachycardia can be a problem because the faster rate increases the workload of the heart muscle so that the heart needs more oxygen. Also, if you remember

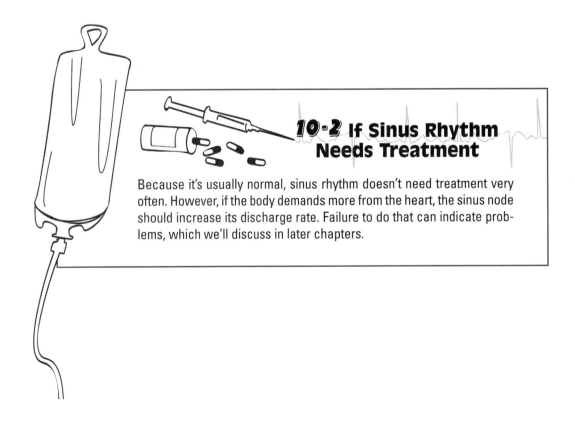

10-2 If Sinus Rhythm Needs Treatment

Because it's usually normal, sinus rhythm doesn't need treatment very often. However, if the body demands more from the heart, the sinus node should increase its discharge rate. Failure to do that can indicate problems, which we'll discuss in later chapters.

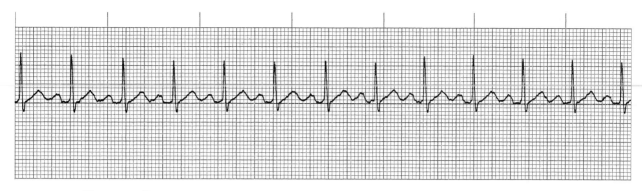

Fig. 10–4 Sinus tachycardia. The rhythm has the same characteristics as sinus rhythm; only the rate is different.

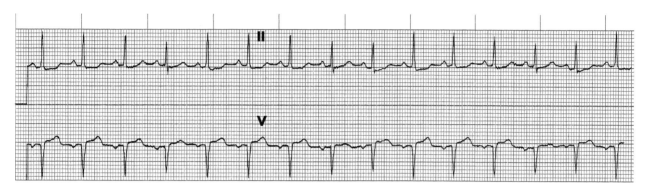

Fig. 10–5 Sinus tachycardia. The QRS direction does not change the interpretation, which relies on the heart rate and the P-wave. The top tracing is in lead II. The bottom tracing is in V1.

from Chapter 1, the ventricles are filled during their rest period (also known as *diastole*). Here's the problem: the tachycardia makes the ventricles contract at a faster rate, decreasing their rest time between beats. Because of this shorter diastolic period, the ventricles can't take in as much blood as they do at a normal rate. In slower tachycardias, 100 to 110 bpm, the difference usually isn't enough to matter. However, at faster rates, the filling time becomes even shorter, and therefore less blood is

ejected with each contraction. This drop in ejection can diminish cardiac output because the increased heart rate isn't enough to offset the decrease in stroke volume. (If you don't remember stroke volume, see the rock-moving discussion in Chapter 1.) The crucial rate varies among individuals, but usually it exceeds 140 to 150. When cardiac output is sufficiently impaired, the patient often experiences dizziness, hypotension, chest pain, and syncope.

Sinus tachycardia does have an upper limit, but this limit is more theoretical and practical than actual. Each person's sinus node has its own built-in maximum rate, usually between 160 and 180 bpm. For this book we'll settle on 160, but keep in mind that this number isn't carved in stone. What does an upper limit of 160 mean? Well, in theory, if a patient has a rhythm with a heart rate of 170, we say that the rhythm can't be originating in the sinus node. The sinus node has limits just like the president—neither can go to extremes. This limit doesn't apply to other tissues, however (we'll discuss those later). If you're in doubt about the origin of a rhythm, get a 12-lead ECG to obtain more information.

Table 10–2 Criteria for sinus tachycardia

Regularity	Regular
Heart Rate	**≥100 bpm** (maximum usually 160 bpm)
P-Wave	1 per QRS, all the same shape
PR Interval	0.12–0.20 seconds (three to five small boxes)
QRS Complex	All the same shape, <0.12 seconds (three small boxes)

10-3 SHIFTING UP

Sinus tachycardia usually begins gradually, with the sinus discharge rate increasing steadily until the heart rate is in the range of 100 to 160 bpm (Fig. 10–6). This process works like gears shifting in a car. To go faster, you press the accelerator (stimulate the sympathetic nervous system). The car doesn't just shift suddenly from first gear to fifth gear. It speeds up gradually and shifts into second, then takes on a little more speed and shifts into third, and so on until the car is in fifth gear and doing 60 miles an hour. In contrast, other *tachydysrhythmias* (the term for any abnormal fast rhythm) tend to start and stop suddenly, jumping from a sinus rate of, say, 70 to a tachycardic rate of, say, 120, with no stops in between.

I know, you're thinking, "What about when someone startles me and my heart rate jumps up immediately?" True, that does happen, but when you calm down, the sinus tachycardia slows gradually back to your resting heart rate. With another type of dysrhythmia, however, the rate would drop as abruptly as it accelerated.

TREAT THE CAUSE, NOT THE SYMPTOMS

Sinus tachycardia is not usually a primary dysrhythmia. In other words, the sinus tachycardia itself isn't usually the problem but a symptom of some other problem (Table 10–3 lists some possible causes). Sure, you can give medications to decrease the heart rate, but that isn't always the treatment of choice for sinus tachycardia. Lowering the heart rate without treating the cause is like giving blood without stopping the bleeding or like giving pain medication without fixing the broken bone causing the pain. In addition, if the problem is a limited stroke volume, then lowering the heart rate can worsen the patient's condition by lowering cardiac output!

Sinus Bradycardia

WHEN LESS SINUS DISCHARGE IS HEALTHY

Sinus bradycardia occurs when the sinus node is the pacemaker site and the heart rate is less than 60 bpm (Figs. 10–7 and 10–8). This rate isn't necessarily bad, although it can be. Remember, the range for sinus rhythms is based on averages from the entire population. Like the athlete we met earlier, many people have heart rates that deviate from the magical range of 60 to 99. Table 10–4 shows the heart rate for sinus bradycardia in bold type to distinguish it from "normal" sinus rhythm.

From Chapter 1 we know that if the stroke volume increases, the heart rate can decrease without affecting

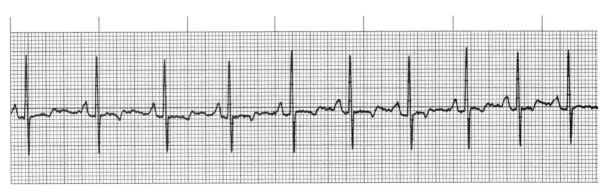

Fig. 10–6 Sinus tachycardia. Notice the gradual change in the spacing between QRS complexes throughout the strip.

Table 10–3 Some causes of sinus tachycardia

Medical Emergencies	Drugs	Other Causes
Acute myocardial infarction	Alcohol in excess	Anxiety
Dehydration	Atropine	Exercise
Heart failure	Caffeine	Fever
Hypoxia	Cocaine	Hyperthyroidism
Pulmonary embolism	Dopamine	Pain
Shock	Tobacco	
Significant blood loss		

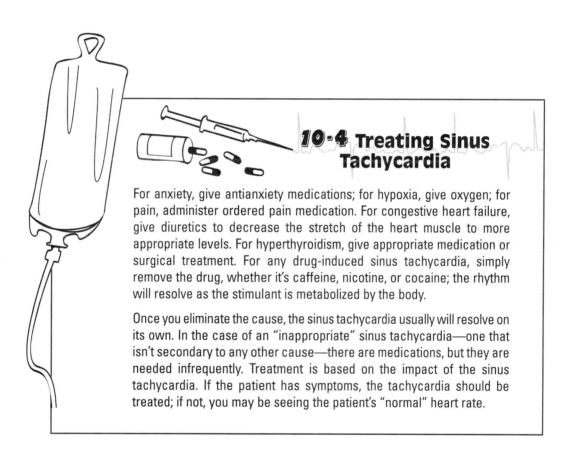

10-4 Treating Sinus Tachycardia

For anxiety, give antianxiety medications; for hypoxia, give oxygen; for pain, administer ordered pain medication. For congestive heart failure, give diuretics to decrease the stretch of the heart muscle to more appropriate levels. For hyperthyroidism, give appropriate medication or surgical treatment. For any drug-induced sinus tachycardia, simply remove the drug, whether it's caffeine, nicotine, or cocaine; the rhythm will resolve as the stimulant is metabolized by the body.

Once you eliminate the cause, the sinus tachycardia usually will resolve on its own. In the case of an "inappropriate" sinus tachycardia—one that isn't secondary to any other cause—there are medications, but they are needed infrequently. Treatment is based on the impact of the sinus tachycardia. If the patient has symptoms, the tachycardia should be treated; if not, you may be seeing the patient's "normal" heart rate.

cardiac output. Healthy people with sinus bradycardia are likely to be in excellent physical condition. As we've seen, a highly trained athlete can have a resting heart rate of less than 40 bpm (Fig. 10–9). The heart muscle is in such good shape that each contraction produces a large stroke volume. When the athlete exercises, the heart rate speeds up to meet the body's increasing metabolic demands.

Once the athlete stops exercising, the heart rate returns to its normal resting level.

WHEN SINUS DISCHARGE ISN'T ENOUGH

However, if the heart rate becomes too low, cardiac output will suffer because the heart can't increase stroke

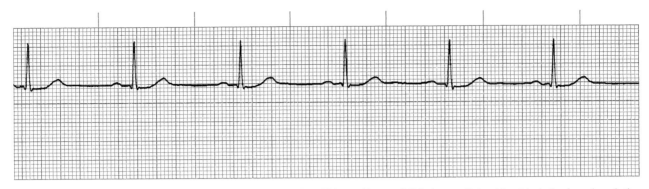

Fig. 10–7 Sinus bradycardia. The P-waves are upright in lead II and the PR interval is normal. Only the rate distinguishes this rhythm from sinus rhythm.

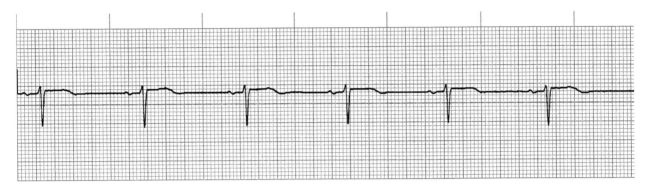

Fig. 10–8 Sinus bradycardia in lead V1. This strip was recorded simultaneously with Fig. 10-7. The P-wave is biphasic, a normal finding in this lead.

Table 10–4 Criteria for sinus bradycardia

Regularity	Regular
Heart Rate	**<60 bpm**
P-Wave	One per QRS, all the same shape
PR Interval	0.12–0.20 seconds
QRS Complex	All the same shape, <0.12 seconds

volume enough to compensate. Like sinus tachycardia, sinus bradycardia can cause dizziness, hypotension, chest pain, and syncope.

Treatment is indicated only if the patient has symptoms. Sinus bradycardia can be caused by many medications, including digoxin, beta-blockers, and calcium channel blockers, to name a few. Withholding the offending medication may be the only treatment the patient needs.

Sinus bradycardia can be secondary to another condition, such as myocardial infarction, stroke, or intracerebral bleeding, or it can be normal. We only treat this rhythm if it produces significant symptoms related to the low cardiac output. Chest pain, low blood pressure, dizziness, and shortness of breath are typical. If treating the primary condition would take a long time, we must improve the

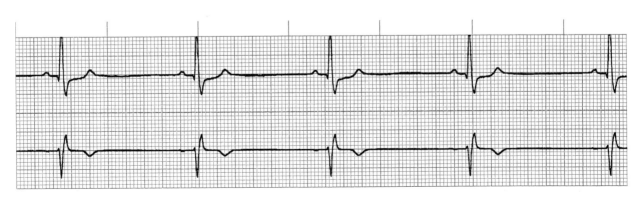

Fig. 10–9 Sinus bradycardia in a triathelete. Although the heart rate is very slow (~40 bpm), the patient was in good health.

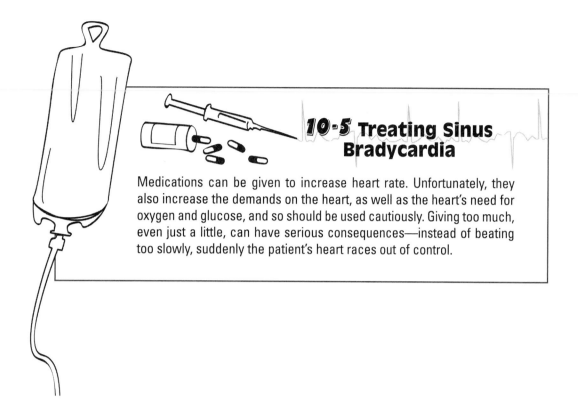

10-5 Treating Sinus Bradycardia

Medications can be given to increase heart rate. Unfortunately, they also increase the demands on the heart, as well as the heart's need for oxygen and glucose, and so should be used cautiously. Giving too much, even just a little, can have serious consequences—instead of beating too slowly, suddenly the patient's heart races out of control.

patient's condition in the meantime by increasing cardiac output using medications or pacemakers which in turn will increase the heart rate. Sometimes the heart rate increases to the point of severe tachycardia. This tends to be self-limiting; as the drug is metabolized, the heart rate decreases. It usually isn't wise to treat the resulting tachycardia.

Sinus Arrhythmia

Sinus arrhythmia is frequently seen with sinus bradycardia and often corresponds to respirations (Figs. 10–10 and 10–11). This type of dysrhythmia is common in children and young adults and usually doesn't need treatment. The heart rate is identical to that of sinus rhythm or sinus bradycardia, but the rhythm is irregular. Table 10–5 shows the outstanding features of the rhythm in bold type.

If the heart rate is slow, we identify this rhythm as sinus bradycardia with sinus arrhythmia. If the heart rate exceeds 99 bpm, the rhythm becomes primarily a tachycardia; we identify it as sinus tachycardia with sinus arrhythmia. The key in naming any rhythm is to identify the most important feature–in this case the excessive speed of the rhythm–and to add more terms if other features need to be clarified.

Although it's irregular, sinus arrhythmia does show a pattern. The rate speeds up for several beats, then slows down for several beats. This cycle repeats continually, usually in response to respiratory rate. In terms of what you see on the strip, the R to R interval varies by at least three small boxes. The discrepancy between the longest and shortest intervals is often much greater than that.

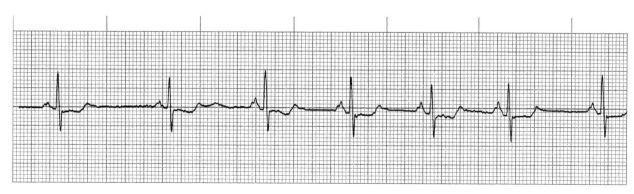

Fig. 10–10 Sinus bradycardia with sinus arrhythmia. The term stresses the slow heart rate.

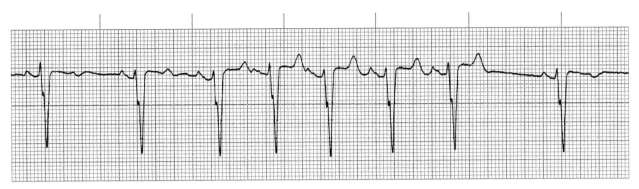

Fig. 10–11 Sinus arrhythmia. The term stresses the irregularity; the heart rate is normal.

Table 10–5 Criteria for sinus arrhythmia

Regularity	Regularly irregular
Heart Rate	<160 bpm, usually <100 bpm
P-Wave	One per QRS, all the same shape
PR Interval	0.12–0.20 seconds
QRS Complex	All the same shape, <0.12 seconds

Sinus Arrest and Sinus Exit Block

A BREAK IN SINUS DISCHARGE

Sometimes, because of an internal problem, the sinus node can't generate a signal to depolarize the atria. When this happens, the P-wave is absent from the ECG strip; remember, you can't have a P-wave without atrial depolarization. An absent P-wave can have either of two primary causes.

Sometimes the sinus node simply fails to generate a signal. This is called *sinus arrest,* or *sinus pause.* The sinus node fires regularly and then suddenly decides to take a

mini-vacation. In failing to discharge, the sinus node breaks its own rhythm; when it begins discharging again, it creates a new rhythm. The cause of sinus arrest is often a mystery.

Sometimes, even if the sinus node depolarizes exactly when it's supposed to, the signal gets trapped in the sinus node. This is called *sinus exit block.* Because the signal can't get out of the sinus node to depolarize the atria, the P-wave again goes missing from the tracing. (If a sinus node discharges in the heart but no one sees it, does it really make a P-wave?)

MARCHING IN AND OUT OF STEP

Superficially these two rhythms seem indistinguishable, but there is a way to differentiate sinus arrest from sinus exit block. Sinus exit block maintains its rhythm, but sinus arrest loses it. Table 10–6 shows the distinguishing feature of the rhythm in bold type for both sinus arrest and sinus exit block.

Comparing the strips in Figures 10–12 and 10–13, you won't see much difference; both rhythms are regular except for the pauses. However, if you try to march out the QRS complexes, you'll see the difference. This is done for you in Figure 10–14. The first strip, Figure 10–14a, shows

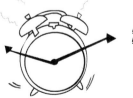

10-6 A Rhythm With a Fingerprint

If the rate of a sinus rhythm is either increasing *or* decreasing, you must be careful not to identify it as a sinus arrhythmia. The unique marker of sinus arrhythmia is that its rate increases *and* decreases over intervals of a few seconds and frequently changes with inhalation and exhalation.

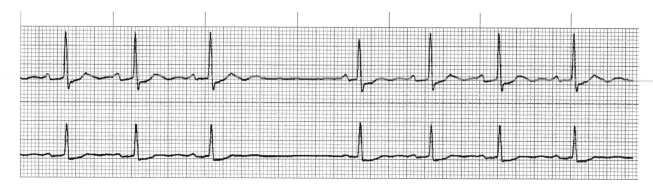

Fig. 10–12 Sinus exit block. The sinus node continues to fire, but the signal is trapped inside it. The underlying regularity is preserved.

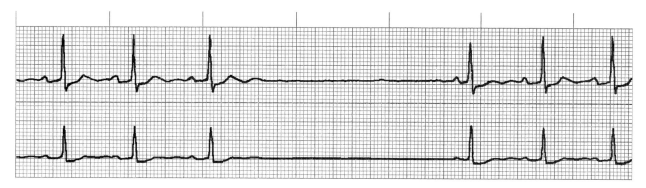

Fig. 10–13 Sinus arrest. The sinus node stops and restarts, disturbing the timing of the next visible P-wave.

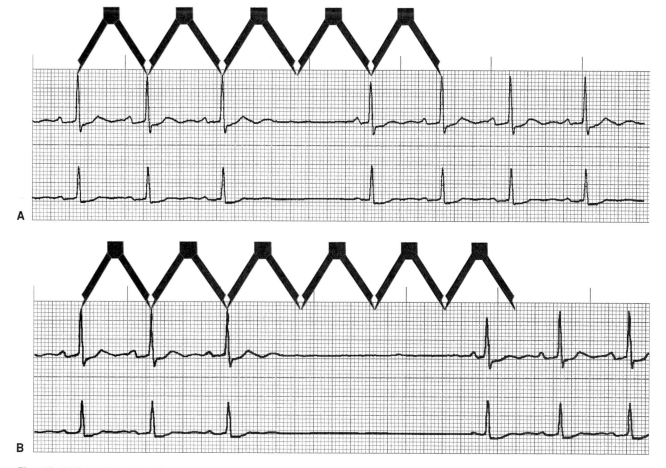

A

B

Fig. 10–14A–B Notice the difference in the timing of the first P-wave after the pause in these two strips. A, Sinus exit block. The calipers march out and the P-wave is in the expected location. B, The calipers do not march out and the P-wave is in a new location.

Table 10-6 Criteria for sinus arrest and sinus exit block

Regularity	Regular except for the pause
Heart Rate	<160 bpm, usually <100 bpm
P-Wave	One per QRS, all the same shape
PR Interval	0.12–0.20 seconds
QRS Complex	All the same shape, <0.12 seconds

an example of sinus exit block. Look at the point where the P-waves return. You can see that the P-wave picks up the beat, continuing exactly where it would have if the signal

hadn't paused. Now look at the second strip, Figure 10–14B, an example of sinus arrest. As you can see, the rhythm doesn't march out–the first QRS after the pause occurs at a different point than it would have if the signal hadn't paused. That happened because the sinus node was reset and then started up again with the timing thrown off.

Pauses tend to occur infrequently, so treatment isn't usually needed. If the pauses become more frequent or the patient develops symptoms *related to the rhythm*, both dysrhythmias are treated like sinus bradycardia. Oxygen therapy can improve oxygen delivery to the malfunctioning sinus node. Intravenous atropine can also be used with pacemaker insertion if necessary.

10-7 A Light Bulb of an Idea

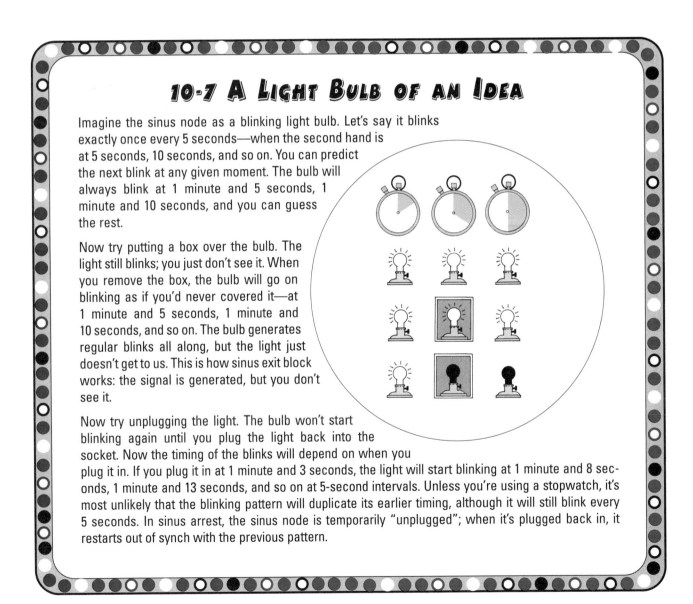

Imagine the sinus node as a blinking light bulb. Let's say it blinks exactly once every 5 seconds—when the second hand is at 5 seconds, 10 seconds, and so on. You can predict the next blink at any given moment. The bulb will always blink at 1 minute and 5 seconds, 1 minute and 10 seconds, and you can guess the rest.

Now try putting a box over the bulb. The light still blinks; you just don't see it. When you remove the box, the bulb will go on blinking as if you'd never covered it—at 1 minute and 5 seconds, 1 minute and 10 seconds, and so on. The bulb generates regular blinks all along, but the light just doesn't get to us. This is how sinus exit block works: the signal is generated, but you don't see it.

Now try unplugging the light. The bulb won't start blinking again until you plug the light back into the socket. Now the timing of the blinks will depend on when you plug it in. If you plug it in at 1 minute and 3 seconds, the light will start blinking at 1 minute and 8 seconds, 1 minute and 13 seconds, and so on at 5-second intervals. Unless you're using a stopwatch, it's most unlikely that the blinking pattern will duplicate its earlier timing, although it will still blink every 5 seconds. In sinus arrest, the sinus node is temporarily "unplugged"; when it's plugged back in, it restarts out of synch with the previous pattern.

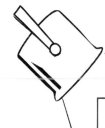

Now You Know

In all types of sinus rhythm, all P-waves are the same shape.

Sinus rhythms differ from each other by heart rate and regularity.

Some sinus rhythms are regular, whereas others are regularly irregular or "regular except."

A sinus rhythm between 60 and 99 bpm is not always normal and can actually warn us that a patient's condition is deteriorating.

Sinus tachycardia is usually between 100 and 160 bpm. The higher figure represents a theoretical limit above which heart rates can quickly harm the patient.

Sinus tachycardia usually is not a primary dysrhythmia but is secondary to some other condition. Treatment of the underlying condition usually corrects the sinus tachycardia.

Sinus arrest occurs when the sinus node stops and restarts.

Sinus exit block occurs when the sinus node discharges normally but doesn't cause a P-wave.

Test Yourself

1. The sinus node has an intrinsic rate of ___ .

2. If the heart rate is less than 60 bpm but otherwise meets the criteria for sinus rhythm, it is called sinus ___ .

3. Sinus tachycardia meets all the criteria for sinus rhythm except the heart rate, which is between ___ and ___ bpm.

4. Name six causes of sinus tachycardia:

    _____   _____

    _____   _____

    _____   _____

5. Fill in the regularity of the following sinus node–generated rhythms:

    Sinus rhythm   _____
    Sinus bradycardia   _____
    Sinus tachycardia   _____
    Sinus arrhythmia   _____
    Sinus exit block   _____
    Sinus arrest   _____

6. What is the effect of atropine on the heart rate?

7. In sinus _____, the P-wave after the pause occurs at the usual interval because the sinus node is not reset.

8. The PR interval for sinus rhythms is between _____ and _____ seconds.

9. Sinus tachycardia usually occurs _____, whereas other tachydysrhythmias usually occur _____.

10. Fill in the information for the following forty rhythm strips, all of which originate in the sinus node:

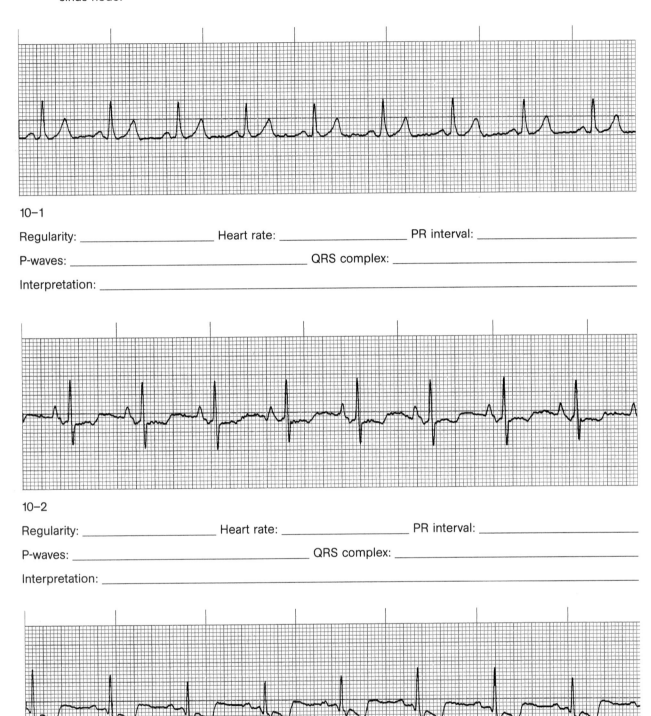

10–1

Regularity: _____ Heart rate: _____ PR interval: _____

P-waves: _____ QRS complex: _____

Interpretation: _____

10–2

Regularity: _____ Heart rate: _____ PR interval: _____

P-waves: _____ QRS complex: _____

Interpretation: _____

10–3

Regularity: _____ Heart rate: _____ PR interval: _____

P-waves: _____ QRS complex: _____

Interpretation: _____

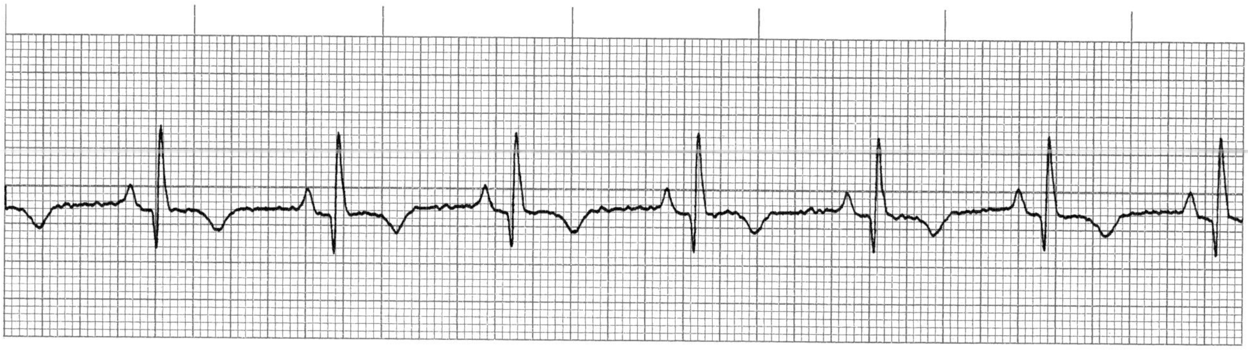

10–4

Regularity: _____ Heart rate: _____ PR interval: _____

P-waves: _____ QRS complex: _____

Interpretation: _____

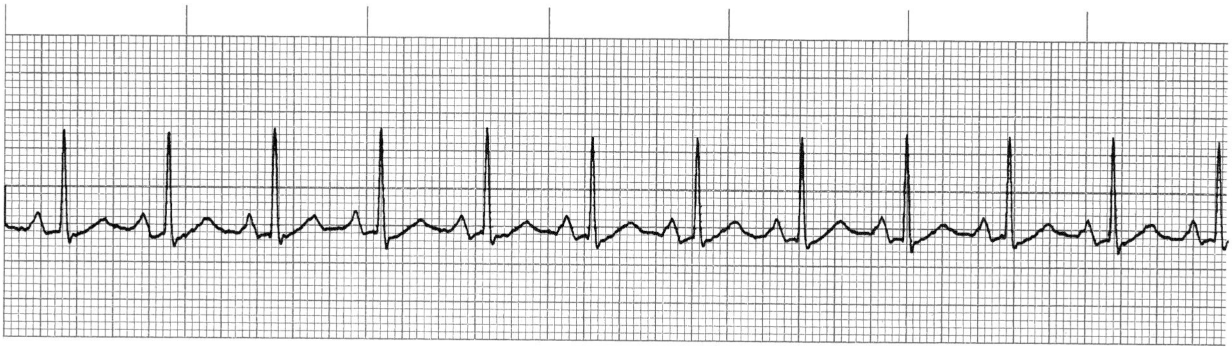

10–5

Regularity: _____ Heart rate: _____ PR interval: _____

P-waves: _____ QRS complex: _____

Interpretation: _____

III

MCL1

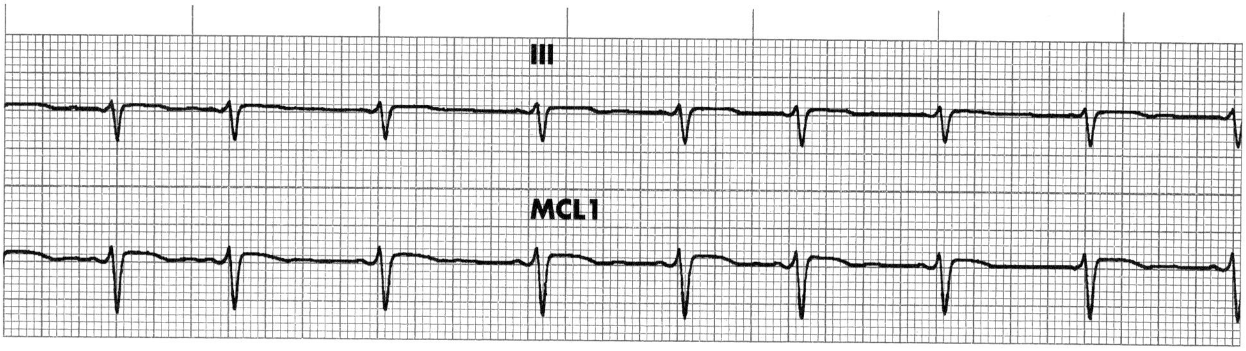

10–6

Regularity: _____ Heart rate: _____ PR interval: _____

P-waves: _____ QRS complex: _____

Interpretation: _____

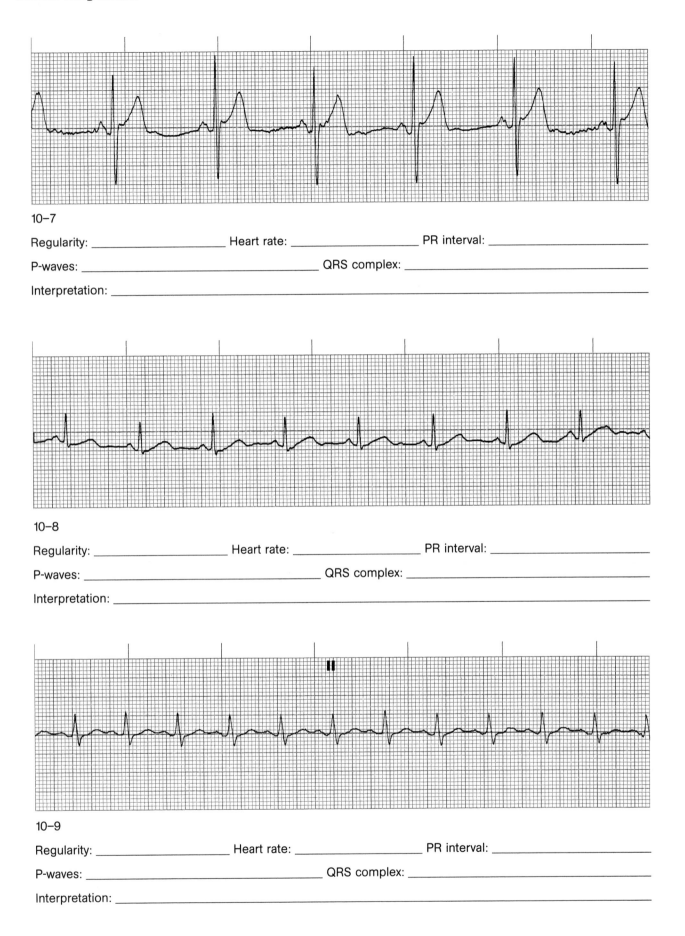

10–7

Regularity: _____ Heart rate: _____ PR interval: _____

P-waves: _____ QRS complex: _____

Interpretation: _____

10–8

Regularity: _____ Heart rate: _____ PR interval: _____

P-waves: _____ QRS complex: _____

Interpretation: _____

10–9

Regularity: _____ Heart rate: _____ PR interval: _____

P-waves: _____ QRS complex: _____

Interpretation: _____

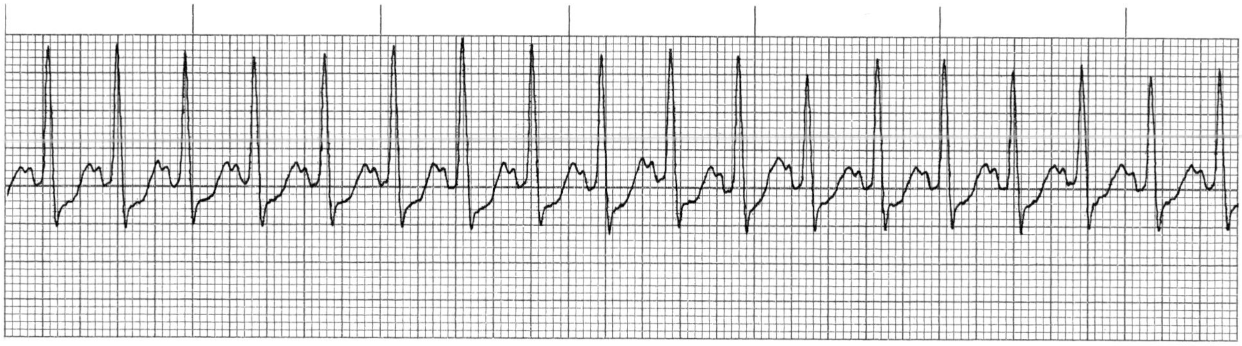

10–10

Regularity: _____ Heart rate: _____ PR interval: _____

P-waves: _____ QRS complex: _____

Interpretation: _____

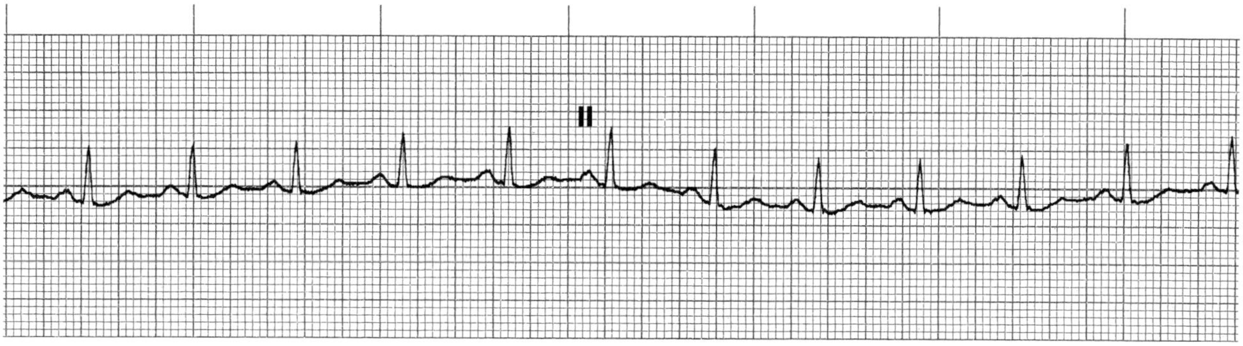

10–11

Regularity: _____ Heart rate: _____ PR interval: _____

P-waves: _____ QRS complex: _____

Interpretation: _____

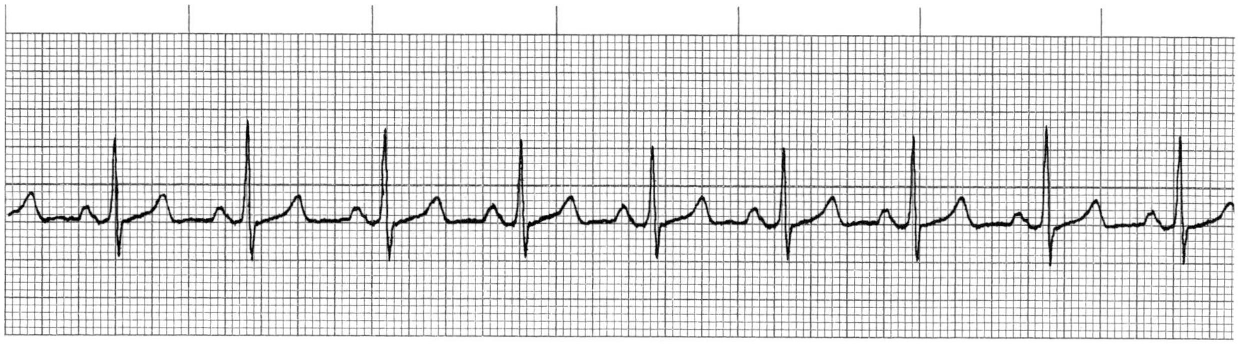

10–12

Regularity: _____ Heart rate: _____ PR interval: _____

P-waves: _____ QRS complex: _____

Interpretation: _____

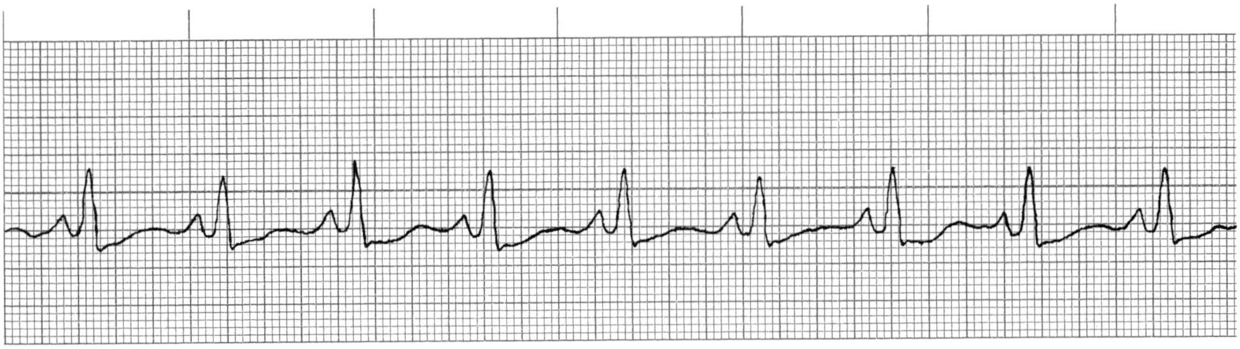

Sinus Rhythms

10–13

Regularity: _____ Heart rate: _____ PR interval: _____

P-waves: _____ QRS complex: _____

Interpretation: _____

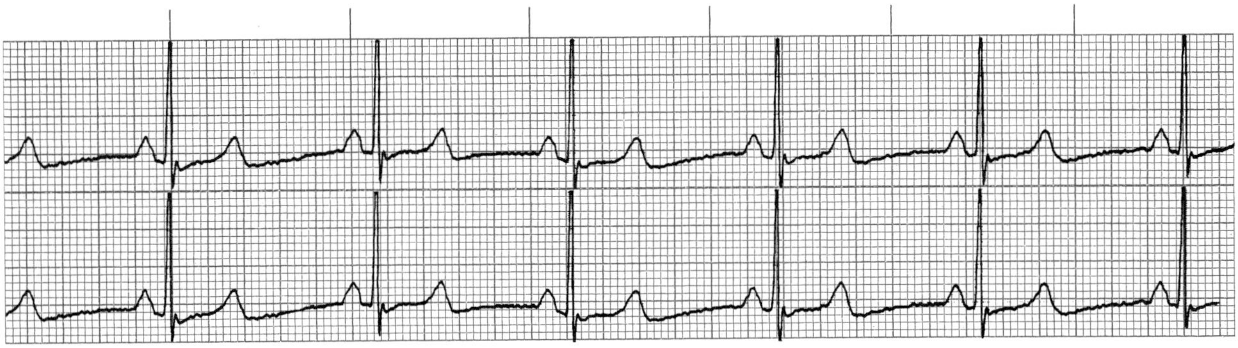

10–14

Regularity: _____ Heart rate: _____ PR interval: _____

P-waves: _____ QRS complex: _____

Interpretation: _____

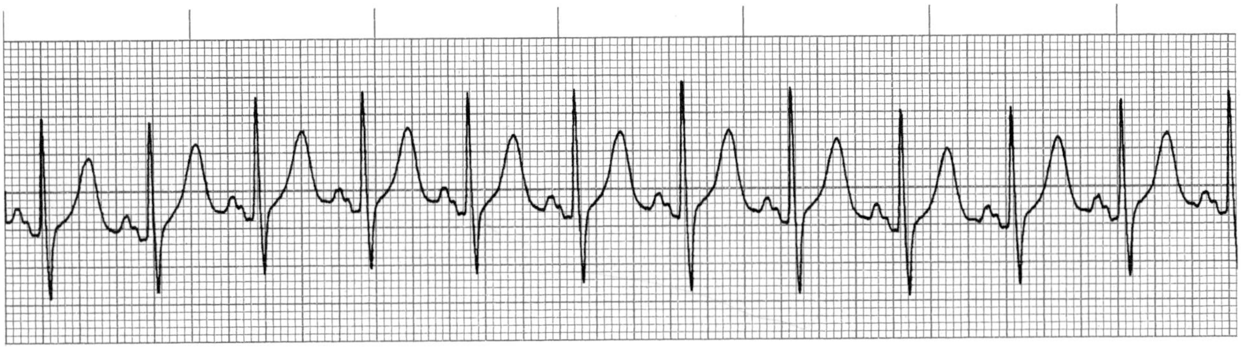

10–15

Regularity: _____ Heart rate: _____ PR interval: _____

P-waves: _____ QRS complex: _____

Interpretation: _____

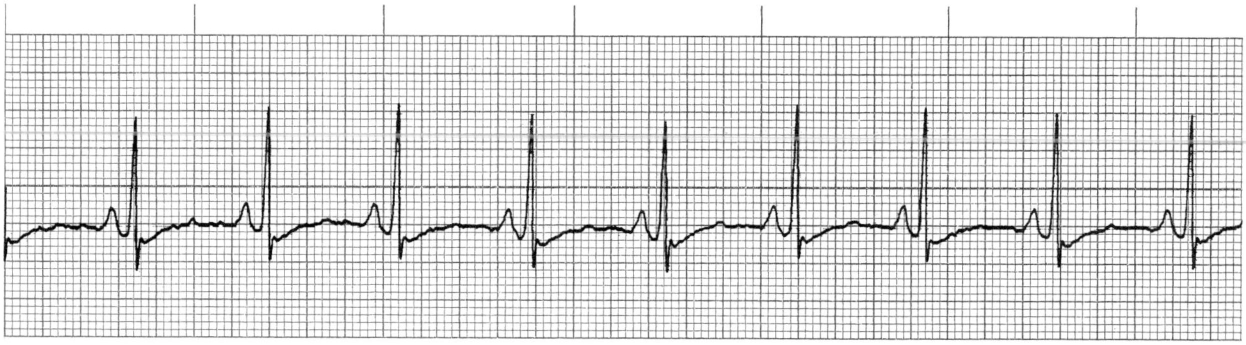

10–16

Regularity: _____ Heart rate: _____ PR interval: _____

P-waves: _____ QRS complex: _____

Interpretation: _____

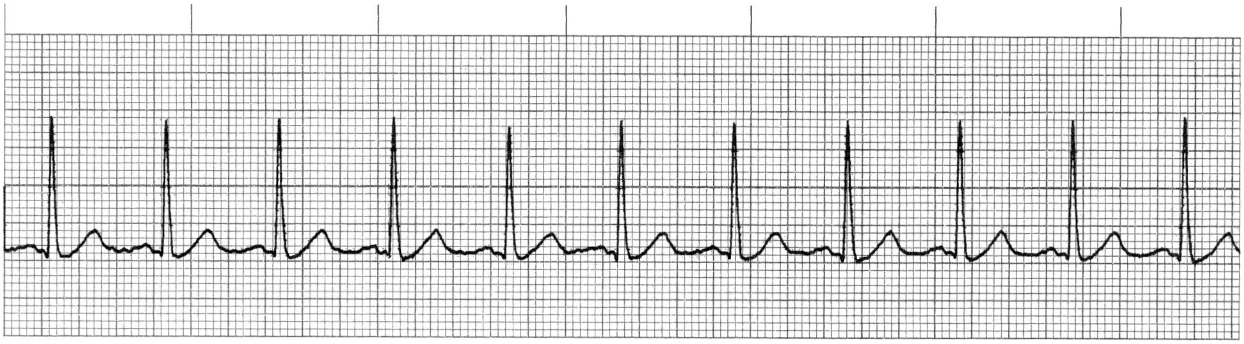

10–17

Regularity: _____ Heart rate: _____ PR interval: _____

P-waves: _____ QRS complex: _____

Interpretation: _____

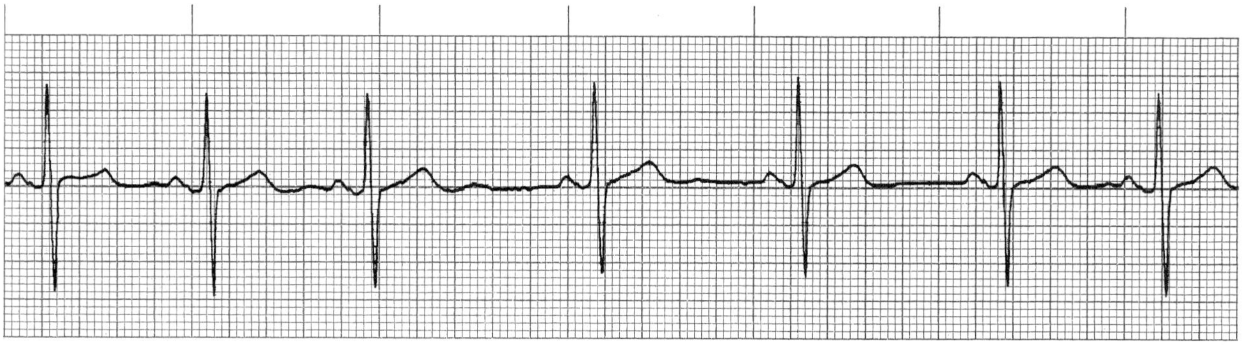

10–18

Regularity: _____ Heart rate: _____ PR interval: _____

P-waves: _____ QRS complex: _____

Interpretation: _____

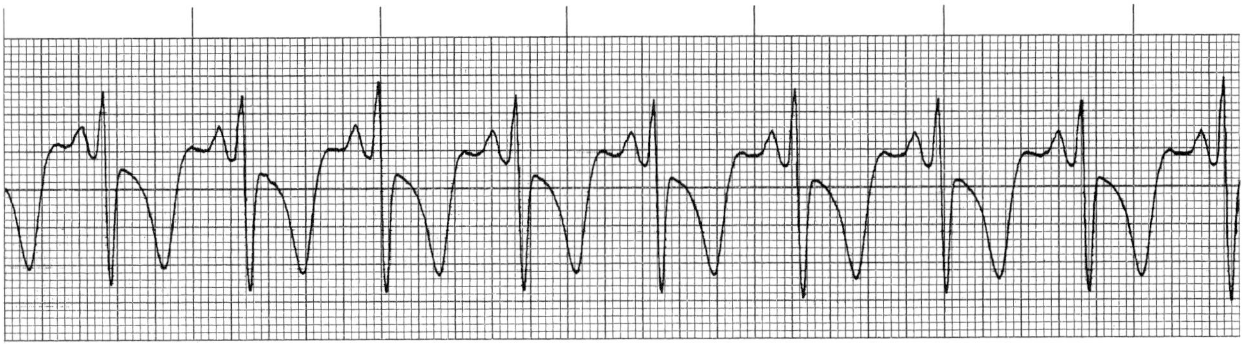

10–19

Regularity: _____ Heart rate: _____ PR interval: _____

P-waves: _____ QRS complex: _____

Interpretation: _____

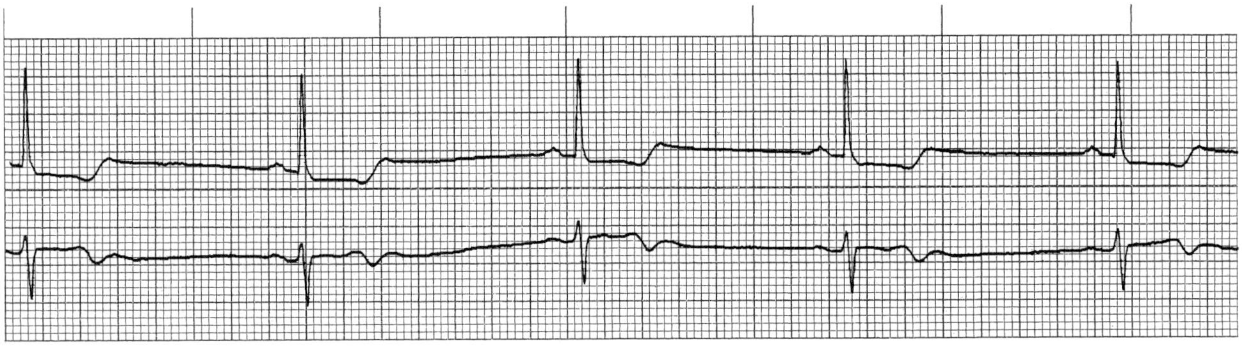

10–20

Regularity: _____ Heart rate: _____ PR interval: _____

P-waves: _____ QRS complex: _____

Interpretation: _____

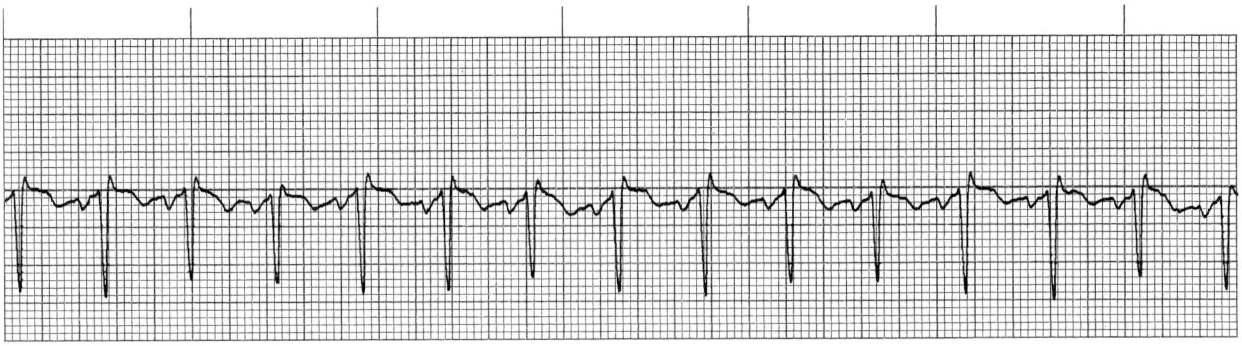

10–21

Regularity: _____ Heart rate: _____ PR interval: _____

P-waves: _____ QRS complex: _____

Interpretation: _____

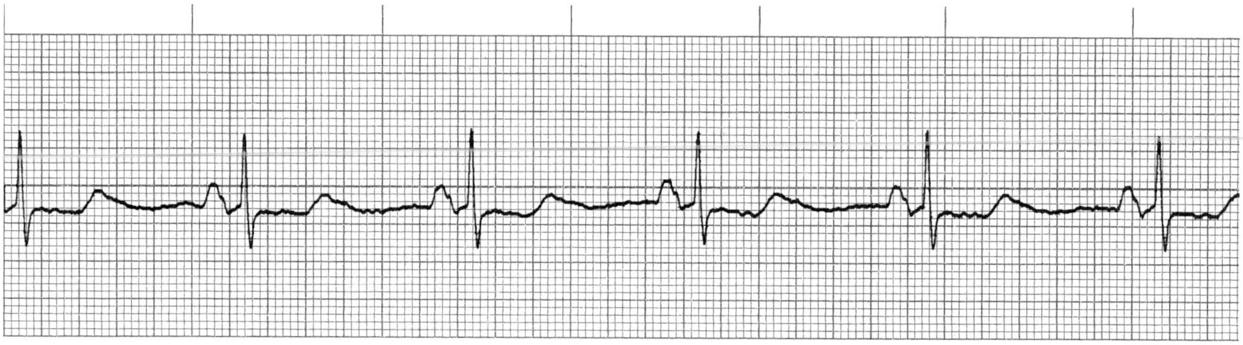

10–22

Regularity: _____ Heart rate: _____ PR interval: _____

P-waves: _____ QRS complex: _____

Interpretation: _____

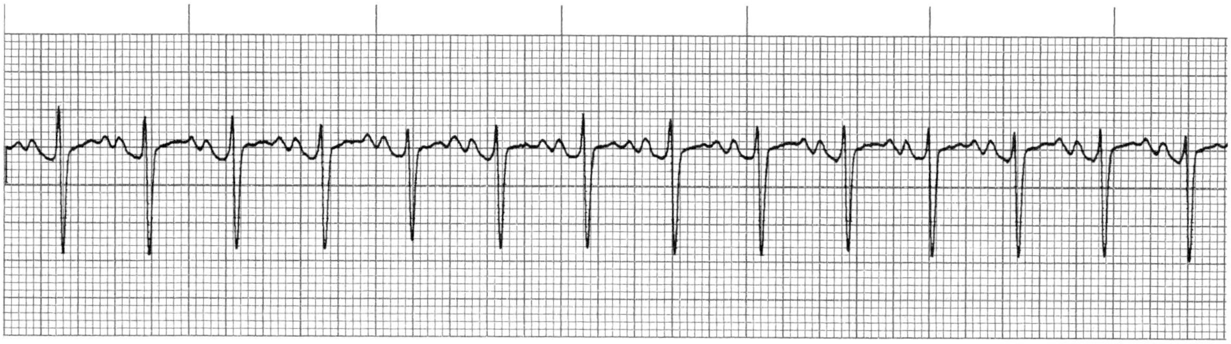

10–23

Regularity: _____ Heart rate: _____ PR interval: _____

P-waves: _____ QRS complex: _____

Interpretation: _____

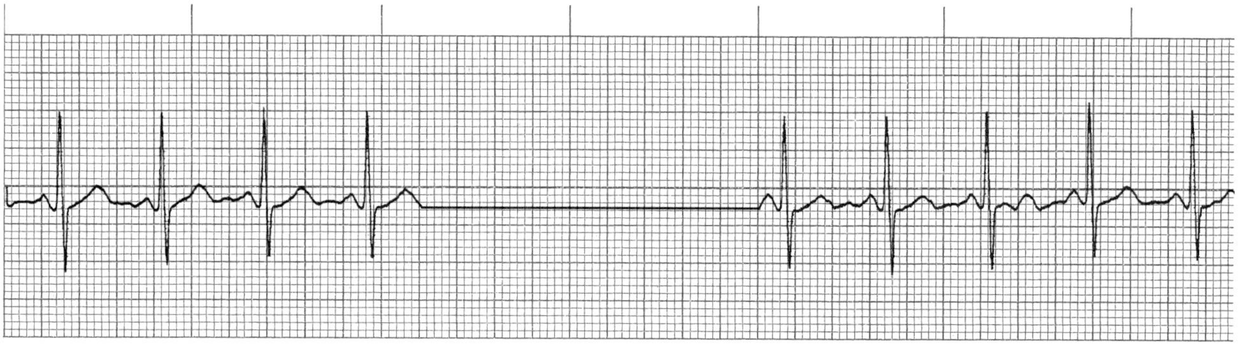

10–24

Regularity: _____ Heart rate: _____ PR interval: _____

P-waves: _____ QRS complex: _____

Interpretation: _____

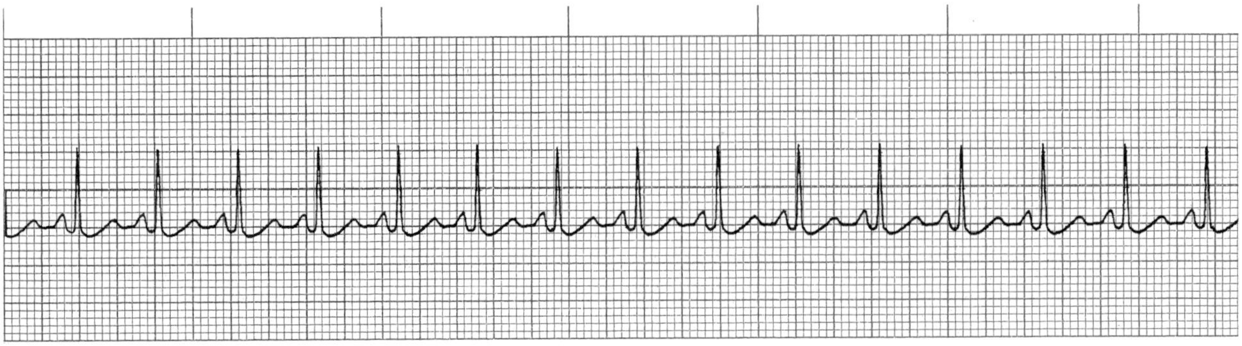

10–25

Regularity: _____ Heart rate: _____ PR interval: _____

P-waves: _____ QRS complex: _____

Interpretation: _____

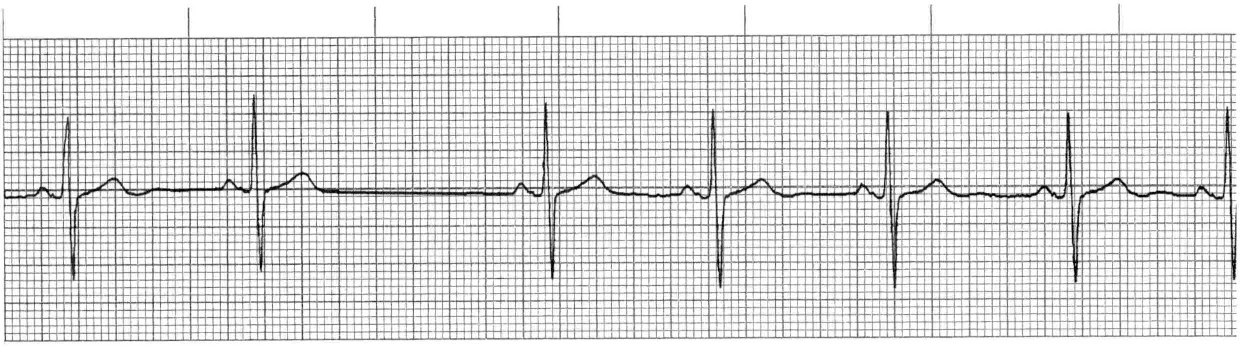

10–26

Regularity: _____ Heart rate: _____ PR interval: _____

P-waves: _____ QRS complex: _____

Interpretation: _____

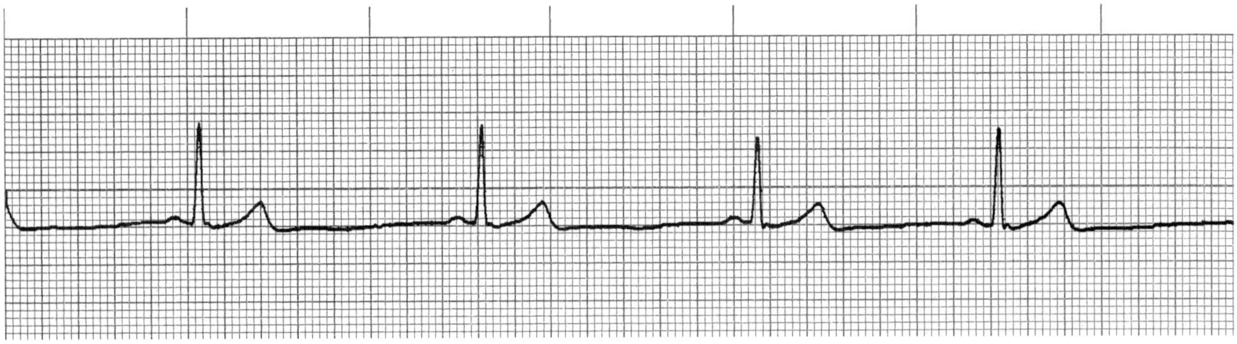

10–27

Regularity: _____ Heart rate: _____ PR interval: _____

P-waves: _____ QRS complex: _____

Interpretation: _____

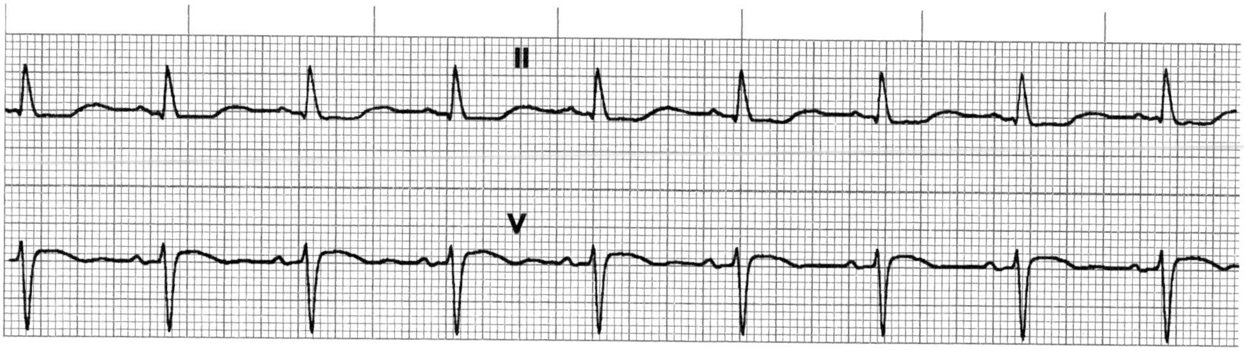

10–28

Regularity: _____ Heart rate: _____ PR interval: _____

P-waves: _____ QRS complex: _____

Interpretation: _____

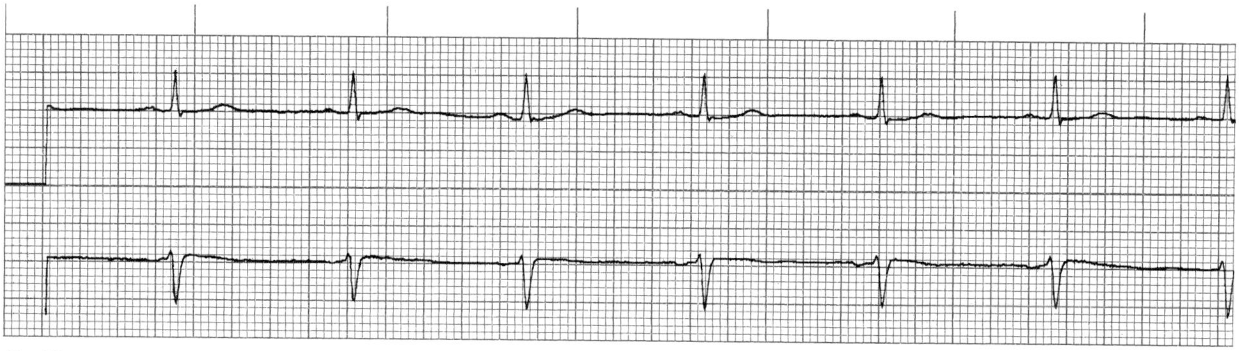

10–29

Regularity: _____ Heart rate: _____ PR interval: _____

P-waves: _____ QRS complex: _____

Interpretation: _____

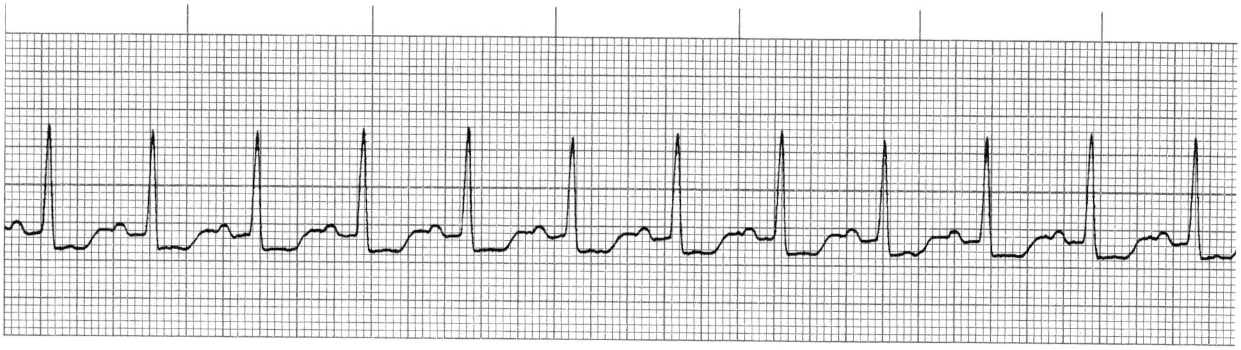

10–30

Regularity: _____ Heart rate: _____ PR interval: _____

P-waves: _____ QRS complex: _____

Interpretation: _____

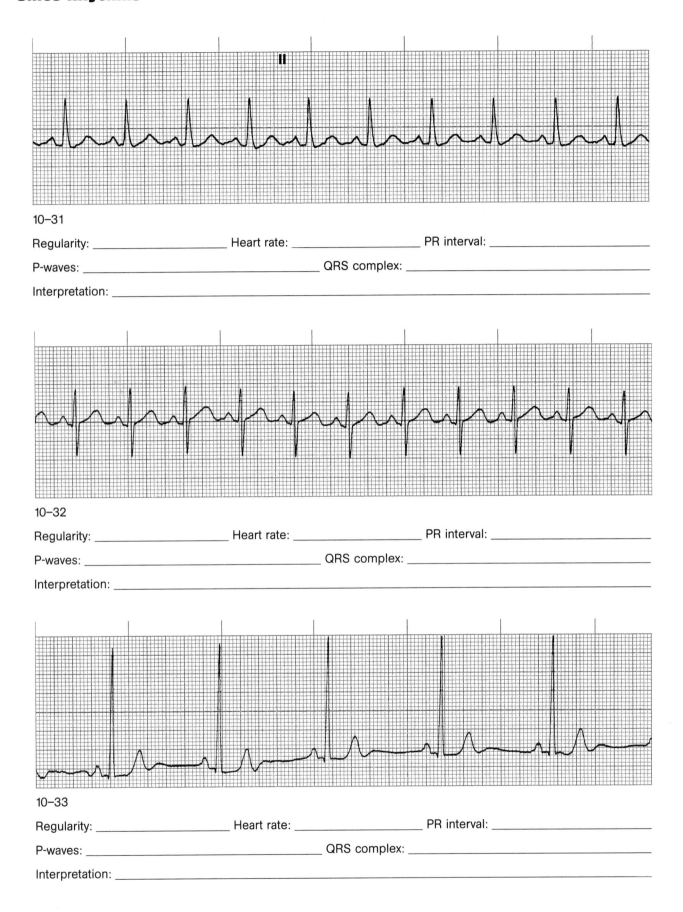

10–31

Regularity: _____ Heart rate: _____ PR interval: _____

P-waves: _____ QRS complex: _____

Interpretation: _____

10–32

Regularity: _____ Heart rate: _____ PR interval: _____

P-waves: _____ QRS complex: _____

Interpretation: _____

10–33

Regularity: _____ Heart rate: _____ PR interval: _____

P-waves: _____ QRS complex: _____

Interpretation: _____

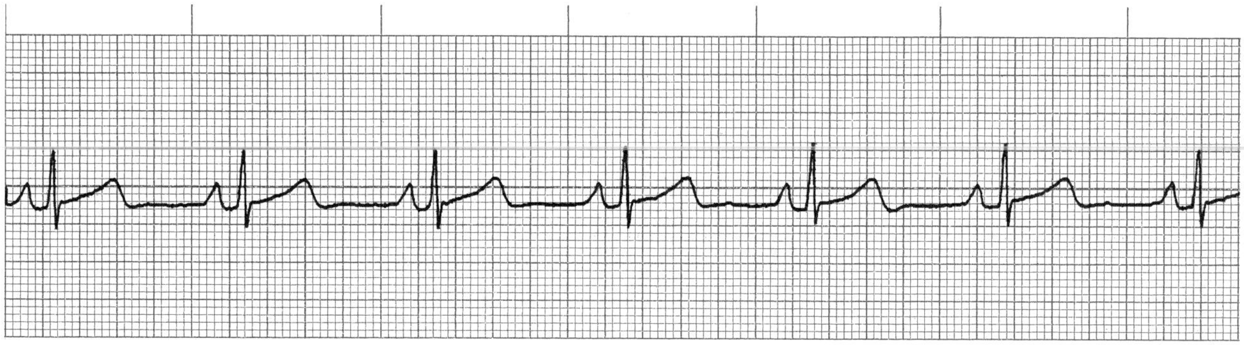

10–34

Regularity: _____ Heart rate: _____ PR interval: _____

P-waves: _____ QRS complex: _____

Interpretation: _____

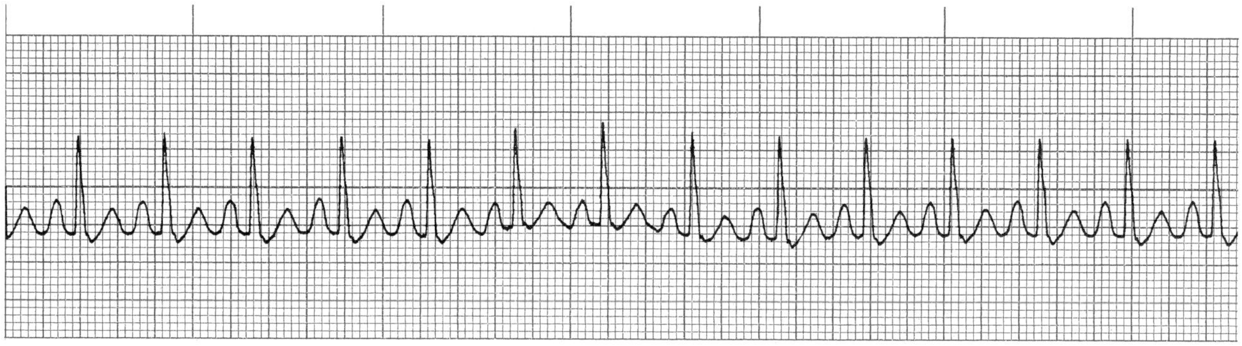

10–35

Regularity: _____ Heart rate: _____ PR interval: _____

P-waves: _____ QRS complex: _____

Interpretation: _____

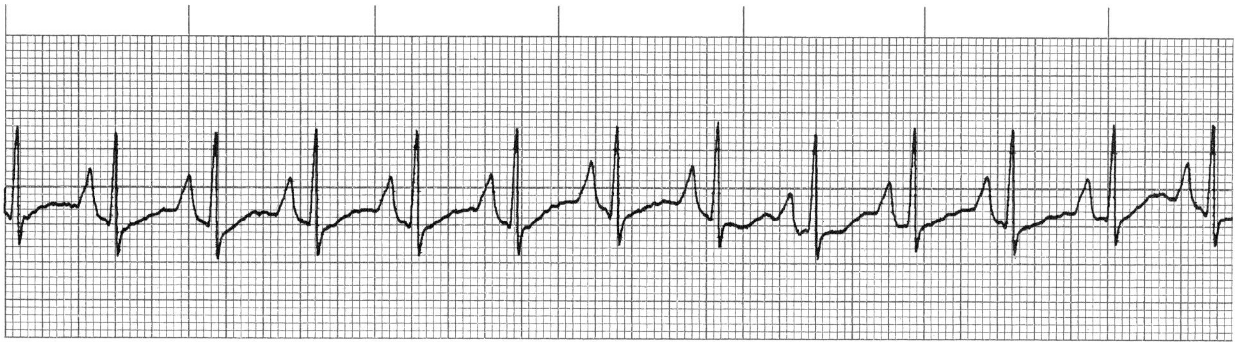

10–36

Regularity: _____ Heart rate: _____ PR interval: _____

P-waves: _____ QRS complex: _____

Interpretation: _____

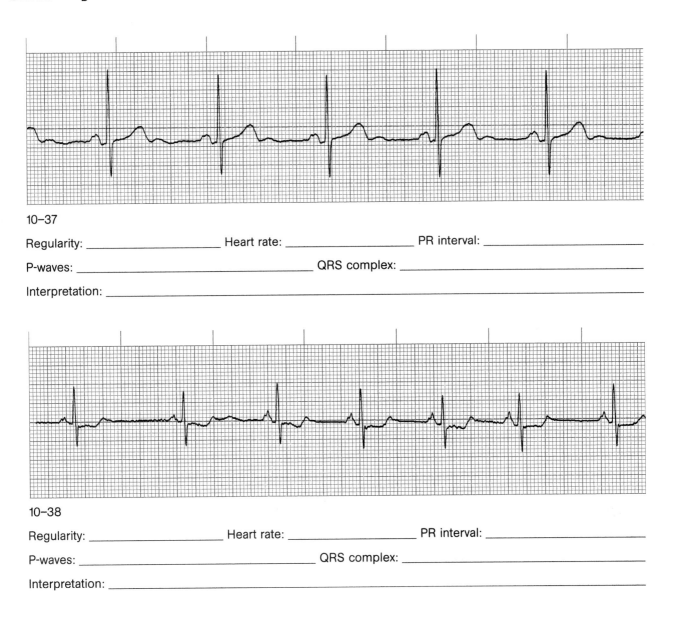

10–37

Regularity: _____ Heart rate: _____ PR interval: _____

P-waves: _____ QRS complex: _____

Interpretation: _____

10–38

Regularity: _____ Heart rate: _____ PR interval: _____

P-waves: _____ QRS complex: _____

Interpretation: _____

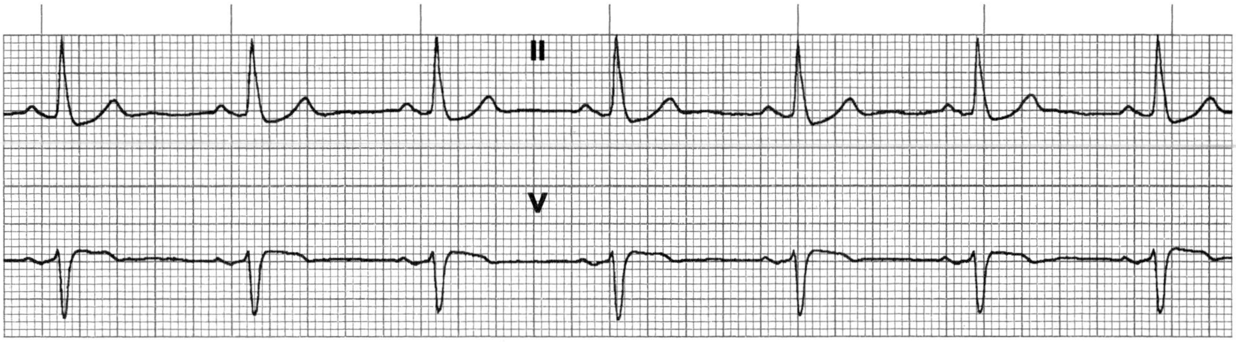

10–39

Regularity: _____ Heart rate: _____ PR interval: _____

P-waves: _____ QRS complex: _____

Interpretation: _____

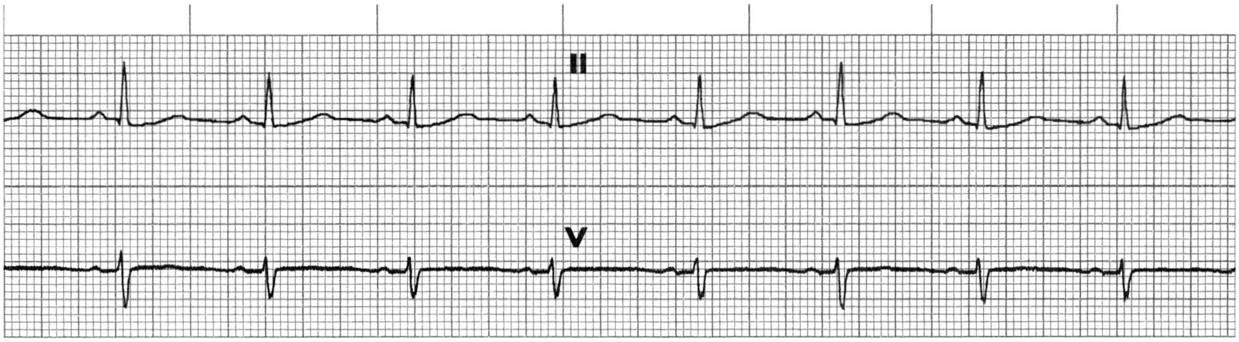

10–40

Regularity: _____ Heart rate: _____ PR interval: _____

P-waves: _____ QRS complex: _____

Interpretation: _____

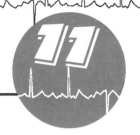

ATRIAL RHYTHMS

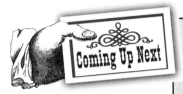

○ Why do the atria sometimes take over the heart's rhythm?

○ Why is atrial fibrillation so dangerous?

○ How does an atrial beat differ from a sinus beat?

○ How do you tell when an atrial pacemaker is wandering?

○ What is meant by slow, controlled, and rapid ventricular response?

○ What two characteristics make atrial fibrillation easy to identify?

○ What medications are given to treat rapid atrial rhythms?

○ What is physiological AV block, and what role does it play in rhythm interpretation?

Atrial Rule: When Leadership Disagrees

In Chapter 8 we crowned the sinus node, declaring it the king of the heart. But don't put unlimited trust in royalty. The sinus node, although reliable, is far from perfect. Normally it leads the heart rhythm, but occasionally the rest of the heart disagrees with its leadership.

Occasionally the sinus node rate falls dangerously low, as in severe sinus bradycardia. In this case, if the atrial tissue takes over at a faster rate, the patient benefits. However, if the sinus node rate provides sufficient cardiac output, an atrial takeover at a faster rate may not be so good. The atria are the revolutionaries of the heart, overturning the existing order to fulfill their own agenda.

Those Irritable Atria

Atrial rhythms are the most common types of dysrhythmia, especially in patients 60 years old or older. Most atrial arrhythmias are benign, but many atrial tachydysrhythmias can be dangerous.

We already know that the sinus node, by convention, can't produce a premature beat, regardless of when it wants to discharge. Atrial beats, however, can be premature. Atrial tissue can discharge before the sinus node,

taking control of the heart's rhythm for one beat. If the atrial tissue continues to discharge faster than the sinus node, it controls the heart for a longer period.

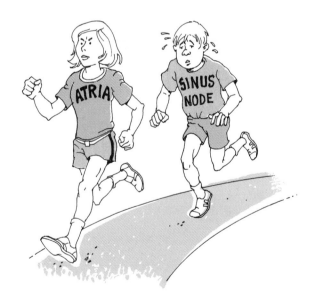

One common reason for the atria to discharge faster than the sinus node is *irritability*, or *increased automaticity*. Remember when we discussed action potentials back in Chapter 2? Each area of the heart has a different action potential curve. That's why the sinus node is the normal pacemaker: because its action potential curve is faster

132

11-1 THE POLITICS OF THE HEART

Let's use the democratic analogy again. The president of the United States doesn't have absolute power but must answer to Congress. If the president vetoes a bill from Congress, that bill can still become law if Congress overrides him. The heart has its own congress, otherwise known as the atrial tissue. If the sinus node doesn't do its job well enough, the atria can step in to take over. Sometimes this is for the best and sometimes it's not.

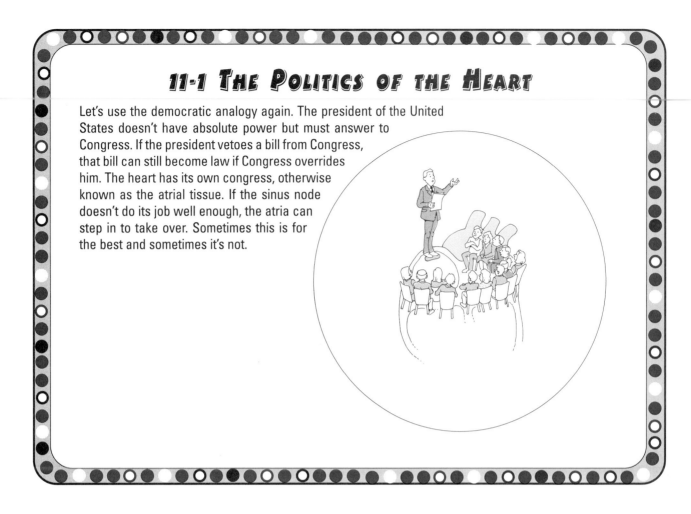

and shorter, the sinus node discharges before the other cells of the heart can reach their particular discharge thresholds.

A PAC Without the Politics

REBELS WITH A CAUSE

When the atrial tissue discharges before the next expected sinus beat, the resulting complex is called a PAC. No, not a political action committee, but a premature atrial complex. It can also be called a premature atrial beat (PAB), atrial premature beat (APB), or atrial premature complex (APC). No matter what you call it, the PAC is lobbying for attention, signaling that at least some of the atrial tissue is irritable and trying to make the heart beat faster.

Even if they're frequent, PACs are generally benign and need no treatment, with certain exceptions. Some PACs occur sporadically, others much more often. Regardless of frequency, the premature beat has replaced a regular sinus beat. Both sinus beats and atrial beats have significant atrial kick. However, because the PAC is premature,

the decreased atrial filling time can produce a modest decrease in cardiac output.

A variety of stimuli can cause PACs. Many of them, including caffeine, tobacco, myocardial ischemia, and hypoxia, can also cause sinus tachycardia. Electrolyte disturbances such as hypokalemia (low potassium) and hypomagnesemia (low magnesium) can easily be investigated. In addition, PACs can result whenever the atrial conduction system is stretched to its limits, as in atrial enlargement from hypertrophy or dilation, or when the atria are stretched abnormally, as in congestive heart failure. Echocardiograms, or in some cases a 12-lead ECG, can indicate dilation or hypertrophy. A diagnosis of congestive heart failure is often based on chest x-ray and clinical presentation as well as laboratory data.

ANATOMY OF A PAC

Where It's Different The key characteristic of a PAC is its P-wave. In sinus beats, all P-waves are shaped identically because they all come from the same place and follow the same path. They also have certain characteristics in particular leads. For instance, sinus P-waves are usually

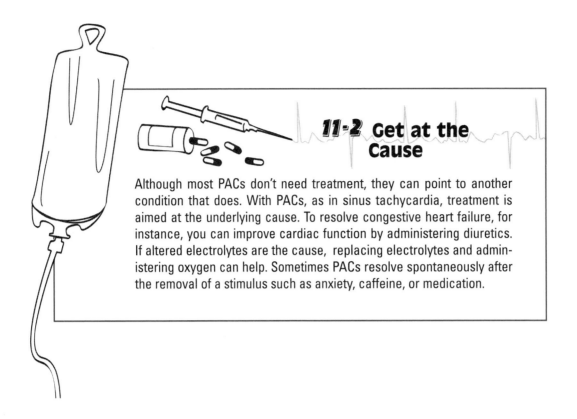

11-2 Get at the Cause

Although most PACs don't need treatment, they can point to another condition that does. With PACs, as in sinus tachycardia, treatment is aimed at the underlying cause. To resolve congestive heart failure, for instance, you can improve cardiac function by administering diuretics. If altered electrolytes are the cause, replacing electrolytes and administering oxygen can help. Sometimes PACs resolve spontaneously after the removal of a stimulus such as anxiety, caffeine, or medication.

upright in leads I, II, and III and in leads V_4, V_5, and V_6. They are inverted in aVR and are frequently inverted or biphasic in V_1.

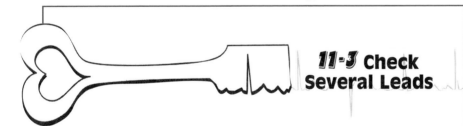

11-3 Check Several Leads

In a PAC, the shape, or morphology, of the P-wave must be different because the wave originates from another location and therefore travels a different path. Remember the morphology discussion in Chapter 9? Two complexes of the same type (P-wave, QRS, or T-wave) can vary for one of two reasons: they start in different places or they follow different paths. The most important thing to do is to check several leads if possible. The atrial P-wave may appear normal in a few leads but abnormal in others. This anomaly can help locate the atrial focus for the P-wave.

In Figure 11–1, you can see that the rhythm is "regular except"; the exceptions are the third and sixth beats. The are PACs. These beats clearly interrupt the regular sinus rhythm, which picks up the rhythm following them. If you analyze the P-wave before the early QRS complexes, you can see that they are tall and pointy, not short and rounded

like all the other P-waves, which originated in the sinus node. That tells us for sure that the distinctive P-wave originated somewhere else.

Where It's Normal In all other aspects, the PAC in Figure 11–1 is identical to the sinus beats (Table 11–1). The PR interval is normal because conduction travels through the AV node as it would in a sinus beat. This aspect of the rhythm is the reason most PACs are benign: a normal PR interval preserves most of the atrial kick. The QRS complexes are normal because conduction travels through the AV node, down the bundle branches, and to the ventricular tissue—the same route as in a sinus beat. Therefore, the amount of blood ejected with each beat (sinus or PAC) is nearly the same, so the cardiac output doesn't suffer. The only difference is the atrial tissue conduction, which changes the shape of the P-wave.

One Focus or Several? Multiple PACs can be either unifocal or multifocal. To differentiate between these two types,

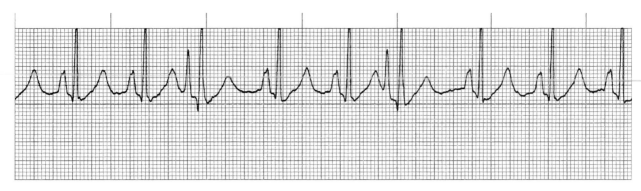

Fig. 11–1 Sinus rhythm with two PACs (the third and sixth beats). The P-wave preceding the PACs is tall, thin, and pointed rather than wide, short, and rounded, indicating that it came from a different location.

Table 11–1 Criteria for premature atrial rhythm

Regularity	Regular except for the premature beats
Heart Rate	Any rate
P-Wave	One per QRS, **different in premature beats**
PR Interval	0.12–0.20 seconds (three to five small boxes)
QRS Complexes	All the same shape, <0.12 seconds (three small boxes)

simply check out their P-waves. Unifocal PACs all have the same morphology because they originate from the same location (one focus) and travel the same path. In multifocal PACs, the premature P-waves will have different morphologies because they start in different places (multiple foci) and therefore travel different paths through the atrial tissue. All other aspects of the rhythm will look the same. This is because the conduction through the AV node and

down the bundle branches is the same for all sinus and atrial foci.

Figure 11–2 shows a rhythm with multifocal PACs. Here the third and sixth beats are early and preceded by two different P-waves that are both different from the other, sinus P-waves in the strip.

Naming the Rhythm If PACs are frequent, they may occur at regular intervals in a specific pattern. In Chapter 8 we encountered bigeminal rhythms. In atrial bigeminy, the rhythm consists of one normal and one abnormal beat in a repeating pattern, as in Figure 11–3A. A trigeminal PAC pattern, shown in Figure 11–3B, consists of two normal beats followed by an abnormal beat, again in a repeating pattern.

Ectopic Atrial Pacemaker

It's difficult, though not impossible, to identify an ectopic atrial pacemaker (EAP) in just one or two leads. In an EAP, a single focus in the atrial tissue discharges at a faster rate than the sinus node. Therefore, because the fastest pacemaker always wins, the atrial focus takes control of the heart. If a patient is admitted to your unit with an EAP,

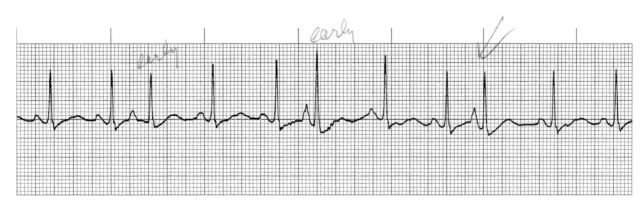

Fig. 11–2 Sinus rhythm with multifocal PACs (third, sixth, and ninth beats). The P-waves associated with the third and sixth beats are different from each other because each PAC originated from a different location.

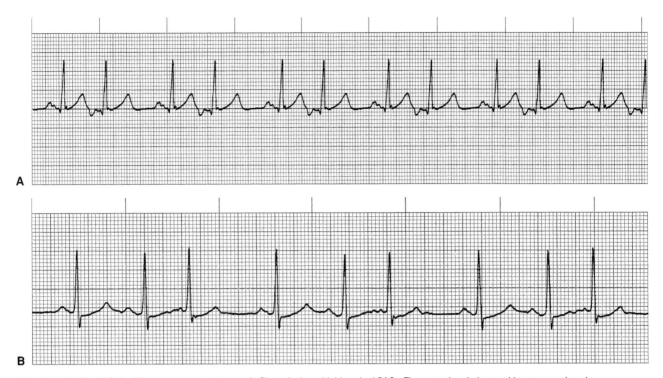

A

B

Fig. 11–3A–B PACs in different recurrent patterns. A, Sinus rhythm with bigeminal PACs. The normal and abnormal beats occur in pairs. B, Sinus rhythm with trigeminal PACs. The normal and abnormal beats occur in groups of three.

you can easily mistake it for sinus rhythm, particularly if the ectopic focus is close to the sinus node. Again, the key is the P-wave.

When the atrial focus is far from the sinus node, recognition becomes easier. This is because the P-wave doesn't look like a sinus P-wave (Table 11–2). Its appearance depends on both the lead and the location in which the P-wave originated. It's important to check as many leads as possible because some leads may show similar P-waves.

Suppose the focus is at the base of the right atrium. To depolarize the right atrium, the signal must travel backward toward the sinus node, moving from the bottom to

the top of the atrium. This path causes an inverted P-wave in leads II and III (see Fig. 11–3A). The P-wave in the PACs is not inverted in Figure 11–3B but is shaped differently from the beats originating in the sinus node. Remember, differently shaped waveforms originate in different locations or follow different paths. The PR interval is normal because of the normal signal delay at the AV node.

Occasionally, if the sinus rate and the atrial ectopic rate are very close, the patient may switch between sinus rhythm and EAP. You can tell when the transition occurs because the P-wave suddenly changes shape.

Figure 11–4 shows an example of EAP. Although the P-wave is upright in lead II. Therefore the rhythm can't be a sinus rhythm because the P-wave changes shape in the middle of the strip, indicating that the P-wave starting point changed.

An ectopic atrial pacemaker rarely causes problems and often is not treated.

Atrial Tachycardia

AT HIGH SPEED

Atrial tachycardia is an uncommon tachydysrhythmia responsible for fewer than 10% of tachycardias with *narrow*

Table 11–2 Criteria for ectopic atrial pacemaker

Regularity	Always regular
Heart Rate	≤99 bpm (usually 60–99 bpm)
P-Wave	One per QRS, all P-waves the same shape and **different from sinus P-waves**
PR Interval	0.12–0.20 seconds (three to five small boxes)
QRS Complexes	All the same shape, <0.12 seconds (three small boxes)

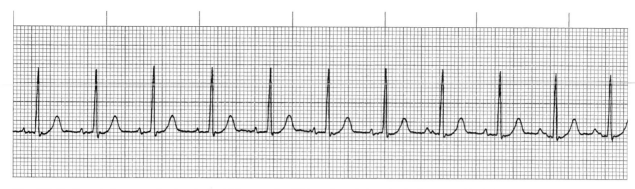

Fig. 11–4 Sinus rhythm converting to ectopic atrial pacemaker. Midway through the strip, the P-wave suddenly changes shape, but the rate changes little or not at all. The sinus node and the atrial tissue are discharging at nearly identical rates. When the sinus node slows or the atrial tissue speeds up, even by a small amount, a different pacemaker takes control.

QRS complexes (the term used to describe QRS complexes of normal duration). It's a frequent cause of accelerated heart rates in patients with digoxin toxicity or digoxin levels significantly above the normal therapeutic range. Like sinus tachycardia, atrial tachycardia has P-waves and narrow QRS complexes. However, there are significant differences.

Although atrial tachycardia can have a rate as low as 100 bpm, it usually exceeds 130 and can go as high as 180. Because atrial tachycardia is relatively rare, most rhythms below 160 (the arbitrarily chosen maximum rate discussed in Chapter 10) are considered sinus tachycardia unless specific evidence to the contrary exists. Such evidence is usually related to the P-wave. Rhythms faster than 160 are usually interpreted as atrial tachycardia if they meet the criteria listed in Table 11–3.

Atrial tachycardia is often distinguished from sinus tachycardia by the shape of the P-waves in certain leads, especially if the atrial focus is far from the sinus node as discussed in the section on PACs. The specific P-wave characteristics depend on the location of the atrial starting point in relation to the lead (Fig. 11–5).

Table 11–3 Criteria for atrial tachycardia

Regularity	Always regular
Heart Rate	100–180 bpm (usually >160 bpm)
P-Wave	One per QRS, all the same shape, **different from sinus P-waves in some or all leads**
PR Interval	0.12–0.20 seconds (three to five small boxes)
QRS Complexes	All the same shape, <0.12 seconds (three small boxes)

Wandering Atrial Pacemaker
PLAYING THE SHELL GAME

Wandering atrial pacemaker (WAP) behaves like an ectopic atrial pacemaker, with one important exception. Instead of having only one atrial focus, the pacemaker site travels, or "wanders," around the atrial tissue. Sometimes the pacemaker actually locates itself in the sinus node (remember, the sinus node is in the right atrium). The pacemaker doesn't stay in one place for long, though; it prefers to pull up stakes and move to different locations throughout the atrial tissue. This rhythm is also referred to as chaotic atrial pacemaker.

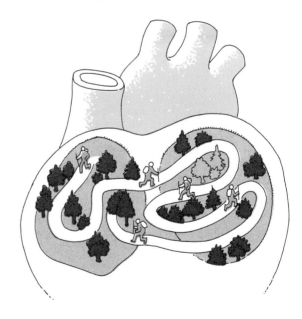

The key to identifying this rhythm is again the P-wave, described in Table 11–4. Its morphology changes as the pacemaker moves to different parts of the atrial tissue. The PR interval and QRS complex are normal because only the atrial conduction is affected, although it can vary slightly from beat to beat.

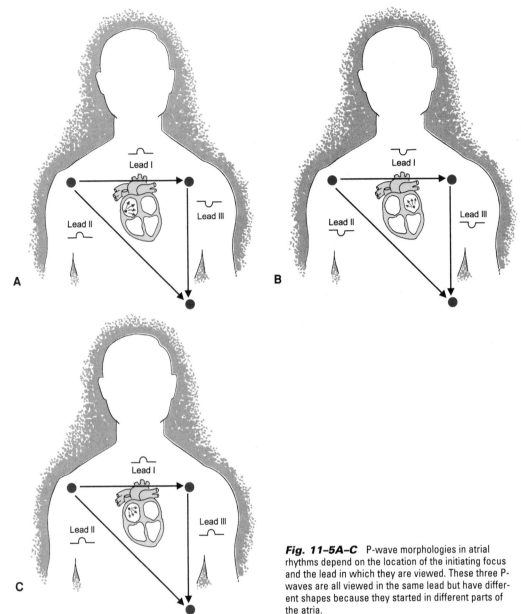

Fig. 11–5A–C P-wave morphologies in atrial rhythms depend on the location of the initiating focus and the lead in which they are viewed. These three P-waves are all viewed in the same lead but have different shapes because they started in different parts of the atria.

A wandering atrial pacemaker rhythm rarely causes problems and is usually not treated. If it is, treatment usually consists of oxygen to reduce irritability and IV fluids to increase blood pressure. If the patient does have symptoms, they're often caused not by the rhythm but by a concomitant medical condition.

READ BETWEEN THE P-WAVES

With WAP, you'll always find at least three different P-wave morphologies on one 6-second strip (see Table 11–4). Be careful, though—this rhythm can look regular to the

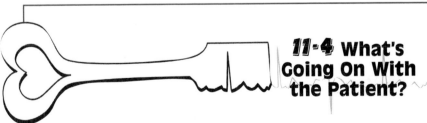

11-4 What's Going On With the Patient?

The symptoms of atrial tachycardia can include (besides a fast heart rate) syncope, nausea, and hypotension. Often they reflect pre-existing cardiac problems. They also show the effects of an increased ventricular rate, with correspondingly shorter filling times, on cardiac output. Be aware that sinus tachycardia causes the same symptoms.

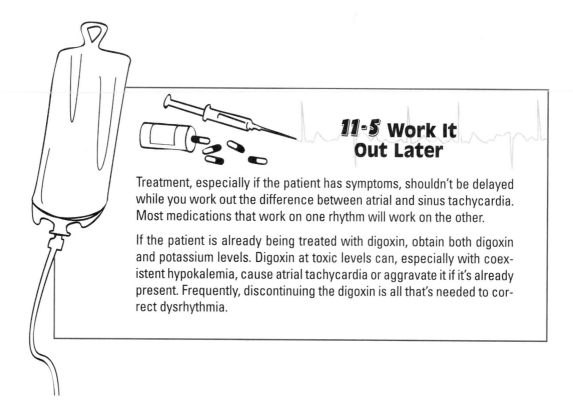

11-5 Work It Out Later

Treatment, especially if the patient has symptoms, shouldn't be delayed while you work out the difference between atrial and sinus tachycardia. Most medications that work on one rhythm will work on the other.

If the patient is already being treated with digoxin, obtain both digoxin and potassium levels. Digoxin at toxic levels can, especially with coexistent hypokalemia, cause atrial tachycardia or aggravate it if it's already present. Frequently, discontinuing the digoxin is all that's needed to correct dysrhythmia.

Table 11–4   Criteria for wandering atrial pacemaker

Regularity	Always irregular, usually only slightly irregular
Heart Rate	≤99 bpm (usually 60–99 bpm)
P-Wave	One per QRS, **at least three different P-wave shapes in one strip**
PR Interval	0.12–0.20 seconds (three to five small boxes)
QRS Complexes	All the same shape, <0.12 seconds (three small boxes)

naked eye, and it can take actual measurement to pick out the sometimes slight irregularities. Because the signals are generated by different foci, they won't be as regular as a signal from a single focus.

In Figure 11–6, the P-waves preceding the first four QRS complexes are dramatically different from each other. The first P-wave is tiny (if present at all), the second is biphasic, the third is "double humped," and the fourth is a small single hump. The heart rate for this rhythm goes as high as 99 bpm, after which the rhythm becomes a tachycardia like all other rhythms. We'll deal with that in the next section.

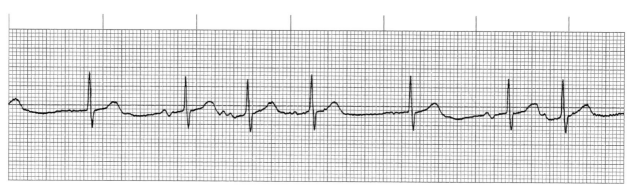

Fig. 11–6   Wandering atrial pacemaker. The P-waves change shape almost continually. This rhythm can be grossly irregular, but commonly it is nearly regular.

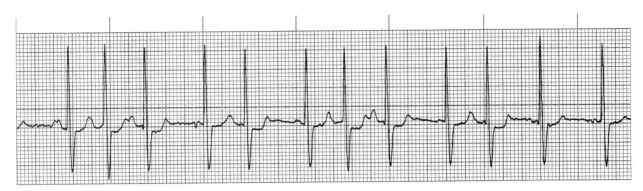

Fig. 11–7 In MAT, the P-waves may be difficult to identify because of the rapid heart rate. This rhythm is simply WAP with a heart rate >100 bpm.

Multifocal Atrial Tachycardia

Multifocal atrial tachycardia (MAT) is essentially a revved-up wandering atrial pacemaker. As the name implies, the focus of the tachycardia moves around the atrial tissue. This rhythm is dangerous. Because it's caused by several irritable foci, not just one, it can deteriorate to more serious dysrhythmias, such as atrial fibrillation.

With multifocal atrial tachycardia, you may find either occasional short runs of sinus tachycardia with multifocal PACs or a changed focus with every beat. Either way, the characteristic feature, as with WAP, is the presence of at least three different P-wave morphologies on a 6-second strip. Usually MAT is more grossly irregular; the higher rate makes it easier to recognize subtle rate differences.

Table 11–5 Criteria for multifocal atrial tachycardia

Regularity	Always irregular
Heart Rate	≥100 bpm
P-Wave	One per QRS, **at least three different P-wave shapes in one strip**
PR Interval	0.12–0.20 seconds (three to five small boxes)
QRS Complexes	All the same shape, <0.12 seconds (three small boxes)

Figure 11–7 shows an example of the different P-wave morphologies in MAT.

As with a wandering atrial pacemaker, the PR interval and QRS complex are normal (Table 11–5). The rate

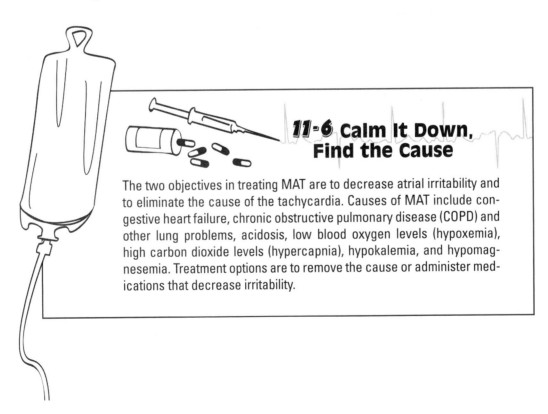

11-6 Calm It Down, Find the Cause

The two objectives in treating MAT are to decrease atrial irritability and to eliminate the cause of the tachycardia. Causes of MAT include congestive heart failure, chronic obstructive pulmonary disease (COPD) and other lung problems, acidosis, low blood oxygen levels (hypoxemia), high carbon dioxide levels (hypercapnia), hypokalemia, and hypomagnesemia. Treatment options are to remove the cause or administer medications that decrease irritability.

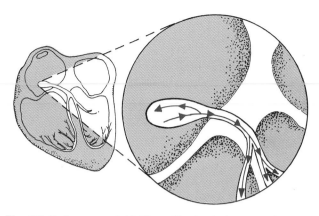

Fig. 11–8 One cause of atrial flutter. The signal takes two paths through the AV node: one to the ventricles to form the QRS complex and one back to the atria to form the next P-wave (F-wave in this rhythm).

must reach 100 bpm or more to meet the criteria for tachycardia.

Atrial Flutter

AT HIGHER SPEED

If one focus in the atrial tissue becomes highly irritable, it can discharge at the phenomenal rate of 250 to 350 bpm. (In rare cases, the atria can discharge more than 400 times per minute.) This type of dysrhythmia is called atrial flutter.

If it's not caused by increased irritability, atrial flutter can reflect an abnormal signal path. The atrial signal may travel to the AV node and split in half (Fig. 11–8). One half travels down the bundle branches to the ventricles, producing the QRS complex; the other half travels a circular path back up to the starting point in the atrium. This type of atrial flutter can have a higher rate than a single

irritable focus, traveling normally through the AV node, would produce.

In atrial flutter, the atrial and ventricular rates are almost never the same. Any idea why? That's right, because of the AV node. Remember how the delay in AV node conduction acts as a gatekeeper, or tollbooth? Some of the atrial impulses arrive at the AV node only to find that it's *refractory,* or unable to conduct an impulse. When this occurs you get a P-wave without a QRS complex. This is called a *physiological AV block* because the AV node is blocking some of the signals from reaching the ventricles. In atrial flutter, this is a protective mechanism, not a problem with the AV node itself. If the ventricles contracted with each of the 300 or so atrial impulses, they would have no time to fill and cardiac output would drop precipitously.

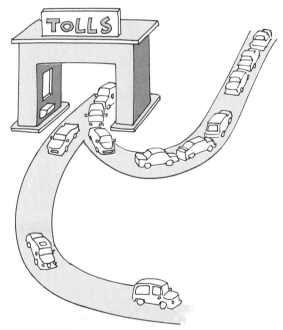

WHAT ARE THE VENTRICLES UP TO?

How Will the Patient Respond?
In atrial flutter, even though the P-waves are regular, the QRS complexes can be regular or irregular. This depends solely on the AV node. If it lets every third atrial impulse through, the resulting rhythm will be regular. If it sometimes lets every third atrial impulse through and sometimes every fourth or fifth, the resulting rhythm will be irregular.

The key to predicting the patient's clinical response to this rhythm is the

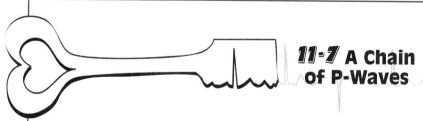

11-7 A Chain of P-Waves

In atrial flutter, the P-waves never stop coming. Because the rate is so rapid, one P-wave starts as the previous one ends. A rate of 300 bpm (the middle of the range) produces five P-waves every second, or one P-wave per large box! Because all the P-waves come from the same focus and travel the same path, they all look identical. However, they come so fast that they can overlap other parts of the PQRSTU complexes. Therefore, they can appear distorted when they show up in the QRS complex or the T-wave.

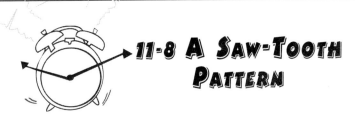

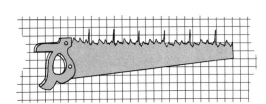

11-8 A SAW-TOOTH PATTERN

The defining characteristics of atrial flutter are the saw-tooth pattern of identical P-waves and the presence of more than one P-wave for each QRS complex (because of the protective AV block). When the P-waves form this saw-tooth pattern, they are called *flutter waves,* or *F-waves,* to distinguish them from normally generated P-waves. Table 11–6 lists the characteristics of atrial flutter.

underlying ventricular rate—how many times the ventricles contract per minute. Symptoms appear when the wrong number of atrial signals—either too few or too many—cause ventricular contractions. If enough atrial signals reach the ventricles and cause them to contract, the patient may not even know there's a problem. In any event, atrial kick is somewhat compromised by the multiple atrial contractions occurring each time the ventricles contract.

Tolerance of this rhythm is determined by two things: how much atrial kick is lost and how often the ventricles respond to the rapid succession of atrial impulses. The AV node, acting as gatekeeper, blocks some of the signals because they arrive before the AV node has repolarized. The AV block is usually expressed as a ratio, such as 3:1 or 4:1.

More Math

To determine the AV block ratio in regular rhythms, divide the atrial rate by the ventricular rate. For instance, if the ventricular rate is 75 bpm and the atrial rate is 300 bpm, the AV node is conducting one out of every four (300/75) atrial impulses. We call this atrial flutter with 4:1 AV conduction block (four atrial beats for every one beat transmitted to the ventricles). If the rhythm is irregular, it's imperative to give a rate range using the small-box method discussed in Chapter 3. Figure 11–9 shows a regular rhythm with 4:1 AV node conduction block.

In Figure 11–10, the irregular rhythm is described as variable AV conduction block; the lowest and highest rates would be recorded for these strips.

Table 11–6 Criteria for atrial flutter

Regularity	Regular or irregular, determined by AV conduction
Heart Rate	**Atrial rate 250–350 bpm,** any ventricular rate
P-Waves (F-waves)	All the same shape but can be distorted by T-wave or QRS
PR Interval	**Not measurable**
QRS Complexes	All the same shape, <0.12 seconds (three small boxes)

A PAC With a Block

A DIFFERENT P-WAVE

Now that we're on the subject of physiological AV block, let's take a look at blocked PACs. Sometimes, when PACs occur very early, the AV node is still refractory. The result, just as in atrial flutter, is a P-wave without a QRS complex. The term "blocked PAC" doesn't describe a rhythm; it's a rhythm modifier, a concept we encountered in Chapter 8.

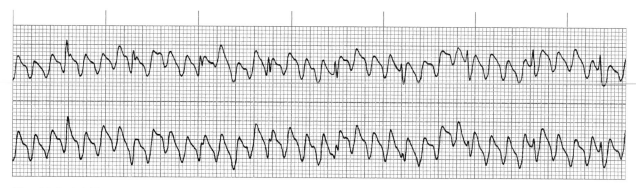

Fig. 11–9 Atrial flutter with a 4:1 AV block: every QRS complex has four F-waves. The presence of the QRS and T-wave make it difficult to count the F-waves. In a regular rhythm, dividing the atrial rate by the ventricular rate determines the conduction ratio.

One criterion for a blocked PAC is the same as for a normal PAC—a differently shaped P-wave that occurs unexpectedly early—but with a variation. In a blocked PAC, there's no normal-looking QRS complex after the offending P-wave. Figure 11–11 shows examples of rhythms with blocked PACs. In Figure 11–11A, the P-wave after the fifth and ninth QRS complexes occurs early, is shaped differently from all the other P-waves on the strip, and is not followed by a QRS. In Figure 11–11B, the blocked PACs come after each of the first three QRSs.

PLAYING DETECTIVE

Though they can look the same on first glance, don't confuse blocked PACs with sinus arrest or sinus exit block. You won't mix them up if the P-wave for the blocked PAC is clearly visible. However, when the P-wave from the PAC occurs in the preceding T-wave, identification can get tricky. Here are a few hints to help you in your quest:

First, blocked PACs are much more common than sinus arrest or sinus exit block. Second, checking different leads can show more clearly the relative sizes and shapes of the T-wave and the P-waves from the blocked PACs. Finally, if in doubt, get a 12-lead ECG. The detailed information from the multiple leads can add a lot of information to your analysis. If you take some time and do what's necessary to investigate, the P-waves from blocked PACs will usually reveal themselves.

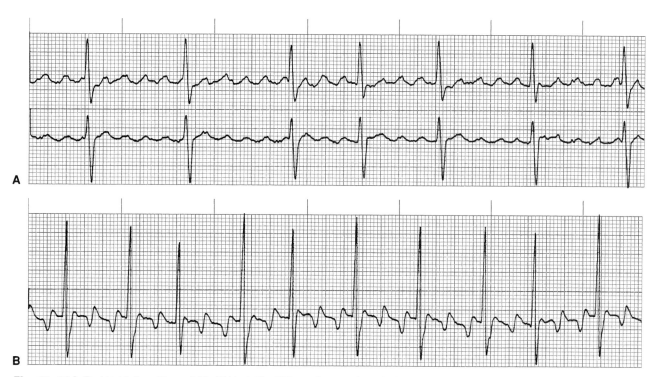

Fig. 11–10A–B Atrial flutter with a variable AV block. The QRS complexes are irregular because the AV node receives a varying number of F-waves before transmitting one to the ventricles.

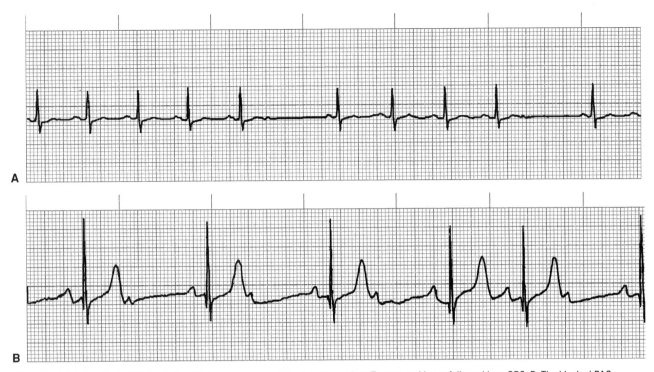

Fig. 11–11A–B Blocked PACs. A, The fifth P-wave is early, distorting the previous T-wave, and is not followed by a QRS. B, The blocked PAC occurs after every QRS; the rhythm has bigeminal blocked PACs then changes to trigominal blocked PACs.

Look back at the sinus arrest and sinus exit block strips in Chapter 10 (Figs. 10–12 and 10–13). You'll see that all the T-waves are the same shape. Compare those strips with the two in Figure 11–12. In the blocked PACs, there's a difference in the shape of the T-waves just before the pause, subtle though that difference may be. Aha—a sure sign of a buried P-wave! In contrast, the T-waves preceding the pause in sinus arrest and sinus exit block aren't deformed at all. Remember, the T-wave can change shape for only two reasons: repolarization started in a different location or the wave followed a different path. So, if the QRS complexes are the same shape, the correlating T-waves should be also.

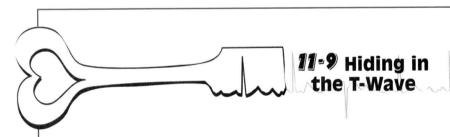

11-9 Hiding in the T-Wave

It's not always easy to identify the P-wave for a blocked PAC. Sometimes the P-wave comes so early that it buries itself in the preceding T-wave. The T-wave changes shape, but the QRS complex doesn't. This is the key to uncovering the early P-wave of the blocked PAC.

The T-wave shape depends solely on the shape of the QRS complex. There are things, such as hypoxemia, that can change T-waves without changing QRS complexes, but all T-waves should change, not just a few. Therefore, if two beats on a strip have identical QRSs, the T-waves should also be the same. If the two T-waves don't look alike, we need to find another reason, such as a buried P-wave. Look at the two strips in Figure 11–12. In both strips, the T-wave just before the pause is different in shape and size from the other T-waves. In Figure 11–12A, it's taller; in Figure 11–12B, it's notched. The culprit in both cases—a buried P-wave from a blocked PAC!

Atrial Fibrillation

THE FASTEST OF ALL

Atrial fibrillation (A-fib) is one of the most common dysrhythmias (Table 11–7). It's often found in patients with chronic lung disorders, such as emphysema or COPD, and in patients with numerous cardiac disorders, including previous heart attacks or heart valve disease. In atrial fibrillation, for the first time, we find a rhythm in which some of the cardiac muscle is depolarized but doesn't contract—the

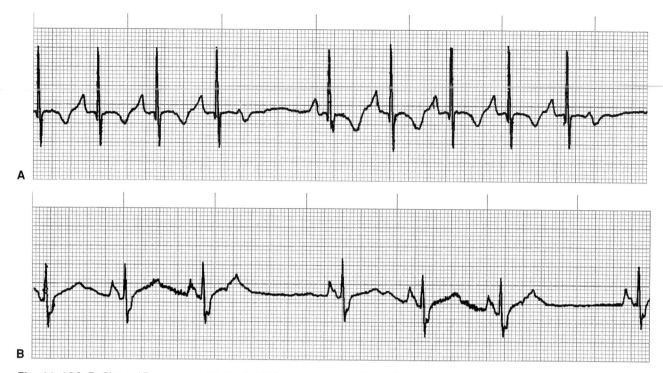

Fig. 11–12A–B Distorted T-waves caused by blocked PACs. In both strips, the T-wave just before the pause is different in morphology from the other T-waves. A, The T-wave before each pause (fourth and ninth QRSs) has an upward deflection not present in the other T-waves. B, The P-wave makes a point in the otherwise rounded T-waves after the second and fifth QRSs.

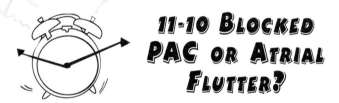

11-10 BLOCKED PAC OR ATRIAL FLUTTER?

Atrial depolarizations without corresponding ventricular depolarizations show up as P-waves (F-waves) without QRS complexes. They have the same cause in blocked PACs and atrial flutter: a P-wave arrives before the AV node is ready. In blocked PACs you'll find an occasional early P-wave from irritable tissue; in atrial flutter, the atria discharge in a rapid, repeating pattern, producing continuous "early" P-waves. You can look for two features to help you distinguish atrial flutter from a blocked PAC. First, in atrial flutter, the P-waves are *always* regular, but in rhythms with blocked PACs, the P-waves are *never* regular, because the PACs P-waves are, by definition, premature. Second, the atrial rates are different. In atrial flutter, the P-waves (F-waves) occur at a rate of 250 to 350 per minute. In a rhythm with blocked PACs, the atrial rate is usually much lower.

Table 11–7 Criteria for atrial fibrillation

Regularity	Irregularly irregular
Heart Rate	Ventricular any rate, **atrial rate >350 bpm, frequently not measurable**
P-Wave	**Wavy baseline,** P-waves rarely or never visible
PR Interval	Not measurable
QRS Complexes	All the same shape, <0.12 seconds (three small boxes)

atrial tissue simply quivers, or *fibrillates.* Many foci are firing simultaneously or one right after another, competing for control of the heart and throwing the atria into chaos.

The atria discharge at least 350 times per minute and sometimes as many as 600 or more. At that speed they can't contract and empty into the ventricles, and so the heart loses atrial kick despite the extremely rapid atrial rate. The cardiac output then drops to as little as 70% of the output in sinus rhythm.

WHERE'S THE QRS COMPLEX?

Atrial fibrillation creates hundreds of partial P-waves. You can't see most of them, and the ones you can see are hard to identify. They're much smaller than normal because just a tiny portion of the atrial tissue can depolarize before the resulting P-wave runs into tissue that's already depolarized from a different P-wave. Because fibrillation occurs at such a phenomenal rate, you can sometimes find 10 or more incomplete P-waves per second. These P-waves, as a group, are known as *fibrillatory waves,* or *f-waves;* don't confuse them with flutter waves, or F-waves. (The upper- and lower-case Fs indicate the relative sizes of the waves they describe and the amount of atrial tissue each depolarizes.)

Figure 11–13 shows two examples of atrial fibrillation. Notice the large number of "mini–P-waves" between QRS complexes, clearly visible in 11–13A, but nearly invisible in 11–13B.

Because the P-waves interfere with each other, many never make it to the AV node and therefore don't generate a QRS complex. The atria are in electrical chaos. As a result, when the P-waves do get through to cause a QRS

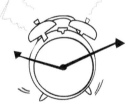

11-11 ATRIAL MISSILES

Atrial fibrillation is potentially dangerous because clots can develop within the heart. Blood clots have their uses—they create the scab that forms over a healing cut—but they don't belong in the heart.

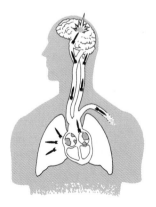

Blood that isn't moving tends to coagulate. Because the atria don't contract and empty regularly, blood clots can form there. Occasionally, when a partial or a rare full contraction occurs (particularly after the rhythm converts to a sinus rhythm), some pieces break off the clotted blood. Once dislodged from their atrial home, they become disabling projectiles capable of causing pulmonary emboli or strokes.

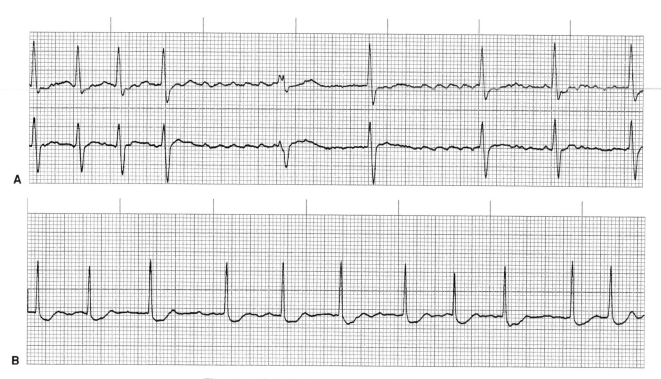

Fig. 11–13A–B Typical examples of atrial fibrillation.

complex, we don't find a pattern as we do in atrial flutter and the ventricular response is irregularly irregular. The QRSs don't follow a cyclical pattern as in sinus dysrhythmia or show any other kind of pattern, such as trigeminal PACs. Their occurrence is truly random, depending on the readiness of the AV node when the atrial impulses get there.

Figure 11–14 shows the random nature of the QRS complexes in two extreme examples of atrial fibrillation. Notice the significant irregularity in Figure 11–14A. In Figure 11–14B, the long pause (greater than 2 seconds) is bracketed by two narrowly spaced QRSs on either side. Such extreme irregularity can compromise cardiac output and cause symptoms such as dizziness, nausea, or loss of consciousness.

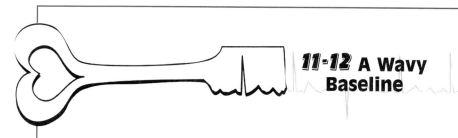

11-12 A Wavy Baseline

With all this chaos, you might think atrial fibrillation is hard to identify. However, the opposite is true. This rhythm is relatively easy to identify because the fibrillatory waves form a characteristic wavy baseline and the rhythm is irregularly irregular. As a matter of fact, no other rhythm has these two characteristics: a wavy baseline with no identifiable P-waves and irregularly irregular QRS complexes.

Therefore, given these two conditions, we presume that the rhythm is atrial fibrillation unless we can prove otherwise. Some conditions, such as artifacts (coming up in Chapter 17), can mimic the wavy baseline, but the rhythm may be regular or regularly irregular. Figures 11–11 through 11–13 show these characteristics in different patients.

ANOTHER RESPONSE FROM THE VENTRICLES

Just as we discussed the average, lowest, and highest heart rates for atrial flutter, we must do so for atrial fibrillation (Table 11–7). In this dysrhythmia, the *ventricular response rate* is usually included in the rhythm identification. Ventricular response is classified as slow, controlled, or rapid (uncontrolled). These rates correspond roughly to the normal ranges for sinus rhythm.

A slow ventricular rate is less than 60 bpm, sometimes less than 50 if the patient is taking digoxin or another medication intended to slow the heart rate (Fig. 11–15A). A controlled rate

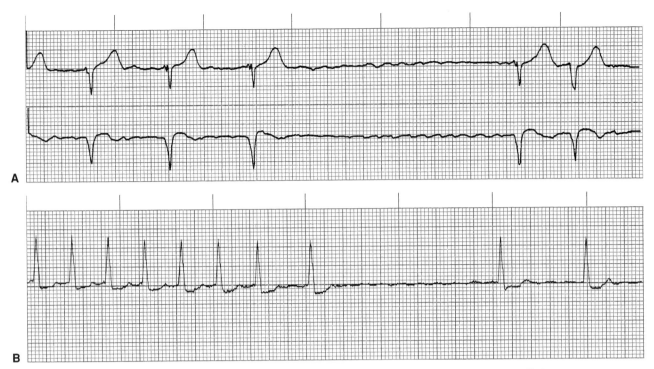

Fig. 11-14A-B These two strips demonstrate the randomness of the AV node conduction in atrial fibrillation.

usually falls between 60 and 100, although some clinicians believe that a controlled rate can reach 120 to compensate for lost atrial kick (Fig. 11–15B).

If the rate exceeds the upper limit, the rhythm is considered a tachycardia, but in atrial fibrillation it's called *rapid ventricular response* (RVR) (Fig. 11–15C). This modifier is the one most used in practice. The reason is simple. In atrial fibrillation, the atria are always discharging at a tachycardic rate; therefore, even when the ventricular response is slow or reasonable, the rhythm is still a tachycardia of sorts. However, because the ventricular rate determines the impact of the rhythm on the patient, we skip the tachycardia moniker in favor of RVR. If no rate modifier is noted, a controlled ventricular response is implied.

Ventricular response categories are based on the average heart rate and reflect how well the atrial fibrillation is meeting the needs of the heart and body. If the rate is too fast, there's an increased risk for adverse cardiac effects such as myocardial ischemia or hypotension. A rate that's too slow, combined with a low stroke volume from loss of atrial kick, can lower cardiac output dangerously. However, a heart rate in the normal range, with an adequate blood pressure, means that the body has compensated enough for the loss of atrial kick to maintain sufficient cardiac output within that range. At a normal rate, the AV node is doing its job, letting the right number of atrial signals through to the ventricles.

TREATING ATRIAL FIBRILLATION IN DEPTH

Anticoagulation Most cases of atrial fibrillation are treated first with anticoagulants. Heparin is a first-line drug because it acts quickly and the effect is easy to test. Also, thanks to a wealth of research, we can adjust the dosages to achieve a therapeutic level quickly and safely. It is important to monitor the patient's response to heparin using the partial thromboplastin time (PTT) and maintain the anticoagulation effect in a narrow range. The exact range depends on the lab, the hospital protocol, the physician's preference, and the patient's response to a given level.

After the patient's condition is stabilized on heparin, warfarin is often substituted. Warfarin must be taken orally, and its half life is long enough for once-a-day dosing. You can monitor the therapy by checking the prothrombin time (PT). The PT will tell you how long the patient's blood takes to clot. Prothrombin time results depend on the reagents the lab uses in testing. Therefore, the international normalization ratio (INR), which converts each lab's PT values to a universally accepted scale, is the usual standard for therapeutic range.

Chemical Cardioversion Once the patient has achieved anticoagulation for a sufficient period (which depends on cardiac history, length of time in atrial fibrillation, and other

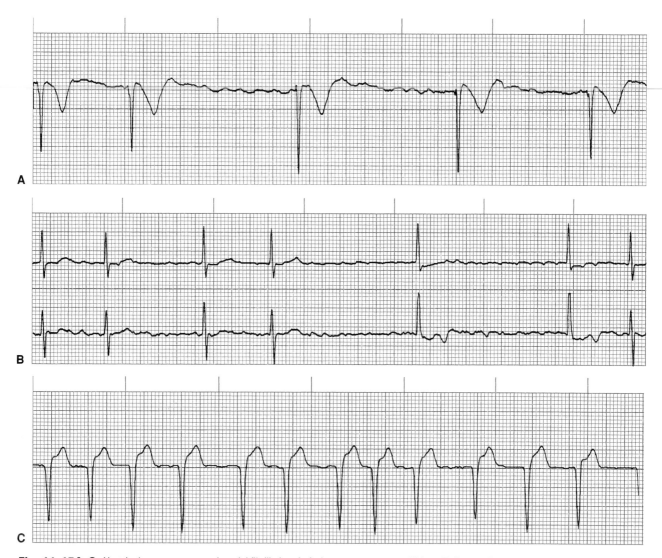

Fig. 11–15A–C Ventricular response rates in atrial fibrillation. A, A slow response rate, <60 bpm. B, A controlled rate, usually 60–100 bpm. C, Rapid ventricular response, considered tachycardic.

factors), you can safely attempt *cardioversion.* That's not as drastic as it sounds, but it is important. Cardioversion is the restoration of a normal sinus rhythm, and it can be done either chemically or electrically. Medications used for chemical cardioversion include, amiodarone, ibutilide, and quinidine. Certain other medications control A-fib but don't produce cardioversion; these include digoxin, calcium channel blockers such as diltiazem or verapamil, and beta blockers such as metoprolol. They can used for patients with chronic A-fib, the kind you get with COPD.

Electrical Cardioversion If chemical cardioversion doesn't work, or if the patient has serious signs or symptoms of inadequate cardiac output (severe hypotension, syncope, chest pain, shortness of breath, change in level of consciousness), try electrical cardioversion right away. Conscious patients should be given oxygen immediately, followed by a sedative if the patient's condition permits.

Synchronized electrical cardioversion begins with lower energy levels than defibrillation and progresses gradually to higher levels. We'll explore cardioversion more thoroughly in Chapter 18.

Final Notes

In practice, you may hear a term—fib/flutter—which is supposed to mean that the rhythm is a combination of atrial fibrillation and atrial flutter. If you think about it, this cannot be. Atrial flutter comes from one atrial focus and atrial fibrillation comes from multiple atrial foci. So, you either have one focus or multiple foci, never both.

If you have a wavy base line and a *regular* rhythm it may be atrial fibrillation in the atria, but it means the AV node is not functional. Atrial fibrillation by itself can *never* be regular.

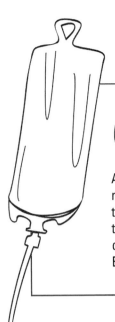

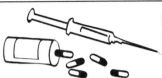

11-13 A Two-step Process?

Atrial fibrillation needs more complicated treatment than any other rhythm we've discussed. The approach depends on the length of time the dysrhythmia has been going on and whether the cause is reversible; the ventricular rate is also a factor. Anticoagulation is the treatment of choice, followed by chemical cardioversion if fibrillation continues. Electrical cardioversion is the next step if drugs don't help.

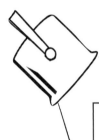

Now You Know

When atrial tissue becomes irritable, it can take over the heart rhythm by discharging at a faster rate than the sinus node.

On the ECG tracing, atrial rhythms differ from sinus rhythms in their P-wave morphology.

Unlike sinus beats, atrial beats can be premature.

Atrial fibrillation is easily identifiable by its irregularly irregular rhythm and wavy baseline.

Rapid atrial fibrillation may be converted by quinidine, procainamide, ibutilide, or amiodarone.

Some cases of chronic A-fib can't be converted, and the rate should be controlled with calcium channel blockers, beta blockers, or digoxin.

Anticoagulants are frequently administered to patients in A-fib because blood clots can form from blood stasis.

Wandering atrial pacemaker and multifocal atrial tachycardia have at least three different P-waves in a 6-second strip.

"Slow," "controlled," and "rapid" are the terms used to describe ventricular response in A-fib.

The AV node helps to control the ventricular response to A-fib and atrial flutter.

Test Yourself

1. _____ has a wavy baseline and an irregularly irregular R to R pattern.

2. Atrial rhythms differ from sinus rhythms in the shape of the _____.

3. In atrial flutter, an irritable atrial focus can discharge from _____ to _____ times per minute.

4. To compute the AV block in atrial flutter, divide the _____ rate by the _____ rate.

5. _____ occurs when a single irritable atrial focus discharges faster than the sinus node.

6. _____, _____, _____, and digoxin are used to control the heart rate in atrial fibrillation.

7. Quinidine, amiodarone are used to convert _____ to _____.

8. _____ has at least three differently shaped _____.

9. _____ toxicity, especially with coexistent _____, can cause atrial tachycardia.

10. Identify the atrial rhythm in the following forty strips:

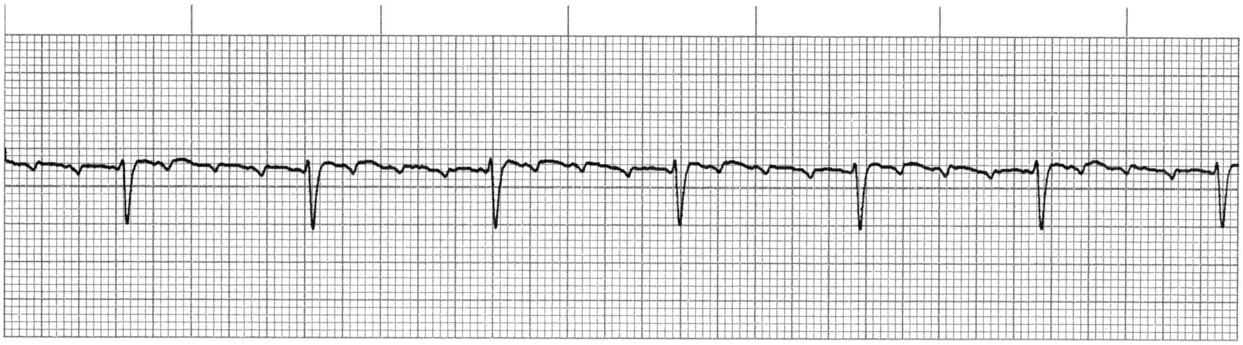

11–1

Regularity: _____   Heart rate: _____   PR interval: _____

P-waves: _____   QRS complex: _____

Interpretation: _____

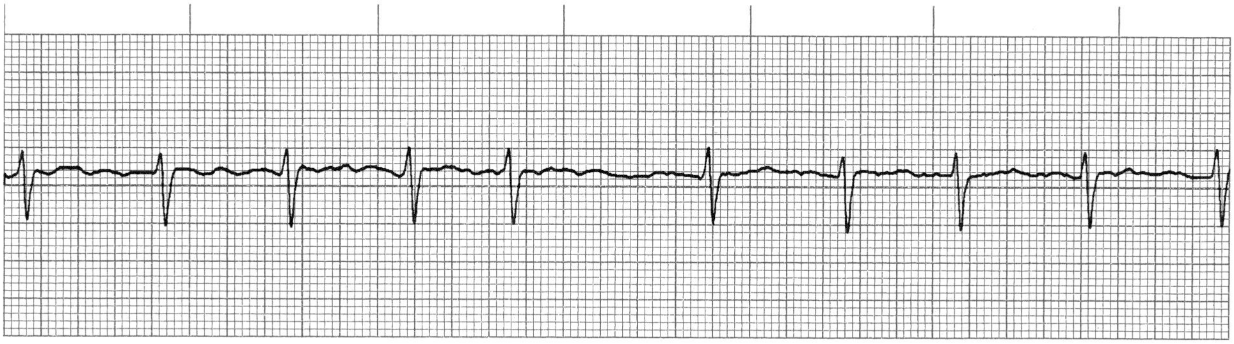

11–2

Regularity: _____   Heart rate: _____   PR interval: _____

P-waves: _____   QRS complex: _____

Interpretation: _____

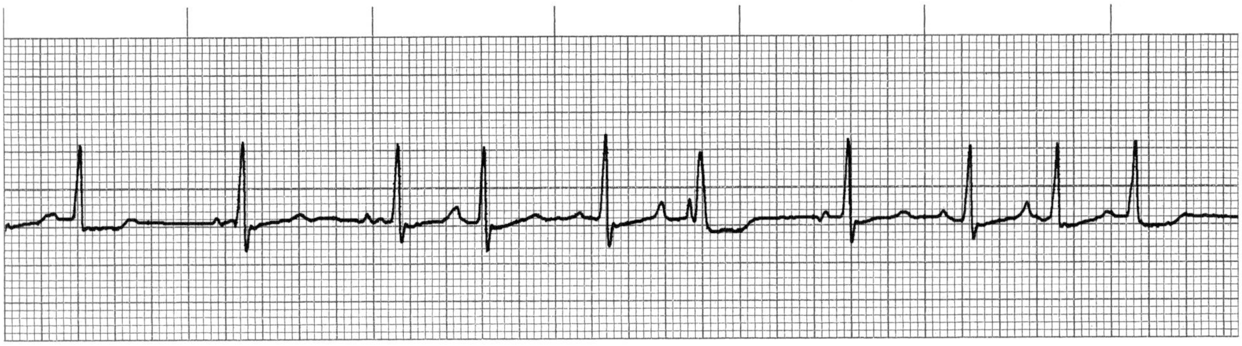

11–3

Regularity: _____

Heart rate: _____

PR interval: _____

P-waves: _____

QRS complex: _____

Interpretation: _____

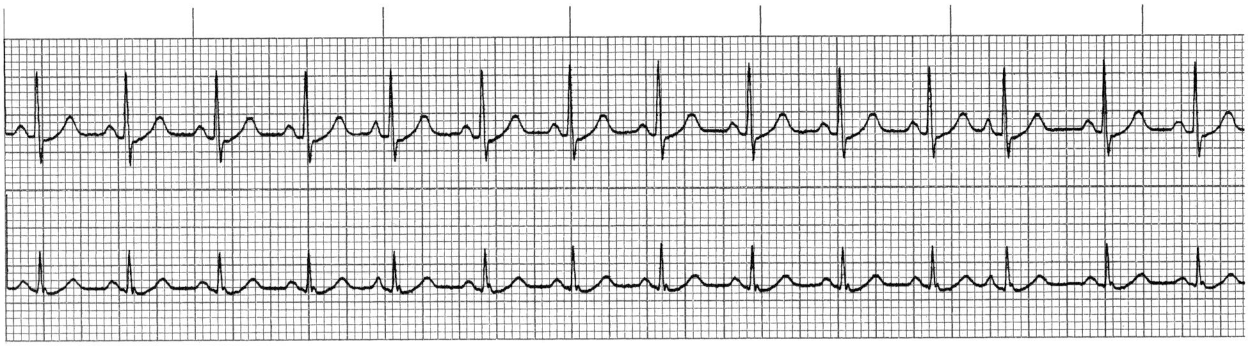

11–4

Regularity: _____

Heart rate: _____

PR interval: _____

P-waves: _____

QRS complex: _____

Interpretation: _____

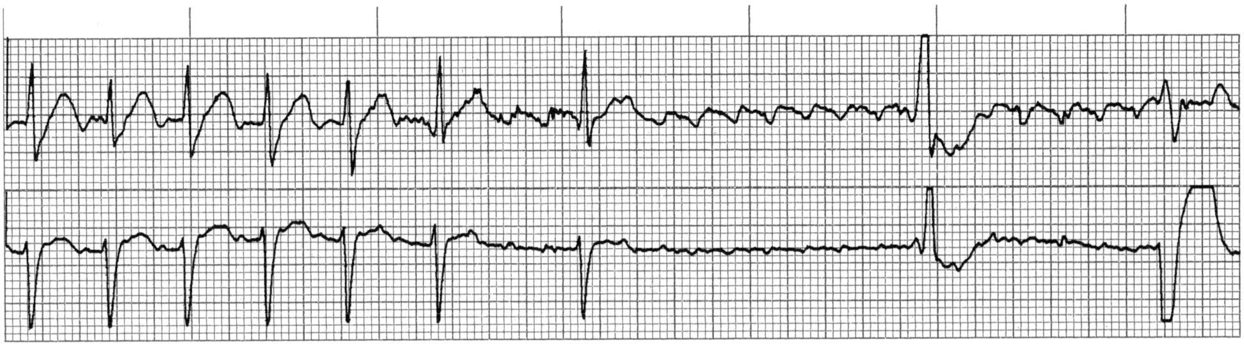

11–5

Regularity: _____

Heart rate: _____

PR interval: _____

P-waves: _____

QRS complex: _____

Interpretation: _____

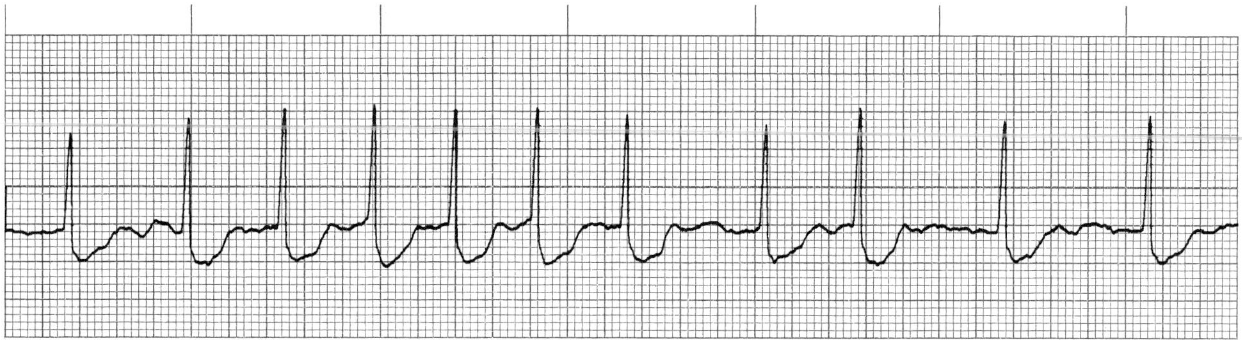

11–6

Regularity: _____

Heart rate: _____

PR interval: _____

P-waves: _____

QRS complex: _____

Interpretation: _____

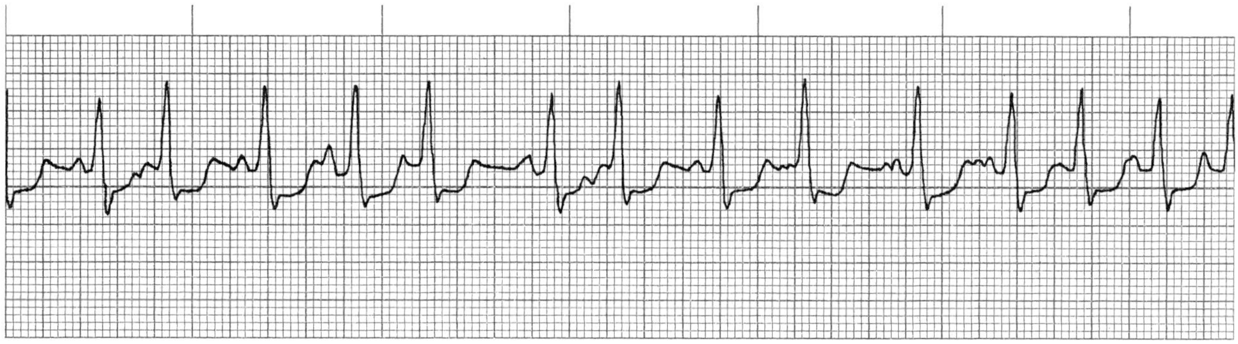

11–7

Regularity: _____

Heart rate: _____

PR interval: _____

P-waves: _____

QRS complex: _____

Interpretation: _____

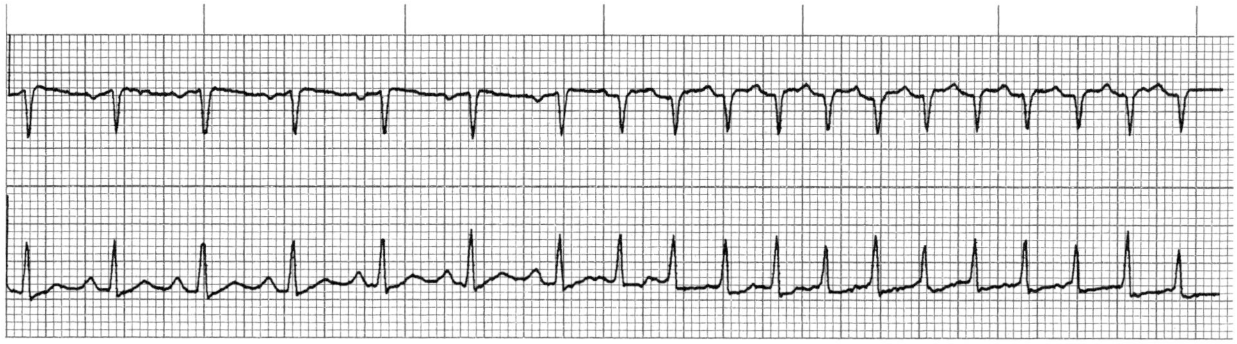

11–8

Regularity: _____

Heart rate: _____

PR interval: _____

P-waves: _____

QRS complex: _____

Interpretation: _____

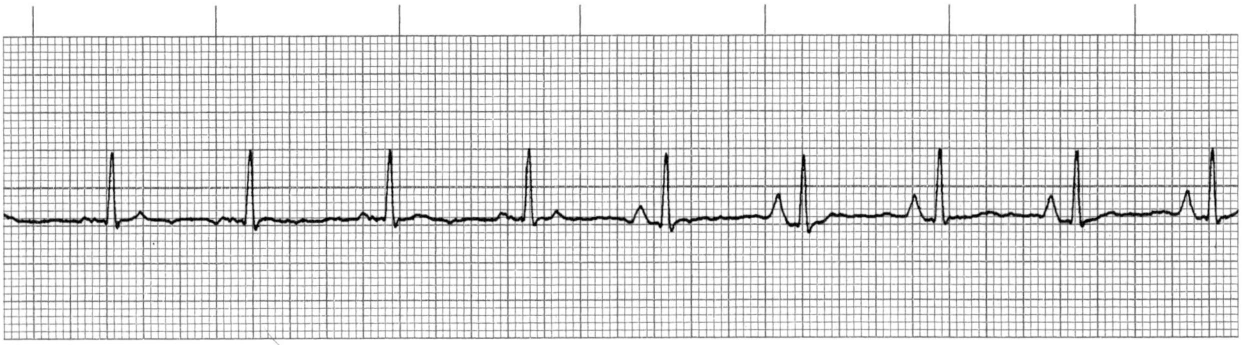

11–9

Regularity: _____

Heart rate: _____

PR interval: _____

P-waves: _____

QRS complex: _____

Interpretation: _____

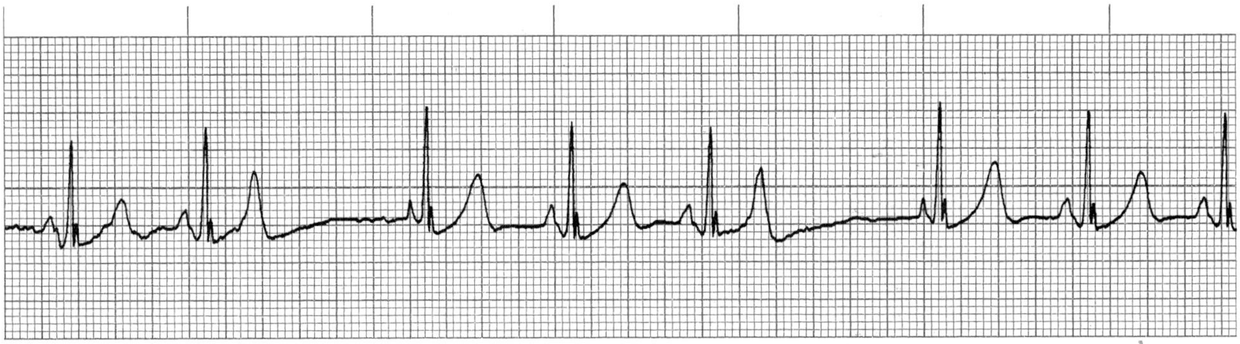

11–10

Regularity: _____

Heart rate: _____

PR interval: _____

P-waves: _____

QRS complex: _____

Interpretation: _____

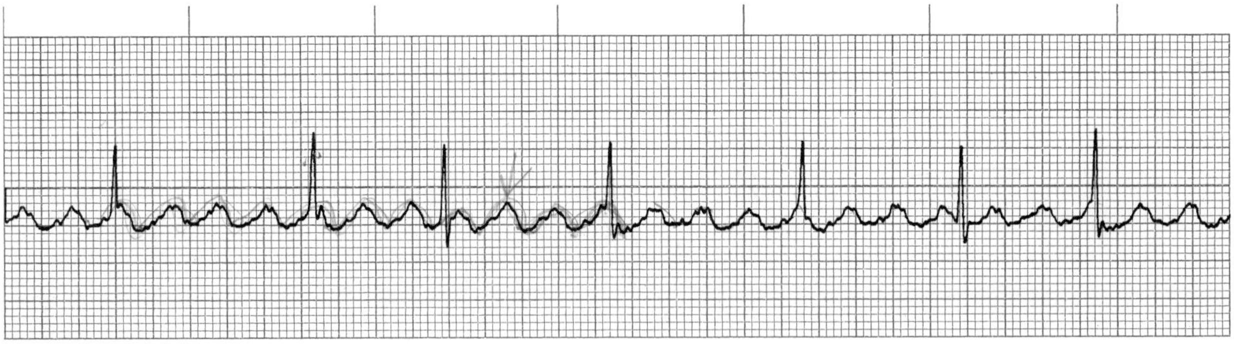

11–11

Regularity: _____

Heart rate: _____

PR interval: _____

P-waves: _____

QRS complex: _____

Interpretation: _____

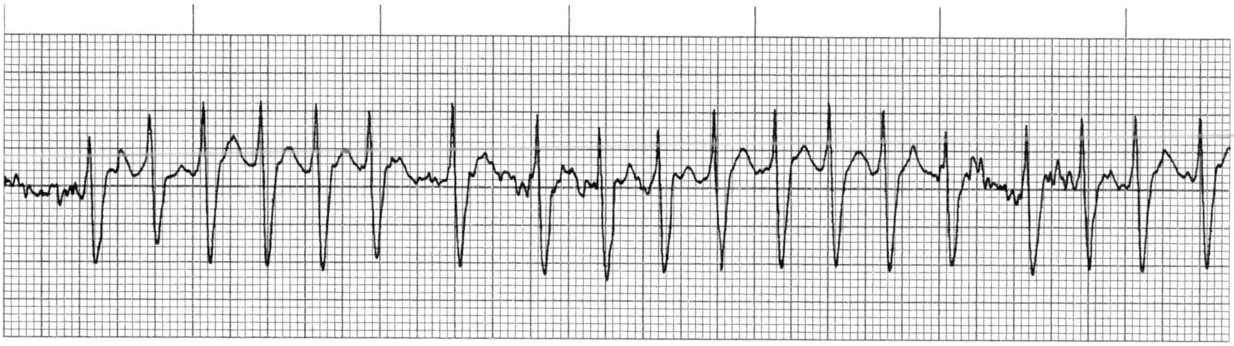

11–12

Regularity: _____

Heart rate: _____

PR interval: _____

P-waves: _____

QRS complex: _____

Interpretation: _____

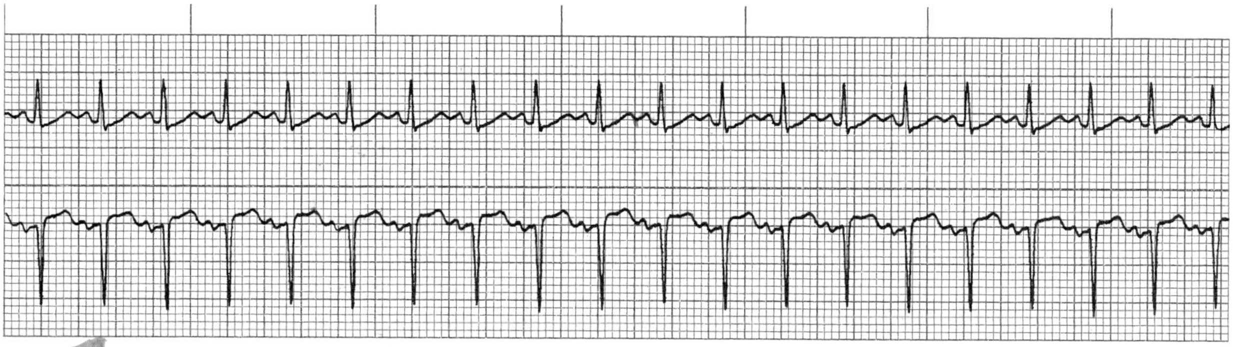

11–13

Regularity: _____

Heart rate: _____

PR interval: _____

P-waves: _____

QRS complex: _____

Interpretation: _____

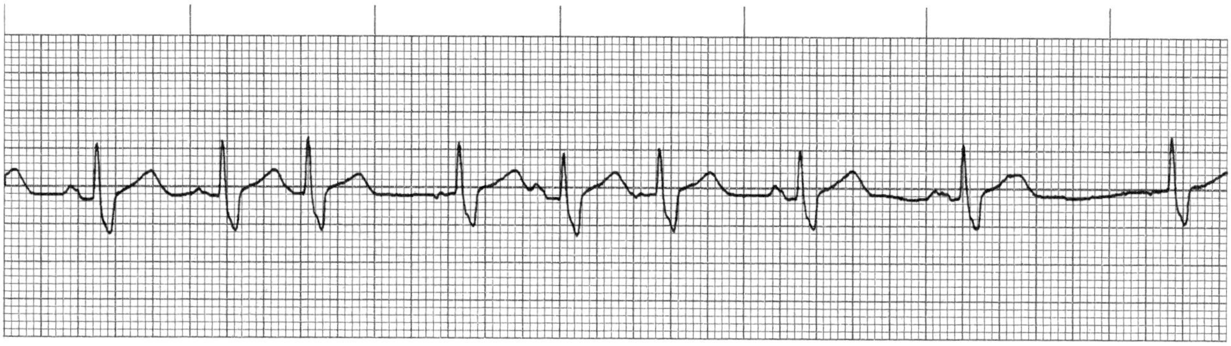

11–14

Regularity: _____

Heart rate: _____

PR interval: _____

P-waves: _____

QRS complex: _____

Interpretation: _____

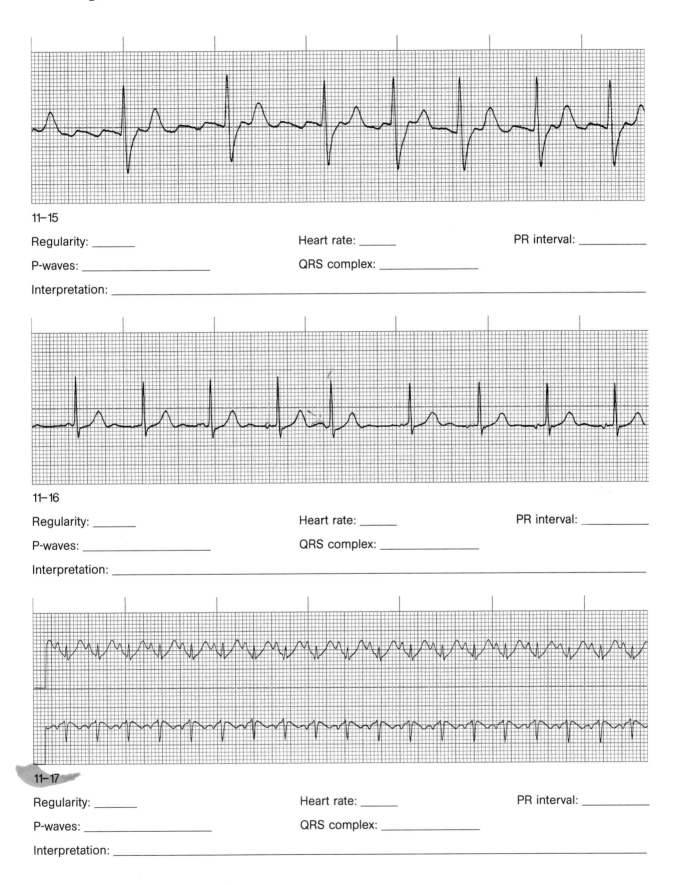

11–15

Regularity: _____

Heart rate: _____

PR interval: _____

P-waves: _____

QRS complex: _____

Interpretation: _____

11–16

Regularity: _____

Heart rate: _____

PR interval: _____

P-waves: _____

QRS complex: _____

Interpretation: _____

11–17

Regularity: _____

Heart rate: _____

PR interval: _____

P-waves: _____

QRS complex: _____

Interpretation: _____

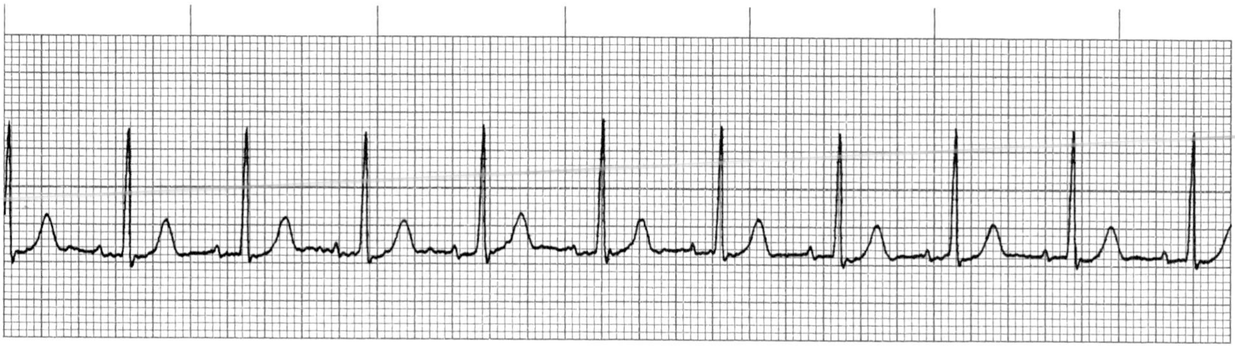

11–18

Regularity: _____

Heart rate: _____

PR interval: _____

P-waves: _____

QRS complex: _____

Interpretation: _____

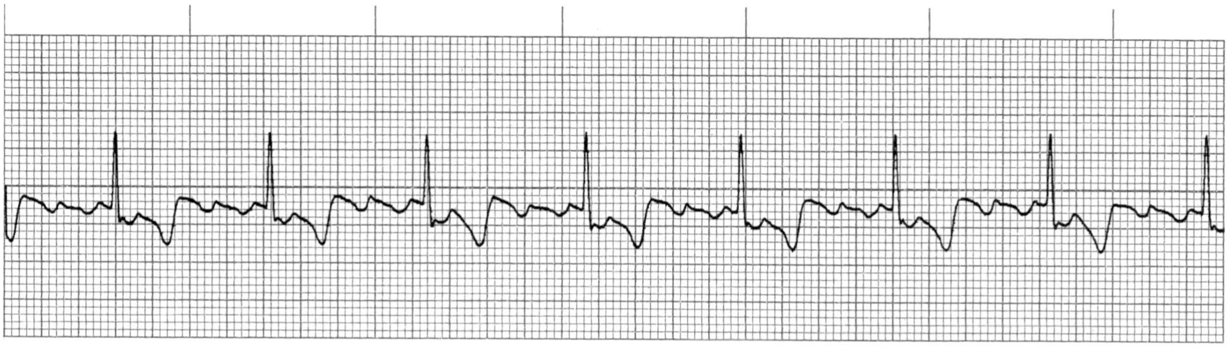

11–19

Regularity: _____

Heart rate: _____

PR interval: _____

P-waves: _____

QRS complex: _____

Interpretation: _____

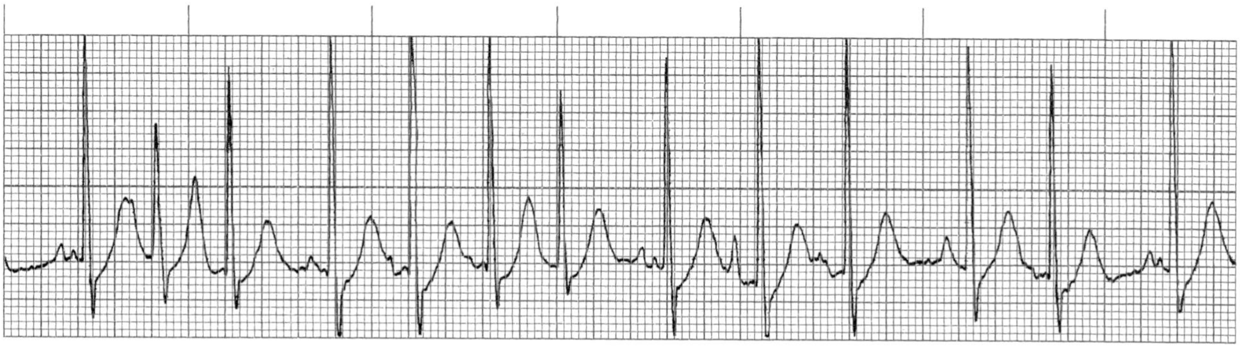

11–20

Regularity: _____

Heart rate: _____

PR interval: _____

P-waves: _____

QRS complex: _____

Interpretation: _____

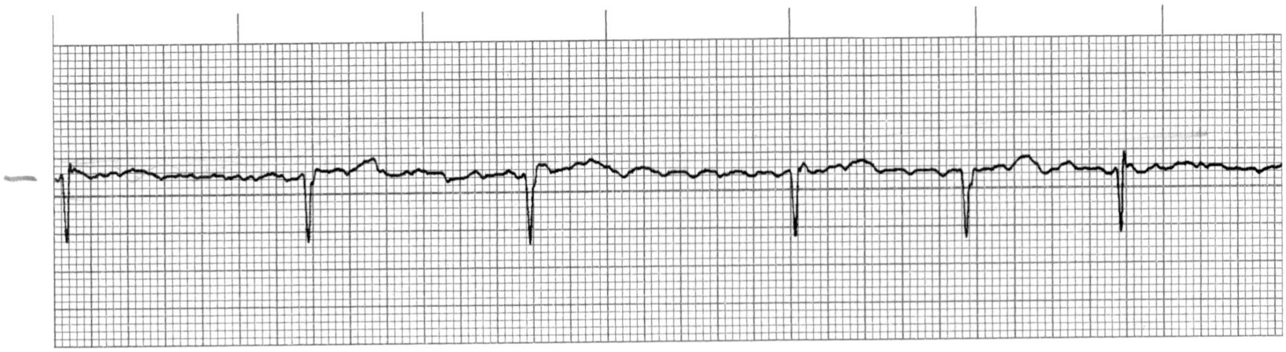

Atrial Rhythms

11–21

Regularity: _____

Heart rate: _____

PR interval: _____

P-waves: _____

QRS complex: _____

Interpretation: _____

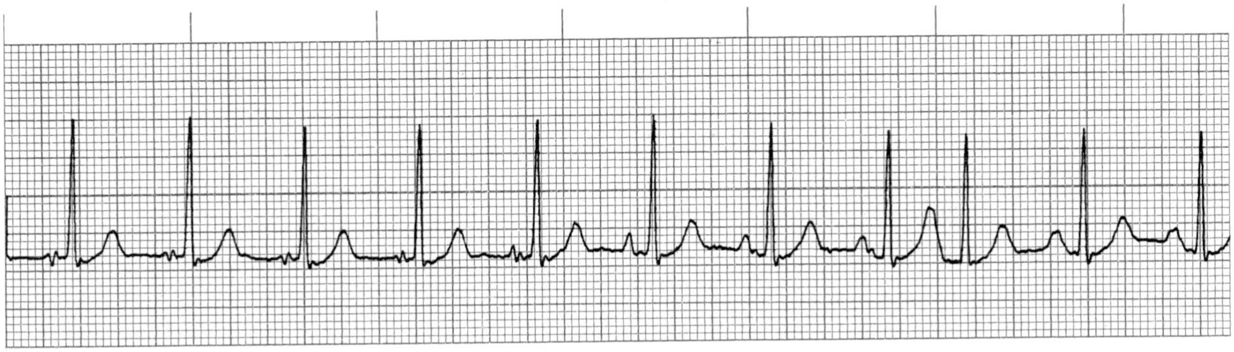

11–22

Regularity: _____

Heart rate: _____

PR interval: _____

P-waves: _____

QRS complex: _____

Interpretation: _____

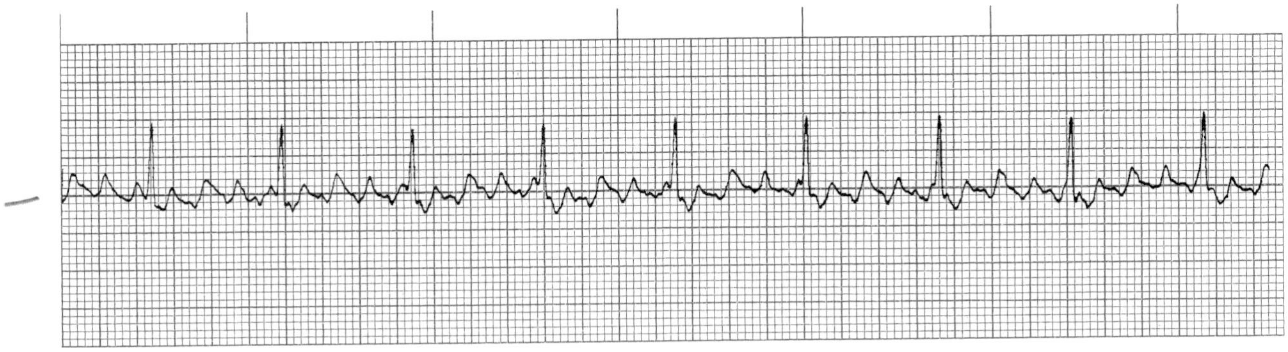

11–23

Regularity: _____

Heart rate: _____

PR interval: _____

P-waves: _____

QRS complex: _____

Interpretation: _____

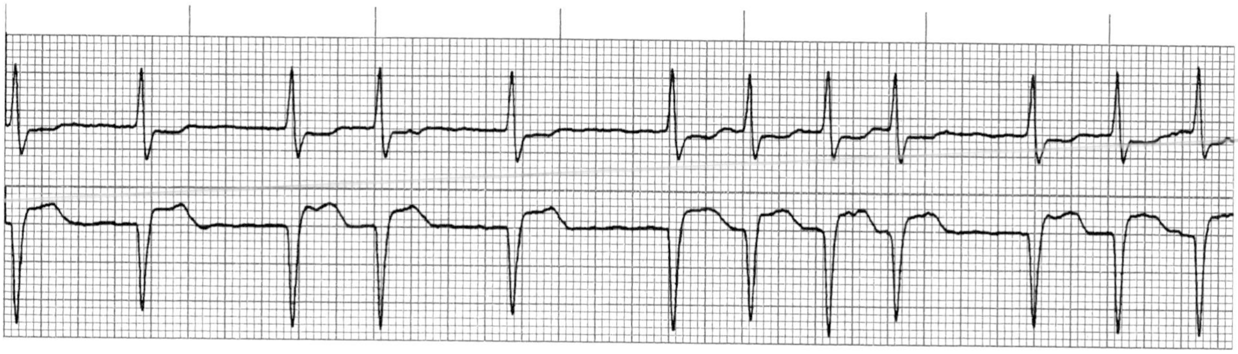

11–24

Regularity: _____

Heart rate: _____

PR interval: _____

P-waves: _____

QRS complex: _____

Interpretation: _____

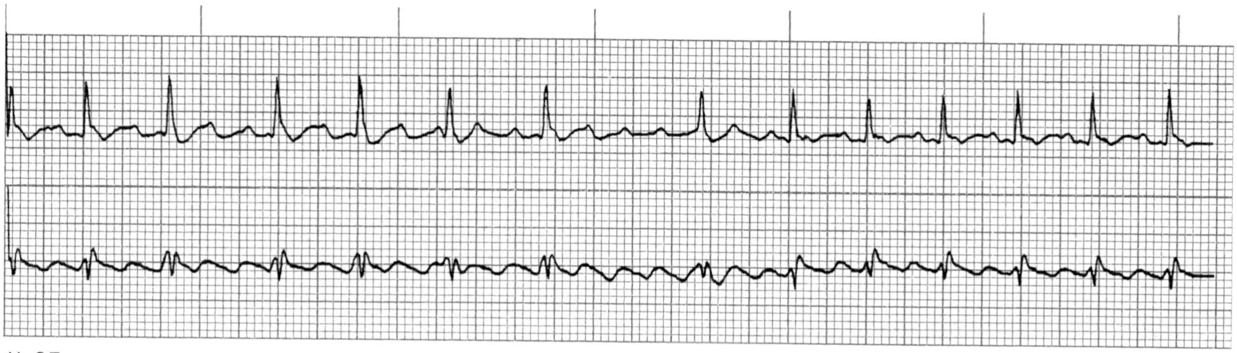

11–25

Regularity: _____

Heart rate: _____

PR interval: _____

P-waves: _____

QRS complex: _____

Interpretation: _____

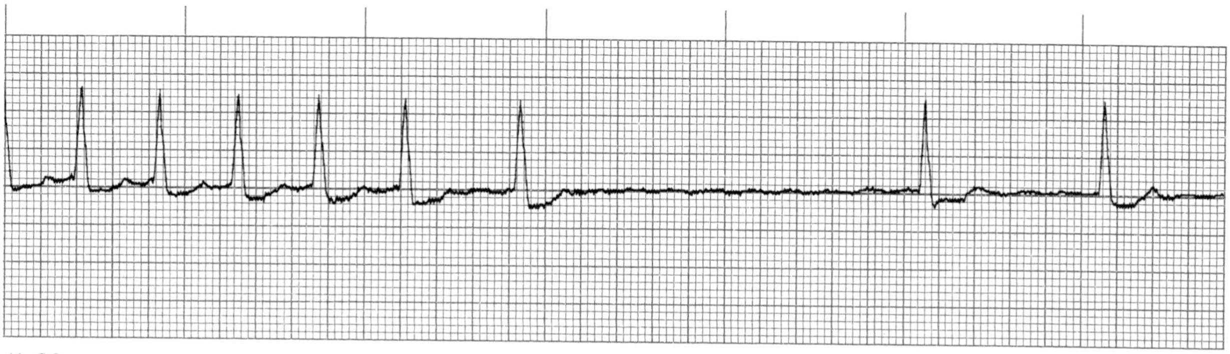

11–26

Regularity: _____

Heart rate: _____

PR interval: _____

P-waves: _____

QRS complex: _____

Interpretation: _____

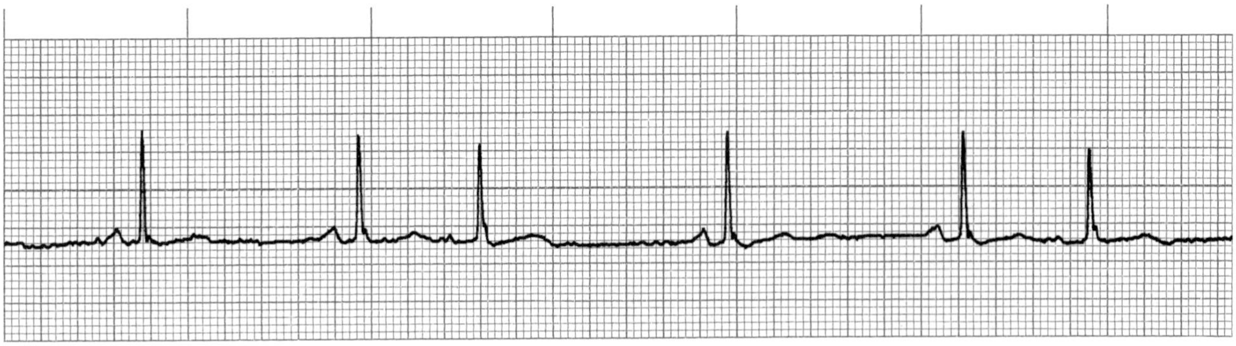

11–27

Regularity: _____   Heart rate: _____   PR interval: _____

P-waves: _____   QRS complex: _____

Interpretation: _____

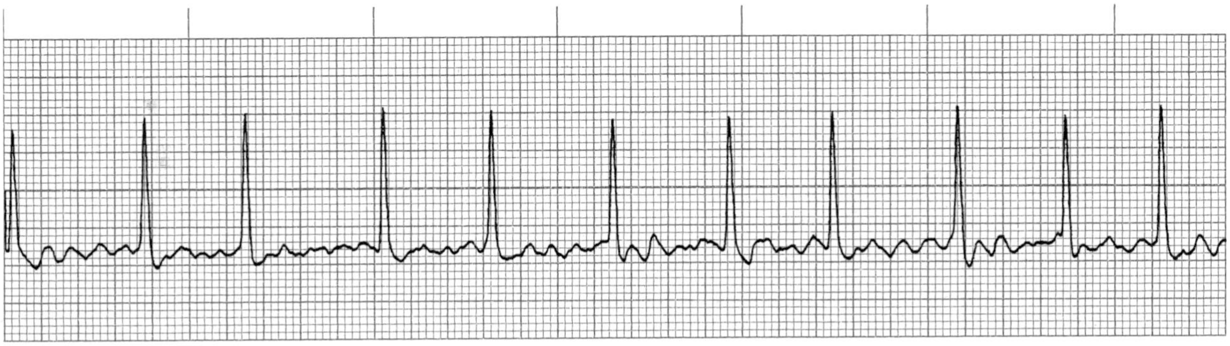

11–28

Regularity: _____   Heart rate: _____   PR interval: _____

P-waves: _____   QRS complex: _____

Interpretation: _____

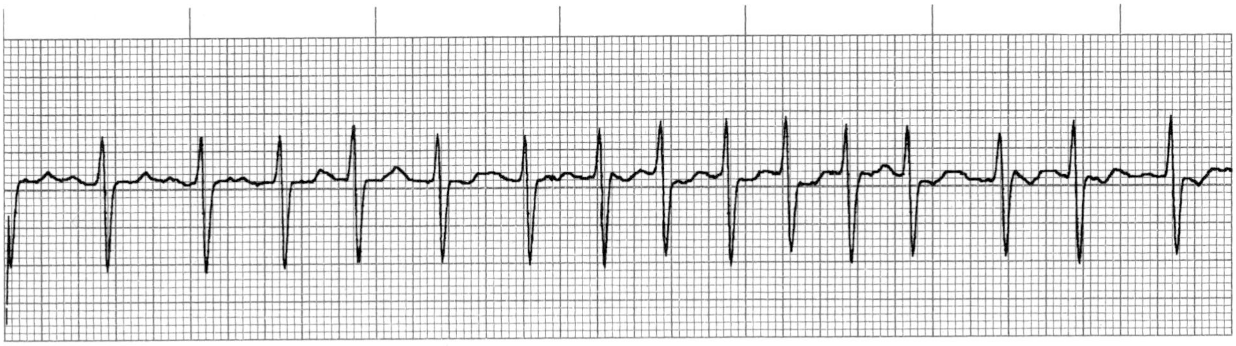

11–29

Regularity: _____   Heart rate: _____   PR interval: _____

P-waves: _____   QRS complex: _____

Interpretation: _____

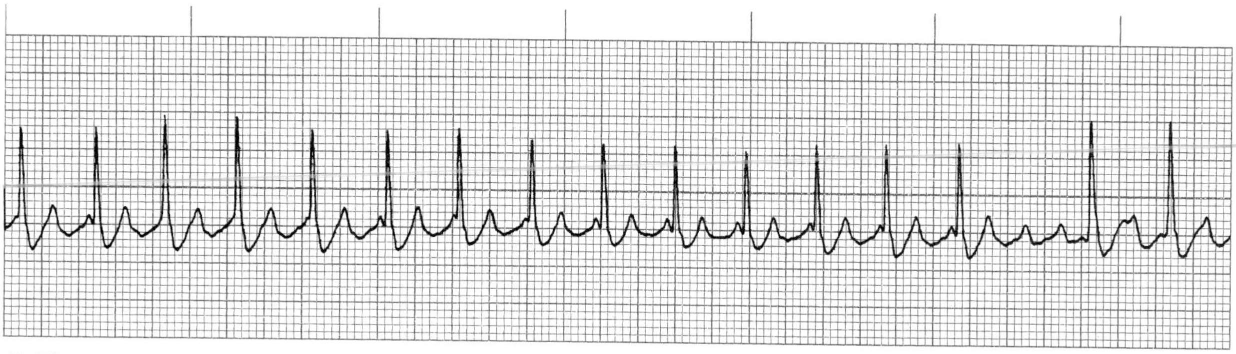

11–30

Regularity: _____

Heart rate: _____

PR interval: _____

P-waves: _____

QRS complex: _____

Interpretation: _____

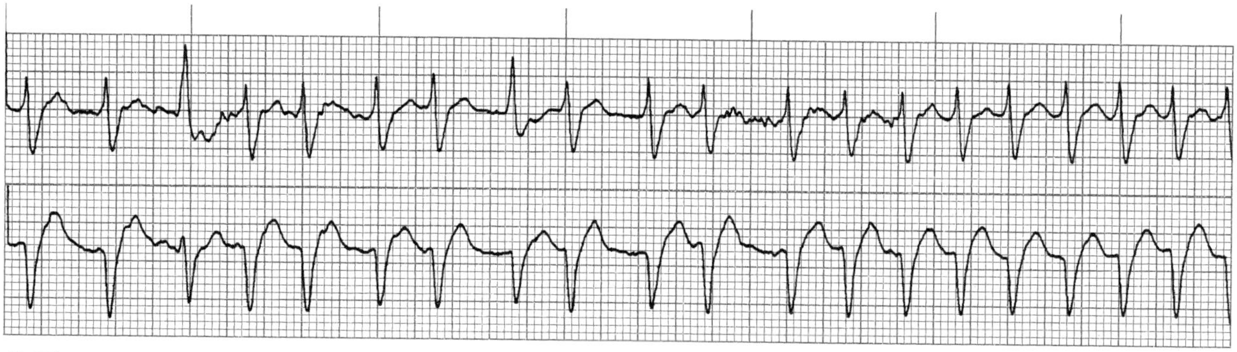

11–31

Regularity: _____

Heart rate: _____

PR interval: _____

P-waves: _____

QRS complex: _____

Interpretation: _____

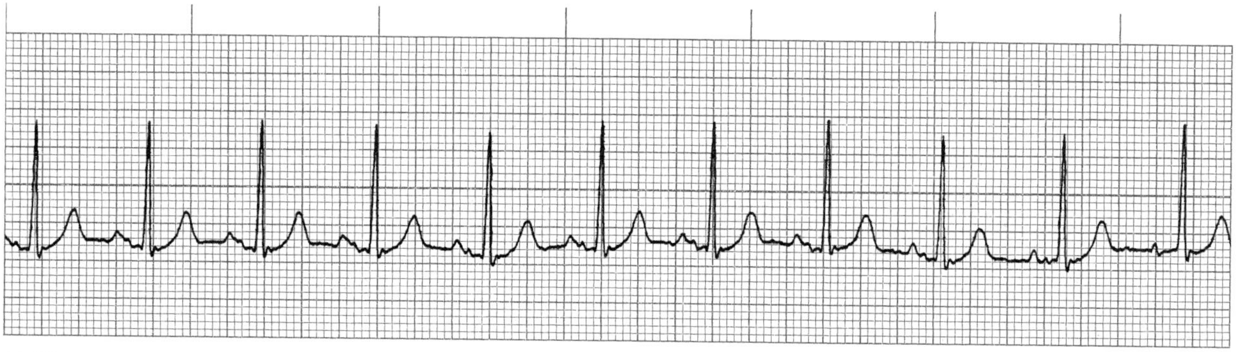

11–32

Regularity: _____

Heart rate: _____

PR interval: _____

P-waves: _____

QRS complex: _____

Interpretation: _____

Atrial Rhythms

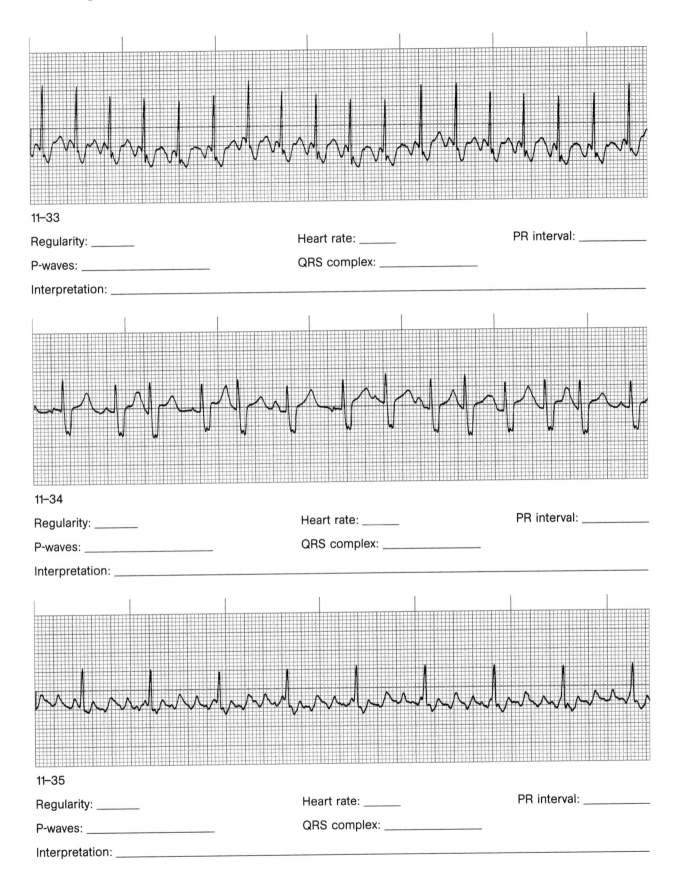

11–33

Regularity: _____

Heart rate: _____

PR interval: _____

P-waves: _____

QRS complex: _____

Interpretation: _____

11–34

Regularity: _____

Heart rate: _____

PR interval: _____

P-waves: _____

QRS complex: _____

Interpretation: _____

11–35

Regularity: _____

Heart rate: _____

PR interval: _____

P-waves: _____

QRS complex: _____

Interpretation: _____

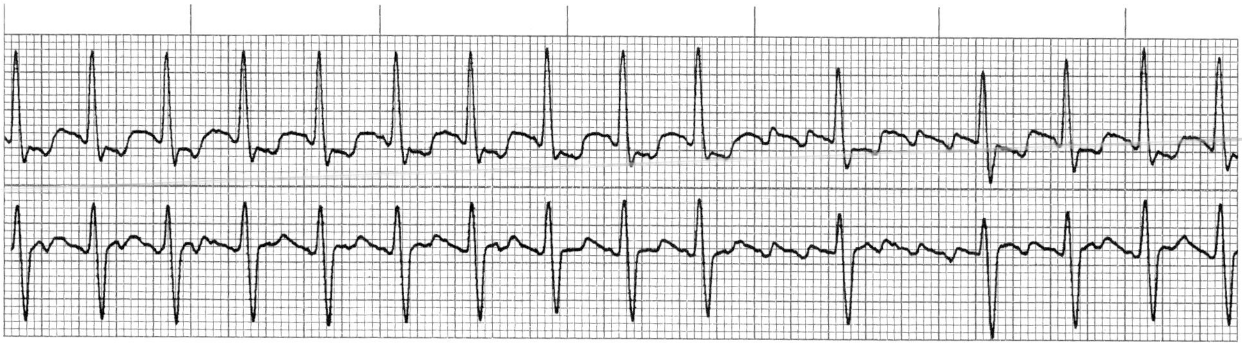

11–36

Regularity: _____   Heart rate: _____   PR interval: _____

P-waves: _____   QRS complex: _____

Interpretation: _____

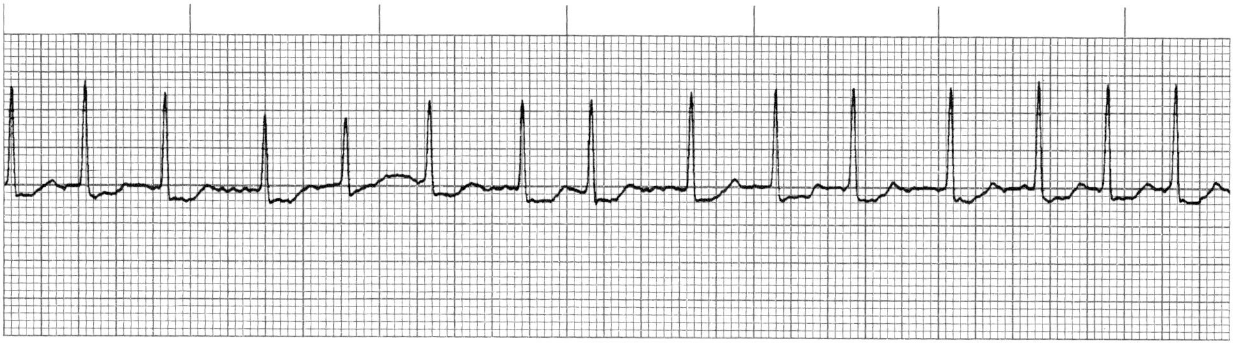

11–37

Regularity: _____   Heart rate: _____   PR interval: _____

P-waves: _____   QRS complex: _____

Interpretation: _____

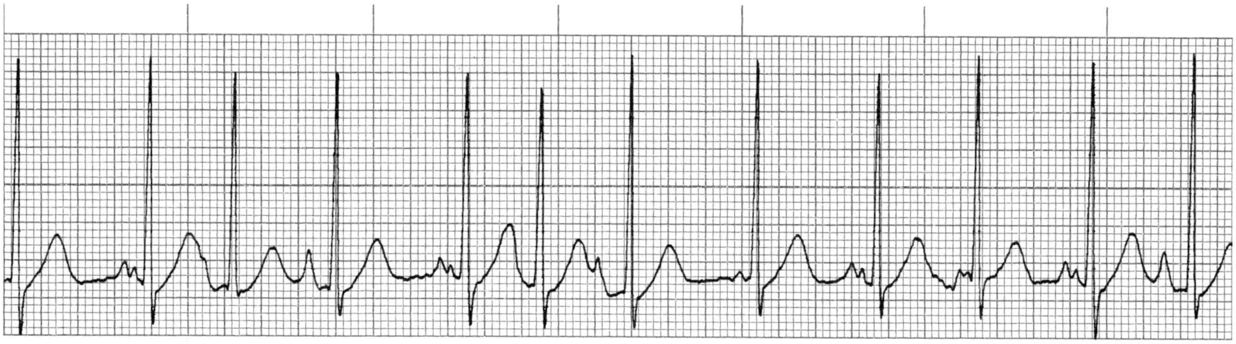

11–38

Regularity: _____   Heart rate: _____   PR interval: _____

P-waves: _____   QRS complex: _____

Interpretation: _____

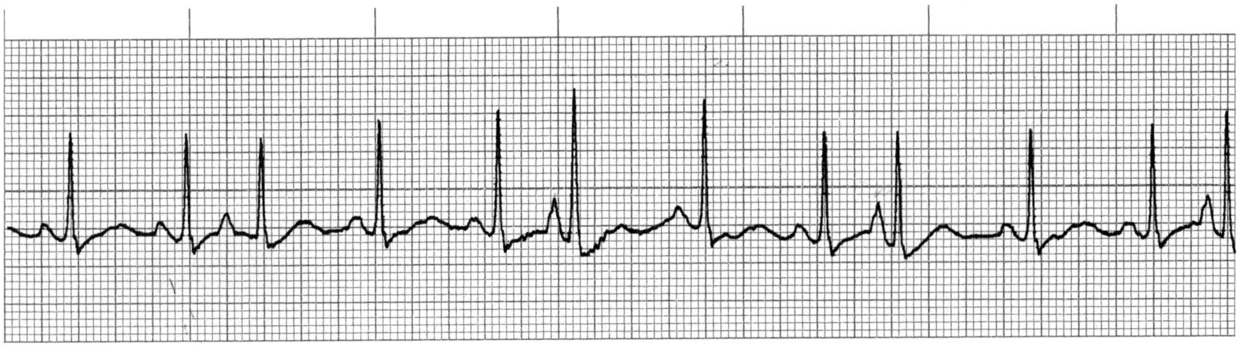

Atrial Rhythms

11–39

Regularity: _____ Heart rate: _____ PR interval: _____

P-waves: _____ QRS complex: _____

Interpretation: _____

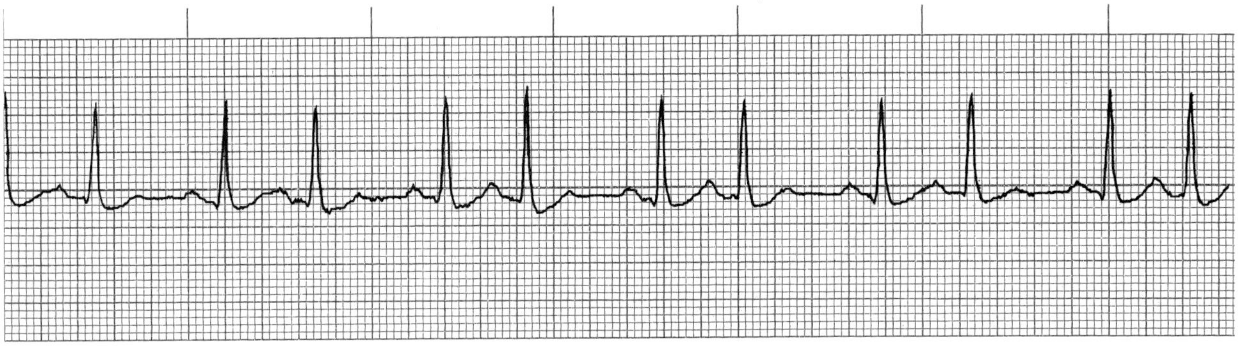

11–40

Regularity: _____ Heart rate: _____ PR interval: _____

P-waves: _____ QRS complex: _____

Interpretation: _____

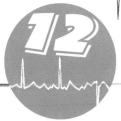

JUNCTIONAL RHYTHMS

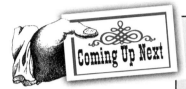
Coming Up Next

○ Why does the AV node sometimes run the heart?

○ What is the intrinsic rate for junctional tissue?

○ Why is accelerated junctional rhythm considered better than junctional rhythm?

○ What does a P-wave look like in junctional rhythms?

○ Why do some junctional rhythms have P-waves and some not?

○ What is supraventricular tachycardia and how is it treated?

Who's Running the Government?

We began the last chapter with a civics review. In our government, the president and Congress make the laws, with Congress putting a brake on the president's power. But as you know, this country has an additional protection in place—the Supreme Court. Supreme Court justices can alter laws if they decide that those laws are not consistent with the rights afforded by the United States Constitution.

The heart has a similar protection in case the sinus node and the atrial tissue can't adequately maintain heart rate. This protection, the heart's Supreme Court, is called the *junctional tissue,* or *nodal tissue.* We use this name because this part of the heart is the junction between the atria and the ventricles and, in normal hearts, is the only path between them.

Junctional tissue has a natural, or intrinsic, rate of approximately 40 to 60 bpm. Normally the sinus node or atrial tissue discharges at a faster rate, suppressing the junctional tissue before it has a chance to discharge. However, junctional tissue is capable of running the heart, either for one beat or as a continuing rhythm. It just has to beat the rush by discharging faster than any other tissue in the heart.

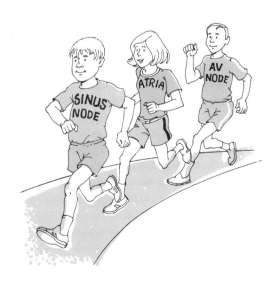

The Supraventricular Jigsaw

ALL PIECES IN PLACE

The junctional tissue represents the final piece of the puzzle we've been putting together. Sinus, atrial, and junctional rhythms all come into the category of *supraventricular rhythms*. The combining form *supra* means "above," so a supraventricular rhythm is generated by tissue located above the ventricles—in other words, the sinus node, atrial tissue, or AV node.

HOW THEY'RE ALIKE

All supraventricular rhythms share a similar characteristic: the QRS complex. Regardless of where the rhythm

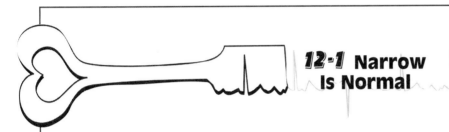

Any QRS complex with a normal duration is called a *narrow QRS complex*. This term tells us that the rhythm originated in the sinus node, atrial tissue, or AV node because the path from the AV node to the terminal Purkinje fibers was normal. Another term for supraventricular rhythms is *narrow–QRS-complex rhythm*. This term tells us that we aren't dealing with the dangerous species of ventricular rhythms, which we'll discuss in the next chapter. Rhythms that start above the ventricles are generally safer.

begins, all supraventricular rhythms pass through the AV node and down the bundle branches in the same way. Because the QRS reflects this passage, all supraventricular rhythms show the same QRS patterns if the ventricular conduction is also normal.

HOW THEY'RE DIFFERENT

The major difference among supraventricular rhythms is the P-wave. The origin of atrial depolarization depends on the tissue generating the rhythm. Just as we rely on the P-wave to determine whether a rhythm is atrial or sinus, we also use it as the key to differentiating junctional rhythms from the other supraventricular rhythms.

In sinus rhythms, all P-waves are the same shape because they all come from the same place and follow the same path. In atrial rhythms, the P-waves can come from

anywhere in either the right or the left atrium, so their shapes and sizes can vary widely even within one lead. If the P-wave originates in the far left atrium, it will be inverted in lead I; a P-wave originating in the right atrium will be mostly positive in the same lead. Junctional beats and rhythms make no secret of their origin: we know within a small, definite area where the depolarization signal originates.

The AV node, unlike the atrial tissue, is small, about the same size as the sinus node. Therefore, all P-waves that originate from the AV node will look the same when viewed in the same lead. All junctional P-waves share two characteristics that make it relatively easy to determine junctional rhythms. The first is probably the most important: inverted P-waves in lead II. Let's examine how they happen.

P-WAVES IN REVERSE

Figure 12–1 shows the heart's conduction system as viewed in lead II. The arrows that connect the pairs of electrodes indicate the approximate normal vectors for P-waves in leads I, II, and III. In lead II, for instance, the atria depolarize from the sinus node to the general area of the AV node. This normal vector inscribes a positive P-wave in lead II, as we discussed in Chapter 6.

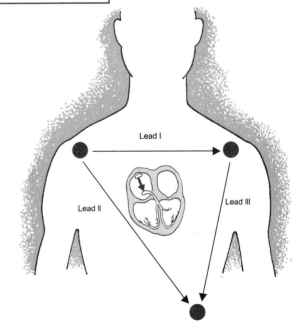

Fig. 12–1 The normal path of atrial depolarization in sinus rhythm in relation to leads I, II, and III.

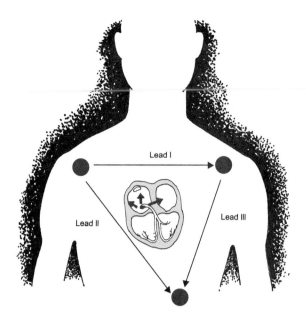

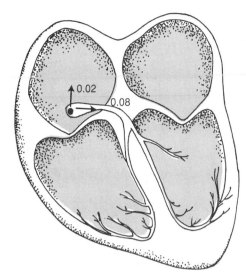

Fig. 12–3 Junctional rhythm originating near the top of the AV node. The signal will take 0.02 seconds to return to the atria, initiating the P-wave, and 0.08 seconds to reach the ventricles, initiating the QRS complex. The P-wave occurs before the QRS.

Fig. 12–2 The normal path of atrial depolarization in junctional rhythms in relation to leads I, II, and III.

But look at atrial depolarization in junctional rhythms (Fig. 12–2). Instead of ending in the AV node, it begins there and ends at the sinus node. Because atrial depolarization is happening in reverse, you might expect the P-wave to be reversed also. That's exactly what happens—the P-wave in junctional rhythms is inverted in lead II. The P-wave can be flat or biphasic in lead I and lead III because half the signal travels away from the lead (negative P-wave) and the other half travels toward it (positive P-wave). In lead aVr, the P-wave will be mostly positive.

A Question of Origin

SHORTCHANGING THE PR INTERVAL

The other important characteristic of junctional P-waves is their location in relation to the QRS complex. If the rhythm starts in the AV node, some of the AV node delay will be lost. Why? Because the signal doesn't have to travel the entire AV node before depolarizing the ventricles. This loss of delay disrupts the PR interval. In fact, the P-wave may actually occur after the QRS in junctional rhythms; this depends on whether depolarization begins in the top, middle, or bottom of the AV node.

If the rhythm originates near the top of the AV node, most of the AV node delay is preserved because the signal started high in the AV node. In Figure 12–3, the signal has taken 0.02 seconds to travel *backwards* to the atrial tissue and initiate the P-wave, a process called *retrograde impulse transmission*. At the same time, the signal has taken 0.08 seconds to travel to the bundle branches and the ventricles, initiating the QRS complex. According to these figures, the signal takes a total of 0.10 seconds (0.02 + 0.08 seconds) to travel in the AV node. This total time delay is normal for the AV node.

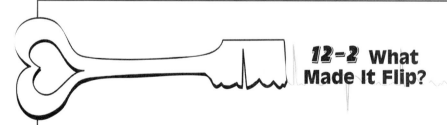

12-2 What Made It Flip?

Don't assume that all inverted P-waves represent junctional beats. You need to make sure that an inverted P-wave isn't normal in the current lead. For instance, inverted P-waves are expected in lead aVr and are common in leads V_1 and V_2. However, we learned in Chapter 10, "Sinus Rhythms," that sinus P-waves in lead II are always upright (positive). Therefore, junctional P-waves should always be inverted in this lead.

Incorrect positioning can also cause inverted P-waves in lead II. Switching the RA wire with the LL wire, for instance, causes this effect. The QRS complex and the P-waves of other leads can indicate a positioning problem, but that discussion belongs at a more advanced level. For now the best method is to physically check the ECG connections for accuracy.

However, because the signal is traveling to the atria and ventricles at the same time, the P-wave and QRS will be only 0.06 (0.08 − 0.02) seconds apart. This number represents the PR interval. To sum up, the PR interval is shorter than normal (less than 0.12 seconds) in junctional rhythms because the signal can depolarize the ventricles without having to travel the full length of the AV node.

THE CASE OF THE DISAPPEARING P-WAVE

In Figure 12–4, we see the consequences of a rhythm that originates in the middle of the AV node. The signal takes 0.05 seconds to reach the atrial tissue and begin the P-wave and takes the same 0.05 seconds to travel forward to the ventricles and generate the QRS complex. As a result, of course, the P-wave and QRS occur at the same time. We know from Chapter 7 that ventricular depolarization generates a much larger waveform than atrial depolarization. Therefore, the QRS often swallows the P-wave, making it invisible.

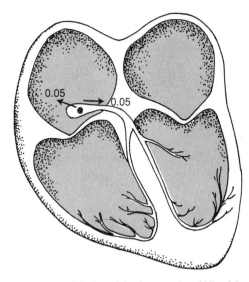

Fig. 12–4 Junctional rhythm originating near the middle of the AV node. The signal will take 0.05 seconds to return to the atria, initiating the P-wave, and 0.05 seconds to reach the ventricles, initiating the QRS complex. The P-wave and QRS occur simultaneously.

12-3 Simultaneous Events

Let's look at what actually happens when the P-wave disappears. Because the signal has reached the atria and the ventricles simultaneously, both these areas are depolarizing at the same time. The atria are forced to contract against contracting ventricles. Because the ventricles contract with much greater force, the net result is a loss of atrial kick and a decrease in stroke volume. Cardiac output drops as much as it does in atrial fibrillation. This can cause significant hypotension, especially if other stresses, such as heart attack or dehydration, are present.

occurs *after* it starts. In the example shown here, the P-wave occurs 0.06 seconds, or about one and one half small boxes, after the QRS begins. If the QRS is narrow enough, the P-wave will even come after it. Sometimes it appears in the ST segment, and sometimes it deforms the T-wave. Because the atria contract when the ventricles aren't ready to receive blood, atrial kick is again lost.

IT'S NOT NICE TO IGNORE THE ATRIA

Regardless of where depolarization begins in the AV node, there's no guarantee that the signal will travel backward to the atrial tissue. When it doesn't, the atrial tissue can't depolarize, so no P-wave is generated from the depolarization of the AV node. There may be P-waves occurring from the sinus node because it isn't being reset and therefore doesn't know what the AV node is doing, because the AV node signal does not depolarize the atria.

Several conditions can keep the signal from traveling back to the atria. It may be blocked by diseased or damaged AV nodal tissue, acute myocardial infarction (MI), or simply an AV node that's incapable of retrograde transmission. We'll revisit AV node conduction in Chapter 14.

BETTER LATE THAN NEVER?

If depolarization begins near the bottom of the AV node, the result is shown in Figure 12–5. Here the travel time to the atrial tissue is 0.08 seconds, and the travel time to the ventricular tissue is 0.02 seconds. The total time signals take to travel through the AV node is still a normal 0.10 seconds (0.08 + 0.02 seconds), but now the PR interval is −0.06 (0.02 − 0.08) seconds—less than zero. This means that the P-wave doesn't come before the QRS complex but

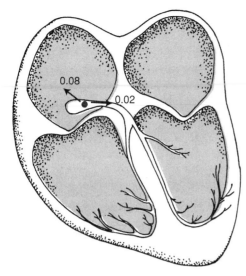

Fig. 12-5 Junctional rhythm originating near the middle of the AV node. The signal will take 0.09 seconds to return to the atria, initiating the P-wave, and 0.02 seconds to reach the ventricles, initiating the QRS complex. The P-wave occurs after the QRS.

Junctional Rhythms in a Nutshell

To recap, junctional beats and rhythms have P-waves that can occur before, during, or after the QRS complex. Junctional rhythms can be divided into two categories: those with identifiable P-waves and those without. When P-waves are present, the PR interval is less than 0.12 seconds and the P-waves are inverted in lead II. When there isn't an identifiable P-wave, the QRS complex should appear normal for the patient. That is to say, a regular rhythm with a QRS of normal duration without P-waves is assumed to be junctional unless it's proved not to be. Now let's get onto specific junctional rhythms.

Premature Junctional Contraction

WHAT CAUSES IT?

When the junctional tissue discharges before the next expected beat, sinus or atrial, the resulting complex is called a premature junctional complex (PJC). The same naming conventions apply to junctional tissue as to atrial tissue: PJC, PJB, JPB, or JPC. No matter what you call it, a premature junctional complex is a cry for attention. It's a signal that at least some of the junctional tissue is irritable and trying to make the heart beat faster.

Premature junctional complexes can occur for many of the same reasons as premature atrial complexes (PACs) and sinus tachycardia. Many causes of sinus tachycardia, such as caffeine, tobacco, myocardial ischemia, and hypoxia, can generate PJCs. Electrolyte disturbances such as hypokalemia and hypomagnesemia are also causes that can be easily investigated. Hypertrophy and dilation have no role here because the AV node tissue isn't stretched in PJCs. Like PACs, PJCs are usually benign, even if they happen frequently, and treatment isn't usually necessary.

WHAT DOES THE P-WAVE TELL US?

A P-wave in a PJC must have a different shape from sinus and atrial P-waves because it originates from a different location and therefore travels a different path. Remember Chapter 9, the morphology chapter? There are only two reasons why one complex (P-wave, QRS complex, or T-wave) looks different from another of the same type: it started in a different place or followed a different path.

In Figure 12–6, you can see that the rhythm is "regular except" for the fifth beat. That beat is the PJC. It clearly interrupts the regular sinus rhythm, which continues with the beat following the PJC. Look closely for the P-wave before the early QRS complex in lead II. You can't see it because it occurs after the QRS complex, in the ST segment. In all other aspects, the PJC is identical to the sinus beats. The QRS and T-wave are the same shape because the conduction has traveled down the bundle

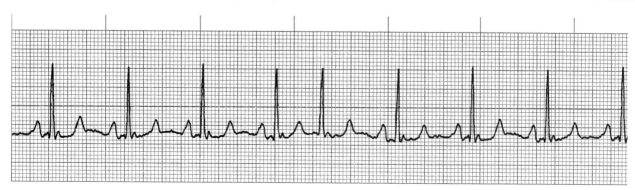

Fig. 12-6 Sinus rhythm with the fifth beat a premature junctional contraction. Notice the inverted P-wave in the ST segment.

Table 12–1 Criteria for premature junctional contraction

Regularity	Regular except for the premature beats
Heart Rate	Any rate
P-Wave	**If present, inverted in leads II, III, aVF. May precede, follow, or be buried in QRS.**
PR Interval	<0.12 seconds or not measurable
QRS Complexes	All the same shape, <0.12 seconds (three small boxes)

branches and to the ventricular tissue as in the sinus beats. The only difference is in the atrial tissue conduction, which changes the shape and location of the P-wave. Table 12–1 lists the characteristics of PJCs.

Like PACs, PJCs can be unifocal or multifocal. To distinguish between these two types, simply observe their P-waves. If the P-waves have the same morphology, they've originated from the same location (one focus) and traveled the same path.

In multifocal PJCs, the P-waves don't change shape significantly. Instead, one is located differently from another in relation to the QRS complex. Junctional P-waves all look the same because they exit the AV node at about the same spot in the atrial tissue and follow the same path (see Fig. 12–3). However, they originate at different points in the AV node and therefore must travel longer or shorter distances to depolarize the atrial tissue. This difference affects the relative timing of the P-waves and QRS complexes, putting the P-waves at varying distances from the QRS (Fig. 12–7).

All other aspects will look normal because conduction through the AV node and down the bundle branches is the same for all sinus and junctional foci.

WHAT DOES THE RHYTHM LOOK LIKE?

Like PACs, PJCs can occur just occasionally or at regular intervals in a specific pattern. If every other beat is a PJC, the pattern is known as *bigeminal PJCs:* two beats, one normal and one abnormal, in a repeating pattern. A rhythm with two normal beats followed by an abnormal beat is called *trigeminal PJCs.* Figure 12–8 shows an example of sinus rhythm with trigeminal PJCs—two regular sinus beats followed by one abnormal beat (the PJC).

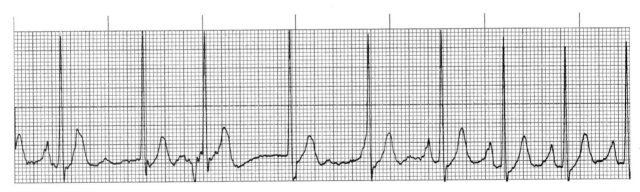

Fig. 12–7 Sinus rhythm with multifocal junctional beats. The morphology of the second, third, and fourth P-waves is different. The second and fourth beat have no P-waves, but are not early, therefore they are junctional escape beats. The third beat has an inverted P-wave in Lead II and IS early, therefore this is a PJC.

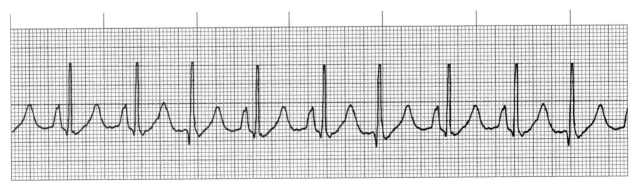

Fig. 12–8 Sinus rhythm with trigeminal premature ventricular contractions. Every third beat has no visible P-wave. (Note—there may be P-waves buried in the previous T-wave as they are slightly wider, but this would have to be verified in other leads.)

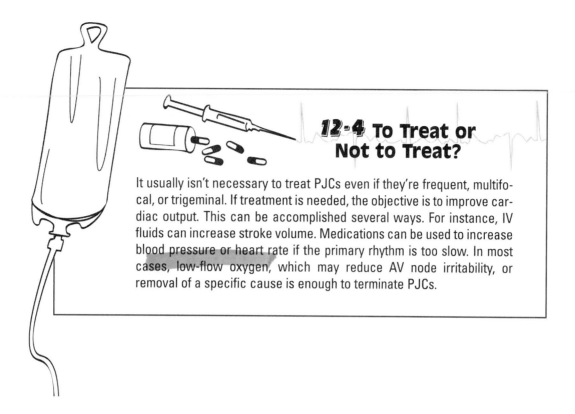

12-4 To Treat or Not to Treat?

It usually isn't necessary to treat PJCs even if they're frequent, multifocal, or trigeminal. If treatment is needed, the objective is to improve cardiac output. This can be accomplished several ways. For instance, IV fluids can increase stroke volume. Medications can be used to increase blood pressure or heart rate if the primary rhythm is too slow. In most cases, low-flow oxygen, which may reduce AV node irritability, or removal of a specific cause is enough to terminate PJCs.

Junctional Rhythm

"Junctional rhythm" refers to a rhythm that's normal for this part of the heart. Technically we could call it "idiojunctional rhythm" and be right, but clinically it's usually called plain "junctional rhythm."

When the sinus node gives out and the atrial tissue doesn't pick up the slack, as it often doesn't, the AV node takes over control of the heart rhythm. However, the junctional tissue is not the sinus node. It's not meant to depolarize as frequently as the sinus node does. If it did, the AV node would take control inappropriately from the sinus node at normal sinus rhythm rates. This would cause a drop in cardiac output from the loss of atrial kick, to the likely detriment of the patient.

The intrinsic discharge rate for the AV node is about 40 to 60 bpm. This rate is fast enough to sustain life with limited activity if injury or illness keeps the sinus node and atrial tissue from functioning properly. Patients with junctional rhythms often don't realize that they have a heart rhythm problem until it shows up on the ECG. Junctional rhythm, especially at rates in the 50s, often allows people to perform normal daily activities in the absence of other conditions, such as lung disease and other heart problems. The patient may show activity intolerance or tire easily because of the moderate drop in cardiac output caused by loss of atrial kick. However, patients often attribute these symptoms to other causes, such as a cold, excessive work, stress, or simply "getting older."

Table 12–2 gives some characteristics of junctional rhythm.

Table 12–2 Criteria for junctional rhythm

Regularity	Regular
Heart Rate	**40–60 bpm**
P-Wave	**If present, inverted in leads II, II, aVF. May precede, follow, or be buried in QRS.**
PR Interval	<0.12 seconds or not measurable
QRS Complexes	All the same shape, <0.12 seconds (three small boxes)

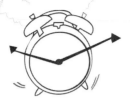

12-5 JUNCTIONAL RHYTHM OR ATRIAL FIBRILLATION?

Junctional tissue is reliable enough to generate a regular rhythm in most cases. That's important to remember. The rhythm most often confused with junctional rhythm is atrial fibrillation. When you think about it, it's easy to understand why. P-waves can be invisible in both rhythms, and both rhythms have normal-looking QRS complexes and T-waves. The key difference, therefore, is regularity. If a rhythm is regular without any visible P-waves, it's considered junctional. If a rhythm is irregularly irregular with no discernible P-waves, it's considered atrial fibrillation, which we discussed in Chapter 11.

Figure 12–9 allows you to compare atrial fibrillation, with an average ventricular response of 55 bpm (Fig. 12–9A), and junctional rhythm with approximately the same rate (Fig. 12–9B). Notice that the most obvious difference is the lack of regularity in Figure 12–9A.

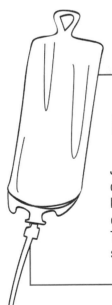

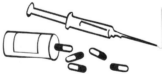

12-6 Increase the Heart Rate

Junctional rhythm may produce symptoms related to decreased cardiac output, caused by both the slower intrinsic rate and the loss of atrial kick. The most common symptoms of junctional rhythm are hypotension, chest pain, altered level of consciousness, and shortness of breath. Treatment, if warranted, is directed at increasing heart rate, or restoring sinus rhythm; which should alleviate most if not all of these symptoms.

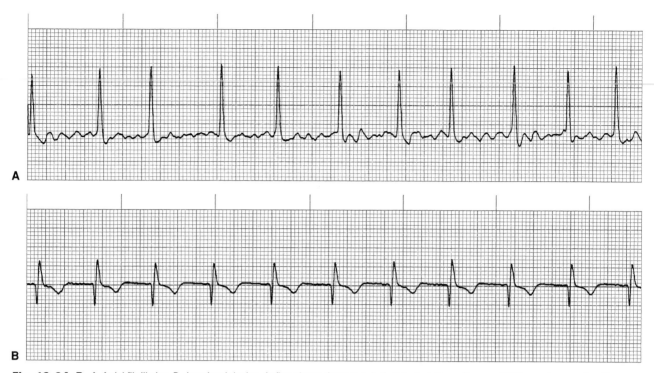

Fig. 12–9A–B A, Atrial fibrillation. B, Junctional rhythm. At first glance these two rhythms look similar, with normal QRS complexes and no P-waves. Closer inspection reveals the major difference: atrial fibrillation is irregularly irregular, whereas junctional rhythm is regular.

Accelerated Junctional Rhythm

NOT A LONG-TERM OPTION?

Accelerated junctional rhythm often develops in patients with a normal AV node when they lose faster pacemakers. A junctional escape rhythm is a good life-sustaining device to have around in case the sinus node and atrial tissue fail. The drawback is that junctional rhythms don't preserve atrial kick. Some patients, especially elderly people or those with pre-existing coronary artery disease or heart damage, need their normal cardiac output to survive. Losing atrial kick is not a viable option for them, even in the short term.

Remember, though, increasing stroke volume isn't the only way for the heart to maintain cardiac output. Another

way is to increase heart rate. The junctional tissue is being stimulated with *catecholamines,* which the body can use to increase heart rate if cardiac output is low. Acceleration of the heart rate makes up, at least partially, for the lost atrial kick and increases cardiac output back to life-sustaining levels.

In accelerated junctional rhythm, the heart rate stays above 60 bpm and below 100 bpm but retains the characteristic P-waves of junctional rhythms (Figs. 12–10, 12–11). Because this rate is faster than normal for the AV node tissue but not fast enough to be considered tachycardia, we need a more specific name than "junctional rhythm." The new name, accelerated junctional rhythm, tells us that the rate is faster than normal for the junctional tissue but not "too fast."

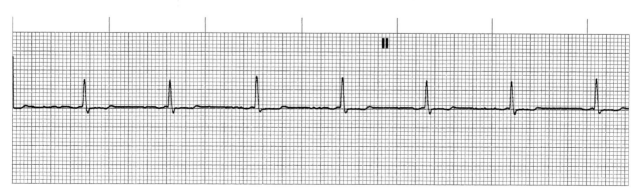

Fig. 12–10 Accelerated junctional rhythm with P-waves.

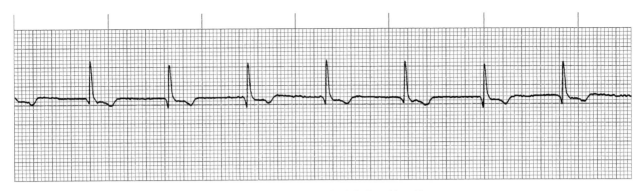

Fig. 12–11 Accelerated junctional rhythm without P-waves.

Except for the rate, all features of accelerated junctional rhythm are the same as in junctional rhythm. The P-wave, if present, is inverted in the inferior leads (leads II, III, and aVF); the PR interval is short, less than 0.12 seconds; and the QRS complex is normal. Table 12–3 lists some criteria for accelerated junctional rhythm.

KEEPING UP THE GOOD WORK

Because accelerated junctional rhythm compensates for a decreased cardiac output and because junctional tissue is reliable in maintaining heart rate and regularity, the patient often needs no treatment. In fact, most patients rarely need intervention of any kind. This rhythm shows

that the heart recognizes the low cardiac output as a problem and responds appropriately. This rhythm can easily remain undetected because the increased heart rate makes up for the loss in stroke volume. That's how the body is supposed to work.

If the cause of the sinus node dysfunction can be corrected, that's ideal, of course. If not, the patient is usually monitored fairly closely by a cardiac specialist to make sure the junctional tissue "keeps up the good work."

Junctional Bradycardia

On the other end of the heart rate spectrum is junctional bradycardia (Fig. 12–12). As we saw in Chapter 8, the term *bradycardia* describes a heart rate slower than the intrinsic rate for the tissue generating the rhythm. Therefore, junctional bradycardia represents a rhythm that originates in the AV node but has an abnormally slow rate for this tissue.

Unlike junctional and accelerated junctional rhythms, junctional bradycardia is usually poorly tolerated. The heart rate is less than 40 bpm, and cardiac output suffers the double insult of low heart rate and decreased stroke volume from lost atrial kick. The symptoms are the same as in other bradycardias: hypotension, confusion, chest pain, and diaphoresis (sweating). This dysrhythmia can

Table 12–3 Criteria for accelerated junctional rhythm

Regularity	Regular
Heart Rate	61–99 bpm
P-Wave	If present, inverted in leads II, II, and aVF. May precede, follow, or be buried in QRS.
PR Interval	<0.12 seconds or not measurable
QRS Complexes	All the same shape, <0.12 seconds (three small boxes)

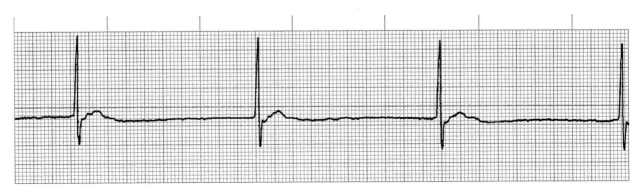

Fig. 12–12 Junctional bradycardia.

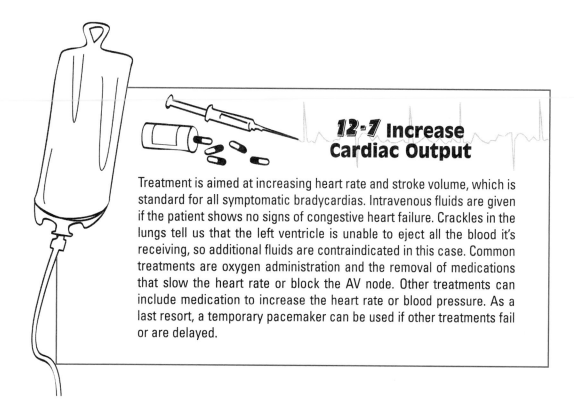

12-7 Increase Cardiac Output

Treatment is aimed at increasing heart rate and stroke volume, which is standard for all symptomatic bradycardias. Intravenous fluids are given if the patient shows no signs of congestive heart failure. Crackles in the lungs tell us that the left ventricle is unable to eject all the blood it's receiving, so additional fluids are contraindicated in this case. Common treatments are oxygen administration and the removal of medications that slow the heart rate or block the AV node. Other treatments can include medication to increase the heart rate or blood pressure. As a last resort, a temporary pacemaker can be used if other treatments fail or are delayed.

occur in digoxin toxicity and acute MI and frequently resolves when these conditions are corrected.

In junctional bradycardia, the heart isn't responding appropriately to the decrease in cardiac output associated with all junctional rhythms. This rhythm indicates significant heart dysfunction. Junctional bradycardia is the most dangerous junctional rhythm because heart rate and stroke volume both decrease severely. Table 12–4 lists some of its characteristics.

All the interventions listed in Box 12–7 above are brief at best. The external pacemaker is temporary because the electricity is generated outside the body, and increased risks have been associated with this method of pacing. The medications are short term because they are rapidly metabolized and can be given only intravenously. We'd have to medicate our patient through an IV site dozens of times a day or else give a continuous drip—clearly an impractical solution for life outside the hospital. Therefore, if the cause can't be corrected (if the patient had a significant MI, for instance) or if you can reasonably expect it to recur, the patient will need a permanent pacemaker.

Junctional Tachycardia

A FAMILIAR RHYTHM

Junctional tachycardia is one of the more common tachy-dysrhythmias. It's responsible for about 30% of supraventricular tachycardias. Junctional tachycardia often occurs

Table 12–4 Criteria for junctional bradycardia

Regularity	Regular
Heart Rate	<40 bpm
P-Wave	If present, inverted in leads II, II, aVF. May precede, follow, or be buried in QRS.
PR Interval	<0.12 seconds or not measurable.
QRS Complexes	All the same shape, <0.12 seconds (three small boxes)

in patients with digoxin toxicity or a digoxin level significantly above the normal therapeutic range. Hypokalemia, a low potassium level, can worsen the symptoms of digoxin toxicity.

Although junctional tachycardia can have a rate as low as 100 bpm, it usually ranges between 130 and 180. Many clinicians actually classify junctional rhythms with heart rates up to 130 as accelerated junctional rhythms. Their rationale is that, in patients who normally have sinus rhythm in the 90s, the junctional tissue needs to accelerate to more than 100 to maintain cardiac output. For our purposes, however, 100 is the beginning rate for junctional tachycardia.

When we see a case of atrial tachycardia at heart rates between 100 and 160 bpm, we may have trouble differentiating between atrial and sinus P-waves. Therefore, atrial rhythms in this range are normally designated sinus tachycardia. However, we usually don't have this problem with junctional rhythms in a similar range. The P-waves of junctional rhythm are easily differentiated from sinus P-waves, particularly at slower rates. Also, a regular rhythm at this accelerated rate is considered junctional, particularly if no P-waves are found in lead II. Therefore, junctional rhythms between 100 and 140 should be easily identifiable.

Table 12–5 lists some characteristics of junctional tachycardia.

Table 12–5 Criteria for junctional tachycardia

Regularity	Regular
Heart Rate	**100–180 bpm**
P-Wave	**If present, inverted in leads II, II, aVF. May precede, follow, or be buried in QRS.**
PR Interval	<0.12 seconds or not measurable
QRS Complexes	All the same shape, <0.12 seconds (three small boxes)

TREAT FIRST, IDENTIFY LATER

The symptoms of junctional tachycardia are the same as those of sinus and atrial tachycardia: syncope, nausea, dizziness, and hypotension. They usually reflect pre-existing cardiac problems as well as the ventricular rate.

Above 140 bpm, atrial or sinus P-waves may be buried in the previous T-wave, and therefore the rhythm can be mistaken for junctional tachycardia. However, this doesn't affect treatment. The Advanced Cardiac Life Support guidelines treat all regular, narrow–QRS-complex tachycardias alike, whether the rhythm is sinus, atrial, or junctional tachycardia, with the exception of atrial fibrillation and atrial flutter, which warrant their own treatment.

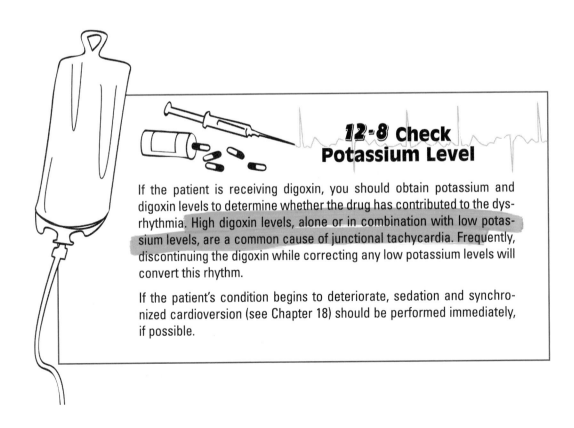

12-8 Check Potassium Level

If the patient is receiving digoxin, you should obtain potassium and digoxin levels to determine whether the drug has contributed to the dysrhythmia. High digoxin levels, alone or in combination with low potassium levels, are a common cause of junctional tachycardia. Frequently, discontinuing the digoxin while correcting any low potassium levels will convert this rhythm.

If the patient's condition begins to deteriorate, sedation and synchronized cardioversion (see Chapter 18) should be performed immediately, if possible.

Therefore, treatment shouldn't be delayed just to find out which type of supraventricular tachycardia the patient has, especially if significant symptoms are present. Most treatments that work for one rhythm will work for the others.

Supraventricular Tachycardia: An Easy Way Out

What happens if we think the rhythm has P-waves but we're not sure? What if the heart rate is too fast to even guess? A 12-lead ECG can help sometimes because it can use computer algorithms to identify P-waves that mere mortals can't pick up. But even with all of this technology, we still run into a lot of very fast rhythms we can't identify. Is it sinus tachycardia, atrial tachycardia, multifocal atrial tachycardia, atrial fibrillation, or junctional tachycardia? Sometimes the only thing we know for sure is that the heart rate is too fast.

In these cases we have a cop-out: supraventricular tachycardia (SVT). Although some clinicians believe the term SVT has a specific definition, the SVT designation in rhythm analysis can be used for rhythms that are hard to distinguish because the heart rate is fast or the P-waves are hard to identify. Figure 12–13 shows three examples of SVT.

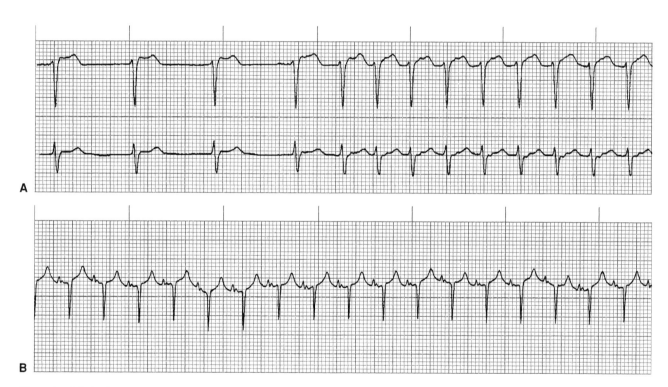

Fig. 12–13A–B Supraventricular tachycardia can come in all shapes and sizes. A, Junctional tachycardia. B, Atrial tachycardia. C, Sinus tachycardia. In all three strips, the QRS complex begins in the AV node.

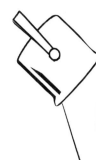

Now You Know

The AV node can take over as pacemaker if it becomes irritated or if the sinus node and atrial tissue fail.

The intrinsic rate for junctional tissue is 40 to 60 bpm.

Because the intrinsic rate of junctional tissue reduces atrial kick, it's important to increase the heart rate in junctional rhythms.

Junctional P-waves can occur before, during, or after the QRS complex. The PR interval should be less than 0.12 seconds.

Junctional P-waves occur only because the signal travels backward through the atria.

If the atria don't depolarize, or depolarize at the same time as the ventricles, there are no visible P-waves.

"Supraventricular tachycardia" is a generic term for any fast rhythm initiated in the sinus node, atrial tissue, or AV node and can be used when a more definitive name can't be obtained.

Test Yourself

1. The main difference among sinus rhythms, atrial rhythms, and junctional rhythms is found in the _____.

2. The main similarity among sinus rhythms, atrial rhythms, and junctional rhythms is found in the _____.

3. The PR interval in junctional rhythms, if measurable, should be less than _____.

4. An important distinction between atrial fibrillation and junctional rhythm is whether or not the rhythm is _____.

5. _____ is the generic term for all rhythms faster than ____ and originating in the sinus node, atrial tissue, or AV node.

6. To compensate for the loss of atrial kick, _____ is the preferred junctional rhythm in most cases.

7. The P-wave in lead II is always _____ in junctional rhythms.

8. _____ PJCs have P-waves that look the same but appear in different locations relative to the QRS complex.

9. The intrinsic rate for junctional tissue is ___ to ___ bpm.

10. Identify the rhythm in the following thirty strips:

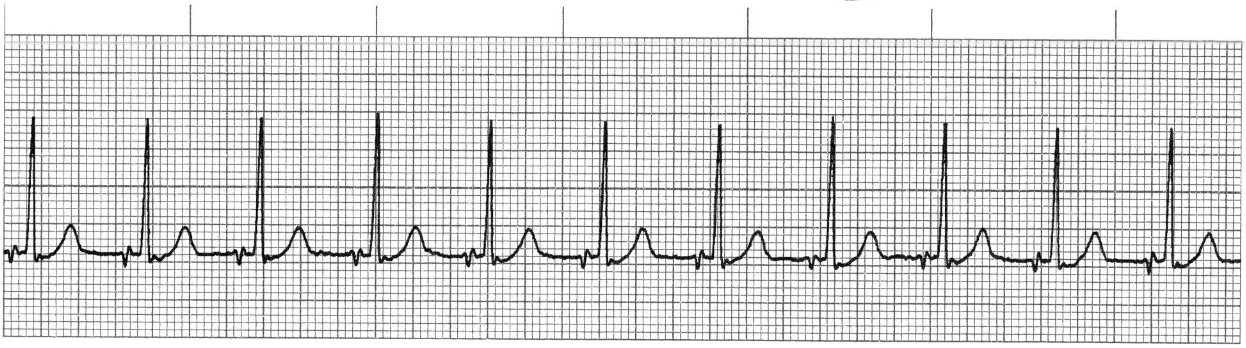

12–1

Regularity: _____ Heart rate: _____ PR interval: _____

P-waves: _____ QRS complex: _____

Interpretation: _____

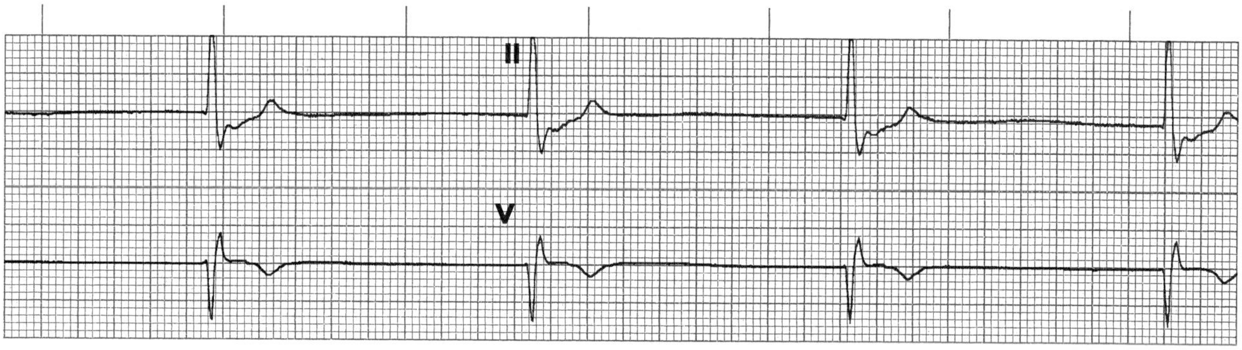

12–2

Regularity: _____ Heart rate: _____ PR interval: _____

P-waves: _____ QRS complex: _____

Interpretation: _____

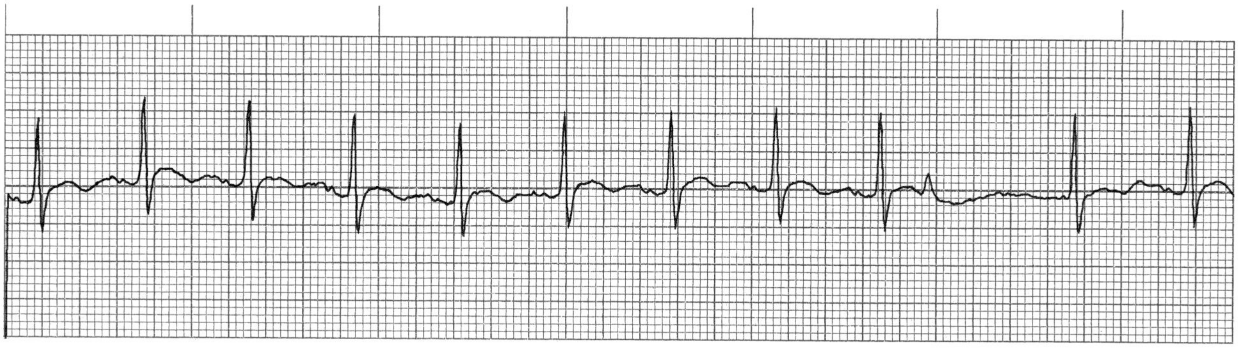

12–3

Regularity: _____ Heart rate: _____ PR interval: _____

P-waves: _____ QRS complex: _____

Interpretation: _____

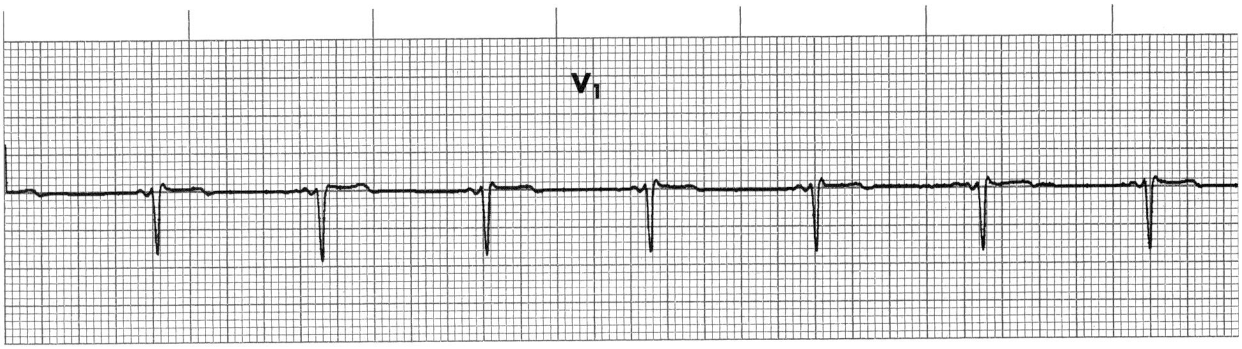

Junctional Rhythms

V_1

12-4

Regularity: _____ Heart rate: _____ PR interval: _____

P-waves: _____ QRS complex: _____

Interpretation: _____

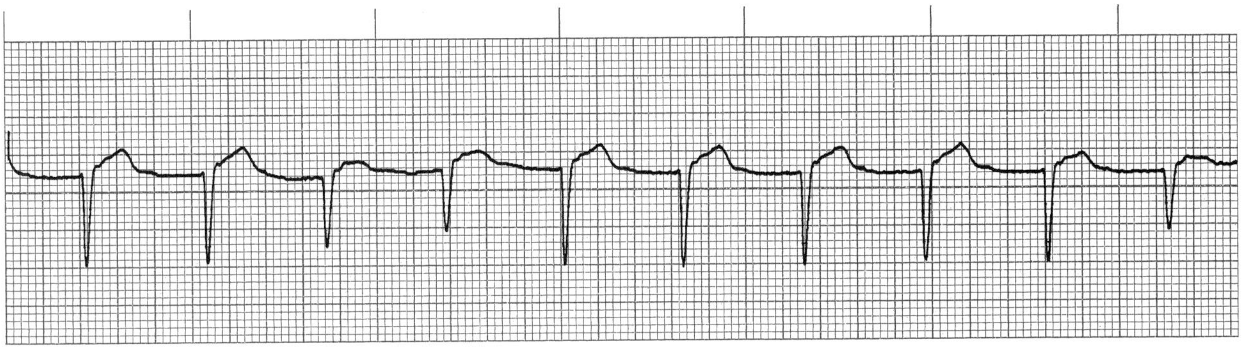

12-5

Regularity: _____ Heart rate: _____ PR interval: _____

P-waves: _____ QRS complex: _____

Interpretation: _____

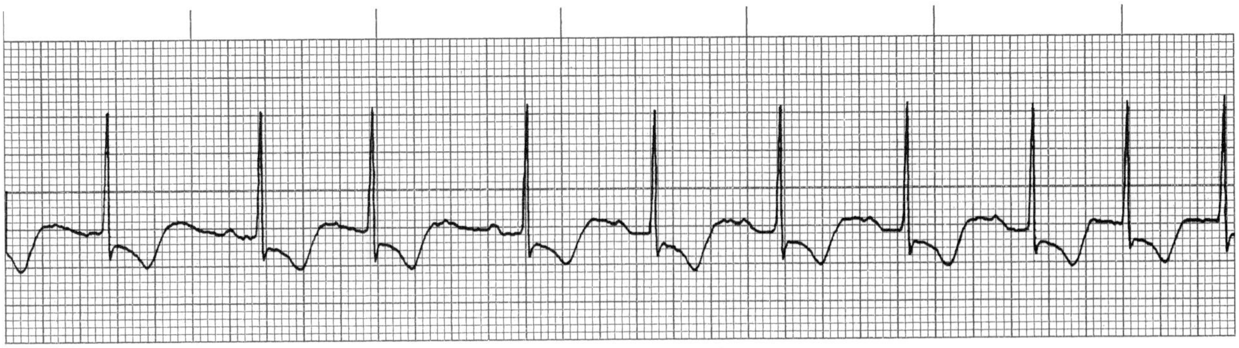

12-6

Regularity: _____ Heart rate: _____ PR interval: _____

P-waves: _____ QRS complex: _____

Interpretation: _____

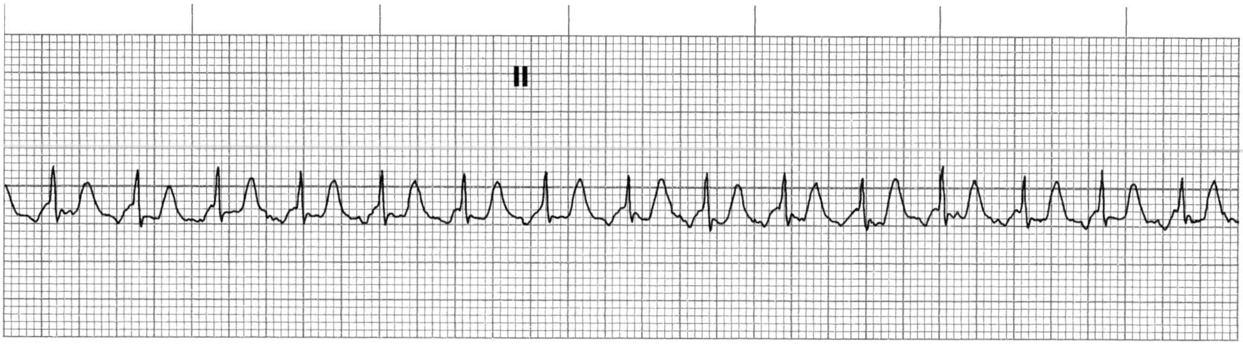

12–7

Regularity: _____ Heart rate: _____ PR interval: _____

P-waves: _____ QRS complex: _____

Interpretation: _____

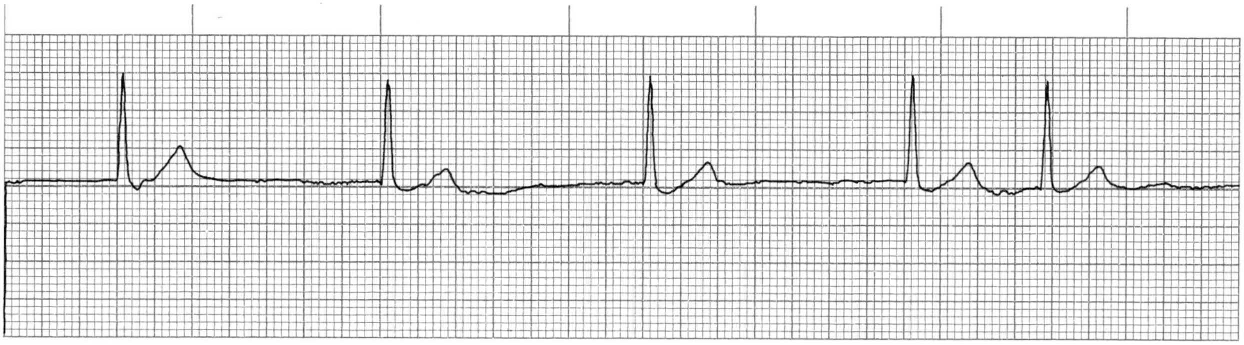

12–8

Regularity: _____ Heart rate: _____ PR interval: _____

P-waves: _____ QRS complex: _____

Interpretation: _____

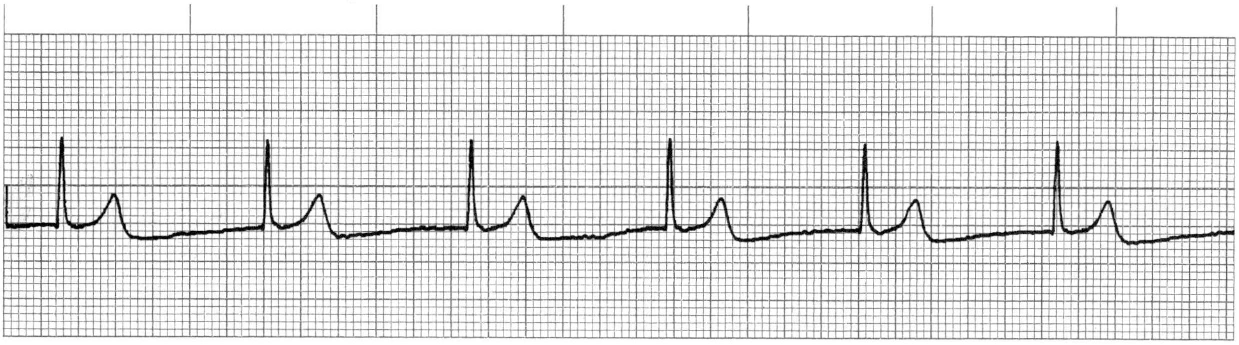

12–9

Regularity: _____ Heart rate: _____ PR interval: _____

P-waves: _____ QRS complex: _____

Interpretation: _____

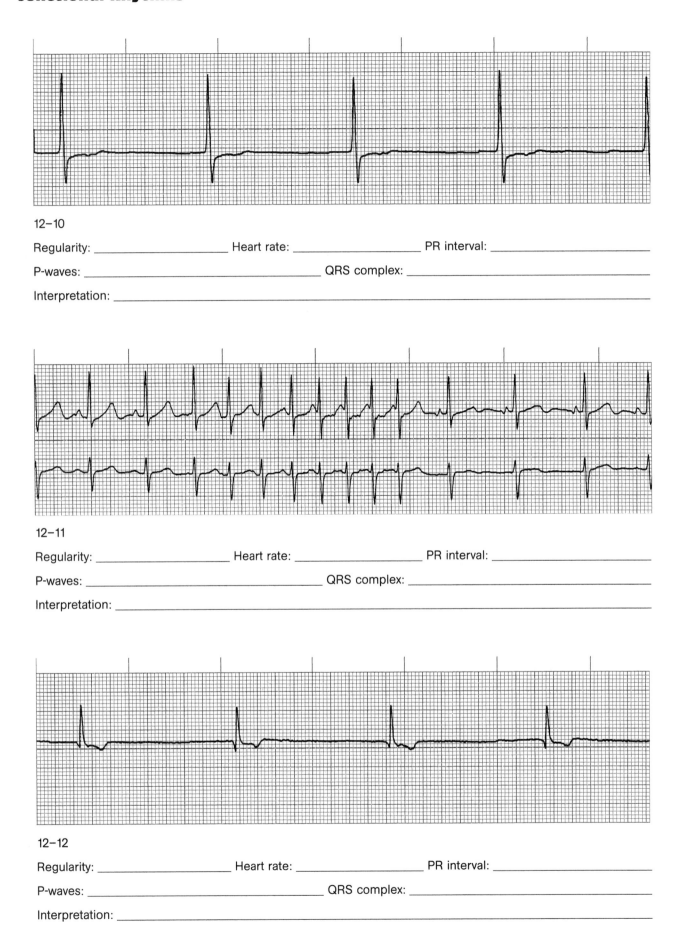

12–10

Regularity: _____ Heart rate: _____ PR interval: _____

P-waves: _____ QRS complex: _____

Interpretation: _____

12–11

Regularity: _____ Heart rate: _____ PR interval: _____

P-waves: _____ QRS complex: _____

Interpretation: _____

12–12

Regularity: _____ Heart rate: _____ PR interval: _____

P-waves: _____ QRS complex: _____

Interpretation: _____

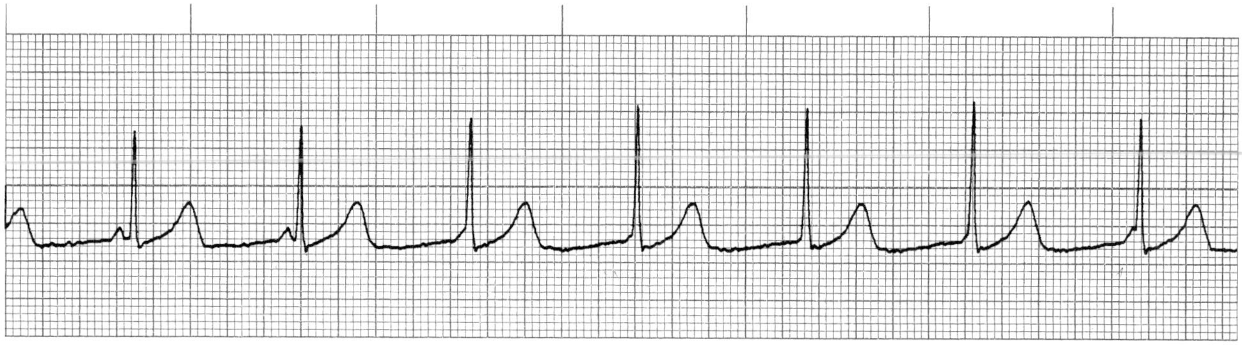

12–13

Regularity: _____ Heart rate: _____ PR interval: _____

P-waves: _____ QRS complex: _____

Interpretation: _____

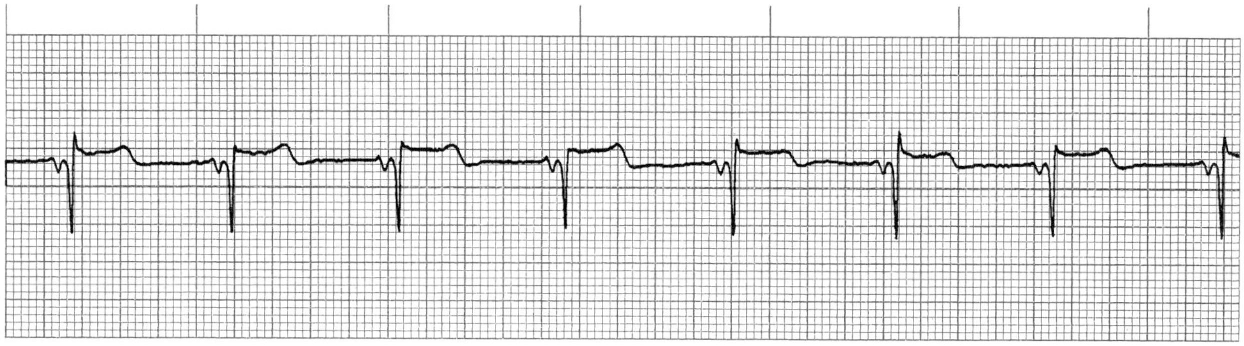

12–14

Regularity: _____ Heart rate: _____ PR interval: _____

P-waves: _____ QRS complex: _____

Interpretation: _____

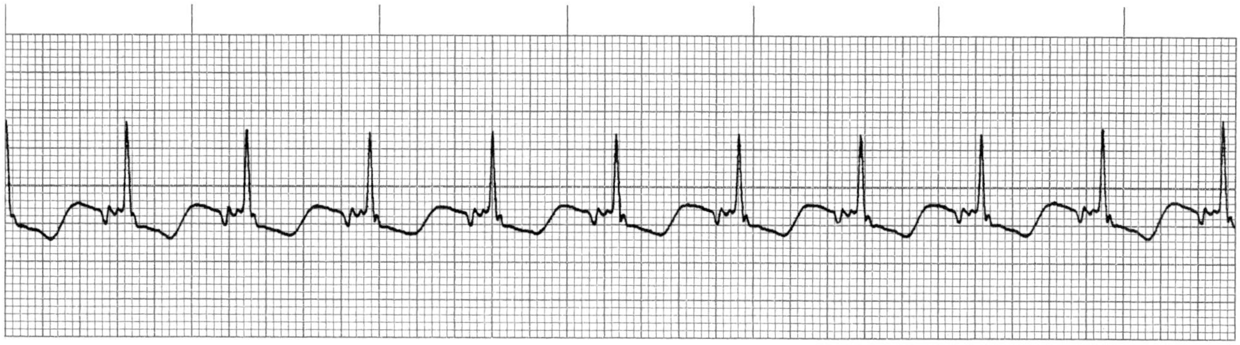

12–15

Regularity: _____ Heart rate: _____ PR interval: _____

P-waves: _____ QRS complex: _____

Interpretation: _____

Junctional Rhythms

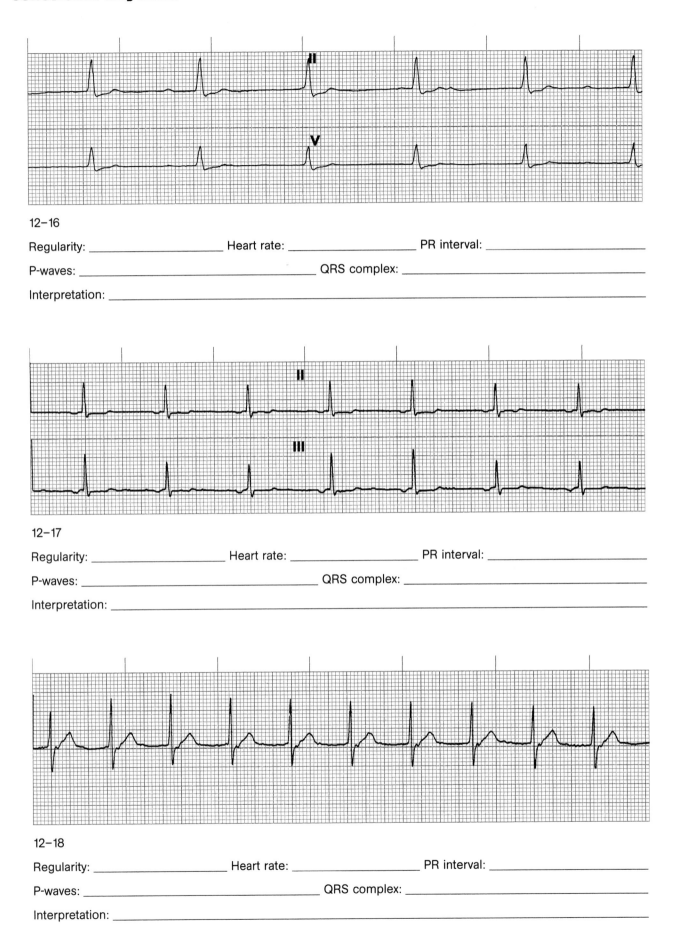

12–16

Regularity: _____ Heart rate: _____ PR interval: _____

P-waves: _____ QRS complex: _____

Interpretation: _____

12–17

Regularity: _____ Heart rate: _____ PR interval: _____

P-waves: _____ QRS complex: _____

Interpretation: _____

12–18

Regularity: _____ Heart rate: _____ PR interval: _____

P-waves: _____ QRS complex: _____

Interpretation: _____

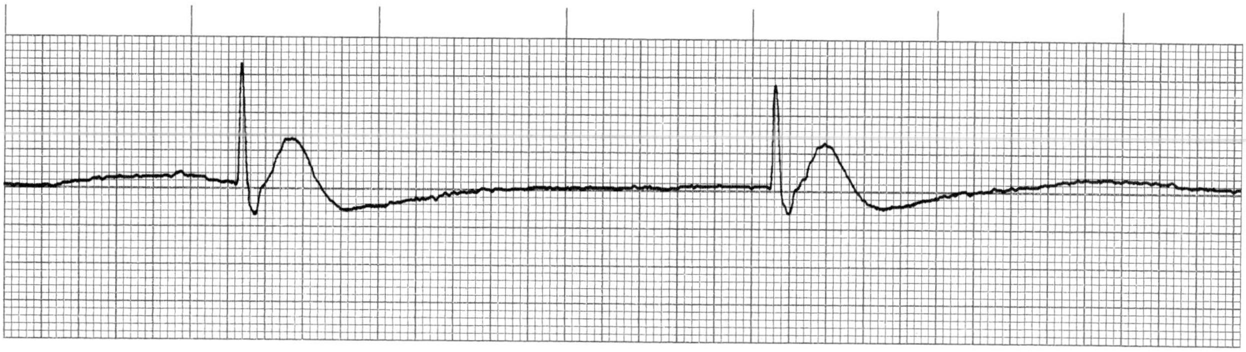

12–19

Regularity: _____ Heart rate: _____ PR interval: _____

P-waves: _____ QRS complex: _____

Interpretation: _____

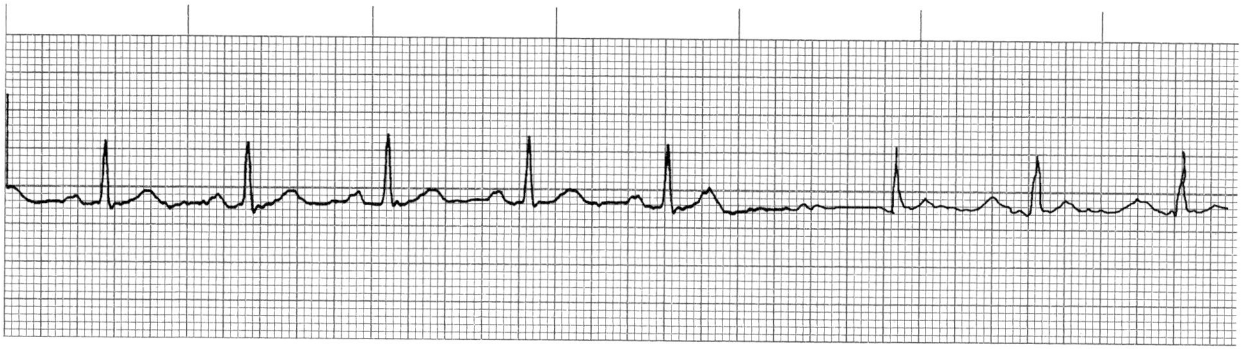

12–20

Regularity: _____ Heart rate: _____ PR interval: _____

P-waves: _____ QRS complex: _____

Interpretation: _____

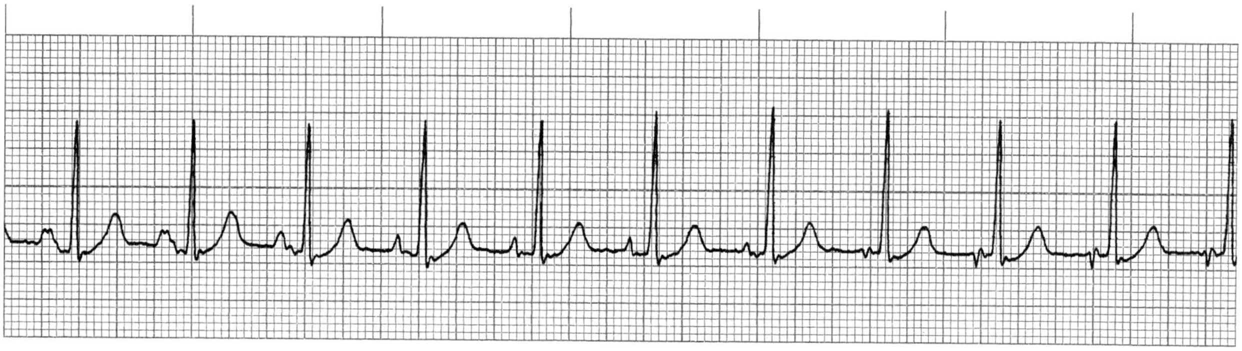

12–21

Regularity: _____ Heart rate: _____ PR interval: _____

P-waves: _____ QRS complex: _____

Interpretation: _____

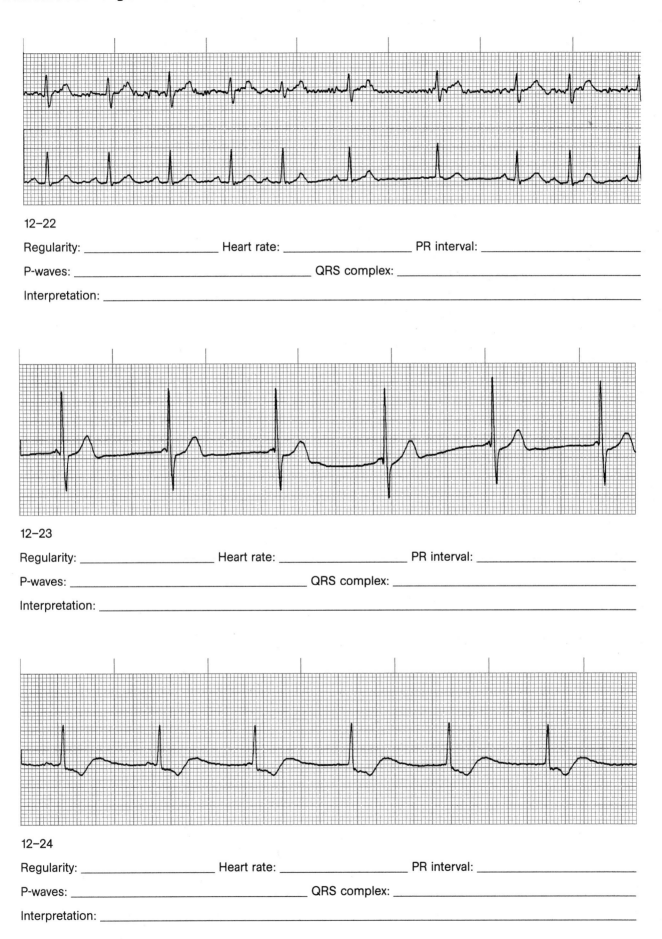

12–22

Regularity: _____ Heart rate: _____ PR interval: _____

P-waves: _____ QRS complex: _____

Interpretation: _____

12–23

Regularity: _____ Heart rate: _____ PR interval: _____

P-waves: _____ QRS complex: _____

Interpretation: _____

12–24

Regularity: _____ Heart rate: _____ PR interval: _____

P-waves: _____ QRS complex: _____

Interpretation: _____

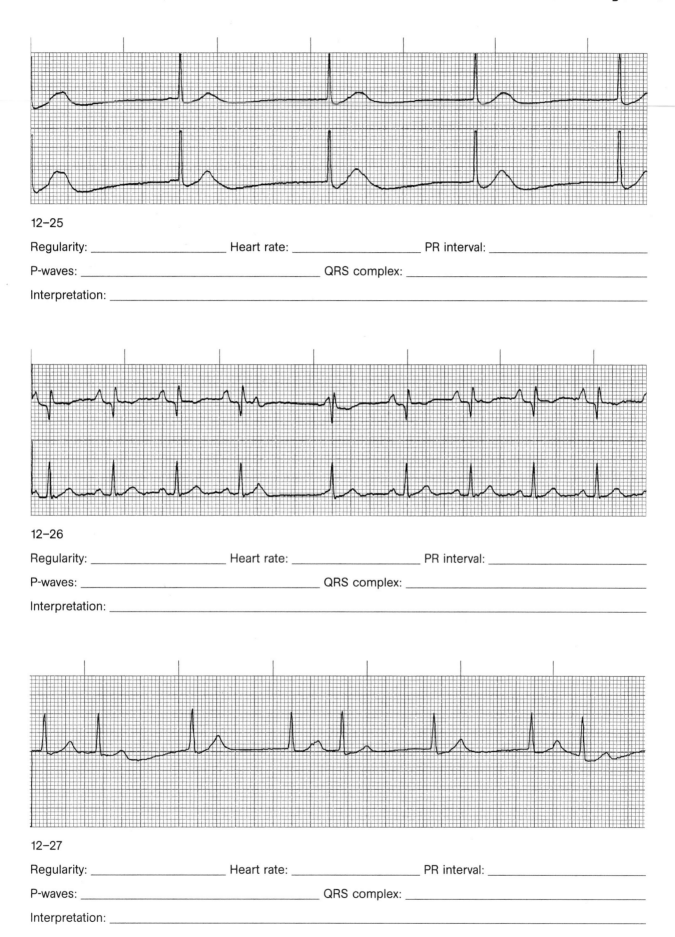

12–25

Regularity: _____ Heart rate: _____ PR interval: _____

P-waves: _____ QRS complex: _____

Interpretation: _____

12–26

Regularity: _____ Heart rate: _____ PR interval: _____

P-waves: _____ QRS complex: _____

Interpretation: _____

12–27

Regularity: _____ Heart rate: _____ PR interval: _____

P-waves: _____ QRS complex: _____

Interpretation: _____

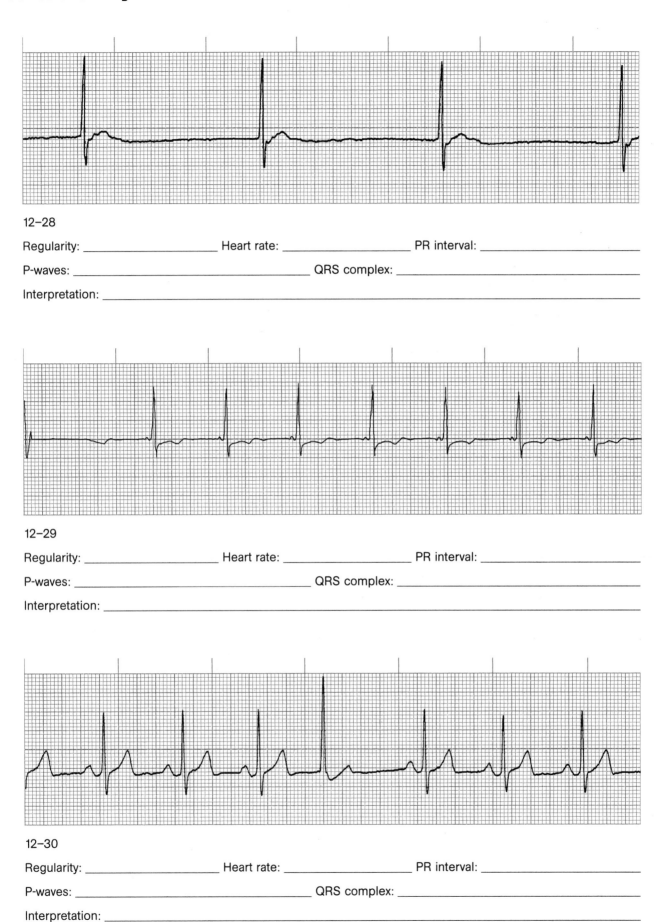

12–28

Regularity: _____ Heart rate: _____ PR interval: _____

P-waves: _____ QRS complex: _____

Interpretation: _____

12–29

Regularity: _____ Heart rate: _____ PR interval: _____

P-waves: _____ QRS complex: _____

Interpretation: _____

12–30

Regularity: _____ Heart rate: _____ PR interval: _____

P-waves: _____ QRS complex: _____

Interpretation: _____

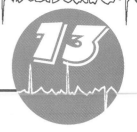

VENTRICULAR RHYTHMS

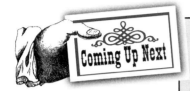

In Revolt

The role of the government is to protect the people and serve their needs. Sometimes the government does the right thing regardless of public opinion, as Abraham Lincoln did with the Emancipation Proclamation. At other times the government goes wrong, supporting racial discrimination or taxation without representation. Then it's the duty of the citizens to rise up and revolt, to take

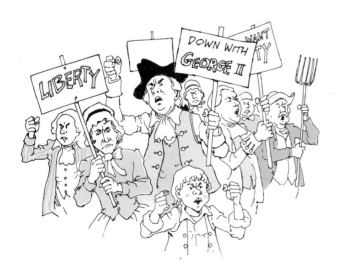

matters into their own hands despite the government's dictates. American history is full of such examples, from the Boston Tea Party to Martin Luther King and Rosa Parks.

In the heart, the pacemaker sites govern. They protect the heart from stopping and they maintain cardiac output to supply the cardiac cells with oxygen. The "people" of the heart are the cells in the ventricles. If all other pacemakers fail in the role of leader, the ventricular tissue can take control of the heart rhythm. As with all pacemakers, the result can be good or bad. Either way, government by "the people" isn't reliable in the long term because it can cause harm and reduce the efficiency of the systems it's trying to run.

Ventricular rhythms differ significantly from the supraventricular rhythms we've focused on up to this point. Let's take a little time to revisit conduction through the ventricles.

From Highways to Back Roads

THE USUAL ROUTE

Back in Chapter 7 we discussed how the ventricles are depolarized. The signal leaves the AV node and travels

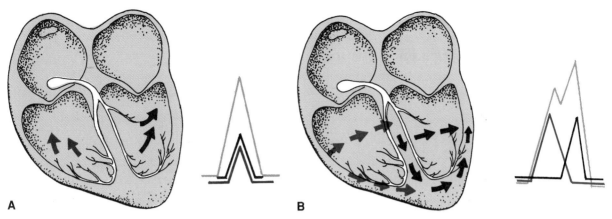

Fig. 13–1A–B QRS complex width depends on whether the left and right ventricles depolarize simultaneously or consecutively. A, Normal depolarization via the bundle branches. B, Depolarization initiated in the ventricles.

through the bundle of His, which delivers the signal to the left and right bundle branches. They in turn divide into smaller and smaller pieces, eventually becoming terminal Purkinje fibers. These fibers are the spark plugs of the conduction system: they deliver the signal to the individual cells of the ventricles, and the ventricles then contract.

This delivery system is designed to send nearly simultaneous signals to the left and right ventricles. As a result, the two QRS complexes (one for each ventricle) occur together, overlap each other, and merge into one QRS of the expected duration, less than 0.12 seconds.

THE BACK ROAD

Sometimes the depolarization of the heart *begins* in the ventricles instead of ending there. What happens to the QRS complex then? Well, the most obvious result is that its duration changes. This happens because the bundle branches are designed to receive the signal from the AV node, not the ventricles. Therefore, if ventricular depolarization begins outside the bundle branches, the signal can't travel its normal "fast" path through the ventricles.

Figure 13–1A shows the heart depolarizing normally, using the bundle branches. Notice that the two individual QRS complexes, one red and the other blue, occur simultaneously and merge to form the narrow QRS that appears on the ECG strip. In Figure 13–1B, however, the two individual QRS complexes, again red and blue, occur sequentially, merging to form a much wider QRS. That wide QRS is the hallmark of ventricular depolarization.

Let's return to our highway analogy. If we think of the bundle branches as intraventricular highways, ventricular

rhythms take the back roads, with all the stop signs, traffic lights, and twists and turns that invariably delay the signal's reaching its destination.

Why Use the Back Roads?

If you're trying to get somewhere and your normal route is closed, do you turn and go home? Not if getting to your destination is important enough. Getting the depolarization signal to all the ventricular tissue is the most important function of the conduction system; if the ventricles don't pump the blood they receive, the patient will die.

Ventricular rhythms can have many causes. One is increased irritability, or increased automaticity, which we encountered in the supraventricular rhythm chapters. In this case, the higher pacemaker foci are *able* to control the heart but the ventricular tissue is discharging at an abnormally fast rate and therefore control the heart. Increased irritability can result from lack of oxygen, blocked coronary arteries, or poor lung function; chemical influences such as nicotine, cocaine, and caffeine; medications; or shortened action potential of the ventricular cells (see Chapter 2).

Another cause of ventricular rhythms is the failure of higher (supraventricular) pacemakers. Sometimes the sinus node, atrial tissue, and junctional tissue all fail to generate a signal, and sometimes they send a signal that never reaches the ventricular tissue. Without that higher pacemaker, the ventricular tissue must generate its own signal or the patient will die.

A major cause of ventricular irritability is acute myocardial infarction (MI). When one or more coronary arteries are blocked, the ventricular tissue doesn't get enough

13-1 Psst, Pass It On

If you want to make a single announcement to a large group of people, the easiest way to do it is over a loudspeaker system. That way everyone receives the message nearly simultaneously. But what happens if the system is broken? Does the message not get out to anyone? It may not, and if the message is as important as the signal telling the ventricles to depolarize, that just won't do.

You can still transmit the message to everyone, although much more slowly than you could over the loudspeaker. Just tell it to all the people standing near you. Then these people can all pass the message to whoever's standing next to them, and so on.

This process goes on until everyone has received the message. It's taken much longer to transmit the message to everyone in the room, but the important point is that everyone heard it. Using the loudspeaker to get the message out is more efficient, but if that doesn't work—psst, pass it on.

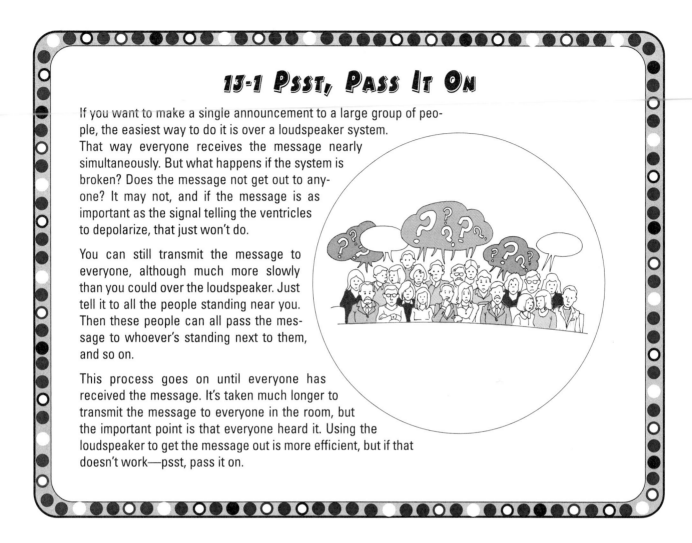

oxygen to function properly. An oxygen-starved heart behaves like an oxygen-starved car engine—it sputters, lacks power, and runs with gross inefficiency.

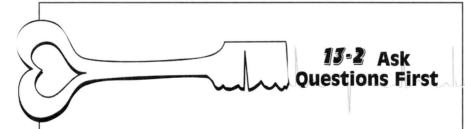

13-2 Ask Questions First

The cause of a ventricular rhythm can determine the way it's treated. For instance, if all higher pacemakers have failed, don't administer medications to get rid of the ventricular rhythm, such as lidocaine. This drug, which makes it more difficult for the ventricular tissue to spontaneously discharge, could prove deadly.

However, if the ventricular rhythm is replacing a normally functioning supraventricular pacemaker, lidocaine may slow the ventricular discharge rate enough to allow the higher pacemaker to take over again. We'll discuss different treatments as we go over each type of rhythm.

Premature Ventricular Contraction

WIDE AND BIZARRE

Weird Interruptions The most common manifestation of ventricular irritability is premature ventricular complexes (PVC). Like their supraventricular brethren, PVCs interrupt the regularity of a rhythm because they occur earlier than they should. However, they look vastly different from supraventricular premature beats such as premature atrial complexes (PAC) and premature junctional complexes (PJC): they're wider than normal and bizarre in shape, with T-waves in the opposite direction of the QRS complex. Table 13–1 lists the criteria for PVCs.

Ventricular Rhythms

Table 13–1 Criteria for premature ventricular contraction

Regularity	Regular except for premature beats
Heart Rate	Any rate
P-Wave	If present, not related to QRS complex
PR Interval	Not measurable
QRS Complex	**Different from supraventricular QRS morphology, ≥ 0.12 sec (3 small boxes).**

Because the signal begins outside the bundle branches, the coordination of the ventricles is lost. That leaves us with a wider than normal QRS complex (in Chap. 15 we'll discover another reason for wide QRS complexes). A wide QRS tells us that the signal didn't follow the normal path through the ventricles. In ventricular rhythms, that happens because the signal originated in the ventricles, outside the fast pathways of the AV node and bundle branches.

If you examine the QRS complex in Figure 13–1B, you'll notice that the total QRS generated by the PVC is different in size than the QRS in which the signal followed the bundle branch path. The QRS can be unusually tall, unusually short, or nearly normal in height—that depends on the lead and on the location of the tissue causing the PVC—but will never look the way it would have if the signal had followed the normal conduction pathways.

Leaning in One Direction Remember the vector discussion back in Chapter 4? In an ECG tracing, the QRS com-

plex represents the average vector formed by the depolarization of both ventricles. Figure 13–2A shows that the signal traveled partly toward the positive patch and partly toward the negative patch in lead I and that both ventricles received the signal nearly simultaneously.

In a PVC, however, the ventricles receive the signal in succession, not together. Figure 13–2B shows what happens when the signal begins in the right ventricle: most of it travels toward the positive patch in lead I, causing a positive deflection on the ECG tracing. The average QRS vector is larger than normal because more of the signal is traveling toward the positive patch than toward the negative.

P-WAVES IN YOUR PVCs

In the last chapter we discussed retrograde impulse transmission, the backward movement of the signal from the AV node to the atrial tissue. As we've seen, the AV node depolarization can generate P-waves when the signal travels backward up to the atria. This can also happen with PVCs, or with any ventricular rhythm for that matter. The signal travels from the ventricular focus to the AV node, and from there up into the atria. These P-waves are inverted in lead II and occur during or after the QRS complex; the speed of the retrograde impulse transmission determines the sequence. Although there are inverted P-waves in lead II in both PJCs and PVCs, the width of the QRS makes differentiating them relatively easy.

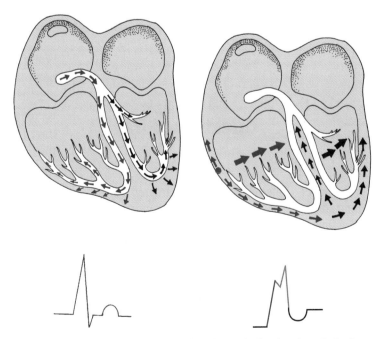

Fig. 13–2A–B QRS complex size depends on the starting location of ventricular depolarization and the lead being viewed. A, Normal depolarization. B, Ventricular depolarization.

13-3 CUTTING THROUGH TERMINOLOGY

Like all the other premature beats we've discussed, PVCs can come occasionally, frequently, or at regular intervals in a specific pattern. If every other beat is a PVC, we have a pattern of bigeminal PVCs: two beats, one normal and one abnormal, in a repeating cycle. We find similar repeating patterns in PACs and PJCs. However, when we name these repeating patterns in ventricular rhythms, we often leave out the "PVC" part. Therefore, the term "bigeminy" used alone refers to PVCs, not to PACs or PJCs. It does make sense to depart from convention: PVCs are usually more dangerous than premature supraventricular beats and therefore are discussed more often.

A pattern of two normal beats followed by a PVC is called "trigeminy." Figure 13–3 shows an example of sinus rhythm with trigeminy: two regular sinus beats followed by one abnormal beat, the PVC. As with bigeminy, it's acceptable to use the term "sinus rhythm with trigeminal PVCs," but the abbreviated terminology is more common.

A PVC occurs before it's supposed to, which means the sinus node hasn't depolarized yet. When the PVC signal reaches the sinus node, it depolarizes the node, resetting it just as if the sinus node had discharged itself. When tissue is reset before it's had a chance to depolarize, we refer to *overdrive suppression.* The tissue is prevented (suppressed) from depolarizing because some other tissue is depolarizing faster (overdrive). Score another victory for "fastest pacemaker wins."

Sometimes the ventricular signal doesn't make it up into the atria. In this case, nothing happens to reset either the sinus node or the atrial tissue. Therefore, the sinus node continues to discharge as usual, not realizing that the ventricles are doing their own thing. So now we've got two rhythms, one sinus and one ventricular. Here the P-waves are upright in lead II. The P-waves and the QRSs don't march out in unison; what's more, P-waves can occur throughout the tracing—before, during, or after the QRS or the T-wave. Therefore, it's important to look everywhere for P-waves, not just where you expect them. We'll continue our hunt for P-waves in odd locations in the next two chapters.

CHECK OUT THE T-WAVE

You can expect PVCs to stand out from the rest of the QRS complexes in the strip—think "wide and bizarre." One other feature you should notice is the T-wave. Normally, if most of the QRS is upright (particularly look at the last portion of the QRS), the T-wave will be upright; if most of the QRS is inverted, the T-wave will be inverted. This rule applies to normal rhythms, but we already know that if a beat starts in the ventricles, the rhythm is far from normal.

Whenever a beat originates in the ventricles, the T-wave moves *away from* the prevailing direction of the QRS complex. Why? Well, one thing leads to another. Because the ventricular depolarization process has been changed, it's only reasonable to expect that repolarization will be altered too.

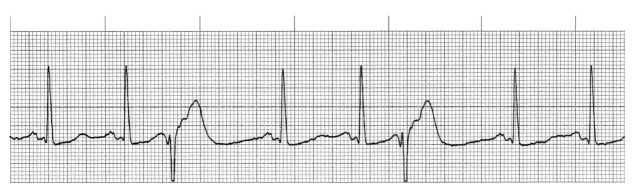

Fig. 13–3 Sinus rhythm with trigeminal PVCs. The size and shape of the QRS complex change with every third beat.

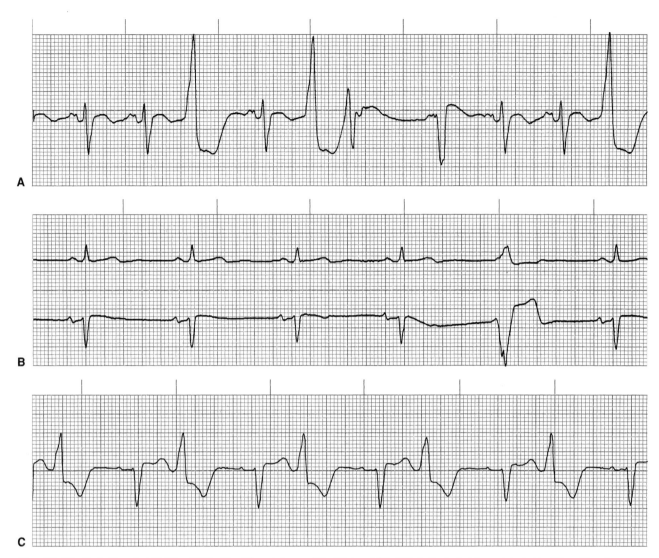

Fig. 13–4A–C A, Bigeminal Multifocal PVCs. The different shapes of the third, and fifth PVCs indicate that they originated in different locations. B, A single PVC. C, Bigeminal PVCs. The pattern of PVCs appears in every other beat.

Figure 13–4 shows three different examples of PVCs. All have wider than normal QRS complexes, a bizarre shape when compared with normal QRSs, and T-waves directed away from most of the QRS complex.

TREATING PREMATURE VENTRICULAR CONTRACTION

How do we treat PVCs? Many approaches exist, and they depend on the circumstances. To begin with, you must determine how much, if any, treatment is needed. Treatment is varied and outside the scope of this book.

Idioventricular Rhythm

What happens when the sinus node gives out, the atrial tissue doesn't pick up the slack, and the AV node fails to take control? Does the heart just stop? It very well

may if it's seriously sick, but the ventricular tissue often comes to the rescue. The intrinsic rate of ventricular tissue is very low, only 20 to 40 bpm. The slow rate, combined with the loss of atrial kick, causes a precipitous drop in cardiac output. This type of rhythm, called idioventricular rhythm, isn't something we like to see; it means that something is seriously wrong with the heart's conduction system. When the higher pacemakers fail completely, you've got a serious situation on your hands.

In idioventricular rhythm, the ventricular tissue takes over at its own intrinsic rate. The *idio-* prefix means "self," "own," or "individual." It indicates that the ventricles are depolarizing on their own, not in response to an outside stimulus as they normally would. This rhythm is dangerous because the low intrinsic discharge rate for ventricular tissue, only 20 to 40 bpm, is usually too slow to sustain life for very long.

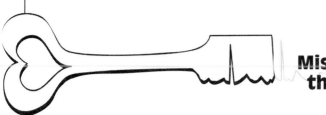

of a rhythm, not a rhythm in themselves. Table 13–2 summarizes the characteristics of idioventricular rhythm.

For treatment of idioventricular rhythms, see the section "Treating Low Cardiac Output" on page **198.**

Accelerated Idioventricular Rhythm

A ventricular escape rhythm can sustain life for a while, but the intrinsic rate of the ventricles usually can't offset the dramatic drop in cardiac output for very long. If the supraventricular pacemakers fail and the ventricles start to discharge at their intrinsic rate, the low cardiac output won't provide enough oxygen to the heart. Enter a new character, accelerated idioventricular rhythm (AIVR).

13-4 Mistreating the Heart

In the not too distant past, PVCs were considered a serious threat to the patient and were treated routinely—symptoms or not. In acute MI, a patient with more than six PVCs per minute usually received a lidocaine bolus followed by a continuous IV drip until the PVCs were suppressed. This treatment was given even if the patient had no symptoms of decreased cardiac output. In recent studies, however, patients receiving this treatment for asymptomatic PVCs were actually more likely to have cardiac complications, up to and including death, than their untreated cohorts!

Any medication has a skeleton in its closet—side effects. Even drugs we take for granted can have serious consequences. For instance, acetaminophen can cause liver failure under certain circumstances, and aspirin and ibuprofen can both cause gastrointestinal bleeding over time, even in reasonable doses. That's why we reserve aggressive treatment unless the patient's health is actually compromised by the PVCs.

This rhythm looks like a series of PVCs (Fig. 13–5), but certain clues tell us that this can't be the case. First, the rhythm is usually regular, so the beats can't be premature. Second, there's no other rhythm, and as we know, PVCs are modifiers

When the ventricular tissue becomes hypoxic, the body uses several mechanisms to stimulate the heart and increase cardiac output. One of the simpler mechanisms is an increased heart rate, which compensates for the low

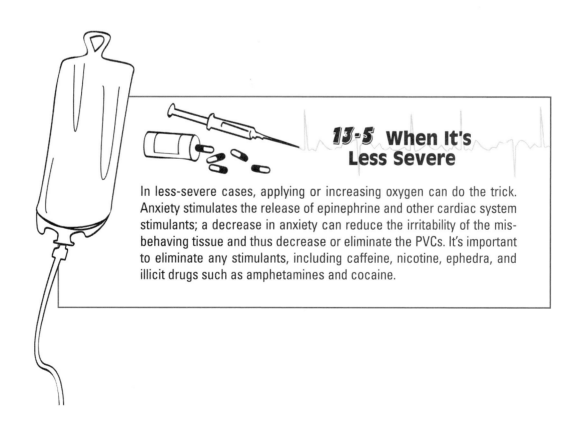

13-5 When It's Less Severe

In less-severe cases, applying or increasing oxygen can do the trick. Anxiety stimulates the release of epinephrine and other cardiac system stimulants; a decrease in anxiety can reduce the irritability of the misbehaving tissue and thus decrease or eliminate the PVCs. It's important to eliminate any stimulants, including caffeine, nicotine, ephedra, and illicit drugs such as amphetamines and cocaine.

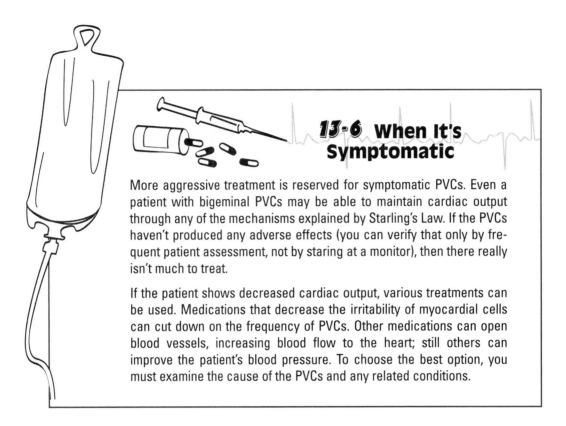

13-6 When It's Symptomatic

More aggressive treatment is reserved for symptomatic PVCs. Even a patient with bigeminal PVCs may be able to maintain cardiac output through any of the mechanisms explained by Starling's Law. If the PVCs haven't produced any adverse effects (you can verify that only by frequent patient assessment, not by staring at a monitor), then there really isn't much to treat.

If the patient shows decreased cardiac output, various treatments can be used. Medications that decrease the irritability of myocardial cells can cut down on the frequency of PVCs. Other medications can open blood vessels, increasing blood flow to the heart; still others can improve the patient's blood pressure. To choose the best option, you must examine the cause of the PVCs and any related conditions.

stroke volume. Because AIVR is initiated in the ventricles, it's still considered idioventricular, but it's faster than the normal ventricular rate. The range for AIVR is 41 to 99 bpm.

Table 13–2 Criteria for idioventricular rhythm

Regularity	Regular
Heart Rate	**20–40 bpm**
P-Wave	If present, not related to QRS complex
PR Interval	Not measurable
QRS Complexes	**All the same shape, ≥ 0.12 sec (3 small boxes). Wide and bizarre, with T-wave opposite deflection of QRS complex.**

Otherwise it's identical to idioventricular rhythm (Fig. 13–6, Table 13–3).

In a ventricular rhythm, the patient is better off with a heart rate that's abnormally fast for ventricular tissue, but not too fast. Like accelerated junctional rhythm, AIVR is considered "normal," compensating for decreased cardiac output when higher pacemakers have failed. If the rhythm is regular, the heart rate is consistent, and there are no symptoms, it's enough to simply to monitor the patient. No other treatment is needed. Recommendations from the North American Society of Pacing and Electrophysiology, the people whose job it is to decide these things, don't even consider AIVR a good reason for inserting a permanent pacemaker unless symptoms are associated with the rhythm.

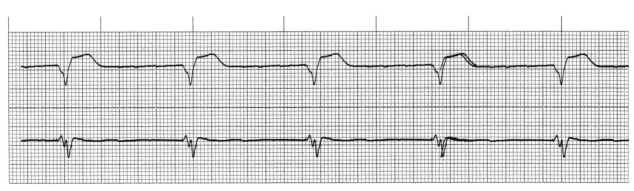

Fig. 13–5 Idioventricular rhythm. Notice the characteristics of ventricular rhythms: wide, bizarre QRS complex, no P-waves, and T-wave in the opposite direction from the QRS.

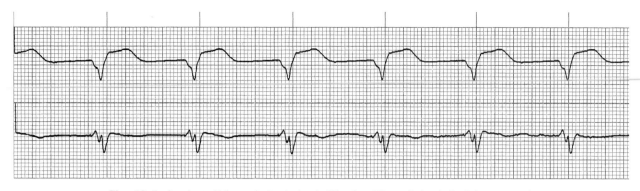

Fig. 13–6 Accelerated idioventricular rhythm. It differs from idioventricular rhythm in heart rate only.

Table 13–3 Criteria for accelerated idioventricular rhythm

Regularity	Regular
Heart Rate	**41–99 bpm**
P-Wave	If present, not related to QRS complex
PR Interval	Not measurable
QRS Complexes	**All the same shape, ≥0.12 sec (3 small boxes). Wide and bizarre, with T-wave opposite deflection of QRS complex.**

Ventricular Bradycardia

On the low end of the heart rate spectrum, we have ventricular bradycardia (Fig. 13–7, Table 13–4). Because the heart rate is below the normal range for ventricular tissue in this rhythm (less than 20 bpm), the patient can't tolerate it. If all the supraventricular pacemakers fail and the ventricular tissue can't muster a heart rate above 20 bpm, death is imminent without treatment.

For treatment of ventricular bradycardia, see "Treating Low Cardiac Output" on page **198.**

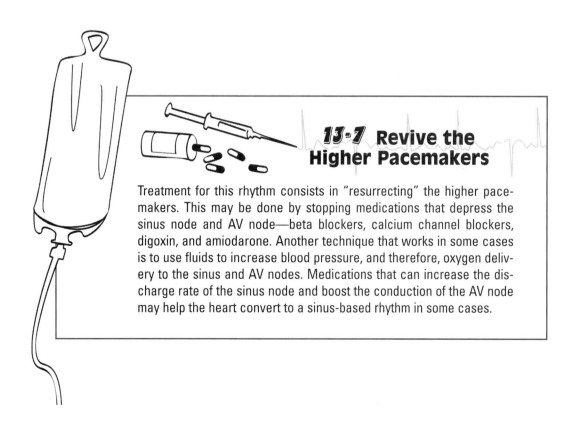

13·7 Revive the Higher Pacemakers

Treatment for this rhythm consists in "resurrecting" the higher pacemakers. This may be done by stopping medications that depress the sinus node and AV node—beta blockers, calcium channel blockers, digoxin, and amiodarone. Another technique that works in some cases is to use fluids to increase blood pressure, and therefore, oxygen delivery to the sinus and AV nodes. Medications that can increase the discharge rate of the sinus node and boost the conduction of the AV node may help the heart convert to a sinus-based rhythm in some cases.

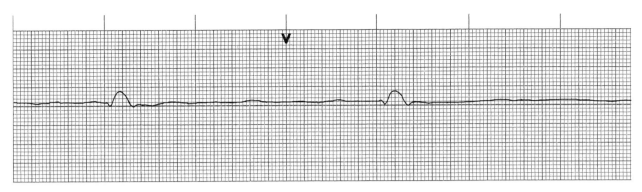

Fig. 13–7 Ventricular bradycardia. This is an ominous rhythm.

Table 13–4 Criteria for ventricular bradycardia

Regularity	Regular
Heart Rate	<20 bpm
P-Wave	If present, not related to QRS complex
PR Interval	Not measurable
QRS Complexes	**All the same shape, ≥0.12 sec (3 small boxes). Wide and bizarre, with T-wave opposite deflection of QRS complex.**

We introduced this rhythm briefly as "agonal rhythm" in Chapter 8. Remember, "agonal" comes from the same Greek root as "agony" (an apt term), which means "death" or "death struggle."

Ventricular bradycardia is frequently seen when the heart is dying. It often begins when an idioventricular rhythm deteriorates further because of low cardiac output and the coronary arteries deliver less oxygen. Usually this rhythm perfuses the heart so poorly that you can't find a pulse, or even heart sounds, because the ventricles are contracting minimally or not at all.

Treating Low Cardiac Output

PICKING UP THE PACE

It's critically important to be careful when treating ventricular bradycardia, idioventricular rhythms, and accelerated idioventricular rhythms. These rhythms don't usually replace a higher-functioning pacemaker, so think about what would happen if you gave a drug that decreased irritability. The ventricular rhythm might stop, leaving no functioning pacemakers in the heart!

The symptoms produced by these rhythms aren't caused by increased irritability but by low cardiac output, usually from a combination of insufficient heart rate, poor ventricular contraction, and insufficient volume from lost atrial kick. The difference between these rhythms and sinus rhythm with PVCs is that the PVCs are interfering with a normal rate and normal rhythm produced by a higher pacemaker.

Occasionally, sinus bradycardia may have PVCs because the decreased cardiac output from the low sinus node rate has increased ventricular irritability. In this case, the treatment objective is to speed up the sinus node rate, increase oxygen delivery, and thus decrease irritability.

The important thing is to be careful with ventricular beats. If they're excessive, treatment is warranted, but if they're simply trying to increase an insufficient heart rate, let them be. When you increase the cardiac output, they will frequently go away.

PICKING UP THE PACE CAUTIOUSLY

Electronic pacemakers can be inserted in patients with a ventricular rhythm who can't maintain an adequate cardiac output. However, it's imperative to thoroughly investigate the failure of the supraventricular pacemakers.

Many drugs can cause conduction problems, especially when used in combination with other drugs or herbal supplements. A simple adjustment in medication may be all that's needed, or the patient may turn out to have increasing compromise in one or more coronary arteries supplying the higher pacemakers. In the latter case, the patient may require treatment up to and including open heart surgery.

Many of these interventions are only short-term. With a temporary pacemaker, the electricity is generated outside the body. Increased risks, including lead movement, power failure, and infection, are associated with this method of pacing. The medications are short-term because they're metabolized quickly and are available only in IV form. They'd need to be given either dozens of times a day or as a continuous drip—clearly an impractical solution.

Ventricular Tachycardia

YELLING, KICKING, AND SCREAMING

Ventricular tachycardia (V-tach or VT) is life threatening. The affected ventricular tissue increases its irritability because it feels the effects of poor oxygen delivery. Causes can include anything that decreases oxygen delivery to the ventricles, or increases calecholamines in the blood stream. V-tach may also be caused by an electrolyte imbalance, such as with the patient's potassium or magnesium level, especially if there are other pre-existing cardiac issues present.

When the ventricular tissue becomes extremely irritable, it may fire a rapid series of impulses (Fig. 13–8). With its very high discharge rate, this ventricular focus becomes the pacemaker of the heart (remember, the fastest pacemaker wins).

The problems with V-tach are frequently associated with its rate. Cardiac output is low because atrial kick has been lost and the ventricular contractions aren't well coordinated. The heart may also have a mechanical problem,

such as pathological enlargement or MI, that reduces cardiac output even further by decreasing stroke volume. To increase cardiac output, especially in ventricular rhythms where stroke volume is low from loss of atrial kick, you'll need to compensate by increasing the heart rate, sometimes even into the tachycardic range.

THE LOW END OF FAST: SLOW VENTRICULAR TACHYCARDIA

It's possible to tolerate V-tach for a long time. Cases of the rhythm have been known to persist for days without serious consequences. V-Tach is easier to live with when the heart rate is at the lower end of the range, approximately 100 to 150 bpm. This range is frequently known by the oxymoron "slow V-tach." That name tells us important things: first, where the rhythm originates; second, that it's faster than normal; and third, that its heart rate is just over the tachycardic line and may be better tolerated than a faster rhythm, at least for a while.

Medical treatment is generally successful because slow V-tach may maintain sufficient cardiac output, and therefore, electrical treatment usually isn't necessary.

THE HIGH END OF FAST: FAST VENTRICULAR TACHYCARDIA

When we refer to V-tach, we're usually talking about fast V-tach because this rhythm is more dangerous at faster

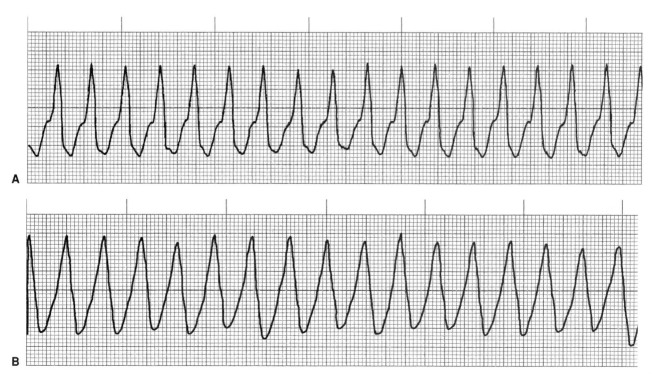

Fig. 13–8A–B Ventricular tachycardia. Only one irritable focus is initiating this rhythm.

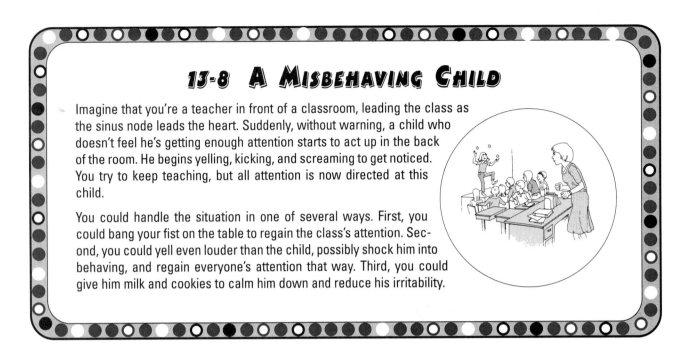

13-8 A MISBEHAVING CHILD

Imagine that you're a teacher in front of a classroom, leading the class as the sinus node leads the heart. Suddenly, without warning, a child who doesn't feel he's getting enough attention starts to act up in the back of the room. He begins yelling, kicking, and screaming to get noticed. You try to keep teaching, but all attention is now directed at this child.

You could handle the situation in one of several ways. First, you could bang your fist on the table to regain the class's attention. Second, you could yell even louder than the child, possibly shock him into behaving, and regain everyone's attention that way. Third, you could give him milk and cookies to calm him down and reduce his irritability.

---

rates. Fast V-tach has a heart rate above 150 bpm and usually isn't tolerated well. The ventricles have much less time to fill so the stroke volume begins to suffer and signs of low cardiac output appear. At this point, we talk about *decompensation,* which means that the heart has tried, but failed, to compensate for the low cardiac output. Now, ironically, the body's compensatory mechanisms are causing more problems.

GOING NOWHERE AT ALL: PULSELESS VENTRICULAR TACHYCARDIA

Finally, V-tach can be pulseless. This type of V-tach is the most dangerous because the heart is not contracting effectively enough to generate a pulse. In this case, the rhythm is immediately treated with defibrillation, not synchronized electrical cardioversion. Time is of the essence; the longer the delay before defibrillation, the less likely recovery becomes.

Multifocal Ventricular Tachycardia

Multifocal ventricular tachycardia (multifocal V-tach) resembles both regular ventricular tachycardia and ventricular fibrillation. In this rhythm, the QRS complexes are clearly identifiable but change shape repeatedly. As in multifocal atrial tachycardia, which we discussed in Chapter 11, the focus of each beat changes; in this case the difference shows in the QRSs, not the P-waves. Because the ventricular signals are so poorly organized, this rhythm can deteriorate quickly and easily into ventricular fibrillation. Figure 13–9 shows two examples of multifocal V-tach.

Treatment is the same as for unifocal V-tach, with the caution that multifocal V-tach is less stable and therefore more dangerous.

Table 13–5 Criteria for ventricular tachycardia

Regularity	Regular
Heart Rate	**100–250 bpm**
P-Wave	If present, not related to QRS complex
PR Interval	Not measurable
QRS Complexes	**All the same shape, ≥0.12 sec (3 small boxes). Wide and bizarre, with T-wave opposite deflection of QRS complex.**

Table 13–6 Criteria for multifocal ventricular tachycardia

Regularity	Regular
Heart Rate	**100–250 bpm**
P-Wave	If present, not related to QRS complex. May be normal or inverted.
PR Interval	Not measurable
QRS Complexes	**All different shapes; no pattern to size changes. ≥0.12 sec (3 small boxes).**

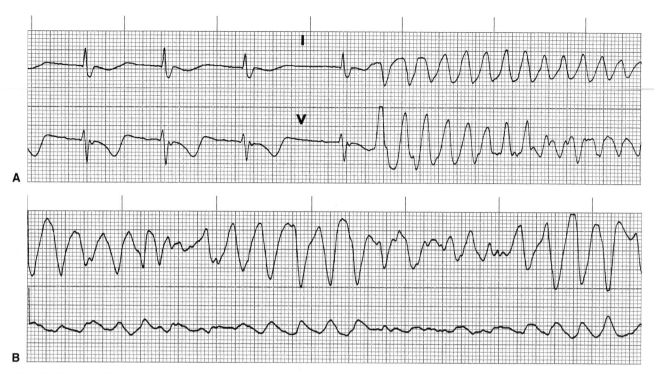

Fig. 13–9A–B Multifocal ventricular tachycardia. The shape of the QRS complex changes constantly. Multiple irritable foci are present in these two rhythm strips. A, The tracing begins with a normal rhythm. A PVC initiates a run of V-tach with a tall, upright QRS, which decreases steadily in size. B, Wide, bizarre QRSs of varying size and shape occur throughout the entire strip.

Ventricular Flutter

Ventricular flutter has a short life span in the heart. In this rhythm the QRS complex and the T-wave fuse into a continuous curved waveform called a *sinusoidal wave*. It

Table 13–7 Criteria for ventricular flutter

Regularity	Regular
Heart Rate	200–350 bpm
P-Wave	Not identifiable
PR Interval	Not measurable
QRS Complex	**QRS and T-wave merge to form one sinusoidal pattern.**

has nothing to do with the sinus node but refers to a mathematical term, *sine*.

Figure 13–10 shows an example of ventricular flutter. Notice that the normally straight lines of the QRS complex are missing, replaced with a continuous curved line. Whenever you see a line like this, you'll know that poor, ineffective contractions are occurring in the ventricles.

Ventricular Fibrillation

WHY IS THIS PATIENT BREATHING?

Ventricular fibrillation should never have a pulse. The ventricles are quivering, or fibrillating, just as the atria do in atrial fibrillation. However, in this scenario, the heart isn't

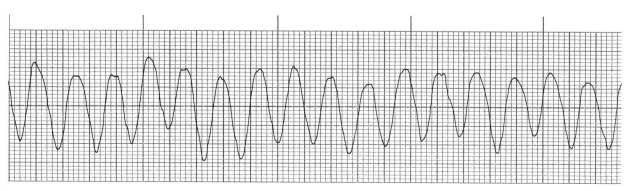

Fig. 13–10 Ventricular flutter. This rhythm causes poor contraction of the ventricles and frequently has no pulse. The entire waveform is smooth and rounded, and the straight lines typical of QRSs are missing.

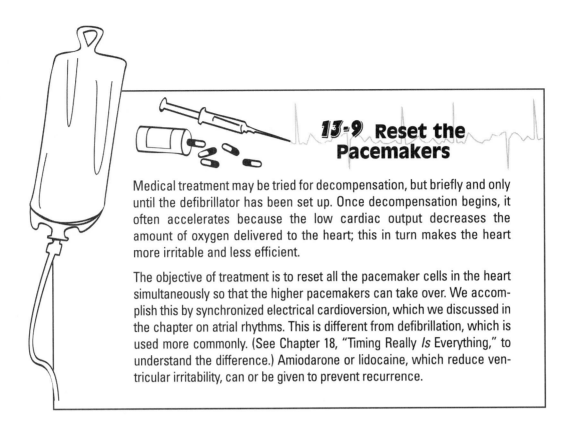

13-9 Reset the Pacemakers

Medical treatment may be tried for decompensation, but briefly and only until the defibrillator has been set up. Once decompensation begins, it often accelerates because the low cardiac output decreases the amount of oxygen delivered to the heart; this in turn makes the heart more irritable and less efficient.

The objective of treatment is to reset all the pacemaker cells in the heart simultaneously so that the higher pacemakers can take over. We accomplish this by synchronized electrical cardioversion, which we discussed in the chapter on atrial rhythms. This is different from defibrillation, which is used more commonly. (See Chapter 18, "Timing Really *Is* Everything," to understand the difference.) Amiodarone or lidocaine, which reduce ventricular irritability, can or be given to prevent recurrence.

just pumping blood inefficiently; it's not pumping any blood at all. The ventricles are discharging at a phenomenal rate, more than 350 times per minute, and the lack of coordinated contraction eliminates cardiac output completely.

Figure 13–11 shows an example of ventricular fibrillation (V-fib). As in atrial fibrillation, there's a wavy baseline, but you won't find any pretty QRS complexes. You'll notice that the QRSs are replaced by small, sharp spikes and rounded bumps on the baseline. Each of those

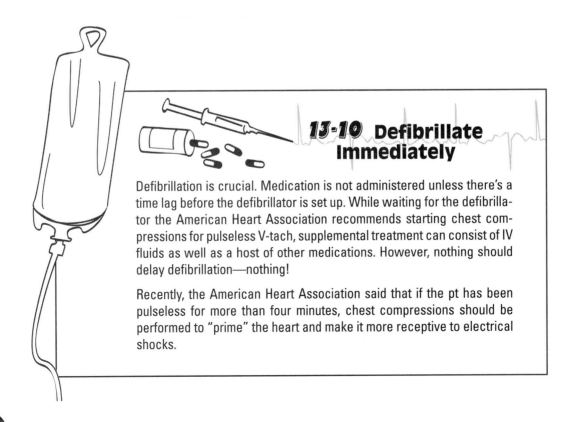

13-10 Defibrillate Immediately

Defibrillation is crucial. Medication is not administered unless there's a time lag before the defibrillator is set up. While waiting for the defibrillator the American Heart Association recommends starting chest compressions for pulseless V-tach, supplemental treatment can consist of IV fluids as well as a host of other medications. However, nothing should delay defibrillation—nothing!

Recently, the American Heart Association said that if the pt has been pulseless for more than four minutes, chest compressions should be performed to "prime" the heart and make it more receptive to electrical shocks.

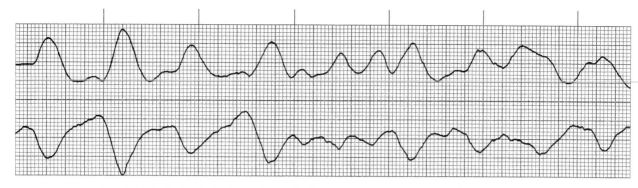

Fig. 13–11 Ventricular fibrillation. This rhythm has no coordinated ventricular conduction or contraction.

bumps and dips in the tracing is a QRS "wannabe"; each represents a partial depolarization of the ventricular tissue.

If you find that a patient with this rhythm is breathing, talking, or exhibiting a pulse, then something isn't right. This rhythm is not compatible with life! Check the patient's patches and the monitoring equipment.

COARSE OR FINE?

Ventricular fibrillation is frequently referred to as "coarse" or "fine." *Coarse V-fib* most often indicates that the rhythm is of recent onset. The ECG strip shows larger baseline undulations, as in Figure 13–11. Remember that larger waveforms indicate a larger signal from a more extensive amount of tissue; this rule also applies to the undulations seen in V-fib.

The lack of cardiac output in V-fib deprives the heart of oxygen. When this first happens, the ventricular cells scream out in their irritable way. When the lack of oxygen persists, the cells become dysfunctional and fewer of them are able to depolarize, each time with less

Table 13–8 Criteria for ventricular fibrillation

Regularity	No waveforms to assess for regularity
Heart Rate	**0 bpm**
P-Wave	Not present
PR Interval	Not measurable
QRS Complexes	**Wavy baseline, no clearly identifiable QRS complexes**

energy. The decreasing strength of the signal causes smaller undulations, which are called *fine V-fib* (Fig. 13–12A–B).

Asystole

WHEN EVERYTHING STOPS

The prefix *a* means "without"; *systole* means "contraction." In asystole there is no contraction because there is no electrical activity. The patient is clinically dead. This rhythm is frequently referred to as *cardiac standstill.* Causes include severe electrolyte disturbances, a large acute MI, a nonfunctioning AV node, and long periods in which the ventricles don't receive adequate oxygen.

Strangely enough, you may find P-waves in asystole; the ECG tracing can show a series of small bumps. In *ventricular standstill,* which is a form of asystole, the sinus node is functioning but the ventricles are too sick to respond. When P-waves are present, as in Figure 13–13, the rhythm is called *sinus rhythm with ventricular standstill* to show that the sinus node is discharging. Because the ventricles are out of commission, this rhythm has no QRS complexes.

True asystole, also called *complete cardiac standstill,* can be literally considered an arrhythmia because there's no rhythm to interpret—no P-waves, no QRS complexes, and no T-waves (Fig. 13–14). The baseline may not be perfectly flat, as you'd expect in the absence of electrical activity, because residual electrical activity in the body may cause minute undulations.

Patients in asystole are rarely resuscitated; this is because the cause persists and is rarely recognized or treated. The American Heart Association provides a list

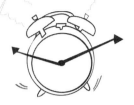

13-11 Torsade de Pointes

A special type of multifocal V-tach is known as *torsade de pointes* (TdP for short), which is French for "twisting of points." That's exactly what this rhythm appears to be doing: twisting the "points" of the QRS complexes around the baseline; the deflection keeps shifting between positive and negative. As you can see in the example here, the QRS size changes as it does in generic multifocal V-tach. However, instead of changing size randomly, in TdP the QRSs grow larger, then smaller, only to repeat the pattern all over again.

Torsade de pointes would be little more than a curiosity if these waveforms were all that distinguished it from multifocal V-tach. However, it's important to note one more thing: TdP is commonly caused by a magnesium deficiency. Therefore, when added to the medications and electrical shocks used in V-tach, a magnesium bolus can frequently help correct the problem. Electrical therapy may convert the rhythm, but it's likely to recur if the magnesium deficiency is left untreated.

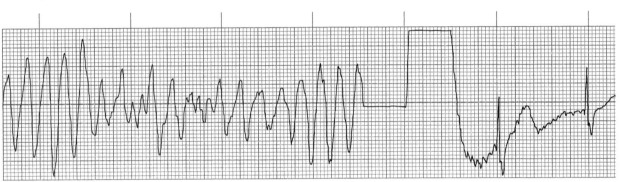

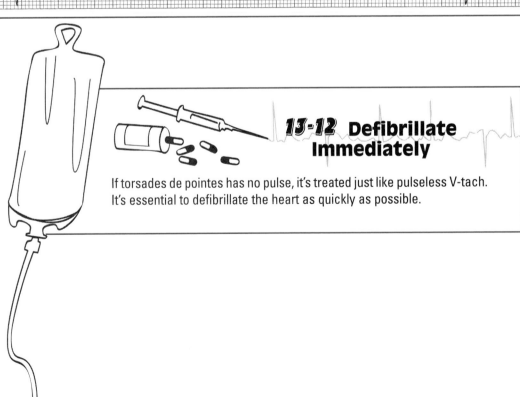

13-12 Defibrillate Immediately

If torsades de pointes has no pulse, it's treated just like pulseless V-tach. It's essential to defibrillate the heart as quickly as possible.

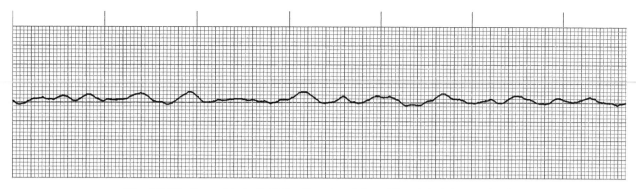

Fig. 13–12 Fine ventricular fibrillation. These two rhythms differ only in their energy levels.

of the more common, more easily assessed causes of asystole. The mnemonic I use to remember these is MATCH($\times$ 5)ED, shown in Table 13–10. The "$\times$ 5" means that the mnemonic uses four different "H" words.

CHECK THE WIRING

Patient assessment is important with asystole. First you need to be sure your equipment is working. What appears to be asystole may be a disconnection in the wires that doesn't allow the cardiac monitor to receive the true rhythm. Finding a pulse in your patient eliminates the diagnosis of asystole.

There's another error that patient assessment can uncover, and believe me, it's happened more often than anyone admits. Don't monitor the wrong patient! In telemetry monitors, a box is attached to the ECG

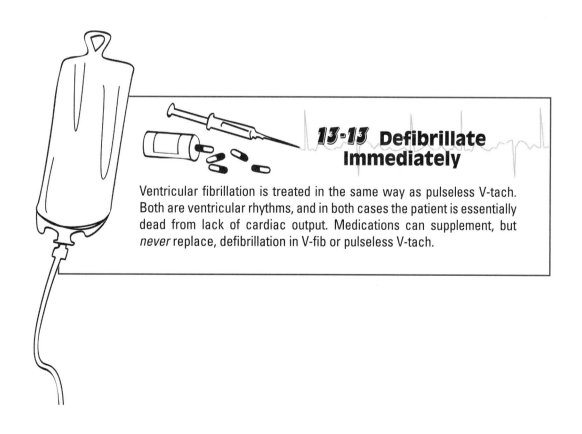

13-13 Defibrillate Immediately

Ventricular fibrillation is treated in the same way as pulseless V-tach. Both are ventricular rhythms, and in both cases the patient is essentially dead from lack of cardiac output. Medications can supplement, but *never* replace, defibrillation in V-fib or pulseless V-tach.

13-14 MANY MISBEHAVING CHILDREN

Imagine yourself back in that classroom, leading the same class. Suddenly, without warning, many children who don't feel they're getting enough attention start to act up at the same moment. They behave horribly, yelling, kicking, and screaming for attention. You can't keep teaching because no one is paying any attention to you.

You can handle this situation the same way you might quiet one misbehaving child: bang your fist and yell louder, then give them all milk and cookies to reduce their irritability. However, this situation is more dangerous because the whole class is out of control—since everybody's involved, you could end up with a riot on your hands.

If you sit back and let the children misbehave to their hearts' content, their energy level will wane and they'll fall asleep eventually. Although this approach takes care of the chaos, you can't teach them anything while they're asleep, so nobody's learning anything. Although this lack of activity may quiet the classroom, in the heart it means death.

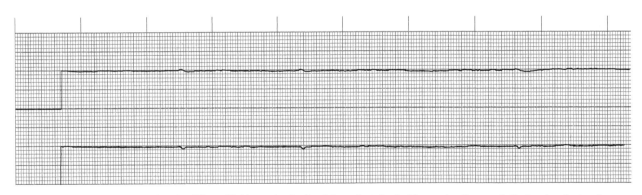

Fig. 13–13 Asystole. This rhythm should be verified in another lead and the patient checked for a pulse. P-waves indicate a functioning sinus node, but without ventricular conduction and contraction there is no cardiac output.

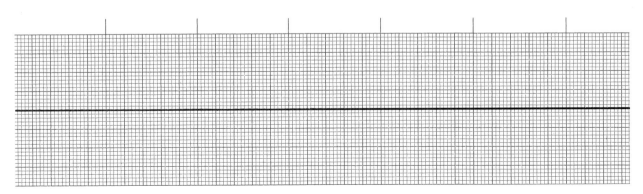

Fig. 13–14 Complete asystole. The lack of waveforms shows that no pacemakers are functioning. If the cause of this rhythm is not found quickly, recovery is nearly impossible.

Table 13–9 Criteria for asystole

Regularity	Not measurable; no identified waves or complexes
Heart Rate	0 bpm
P-Wave	Not present in true asystole
PR Interval	Not measurable
QRS Complex	None

Table 13–10 Mnemonic for causes of asystole

Letter	Condition
M	Myocardial infarction
A	Acidosis
T	Tension pneumothorax
C	Cardiac tamponade
H × 5	Hyperkalemia Hypothermia Hypotension Hypoxia Hyvolemia
E	Embolus (pulmonary)
D	Drugs or drug overdose

patches and sends the signal via radio waves to a distant monitoring station, sometimes on a different unit or even a different floor. Each box has a unique identifying number. If the wrong number is paired with a patient's name and room number on the monitoring equipment, you may have difficulty finding the patient who truly needs assistance.

The old adage "Treat the patient, not the equipment," was never truer than in cardiac care.

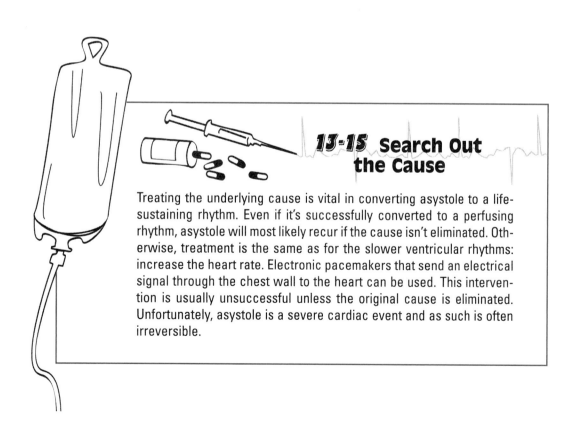

13-15 Search Out the Cause

Treating the underlying cause is vital in converting asystole to a life-sustaining rhythm. Even if it's successfully converted to a perfusing rhythm, asystole will most likely recur if the cause isn't eliminated. Otherwise, treatment is the same as for the slower ventricular rhythms: increase the heart rate. Electronic pacemakers that send an electrical signal through the chest wall to the heart can be used. This intervention is usually unsuccessful unless the original cause is eliminated. Unfortunately, asystole is a severe cardiac event and as such is often irreversible.

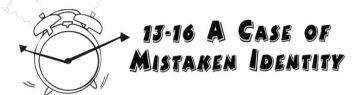

13-16 A Case of Mistaken Identity

Fine ventricular fibrillation is often confused with asystole. Because these two rhythms need different types of treatment, it's crucial to differentiate between the two. Asystole must be verified *quickly* in at least two leads and preferably in as many leads as possible. Remember, a change in perspective can alter the size and shape of the ECG tracing. Even if one perspective appears to show asystole, a different perspective can reveal fine V-fib.

Remember, defibrillation "resets" all the pacemaker cells, allowing the sinus node to take control of the heart. In asystole, there are no discharging pacemaker cells to reset; all of the pacemaker cells are already "stunned." So, although defibrillation works for fine V-fib, defibrillation in asystole can stun the heart further, making recovery from asystole more difficult or impossible.

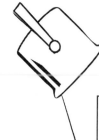

Now You Know

Ventricular tissue can take over the heart rhythm for several reasons: the higher pacemakers fail to generate a signal, the signal doesn't reach the ventricles, or the ventricles generate a faster heart rate than the higher pacemakers do.

In ventricular rhythms, the QRS complexes are wide and bizarre and the T-waves are in the direction opposite that of the QRS complex.

Some ventricular rhythms have no QRS complexes, or the QRS complexes are indistinguishable from the T-waves.

The intrinsic rate for ventricular tissue is 20 to 40 bpm.

Ventricular rhythms are dangerous because atrial kick and coordinated ventricular contractions are lost. Cardiac output drops significantly, and there are no back-up pacemakers to save the heart if the ventricular pacemakers fail.

Slow ventricular tachycardia (slow V-tach) has a heart rate about 100 to 150 bpm. This rhythm is well tolerated because the increased heart rate makes up for the loss of cardiac output inherent in ventricular rhythms.

In ventricular fibrillation (V-fib), the heart is quivering without effective contractions; because there is no cardiac output, there is also no pulse.

Symptomatic V-tach with a pulse is treated with synchronized cardioversion; V-tach without a pulse and V-fib are treated with defibrillation.

Coarse V-fib is present when the baseline undulations are relatively large; fine V-fib shows smaller peaks and valleys on the ECG tracing the longer it persists. The two rhythms are treated identically.

It's important to verify asystole in two or more leads to make sure that the rhythm is not fine V-fib or a faulty reading from a loose patch.

It's important to find and eliminate the cause of asystole, or resuscitation will be unsuccessful.

Ventricular Rhythms

Test Yourself

1. Increased _____ of the ventricular cells is one cause of ventricular rhythms.

2. Unless verified in at least one other lead, _____ can be mistaken for asystole, leading to improper treatment.

3. The QRS duration is _____ in ventricular rhythms.

4. Key characteristics of ventricular beats are _____ and _____ QRS complexes, with the _____ in the direction opposite to most of the QRS complex.

5. The _____ prefix indicates that the ventricles are depolarizing on their own, not being triggered by another pacemaker site.

6. List at least four causes of asystole.

7. The intrinsic rate for ventricular tissue is _____ bpm to _____ bpm.

8. Why is slow ventricular tachycardia sometimes treated differently from fast V-tach?

9. V-Fib can be described as _____ or _____.

10. In addition to decreasing atrial kick, fast V-tach decreases cardiac output by reducing _____.

11. Ventricular fibrillation is a dangerous rhythm because no effective _____ are occurring, and therefore there is no cardiac output.

12. When V-tach has a pulse, _____ cardioversion is used, but when it doesn't have a pulse, _____ is used.

13. Identify the rhythm for the following 40 ECG strips:

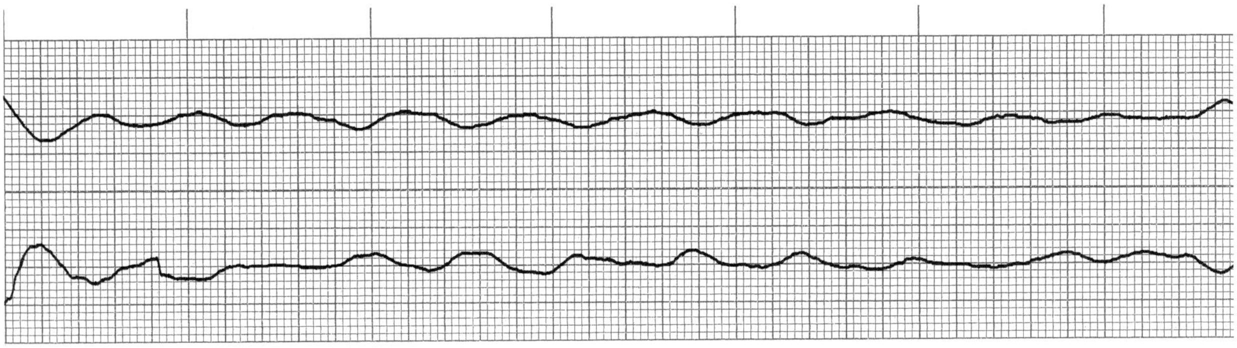

13–1

Regularity: _____ Heart rate: _____ PR interval: _____

P-waves: _____ QRS complex: _____

Interpretation: _____

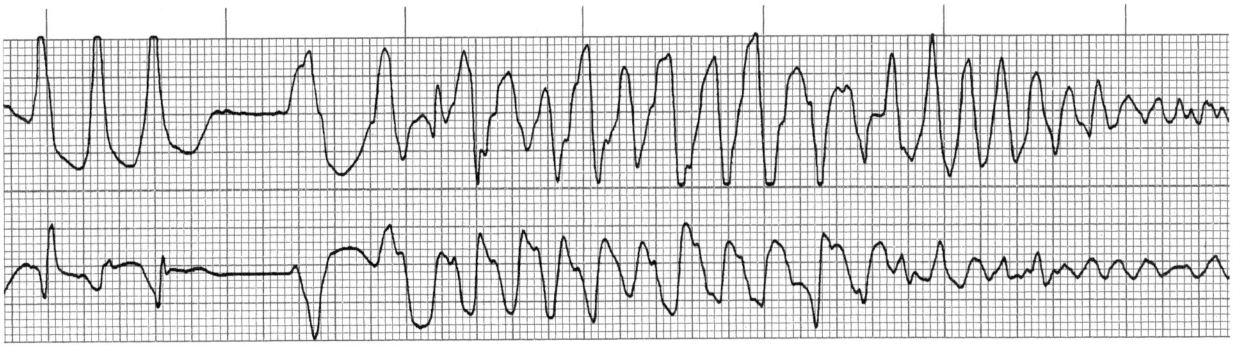

13–2

Regularity: _____ Heart rate: _____ PR interval: _____

P-waves: _____ QRS complex: _____

Interpretation: _____

210

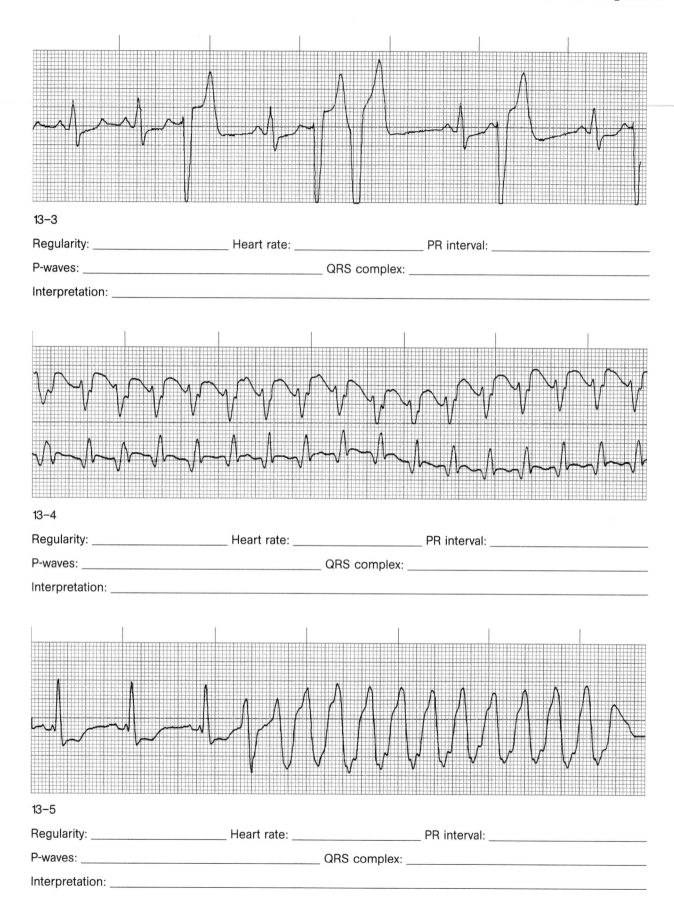

13–3

Regularity: _____ Heart rate: _____ PR interval: _____

P-waves: _____ QRS complex: _____

Interpretation: _____

13–4

Regularity: _____ Heart rate: _____ PR interval: _____

P-waves: _____ QRS complex: _____

Interpretation: _____

13–5

Regularity: _____ Heart rate: _____ PR interval: _____

P-waves: _____ QRS complex: _____

Interpretation: _____

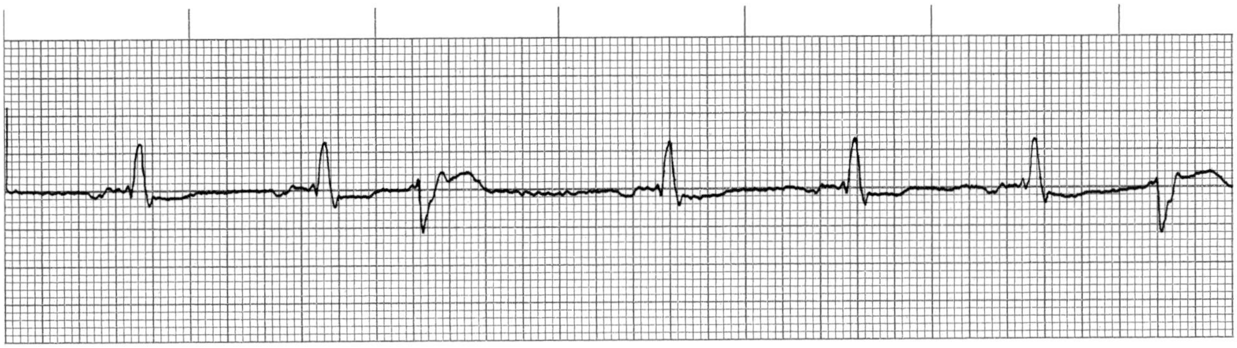

13–6

Regularity: _____ Heart rate: _____ PR interval: _____

P-waves: _____ QRS complex: _____

Interpretation: _____

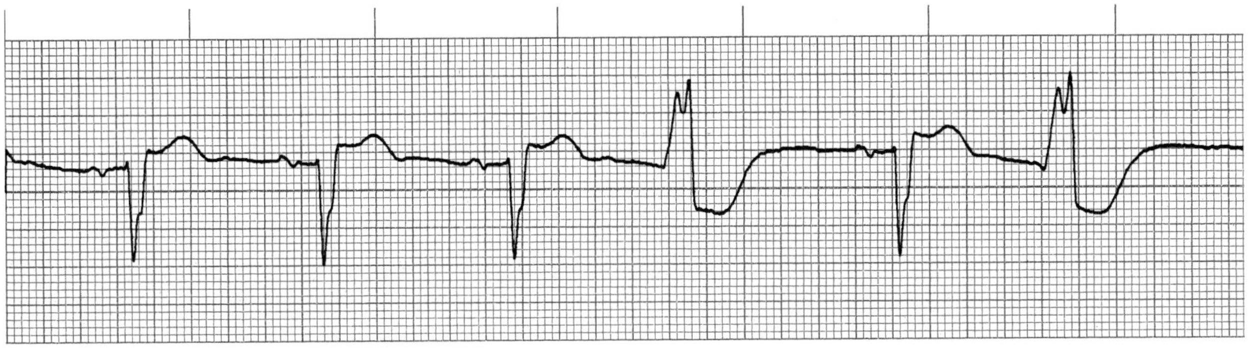

13–7

Regularity: _____ Heart rate: _____ PR interval: _____

P-waves: _____ QRS complex: _____

Interpretation: _____

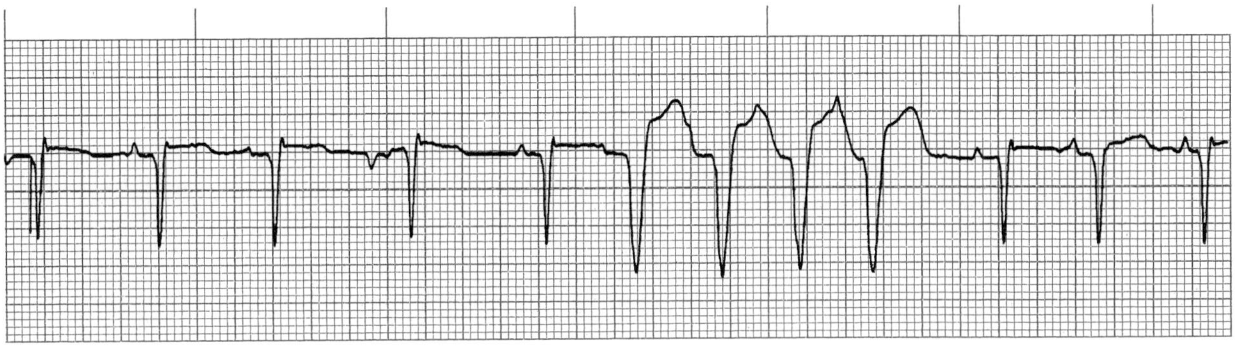

13–8

Regularity: _____ Heart rate: _____ PR interval: _____

P-waves: _____ QRS complex: _____

Interpretation: _____

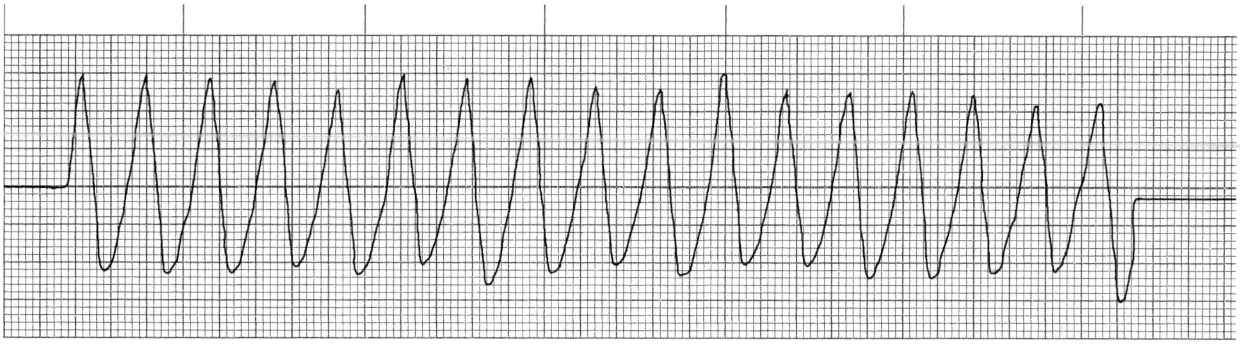

13-9

Regularity: _____ Heart rate: _____ PR interval: _____

P-waves: _____ QRS complex: _____

Interpretation: _____

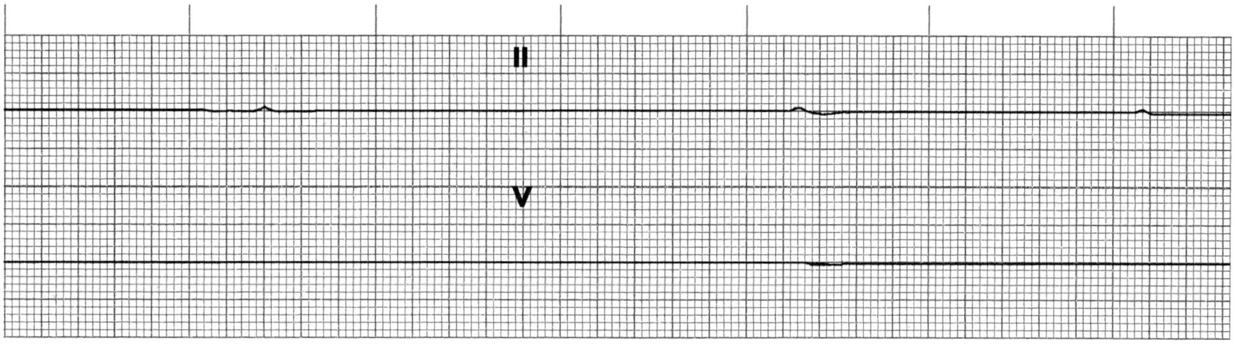

13-10

Regularity: _____ Heart rate: _____ PR interval: _____

P-waves: _____ QRS complex: _____

Interpretation: _____

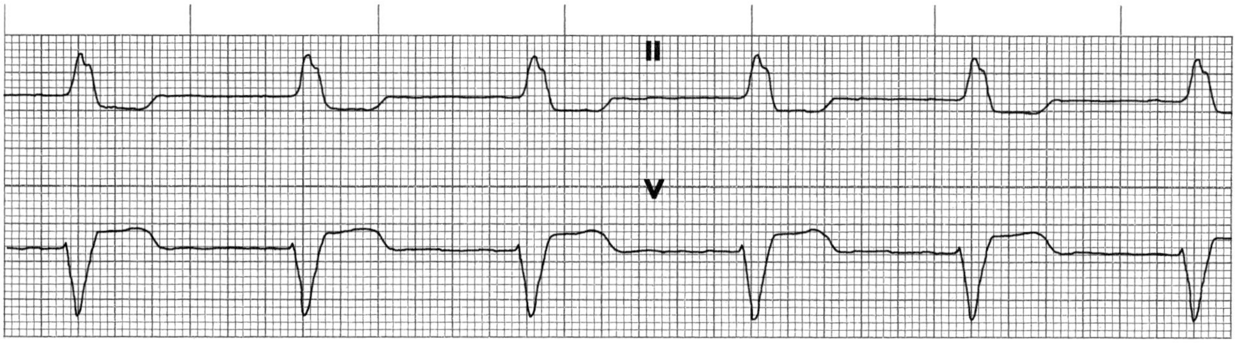

13-11

Regularity: _____ Heart rate: _____ PR interval: _____

P-waves: _____ QRS complex: _____

Interpretation: _____

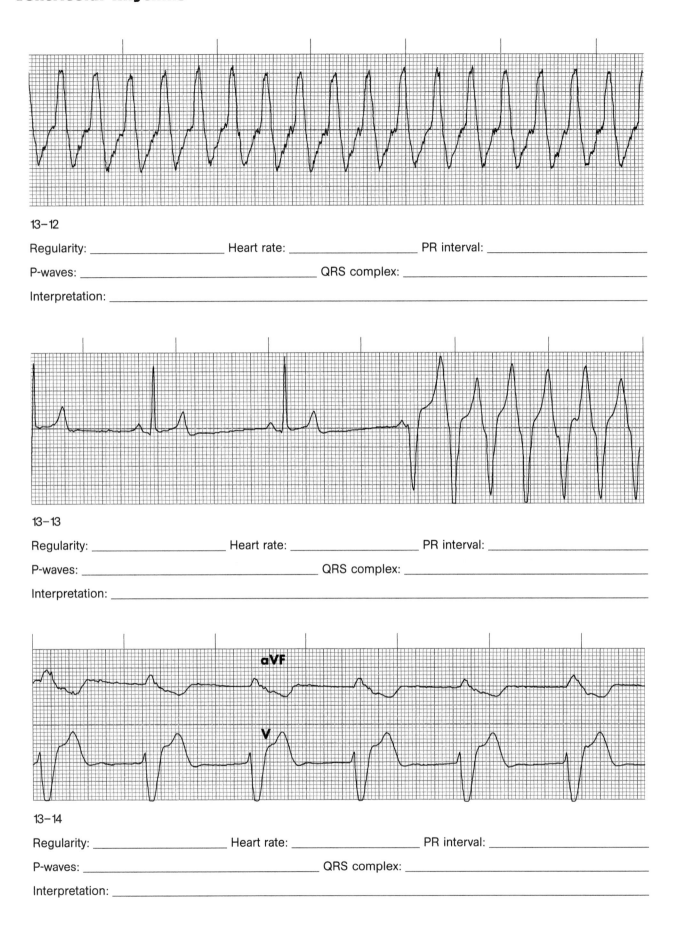

13–12

Regularity: _____ Heart rate: _____ PR interval: _____

P-waves: _____ QRS complex: _____

Interpretation: _____

13–13

Regularity: _____ Heart rate: _____ PR interval: _____

P-waves: _____ QRS complex: _____

Interpretation: _____

aVF

V

13–14

Regularity: _____ Heart rate: _____ PR interval: _____

P-waves: _____ QRS complex: _____

Interpretation: _____

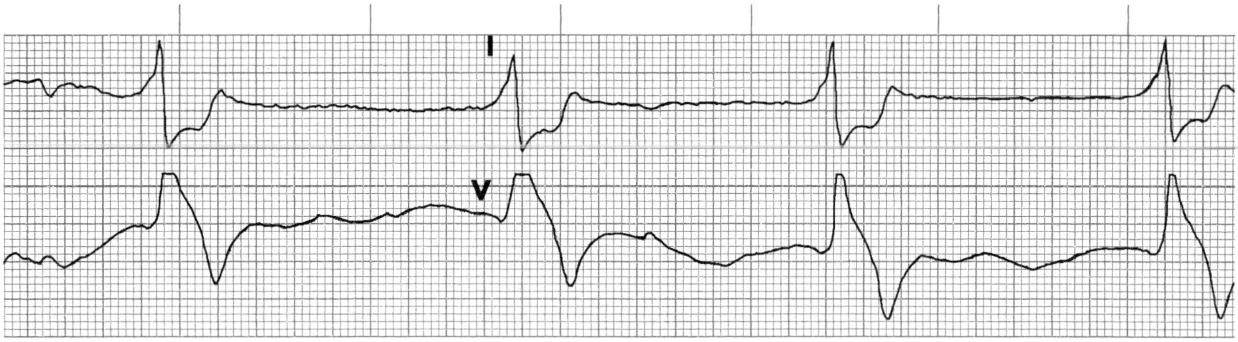

13–15

Regularity: _____ Heart rate: _____ PR interval: _____

P-waves: _____ QRS complex: _____

Interpretation: _____

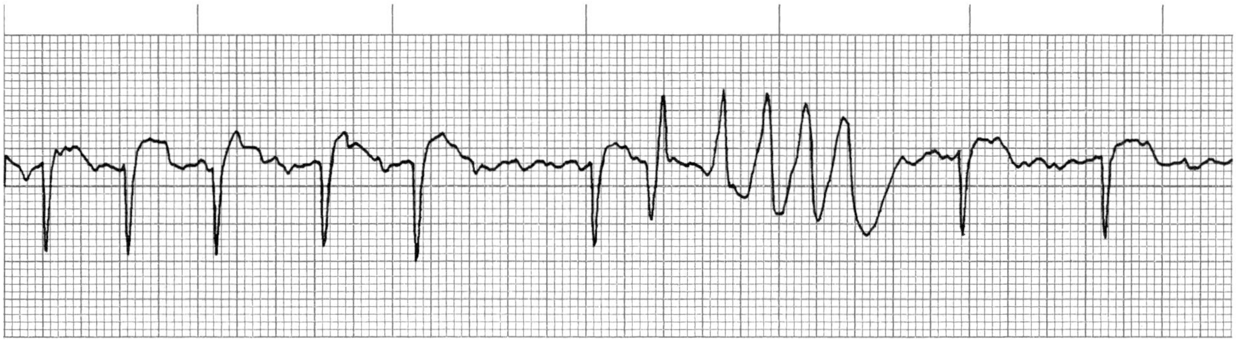

13–16

Regularity: _____ Heart rate: _____ PR interval: _____

P-waves: _____ QRS complex: _____

Interpretation: _____

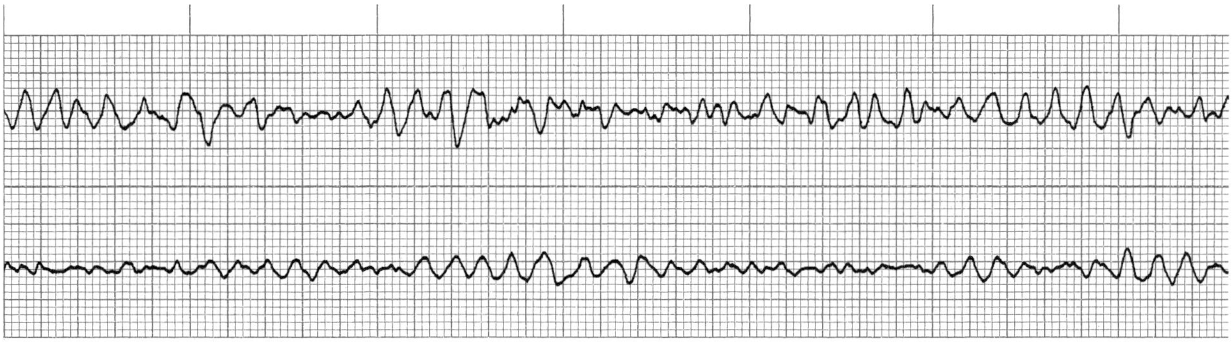

13–17

Regularity: _____ Heart rate: _____ PR interval: _____

P-waves: _____ QRS complex: _____

Interpretation: _____

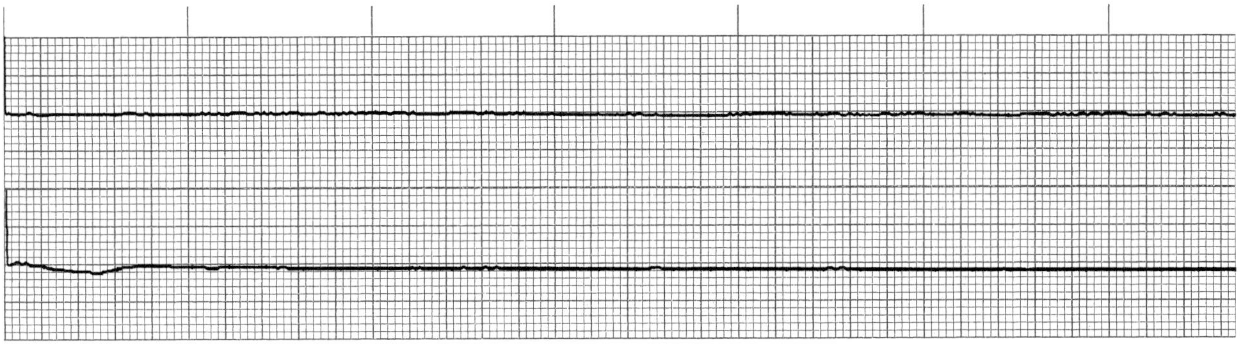

Ventricular Rhythms

13–18

Regularity: _____ Heart rate: _____ PR interval: _____

P-waves: _____ QRS complex: _____

Interpretation: _____

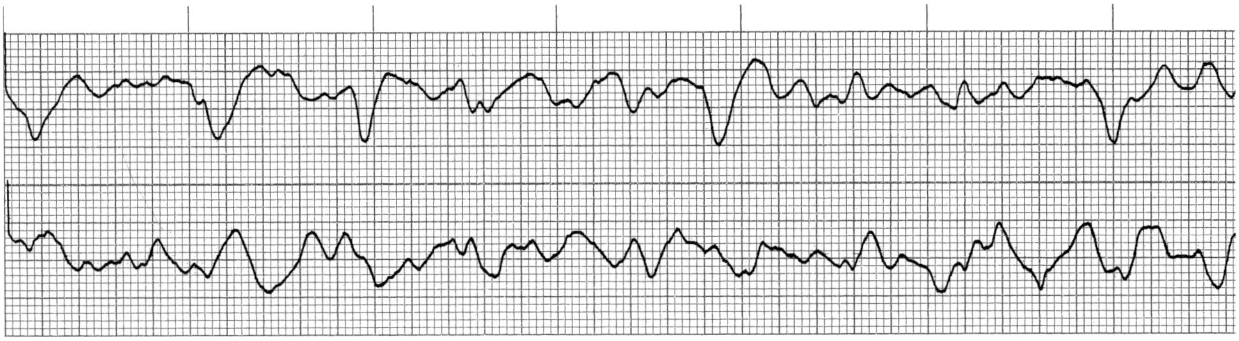

13–19

Regularity: _____ Heart rate: _____ PR interval: _____

P-waves: _____ QRS complex: _____

Interpretation: _____

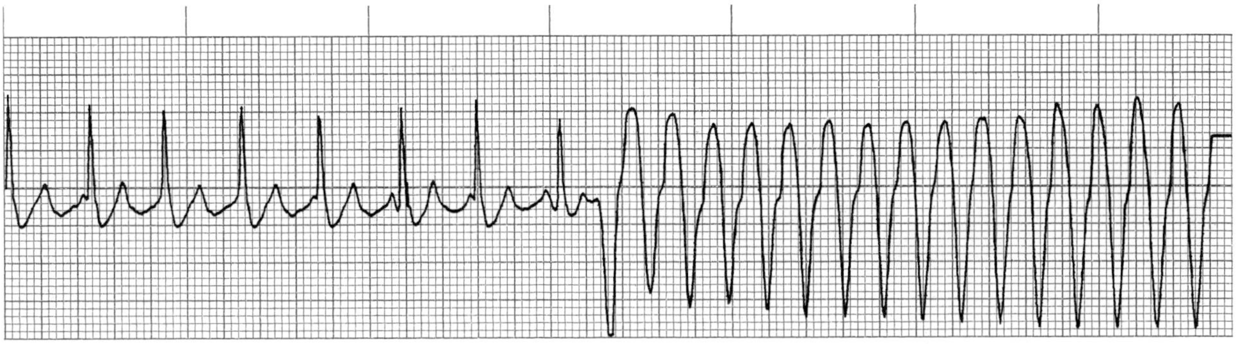

13–20

Regularity: _____ Heart rate: _____ PR interval: _____

P-waves: _____ QRS complex: _____

Interpretation: _____

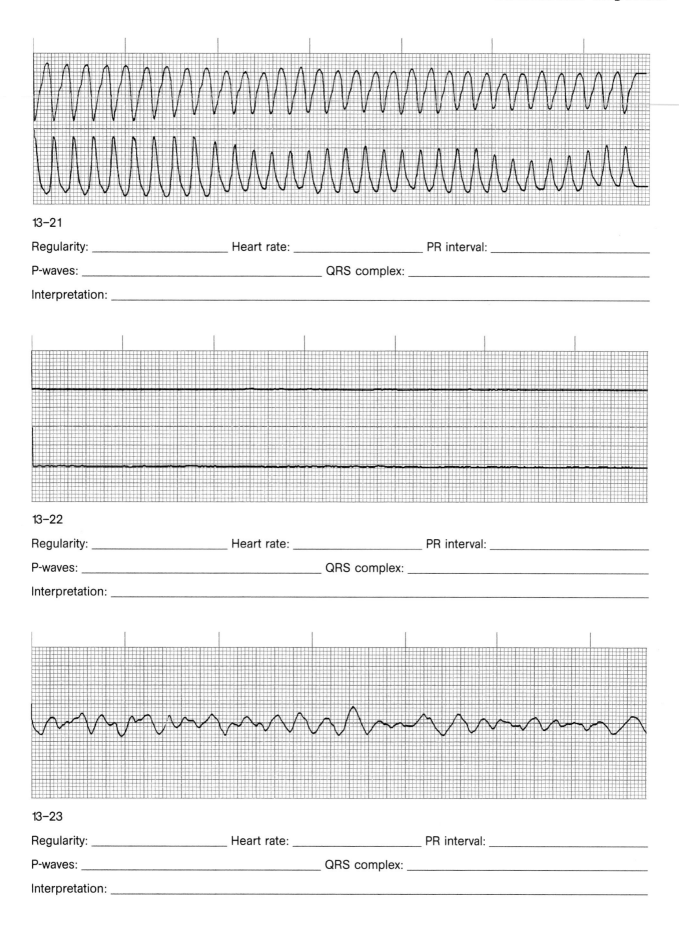

13–21

Regularity: _____ Heart rate: _____ PR interval: _____

P-waves: _____ QRS complex: _____

Interpretation: _____

13–22

Regularity: _____ Heart rate: _____ PR interval: _____

P-waves: _____ QRS complex: _____

Interpretation: _____

13–23

Regularity: _____ Heart rate: _____ PR interval: _____

P-waves: _____ QRS complex: _____

Interpretation: _____

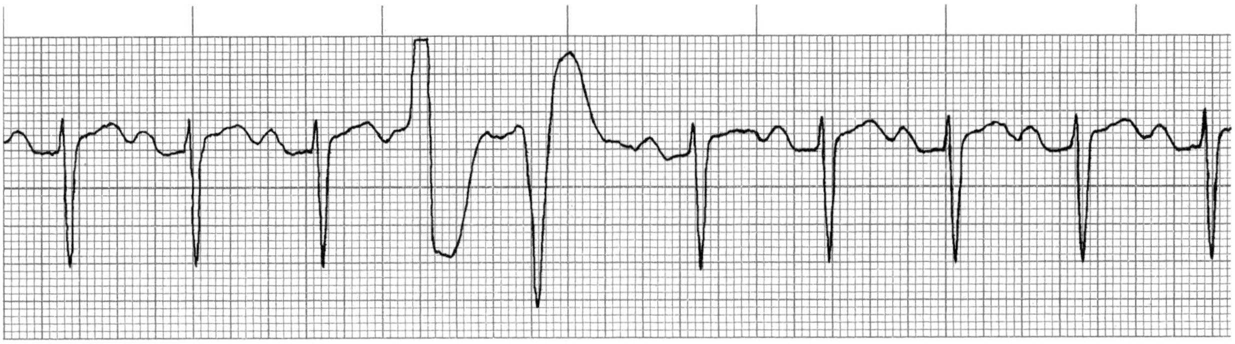

Ventricular Rhythms

13–24

Regularity: _____ Heart rate: _____ PR interval: _____

P-waves: _____ QRS complex: _____

Interpretation: _____

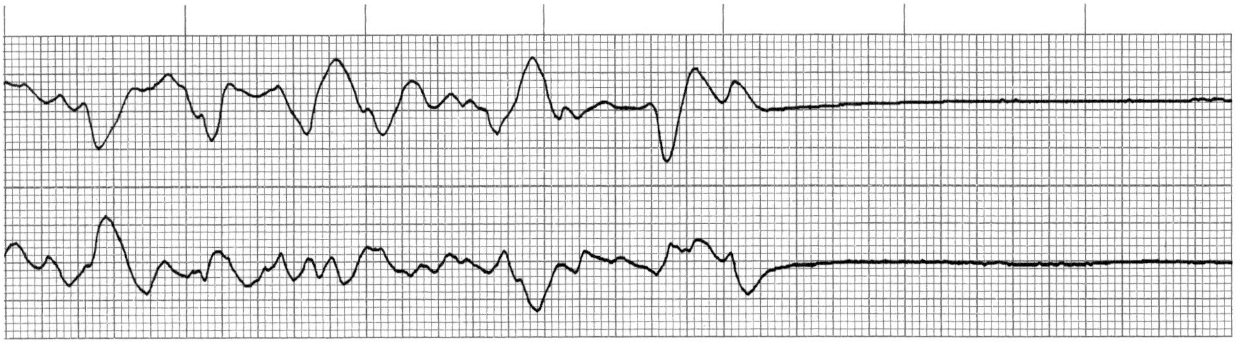

13–25

Regularity: _____ Heart rate: _____ PR interval: _____

P-waves: _____ QRS complex: _____

Interpretation: _____

V

MCL 1

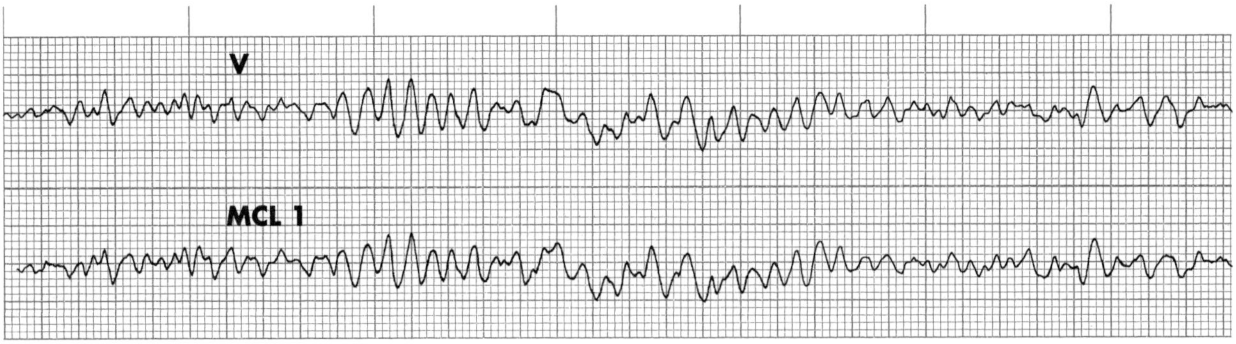

13–26

Regularity: _____ Heart rate: _____ PR interval: _____

P-waves: _____ QRS complex: _____

Interpretation: _____

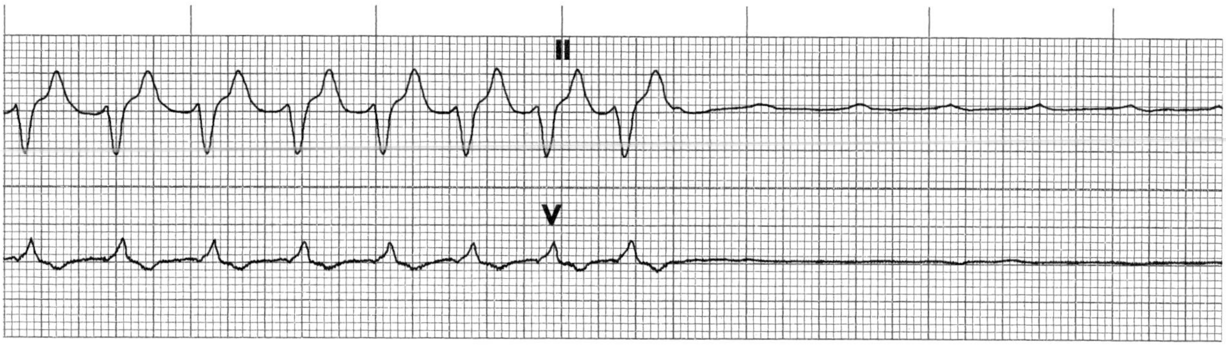

13–27

Regularity: _____ Heart rate: _____ PR interval: _____

P-waves: _____ QRS complex: _____

Interpretation: _____

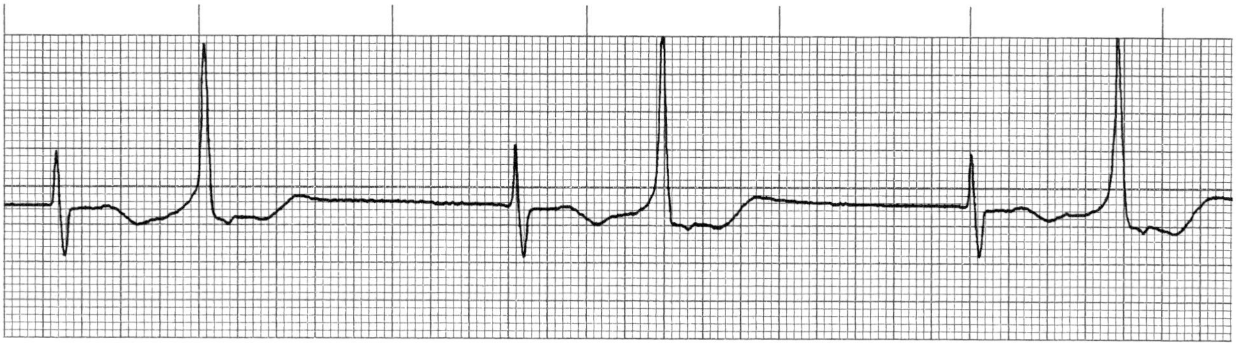

13–28

Regularity: _____ Heart rate: _____ PR interval: _____

P-waves: _____ QRS complex: _____

Interpretation: _____

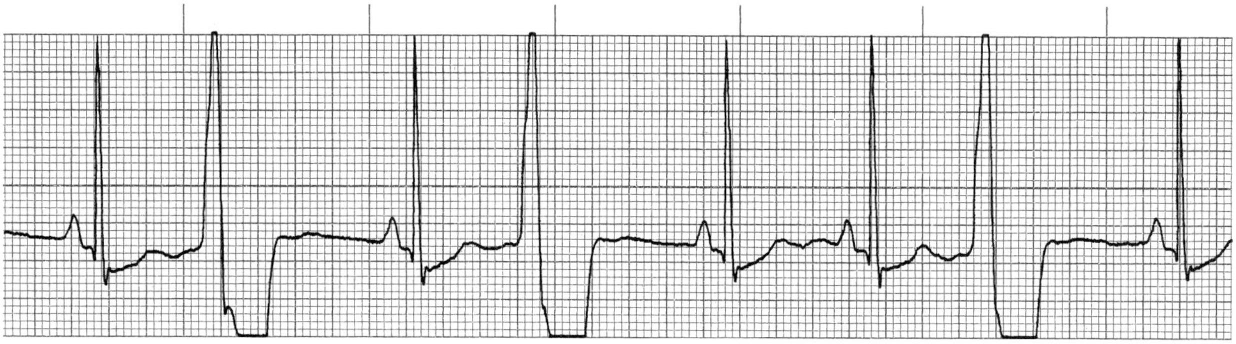

13–29

Regularity: _____ Heart rate: _____ PR interval: _____

P-waves: _____ QRS complex: _____

Interpretation: _____

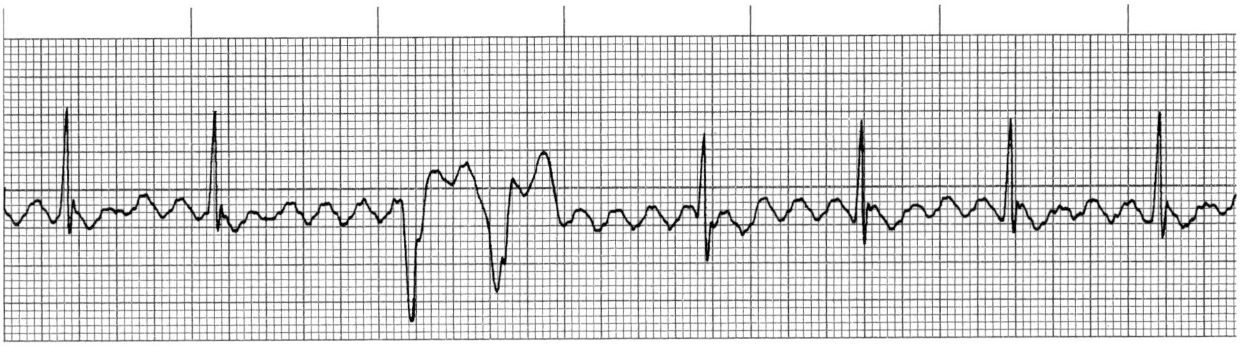

Ventricular Rhythms

13–30

Regularity: _____ Heart rate: _____ PR interval: _____

P-waves: _____ QRS complex: _____

Interpretation: _____

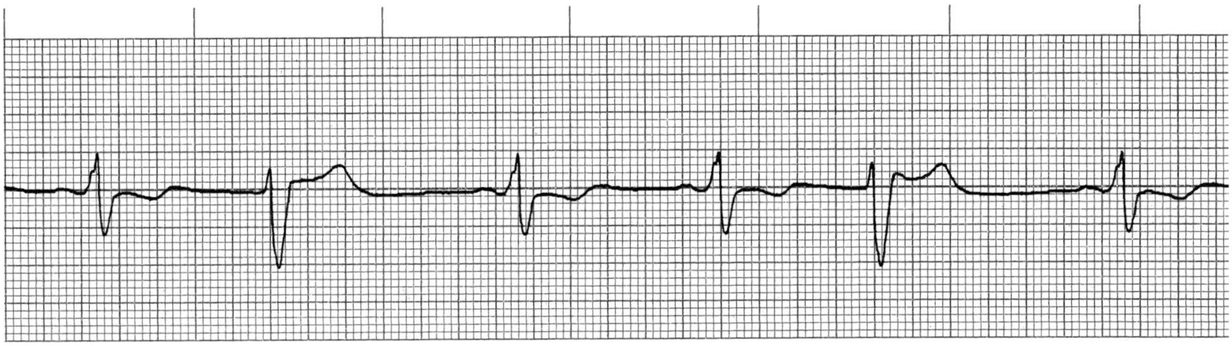

13–31

Regularity: _____ Heart rate: _____ PR interval: _____

P-waves: _____ QRS complex: _____

Interpretation: _____

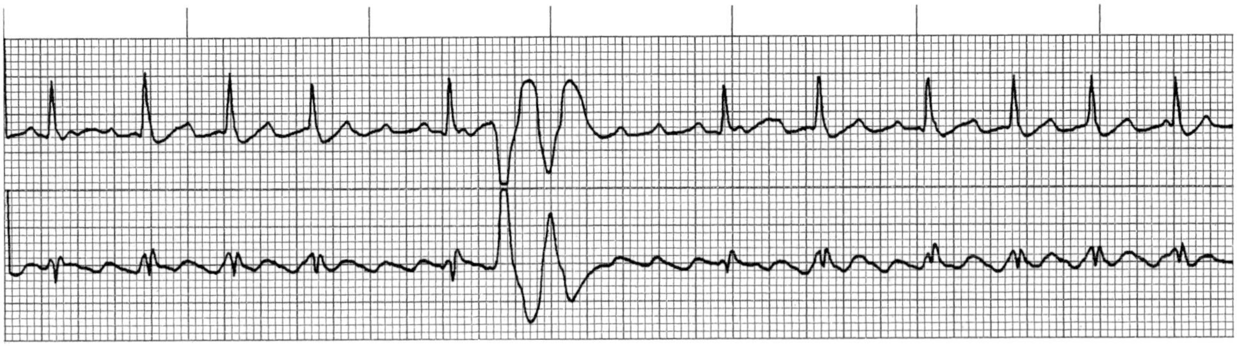

13–32

Regularity: _____ Heart rate: _____ PR interval: _____

P-waves: _____ QRS complex: _____

Interpretation: _____

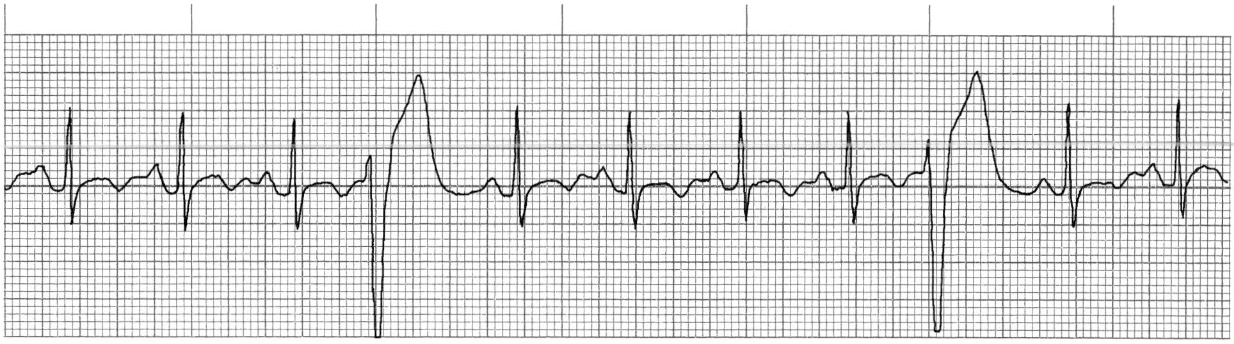

13–33

Regularity: _____ Heart rate: _____ PR interval: _____

P-waves: _____ QRS complex: _____

Interpretation: _____

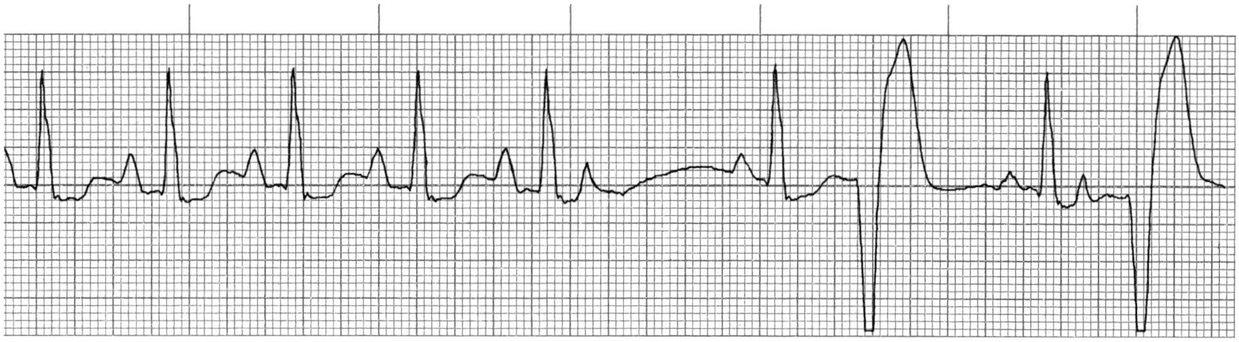

13–34

Regularity: _____ Heart rate: _____ PR interval: _____

P-waves: _____ QRS complex: _____

Interpretation: _____

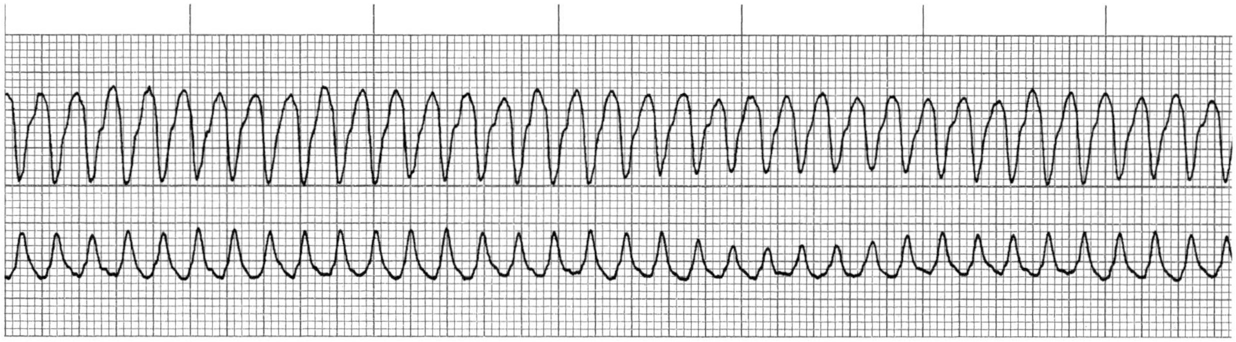

13–35

Regularity: _____ Heart rate: _____ PR interval: _____

P-waves: _____ QRS complex: _____

Interpretation: _____

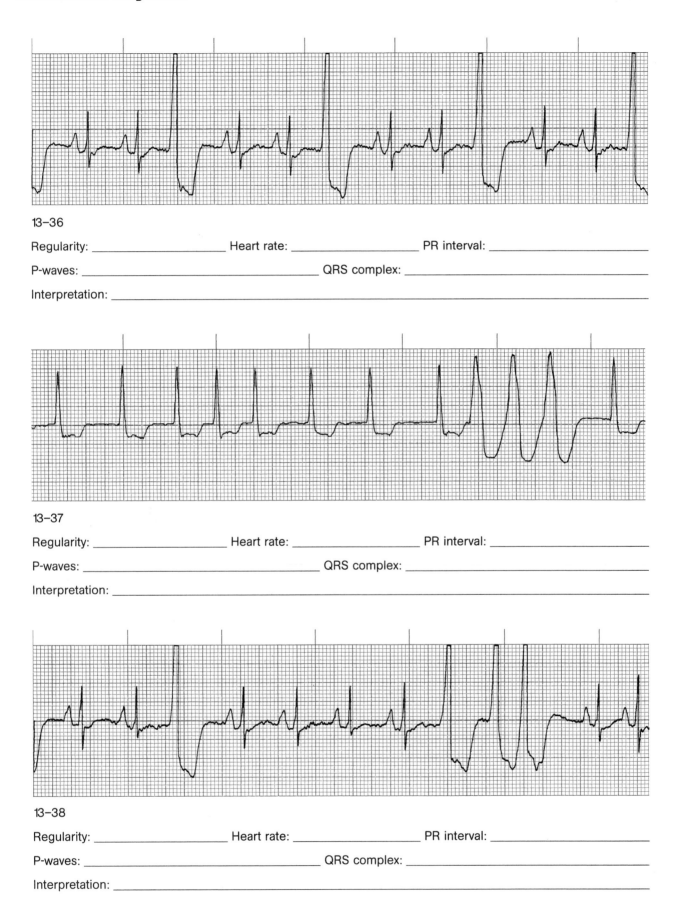

13-36

Regularity: _____ Heart rate: _____ PR interval: _____

P-waves: _____ QRS complex: _____

Interpretation: _____

13-37

Regularity: _____ Heart rate: _____ PR interval: _____

P-waves: _____ QRS complex: _____

Interpretation: _____

13-38

Regularity: _____ Heart rate: _____ PR interval: _____

P-waves: _____ QRS complex: _____

Interpretation: _____

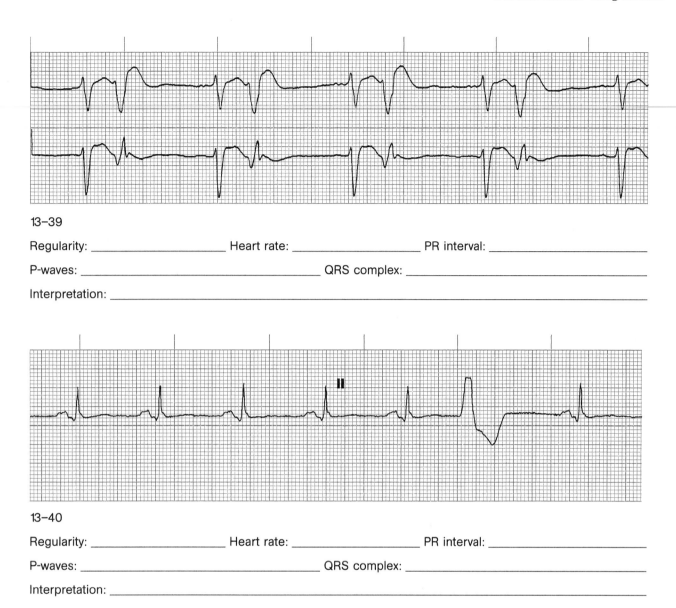

13–39

Regularity: _____ Heart rate: _____ PR interval: _____

P-waves: _____ QRS complex: _____

Interpretation: _____

13–40

Regularity: _____ Heart rate: _____ PR interval: _____

P-waves: _____ QRS complex: _____

Interpretation: _____

SECTION

Contemplating Conduction

THE MENTAL BLOCK
OF AV BLOCKS

14

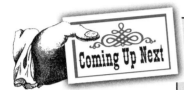
Coming Up Next

- ○ What happens if the AV node does not conduct an atrial signal?
- ○ Why is the AV node called the gatekeeper?
- ○ Which is more serious, first-degree or third-degree AV block, and why?
- ○ What part of the ECG tracing tells us about the functioning of the AV node?
- ○ What is the major difference between the types of second-degree AV block?
- ○ When can it prove deadly to make the ventricles less irritable?

Dissolving the Mental Block

SIMPLE YET VITAL

A long time ago, when I was just knee-high to a T-wave in my ECG interpretation skills, I found atrioventricular blocks the most perplexing to identify. I studied, analyzed, and questioned educators, RNs, CCRNs, even MDs, but I was still having trouble. It wasn't until I thought about what happens in AV block, instead of what the strip should look like, that I began to get a grip on these dysrhythmias. Suddenly, in a flash of insight, I understood the trick to getting them right almost all the time. Later in this chapter I'll share that trick with you, and you too will be able to count AV blocks among your conquered rhythms.

As you remember from earlier discussions of the conduction system, the AV node is the gatekeeper between the atria and the ventricles. Its role is simple yet vital. It receives signals from the atria, holds them briefly to allow the atria time to contract and empty completely, and then sends the signals down to the ventricles. Sounds simple enough: get the signal, wait a moment, and send the signal on its way. But, as we already know, "simple" doesn't mean "infallible"!

FOCUS ON THE PR INTERVAL

Many things can cause trouble with the AV node. This chapter will give you the basics of potential AV node

conduction problems. The area of the strip we're concentrating on here is the PR interval. As you recall, the PR interval reflects the time the signal takes to leave the sinus node, traverse the atria to the AV node, speed down the bundle branches, and arrive at the terminal Purkinje fibers. Once there, the signal produces the QRS complex.

We already know what the P-wave gives us—a look at atrial depolarization. But what about the PR interval? You may ask, "What information can we get from a flat isoelectric line?" Well, actually quite a lot. Instead of looking at shape, height, or direction, we're concerned with the relation of the P-wave to the QRS complex (actually the distance between them), and that flat baseline is the string that binds them together.

The length of the PR interval is an important determinant of AV node function. Remember that the normal PR interval for sinus rhythm is between 0.12 and 0.20 seconds. Two things are involved in this interval. One is the P-wave; the other is the conduction through the AV node and bundle branches. However, as we'll see in Chapter 15, the delays in the bundle branches show up in the QRS complex, not the PR interval. So, by elimination, we know that the PR interval simply measures any delay or any problem with P-wave conduction or with the AV node (and technically the bundle of His, but that discussion is too complex for this book). A longer P-wave can also lengthen the PR interval, but we'll save that thought, too.

THE TOLLBOOTH REVISITED

We learned in Chapters 6 and 7 that the AV node behaves like a tollbooth. Let's re-examine that analogy. How does a tollbooth work? Cars enter it from one or more roads, slow down to pay the toll, and drive through onto the highway. Because of the brief delay, only a certain number of vehicles can get through a tollbooth at any given time.

In the heart, signals coming from the atria slow down briefly in the AV node and then continue on their way to the bundle branches and the ventricles to produce the QRS complex. If too many signals approach the AV node, it allows only a certain number to get through at any one time. The delay in the AV node is vital to the normal functioning of the heart. That extra fraction of a second delay lets the ventricles fill with as much blood as possible before they contract, allowing them the greatest possible efficiency. The more blood the ventricles contain, the more blood they can pump out with each contraction, and the fewer contractions are necessary to meet the body's needs.

For the purposes of this book, AV node conduction problems begin with too long a wait at the tollbooth. When that happens, what's going on? The answer is a blocked signal: when the PR interval is too long, the signal is "blocked" in the AV node. It may just be delayed longer than usual, or the AV node may be letting some signals through and holding others back, or all the signals may be blocked completely.

Tollbooth Trouble

WHAT CAUSED THE TIE-UP?

When you lay all your ECG strips on the table, there are four basic types of AV block. These blocks are divided into three different categories, which we call *degrees.* The degree of AV block is a general guide to the severity of the problem. First-degree block is the least severe, and third-degree block is the most serious.

The degree of block also indicates the functioning level of the AV node. In first-degree AV block, all atrial signals get through to the ventricles. In second-degree blocks, some signals get through but others are completely blocked at the AV node. And in third-degree block, also known as *complete heart block,* no atrial signals reach the ventricles.

Each type of AV block has certain distinguishing characteristics, but it's not enough to just recognize them. Before you can treat them, you need to understand what produces them. To that end, let's review the conduction system.

SHORT BUT CRITICAL

In the "normal" heart, conduction begins with an automatically generated signal from the sinus node. The signal travels through the intra-atrial pathway to the left atrium while simultaneously traveling through the internodal pathways to the AV node. When it arrives at the AV node, the signal is delayed. This delay is vital. It gives the atria a chance to depolarize fully, contract, and empty as much blood as possible into the ventricles before the ventricles contract. Figure 14–1 shows a simplistic overview of the relationship between the conduction system and the ECG strip.

The signal usually spends about 0.10 seconds at the AV node tollbooth. Doesn't sound like much of a delay, does it? Well, it may be short, but it's important. The amount of blood pumped into the ventricles determines the amount

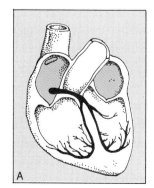
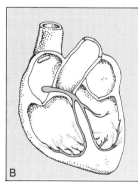
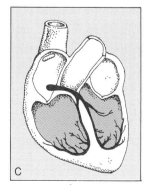

Fig. 14–1A–C The conduction system. A, The P-wave reflects conduction through and depolarization of the atrial tissue. B, The PR segment reflects conduction through and depolarization of the AV node and conduction through the bundle branches. C, The QRS complex reflects conduction through and depolarization of the ventricular tissue.

of atrial kick (if you need to review the mechanical aspects of the heart, look back at Chapter 1). Without this atrial kick, the amount of blood ejected from the ventricles would decrease by as much as 30%! So, even though it is short, that delay is critically important.

As you recall, in Chapter 11 I referred to the AV node as the "gatekeeper," a commonly used term. "Gatekeeper" is an appropriate name because, in almost all cases, the AV node is responsible for transmitting all sinus and atrial signals to the ventricles. If it didn't, the atrial and ventricular contractions would lose their coordination, with potentially serious consequences.

A Matter of Degree

Usually it's easy to recognize an AV block. Check the rhythm strip for either of two clues that you may be dealing with an AV block: a PR interval that's longer than 0.20 seconds or a P-wave without a QRS complex. The difficult part comes in identifying the type of block. As we've already seen, it's not always possible to name a rhythm precisely. However, it's important to do that with AV blocks.

First-degree AV block and second-degree AV block type I (also called Wenckebach block or just Wenckebach) are usually benign; they either correct themselves or cause minimal or no detectable problems. Treatment is usually limited to rest or oxygen therapy. On the other hand, second-degree AV block type II is usually a source of concern and can be a poor prognostic sign in the presence of other conditions, such as acute myocardial infarction (MI). Third-degree AV block is often ominous and frequently indicates the need for at least a temporary pacemaker.

Third-degree AV block is frequently confused with the benign Wenckebach. If we mistake third-degree block for Wenckebach, the patient may die. However, if the rhythm is Wenckebach and we call it third-degree block, the patient may be exposed to unnecessary tests and inappropriate treatments. The second-degree AV blocks are often identified as less problematic rhythms—Wenckebach is confused with sinus arrhythmia and wandering atrial pacemaker, and second-degree block type II is mistaken for sinus rhythm with blocked premature atrial contractions. Therefore, to assess and treat AV blocks, it's critical to name them correctly.

First, let's try to understand why each type of AV block behaves the way it does.

This is a good time to introduce some shorthand. When we note the type of AV block on a strip or in a patient's

chart, we usually use the number and degree symbol: 1° AVB (first-degree AV block), for instance. We do this for brevity when we're writing in a limited space.

First-Degree Block

First-degree AV block is the simplest of them all. In fact, it isn't a true block, but a longer-than-normal delay of the signal as it travels from the atria to the ventricles. First-degree block has two important identifying characteristics: the delay is always the same and the signal always gets through. On the strip, you see that the PR interval doesn't change (because all beats are equally delayed). You also find only one P-wave per QRS complex and a QRS following every P-wave (because the signal gets to the ventricles each time).

First-degree block affects the PR interval, as do all of the AV blocks. In first-degree block, the PR interval is longer than 0.20 seconds. The AV node tissue is stunned but still functioning, although a little sluggishly. What stunned it? You can't determine the cause from the ECG strip. Although the answer won't affect your interpretation of the tracing, it may influence the choice of treatment. What's important is that the AV node can't conduct its electrical traffic efficiently, but if you want to fix the problem, you also need to look for the cause.

The same thing happens a lot on the highway. If unusually few cars are getting through the tollbooth in a given amount of time, there may not be enough toll takers, or all the slow ones may be working that day. Or the problem could be traffic: too many cars trying to get through all at once. Whatever the reason, the cars are delayed longer than they should be, even if they all get through eventually. However, it's one thing to notice a traffic tie-up and another to understand what caused it, and still another to use the correct method to fix it.

The more stunned the AV node, the slower the conduction through it and the longer the PR interval (Fig. 14–2). The PR interval can be as long as 0.40 seconds or more. Although that can be startling, it usually isn't serious. The ventricles don't contract until after the atria contract and empty. Therefore, the ventricles still function at near-normal efficiency, and all the heart's contractions are coordinated from the sinus and AV nodes the way they're supposed to be. For the most part, first-degree AV block is a signal that *something* is wrong with the heart's conduction system. If the onset is new or sudden, you may need to investigate the cause, but if it's been going on a long time, often it's simply noted.

14-1 BOXING TO THE FIRST DEGREE

Imagine a boxing match. One of the boxers is getting the worst of it; his opponent is fighting hard and getting in a lot of hits (many signals are coming from the atria). Our boxer continues to fight, although he's getting a little sluggish and his reaction time is slow (the PR interval becomes longer than normal). His reaction time depends on how stunned he is, just as the length of the PR interval depends on how stunned the AV node is.

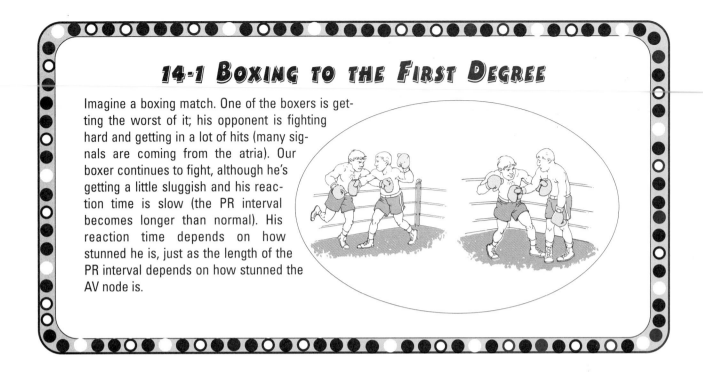

Why even bother naming a dysrhythmia if it's usually not serious? Just like sinus bradycardia, first-degree AV block is often benign. However, because it's still different from the normal rhythm, we name it so we can differentiate the normal from the abnormal. Also, naming this type of block helps us to contrast it with the more serious blocks that we'll be discussing soon.

Second-Degree Block Type I (Wenckebach)

Second-degree AV block type I, also called *Wenckebach* or *Mobitz I block,* can be tricky to understand. On the ECG strip, the first PR interval in the cycle is usually normal or slightly elongated (Fig. 14–3). The first P-wave going

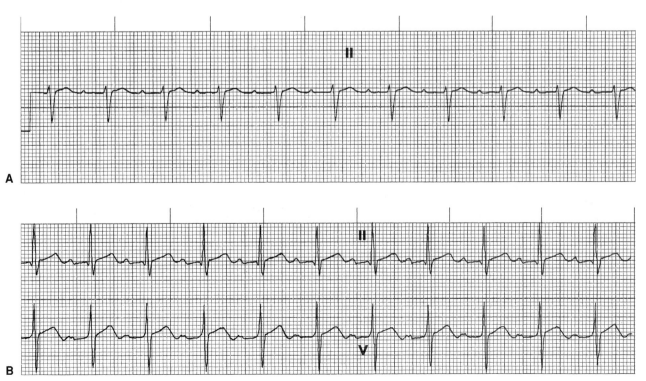

Fig. 14–2A–B Sinus rhythm with 1° AVB. The increased length of the delay in the AV node lengthens the PR segment and therefore the PR interval.

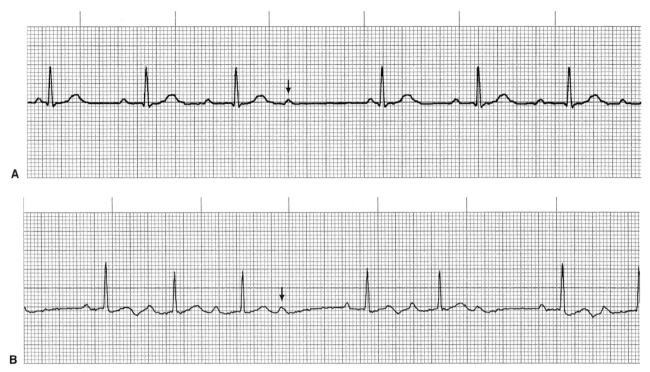

Fig. 14–3A–B In 2° AVB type I, the P-waves march out and the R to R intervals are irregular. Arrows indicate P-waves that are missing QRS complexes.

through slightly stuns the AV node and taxes the ability of the AV node to conduct the subsequent signals as they pass through. When the next signal does come through, the AV node is less responsive and takes longer to conduct the signal. The result is a slightly longer PR interval and a slightly more stunned AV node.

The next PR interval is longer still. The AV node, already stunned, takes another hit from having to transmit a signal before it's ready, and the progression of longer PR intervals continues. Finally, after a string of lengthening PR intervals, one signal comes from the atria and the AV node takes a rest by not conducting the signal at all. That's where the ECG strip shows a dropped beat (see the arrows in Fig. 14–3).

In Wenckebach, the R to R interval is irregular because of the P-wave that is not followed by a QRS complex. Because the P to P interval is regular, the lengthening PR intervals increase the distances between consecutive QRS complexes. Measure the P to P and the R to R intervals in Figure 14–3 and see for yourself.

14-2 BOXING TO THE SECOND DEGREE

In second-degree block type I (Wenckebach or Mobitz I), our boxer is initially spry and energetic, not sluggish at all. Again he becomes more stunned and sluggish with each successive blow from his opponent. Finally, after taking numerous hits in his stunned state, he falls to the canvas (a signal from the atrial signal is completely blocked). The referee comes over and starts counting, "One, two, three. . . ." The boxer takes a break and clears his head as the referee continues to count, "Four, five, six. . . ." Finally he gets up, clear headed and no longer sluggish after his brief but rejuvenating rest. He feels fine until his opponent starts hitting him and the cycle starts all over again.

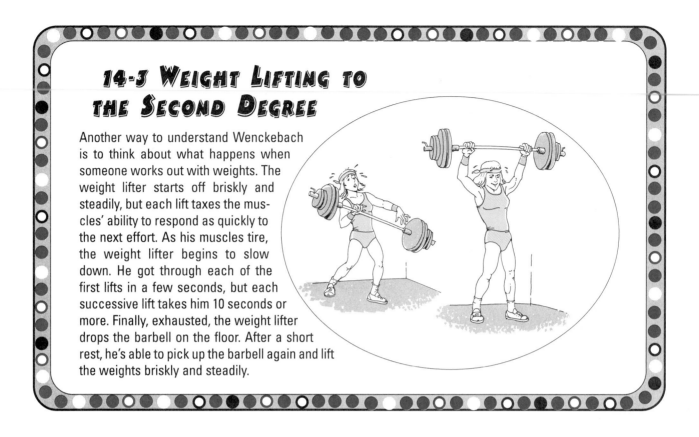

14-3 WEIGHT LIFTING TO THE SECOND DEGREE

Another way to understand Wenckebach is to think about what happens when someone works out with weights. The weight lifter starts off briskly and steadily, but each lift taxes the muscles' ability to respond as quickly to the next effort. As his muscles tire, the weight lifter begins to slow down. He got through each of the first lifts in a few seconds, but each successive lift takes him 10 seconds or more. Finally, exhausted, the weight lifter drops the barbell on the floor. After a short rest, he's able to pick up the barbell again and lift the weights briskly and steadily.

Second-Degree Block Type II (Classic Second-Degree)

Second-degree AV block type II, also called *classic second-degree AV block* or *Mobitz II block,* can resemble Wenckebach. The two types of block are similar; however, in second-degree type II, the PR interval doesn't change.

Wait a minute, you're asking. If the PR interval doesn't change, where's the resemblance to Wenckebach? In both types of second-degree AV block, some P-waves occur without a QRS complex, in which case there can't

be a PR interval. Any time we see a P-wave without a QRS, we know that the AV node didn't conduct the atrial signal to the bundle branches and the ventricles (Fig. 14–4).

In second-degree block type II, the AV node is functioning normally, then is suddenly stunned so severely that it can't conduct the atrial signal at all. In fact, it can remain stunned for several conduction cycles (more about this later). You may see several P-waves in a row that are not followed by QRS complexes. The AV node conducts normally and regularly until, like an overwhelmed parent, it

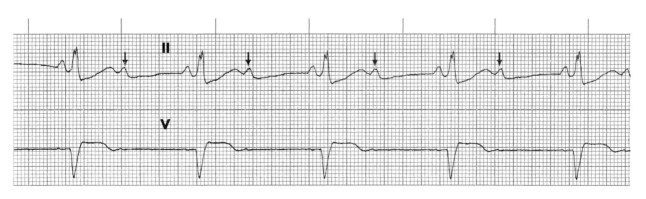

Fig. 14–4 In 2° AVB type II, the P-waves are regular and the PR interval stays the same, but some P-waves (with the arrows) are not followed by QRS complexes. (The wide QRS complexes are also suggestive of type II.)

231

14-4 BOXING TO THE SECOND DEGREE TYPE II

The boxing analogy is almost the same for second-degree block type II as it is for Wenckebach. The main difference is that both boxers are fighting normally and then one boxer suddenly lands a lucky punch: the stunned boxer goes right down even though he wasn't previously stunned. The referee stops the fight for a short time to let the stunned boxer recuperate; he then gets up and fights normally again.

screams, "Enough!" and then does nothing. Then, just as suddenly as the AV node was stunned, conduction returns to normal and signals pass through the AV node as if nothing were wrong—until next time.

The cycle repeats itself over and over again. Sometimes every third QRS complex is dropped, sometimes every fifth. The more frequently the QRS is dropped, the more likely the patient is to exhibit symptoms.

In second-degree block type II, the stunned AV node is having the same kind of trouble as the boxer. Unless the problem with the AV node is corrected, the stunned periods can increase in frequency and length and the patient's condition can go on deteriorating.

Third-Degree Block

WHEN NOTHING GETS THROUGH

Finally, we have third-degree AV block, also referred to as *complete heart block.* The first term is preferred over the second and is more accurate. It isn't the heart that's completely blocked, just conduction through the AV node. In third-degree AV block, the lanes of the tollbooth are all closed and no one can get around them. Not one signal is getting through the AV node; therefore, the atria and the ventricles can't communicate at all.

On the ECG strip, we often find QRS complexes that originate beyond the blockage. They tell us that the heart is contracting, although its ability to function is severely compromised (Fig. 14–5). Sometimes, however, no QRSs occur at all. This type of dysrhythmia, which we covered in Chapter 13, is called ventricular asystole or ventricular standstill. Ventricular asystole is always fatal if untreated and needs immediate attention.

If the conduction system below the block doesn't start the ventricles contracting on their own, the patient will die. Although the ventricles are able to function independently, the rhythm they generate is usually much slower and less reliable than a sinus, atrial, or even junctional rhythm. Therefore, even if the patient has sufficient QRS complexes, this rhythm deserves *immediate* attention. If you find it, you must document it and then notify the doctor immediately. If the patient is stable enough, it is a good idea to document this rhythm with a 12-lead ECG to assist in possibly identifying the cause. This rhythm, especially if newly discovered, may indicate severe damage may be occurring. Such damage can become irreversible in hours if it's not treated.

HIDE AND GO SEEK THE P-WAVES

Third-degree AV block is often missed because some of the P-waves aren't identified. For example, the strip in Figure 14–6 has four obvious P-waves—before the second, fourth, and sixth beats and just before the end of the strip. You could easily misidentify this rhythm as sinus rhythm with a first-degree AV block with bigeminal junctional beats. However, look closely at the T-wave after the sixth beat—that's probably a P-wave hiding there. If you can find one hidden P-wave, more may be lurking.

To find out, take your calipers (or paper edge) to Figure 14–6 and measure the interval from the P-wave before the sixth QRS to the buried P-wave. Then, to check for additional P-waves, place that measure at the end of the P-waves you already know are there. The obvious P-waves are marked "P," and the buried ones are marked "*."

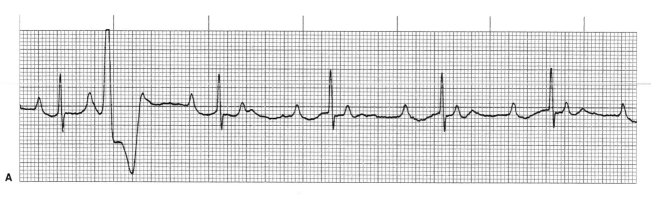

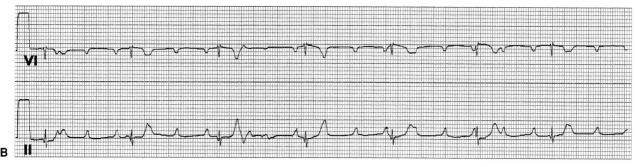

A

B   VI   II

Fig. 14–5A–B In 3° AVB, the P-waves and the R to R interval are regular. In (a), both the P-waves and the R-to-R interval are regular (except for the PVC), but the PR interval are different. The PR interval varies—the atria and ventricles are depolarizing independently because the AV node has failed.

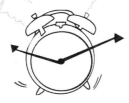

14-5 Boxing to the Last Degree

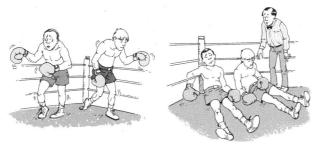

To finish with the boxing analogy, in third-degree AV block, both boxers are clueless. Our friend is too groggy to fight at all. He's so stunned he doesn't even realize there's another boxer in the ring. It's almost as if the boxers were trying to fight each other from separate rings in separate stadiums in different cities! Although he's come back from all his earlier beatings, this time our poor friend never recovers his wits.

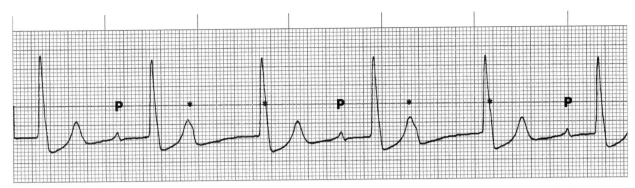

Fig. 14–6 Sometimes the regular P-waves are hidden and difficult to see. It may be necessary to "guess" where two consecutive P-waves are and then march out to find other hidden P-waves. (Obvious P-waves are marked "P" and hard-to-find ones are marked with an asterisk.)

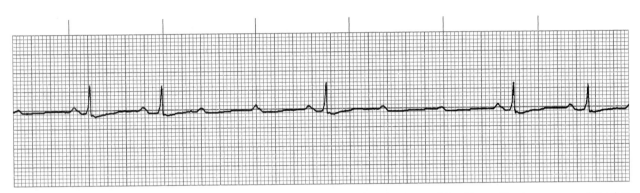

Fig. 14–7 High-grade 2° AVB. Because several successive P-waves are not conducted to the ventricles, this condition is more severe than other forms of 2° AV block.

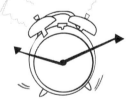

14-6 RARE AND DANGEROUS

High-grade second-degree AV block is a more advanced version of second-degree block type II—more a merging of second- and third-degree blocks. In this rhythm, multiple, *consecutive* P-waves are missing QRS complexes; Figure 14–7 shows an example. Notice the long pause between the QRSs and the five P-waves not followed by QRS complexes. This pause, which is identical to a period of ventricular asystole, almost universally produces symptoms of low cardiac output. High-grade second-degree AV block is rare, not nearly as common as the other four AV blocks discussed in this chapter, but it's important for you to be aware of it. This heart is very sick and may require a permanent pacemaker.

Measuring makes it easier to see the subtle changes in the T-waves that harbor the hidden P-waves. Because the P-waves march out, the patient has a sinus rhythm. Because the QRS complexes also march out, but at a different rate, we're looking at third-degree AV block, and the QRSs are generated by a junctional escape rhythm Therefore, we can identify this rhythm as sinus rhythm with third-degree AV block and a junctional escape rhythm.

Now you know why it's so important to be able to differentiate the various AV blocks from one another. Some, like first-degree block and Wenckebach, are benign and rarely require treatment. Others, like second-degree type II and third-degree blocks, may warn of imminent heart damage or even death.

Table 14-1 recaps the major characteristics of the different types of AV block.

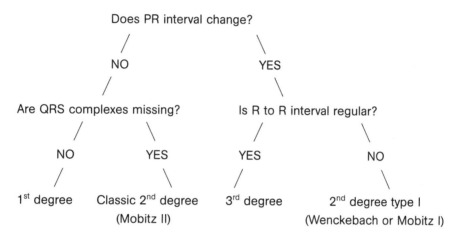

Now, I promised an almost surefire way of correctly identifying these complex rhythms. I am a man of my word! Here it is—get ready, get set. . . .

The AV block interpretation tree is easy to use, and when it's used properly, it's a powerful tool for identifying rhythms. Whenever you suspect an AV block because of an abnormally long PR interval or missing QRS complexes, turn to this decision tree and discover which type of AV block you're dealing with, but remember in AV blocks the P-waves should be regular. If they are not, it may be a blocked PAC. But first do yourself a favor. Try to determine the type of AV block by yourself, and only then use the tree to confirm your conclusions. That way you'll

The Interpretation Tree

FROM THE TOP DOWN

Table 14-1 Types of atrioventricular block

Type of AV block	PR interval	Does PR interval change?	Is RR interval regular?	1 P-wave for each QRS?
1° AV Block	>0.20 sec	Never	Yes	Yes
2° AV Block type I	Variable	Yes, in a pattern	No	No
2° AV Block type II	Normal	Never	Sometimes	No
3° AV Block	Not measurable	Yes, randomly	Yes	No

learn to understand the rhythms instead of just memorizing rules.

AT ITS ROOTS: THE UNDERLYING QUESTIONS

Does the PR Interval Change? To answer the first question, measure all the PR intervals on the strip. Only two types of AV block have a PR interval that changes. They are second-degree block type I (Wenckebach) and third-degree block.

In Wenckebach, the P-waves march out but the QRS complexes don't. That's because the PR interval increases until one P-wave doesn't have a QRS at all. However, in third-degree block, conduction through the AV node has stopped completely, so there isn't any PR interval in the usual sense. The signal generating the QRSs doesn't begin in the atria but in tissue beyond the AV block. It may originate in one of several areas, including the AV node below the point of the block, the bundle of His, or the ventricular tissue. The QRSs may be wide and bizarre or narrow and normal, but either way they don't rely on sinus node–AV node conduction.

Third-degree AV block rhythms are generally regular. As (I hope) you remember, the same is true of junctional and ventricular rhythms. All three types of rhythm—third-degree AV block, junctional, and ventricular—are escape rhythms. All of them are regular because they're generated by a lower pacemaker, independently of the dysfunctional AV node.

Now that we've lopped some branches off the interpretation tree, we're left with only two possible rhythms instead of four.

Is the R to R Interval Regular? To answer the second question, put it more simply: do the QRS complexes march out or not? If the PR interval changes and the rhythm is regular, our previous reasoning tells us that the rhythm must be third-degree AV block. If the PR interval changes and the QRSs are irregular, we must have a second-degree type I block, or Wenckebach.

Are QRS Complexes Missing? What if the PR interval doesn't change? Now we're seeing a different bird altogether. Only two types of AV block have a consistent PR interval: first-degree block and second-degree type II

(classic second-degree) block. The P-waves march out in both rhythms. However, only one rhythm has P-waves that are missing QRS complexes, which makes it easy to distinguish between the two. If some P-waves are missing QRSs, you're looking at second-degree block type II. If every P-wave has a QRS, you're looking at first-degree block.

Time for a solo flight: go back to all the strips in this chapter and use the decision tree to interpret each type of AV block.

Treating AV Blocks

[Note: This section is more advanced than the rest of the book and may be considered optional reading.]

AN OVERALL VIEW

In general, treatment of AV blocks is aimed at maintaining cardiac output by increasing either heart rate or stroke volume. Atropine and epinephrine both increase heart rate. Dopamine, dobutamine, and intravenous fluids increase stroke volume. If nothing else works and bradycardia is the primary problem, the patient will need a temporary pacemaker, or possibly a permanent one.

FIRST-DEGREE BLOCK

Treatment of AV blocks is based on how much the rhythm affects the patient. First-degree block usually doesn't warrant treatment. The AV node conducts all signals, so the heart rate doesn't suffer. If the onset is new, any treatment that decreases the oxygen needs of the heart may help. Alternatively, low-flow oxygen may fill the same demand and restore normal conduction to the AV node.

SECOND-DEGREE BLOCK TYPE I

Second-degree type I (Wenckebach or Mobitz I) block is usually both benign and transient. If the rhythm is of recent onset, it may indicate worsening coronary artery disease and should be investigated, at least initially. Low-flow oxygen, rest, or relief of stress—physical, mental, or emotional—can decrease the heart's need for oxygen and improve AV node conduction. Neither first-degree block nor Wenckebach usually progresses to a worse type of

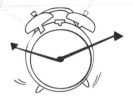

14-7 Avoid Antiarrhythmics

One major caution: when dealing with third-degree AV block, you must stay away from antiarrhythmic drugs, such as lidocaine, that decrease ventricular irritability. A patient with third-degree AV block may depend on that irritability to keep the heart going. Complete AV block leaves only two possible places that can generate a life-saving escape rhythm: the AV node below the level of the block, and the ventricles. If the only rhythm keeping the patient alive is a ventricular escape rhythm, lidocaine will eliminate it and the patient may die.

block. However, both need continued monitoring, especially if the patient has another cardiac or significant medical condition.

SECOND-DEGREE BLOCK TYPE II

Second-degree type II (classic second-degree or Mobitz II) block is more serious and can progress to third-degree AV block. This rhythm disturbance often accompanies an MI, and if so, that's a poor prognostic sign. Studies have shown that a much larger percentage of patients will die if an MI involves second-degree type II block than if it involves Wenckebach. This statistic reflects differences in the types of MI that cause each of these blocks.

Treatment of second-degree type II is based on the patient's heart rate and symptoms. If the number of missing QRS complexes has lowered the heart rate (and therefore the cardiac output) dangerously, treatment is aimed at restoring a faster rate. You can do this by following the symptomatic bradycardia decision tree in the ACLS algorithm. The drug of choice is atropine, which stimulates the AV node to conduct the signals more effectively. Other treatments may include fluid challenges to help alleviate hypotension. If all else fails, which it may if

the patient has high-grade AV block, a temporary or permanent pacemaker may be necessary to maintain an adequate heart rate.

THIRD-DEGREE BLOCK

Third-degree block is the most serious kind of AV block and the one most often in need of treatment. Again the major concern is cardiac output. Many factors can affect ventricular heart rate, but it's critical to pay attention to the lack of atrial and ventricular coordination, which causes a significant drop in cardiac output because atrial kick has been lost. Therefore, treatment is aimed at increasing the cardiac output.

Administering atropine or epinephrine can speed up the heart rate. Fluid challenges, which increase stroke volume, can also increase pressure throughout the cardiovascular system. Greater pressure increases the stretch of the left ventricle; according to Starling's Law, this increases the strength of contraction and finally the stroke volume. If symptoms continue after treatment or if the patient's condition deteriorates rapidly, the next step is external pacing. If the escape rhythm is ventricular, pacing is the treatment of choice, with transvenous or permanent pacemaker placement as soon as possible.

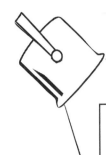

Now You Know

The AV node is called the gatekeeper because it controls the atrial signal's access to the ventricles.

The AV node regulates the number and frequency of signals that are transmitted to the ventricles.

When the AV node does not conduct a signal from the atrial tissue, QRS complexes or ventricular contractions will be missing.

In third-degree AV block, the atria and ventricles are unable to coordinate their contractions. This condition is far more serious than first-degree AV block.

The PR interval tells us how well the AV node is functioning.

In second-degree AV block type I, or Wenckebach, the AV node is stunned progressively through several beats before it stops conducting the signal. In second-degree AV block type II, the AV node conducts all signals normally, then suddenly fails to conduct one signal.

Test Yourself

1. The AV node normally holds on to signals from the atria for approximately _____ seconds before sending them to the ventricles.

2. _____ degree and second-degree type _____ are the types of AV block in which the PR interval does not change.

3. The two types of AV block that most frequently have regular ventricular rhythms are _____ and _____.

4. Lidocaine, and other medications that reduce ventricular irritability, should be avoided in patients exhibiting _____ AV block.

5. _____ is not really a true block but simply an abnormally long delay of the signal in the AV node.

6. The criteria for second-degree type I AV block include _____ P-waves, _____ PR intervals, and _____ P-waves than QRS complexes.

7. Which part of the ECG tracing do AV blocks affect?

8. Identify the rhythm and type of AV block
present in the following 20 ECG strips:

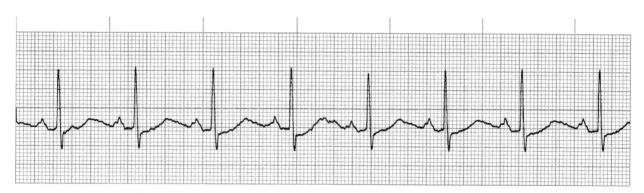

14-1

Regularity: _____ Heart rate: _____ PR interval: _____

P-waves: _____ QRS complex: _____

Interpretation: _____

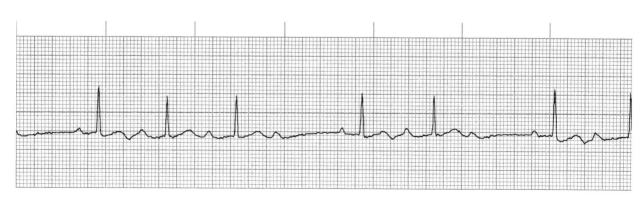

14-2

Regularity: _____ Heart rate: _____ PR interval: _____

P-waves: _____ QRS complex: _____

Interpretation: _____

14-3

Regularity: _____ Heart rate: _____ PR interval: _____

P-waves: _____ QRS complex: _____

Interpretation: _____

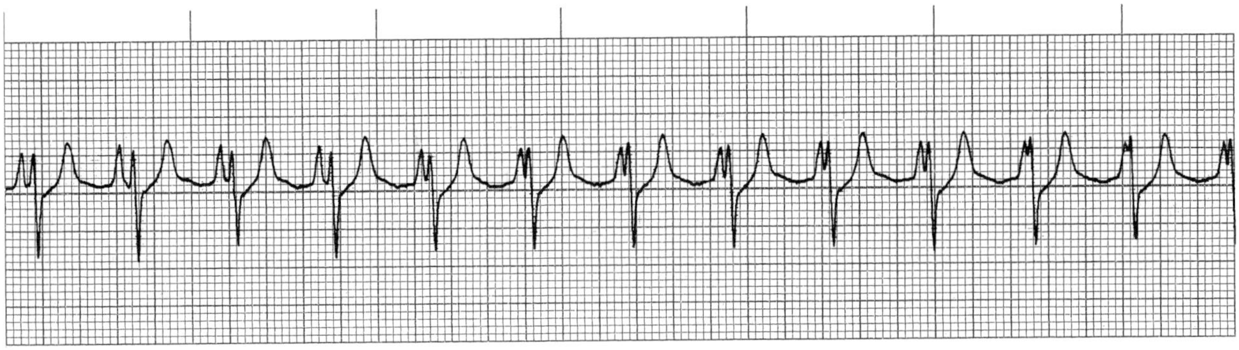

14-4

Regularity: _____ Heart rate: _____ PR interval: _____

P-waves: _____ QRS complex: _____

Interpretation: _____

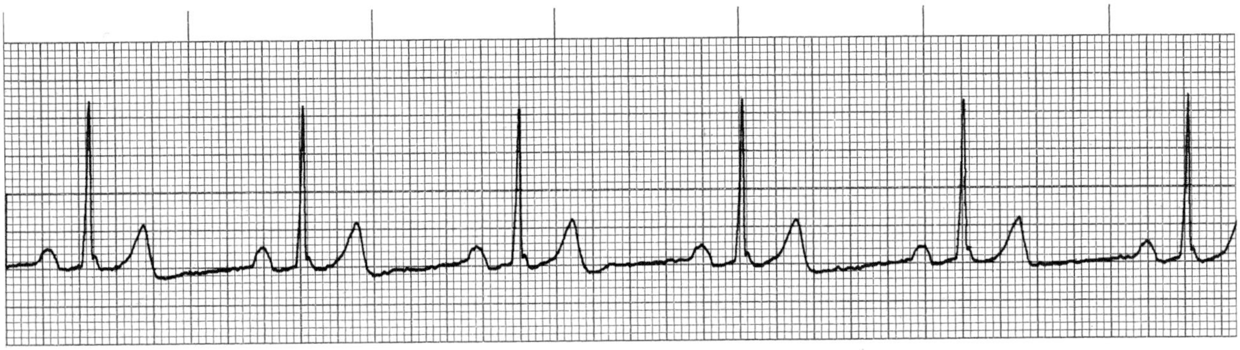

14-5

Regularity: _____ Heart rate: _____ PR interval: _____

P-waves: _____ QRS complex: _____

Interpretation: _____

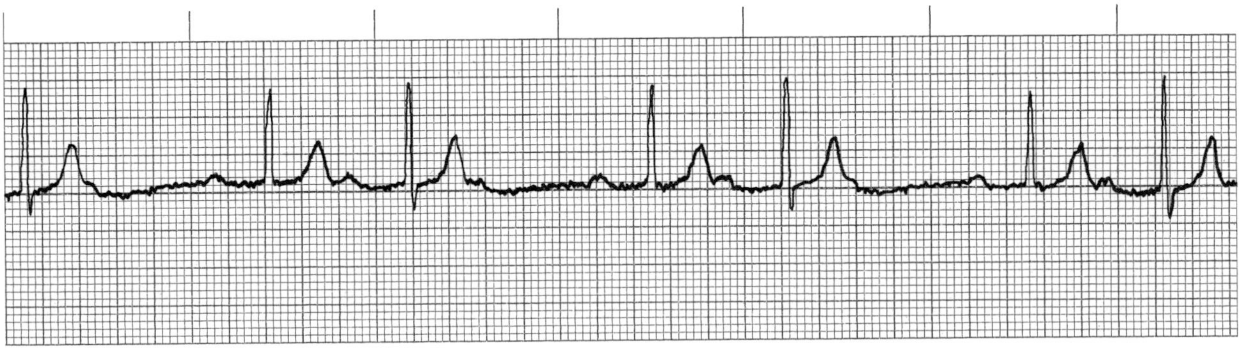

14-6

Regularity: _____ Heart rate: _____ PR interval: _____

P-waves: _____ QRS complex: _____

Interpretation: _____

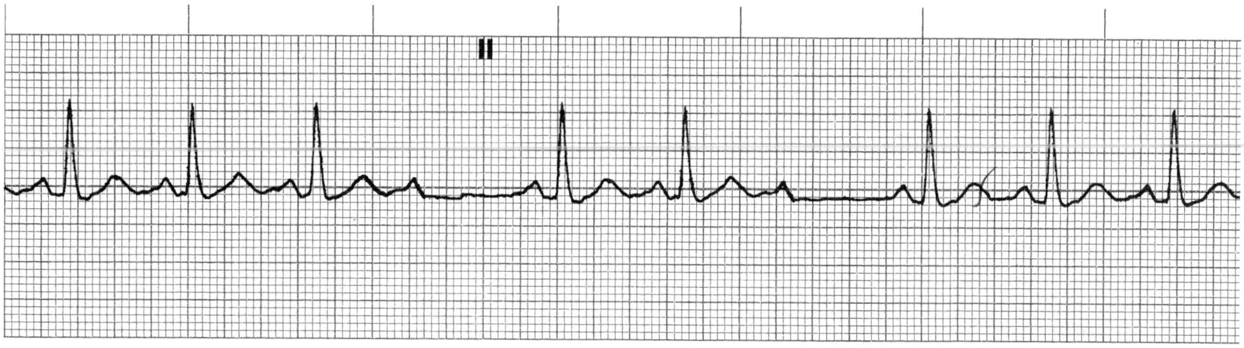

14-7

Regularity: _____ Heart rate: _____ PR interval: _____

P-waves: _____ QRS complex: _____

Interpretation: _____

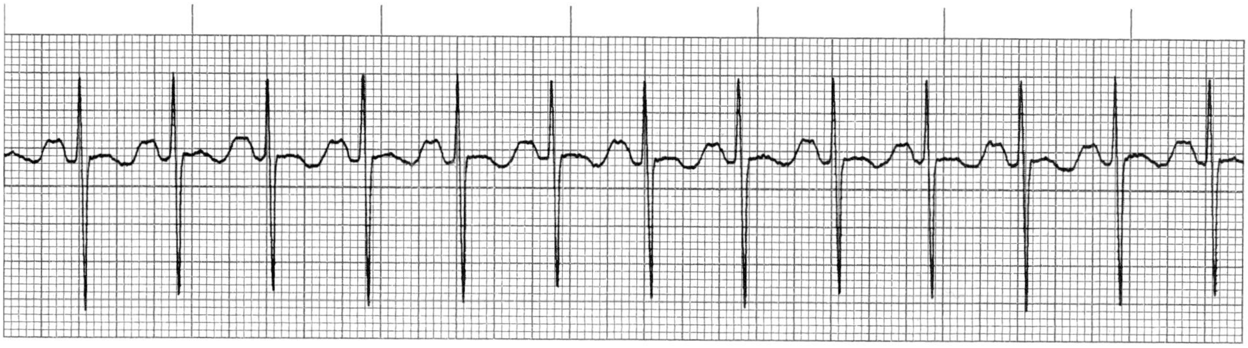

14-8

Regularity: _____ Heart rate: _____ PR interval: _____

P-waves: _____ QRS complex: _____

Interpretation: _____

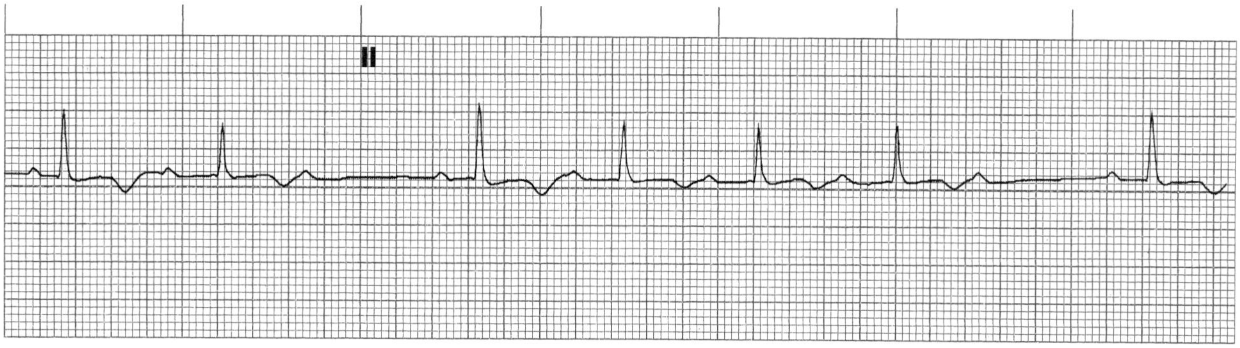

14-9

Regularity: _____ Heart rate: _____ PR interval: _____

P-waves: _____ QRS complex: _____

Interpretation: _____

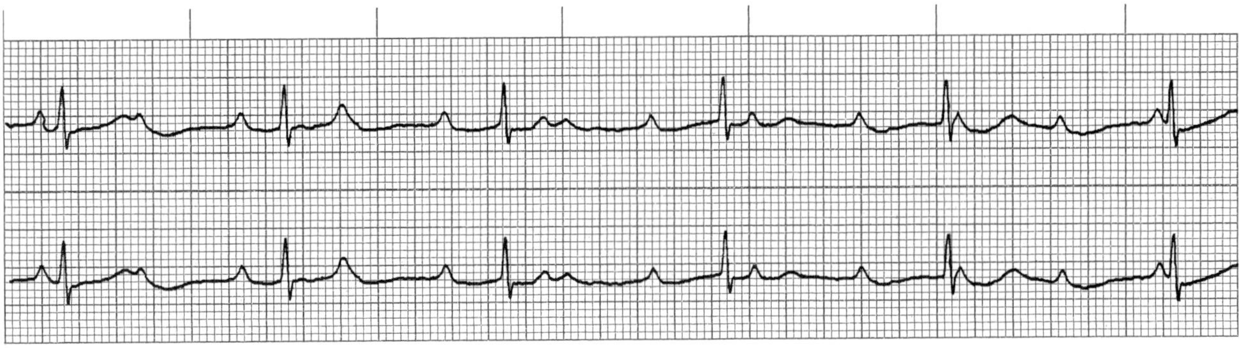

14-10

Regularity: _____ Heart rate: _____ PR interval: _____

P-waves: _____ QRS complex: _____

Interpretation: _____

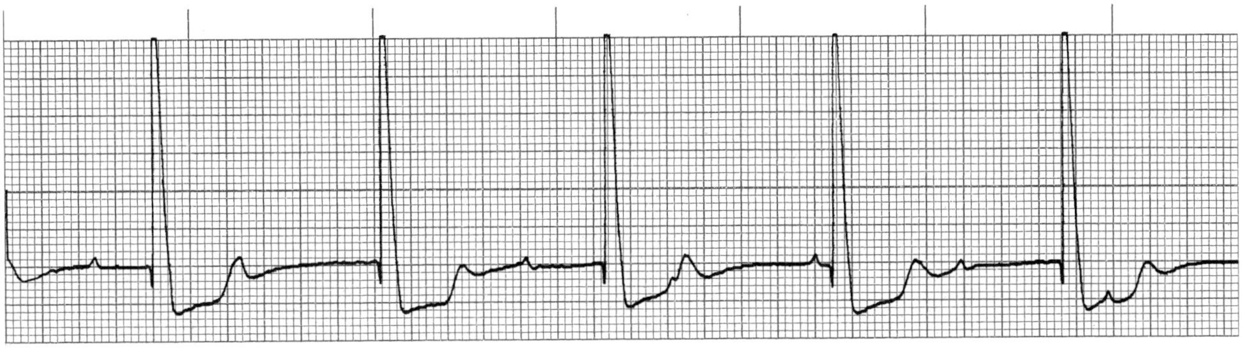

14-11

Regularity: _____ Heart rate: _____ PR interval: _____

P-waves: _____ QRS complex: _____

Interpretation: _____

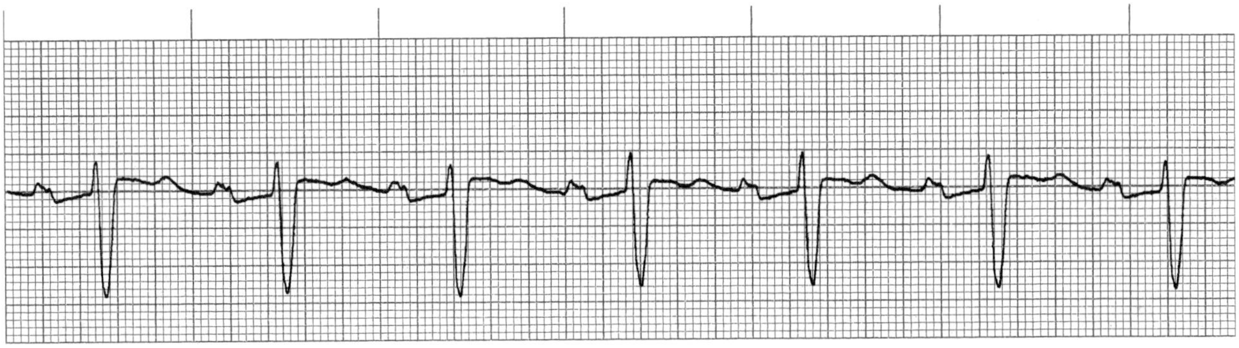

14-12

Regularity: _____ Heart rate: _____ PR interval: _____

P-waves: _____ QRS complex: _____

Interpretation: _____

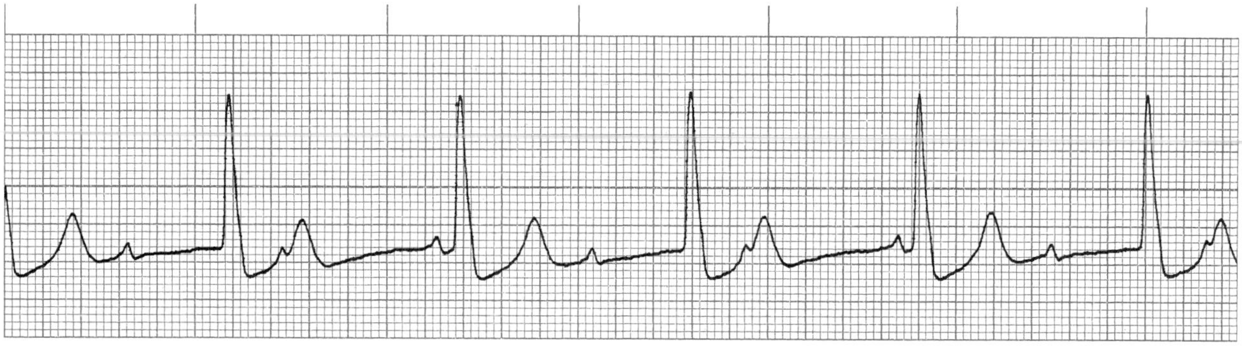

14–13

Regularity: _____ Heart rate: _____ PR interval: _____

P-waves: _____ QRS complex: _____

Interpretation: _____

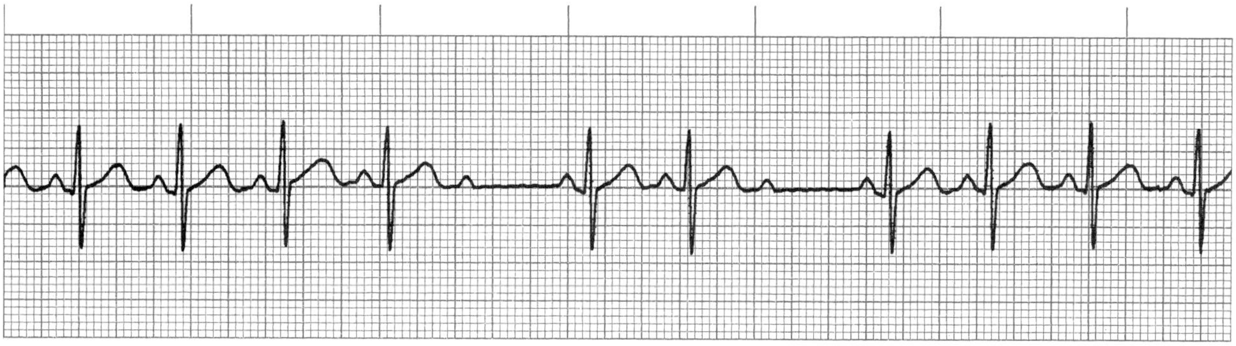

14–14

Regularity: _____ Heart rate: _____ PR interval: _____

P-waves: _____ QRS complex: _____

Interpretation: _____

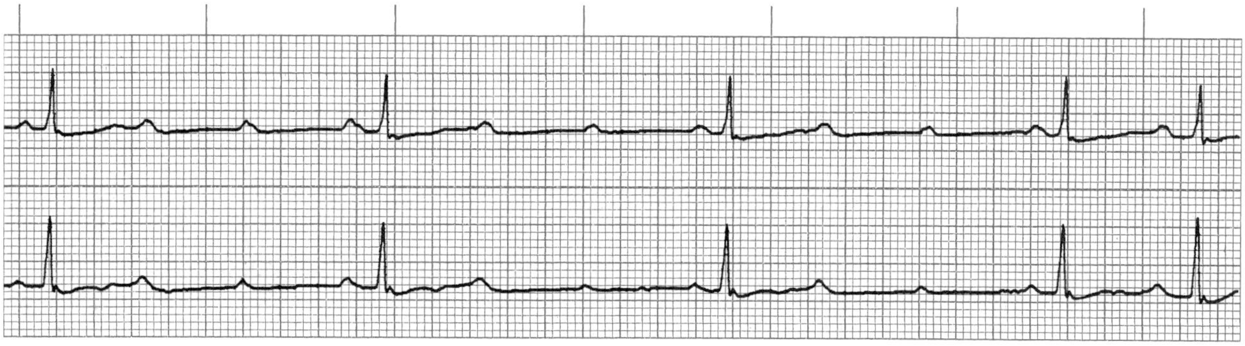

14–15

Regularity: _____ Heart rate: _____ PR interval: _____

P-waves: _____ QRS complex: _____

Interpretation: _____

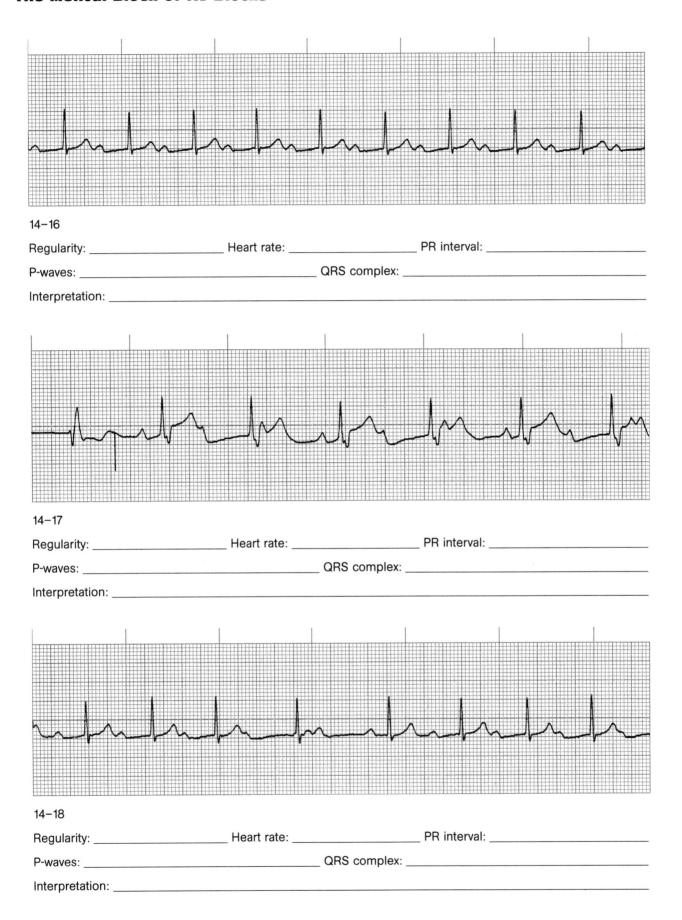

14–16

Regularity: _____ Heart rate: _____ PR interval: _____

P-waves: _____ QRS complex: _____

Interpretation: _____

14–17

Regularity: _____ Heart rate: _____ PR interval: _____

P-waves: _____ QRS complex: _____

Interpretation: _____

14–18

Regularity: _____ Heart rate: _____ PR interval: _____

P-waves: _____ QRS complex: _____

Interpretation: _____

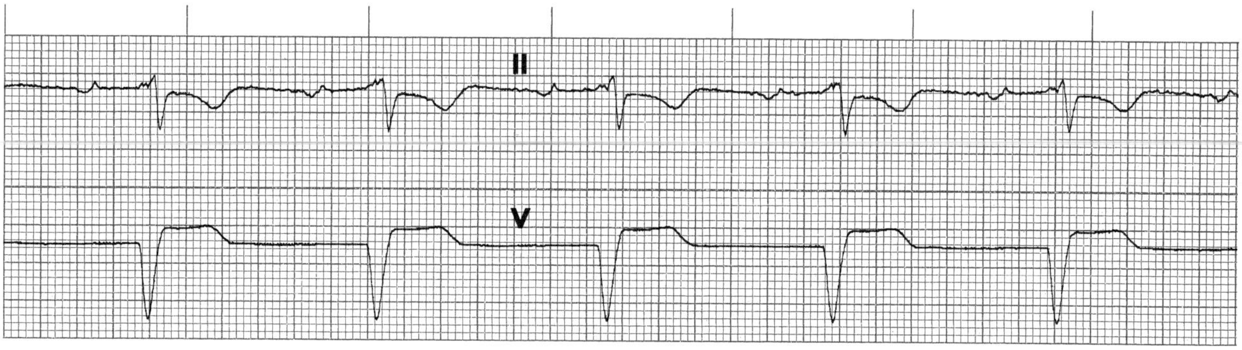

14-19

Regularity: _____ Heart rate: _____ PR interval: _____

P-waves: _____ QRS complex: _____

Interpretation: _____

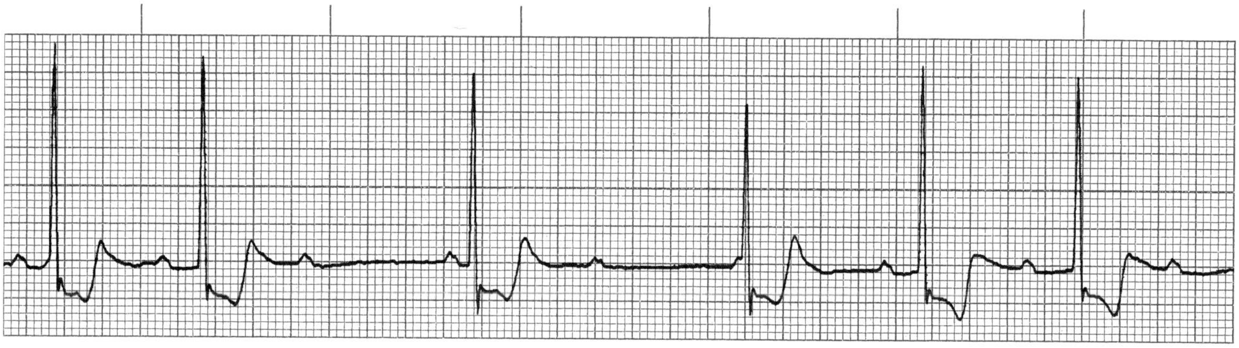

14-20

Regularity: _____ Heart rate: _____ PR interval: _____

P-waves: _____ QRS complex: _____

Interpretation: _____

DETOURS ON THE
INTRAVENTRICULAR HIGHWAYS

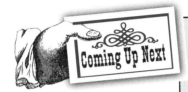

Coming Up Next

- ○ What is a bundle branch block?
- ○ What are some characteristics of a rhythm with a bundle branch block?
- ○ Is a bundle branch block dangerous?
- ○ Can more than one bundle branch be blocked?
- ○ How can supraventricular rhythms with bundle branch blocks be differentiated from ventricular rhythms?
- ○ Why is it important to differentiate supraventricular tachycardia with a bundle branch block from ventricular tachycardia?
- ○ What do we do if we can't differentiate between the two types of tachycardia?

Frustration on the Highway

A ROAD CREW

You're driving through rush-hour traffic to get to work and you see a sign that says "Construction Ahead." What do you think? Well, if you're like me, your first thought is, "It's going to take me longer to get to work." Just like asphalt highways, the intraventricular highways are subject to delays, breakdowns, and detour signs. In this chapter we'll learn to recognize the detours and delays and to understand where their characteristics originated.

In Chapter 7 you learned how to measure the width of the QRS complex. As you recall, I hope, the normal QRS interval is 0.06 to 0.10 seconds. But, as you already know, sometimes the QRS complex is wider than that (Fig. 15–1). When you see a wide QRS, you know that the signal isn't traveling on the fast paths—the bundle branches. Something has forced it to take a detour.

When you ride the intraventricular highways to the terminal Purkinje fibers, sometimes the route isn't direct. If you're trying to get from the AV node to the right ventricle and encounter an obstacle on the right bundle branch highway, the signal can't make it through to the ventricle. By this time we know the signal won't just sit there abandoned and ignored, feeling sorry for itself. Although the bundle branches may be the quickest path through the ventricles, they are not the only way.

When you come up against road construction, you don't just give up, turn around, and head home, and neither does the signal. You get off the fast interstate highway and take the slower back roads, which twist and turn. These back roads will get you to your destination, in this case the right ventricle, but not at the breakneck speed you're accustomed to.

BROKEN BRANCHES

We've already learned that all myocardial cells, not just the ones in the preferred conduction system, can transmit a signal. The bundle branches are the preferred route because they're designed for efficient signal transmission. If one bundle branch, or a portion of one, is blocked, the other, working branches still transmit the signal normally to the terminal Purkinje fibers. But what happens to the myocardial cells served by the "broken" bundle branch, which has turned into a roadblock? Obviously they don't receive the signal directly from the working bundle branches.

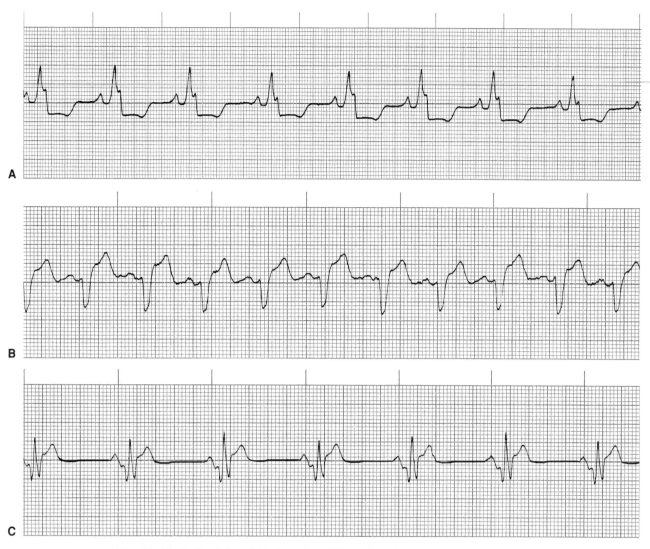

Fig. 15–1A–C Bundle branch blocks produce QRS complexes that last longer than 0.10 seconds.

Like good neighbors, adjacent myocardial cells take over. The cells that have received the signal (from the working bundle branch) transmit it to the neighboring "neglected cells" (the ones normally depolarized by the "broken" bundle branch). However, the signal takes a while to traverse this awkward new path. While it's finding its way, the cells served by the working bundle branches depolarize

rapidly together, beginning the QRS complex. Because the two ventricles are no longer contracting in unison, this new QRS won't look like the normal ones that travel the intraventricular highway—remember "wide and bizarre"? As you know, the elements of the ECG tracing change shape for only two reasons—a different point of origin or, as we're seeing here, a different path through the heart.

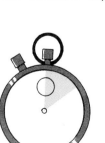

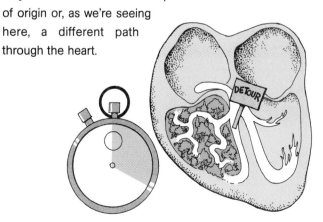

15-1 PSST, ANOTHER MESSAGE....

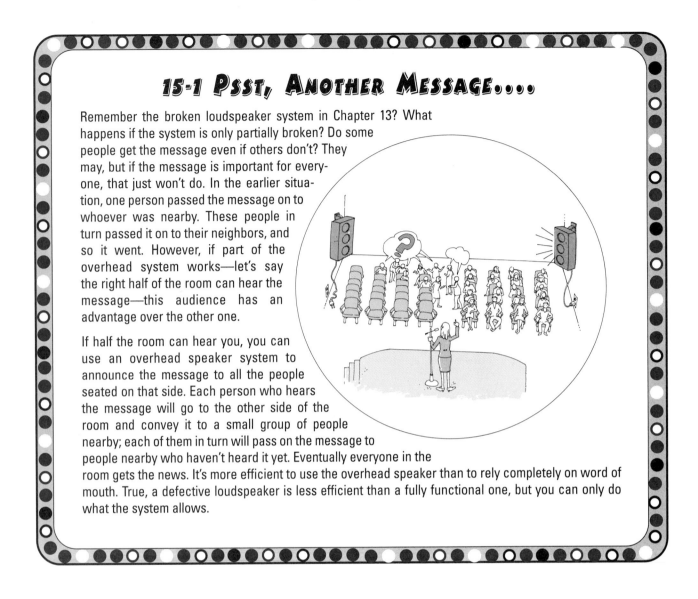

Remember the broken loudspeaker system in Chapter 13? What happens if the system is only partially broken? Do some people get the message even if others don't? They may, but if the message is important for everyone, that just won't do. In the earlier situation, one person passed the message on to whoever was nearby. These people in turn passed it on to their neighbors, and so it went. However, if part of the overhead system works—let's say the right half of the room can hear the message—this audience has an advantage over the other one.

If half the room can hear you, you can use an overhead speaker system to announce the message to all the people seated on that side. Each person who hears the message will go to the other side of the room and convey it to a small group of people nearby; each of them in turn will pass on the message to people nearby who haven't heard it yet. Eventually everyone in the room gets the news. It's more efficient to use the overhead speaker than to rely completely on word of mouth. True, a defective loudspeaker is less efficient than a fully functional one, but you can only do what the system allows.

Landmarks on the Long Way Home

A WIDENING OF THE WAYS

You've gotten pretty familiar with the bundle branches by now, but let's review them anyway. Three main bundle branches emerge from the bundle of His. The right bundle branch carries the signal to the right ventricle. The two others carry the signal to the left ventricle—the left anterior fascicle to the front of the ventricle, and the left posterior fascicle to the rear.

Each of these three main branches is capable of being blocked. In fact, two or even all three can be blocked at the same time and at any point along their length. When this happens, it's often hard for us to determine which paths are blocked. If the QRS complex is too wide it is referred to as an intraventricular conduction defect. It usually lets you know that there is a blockage in *some* part

of the bundle branches. If it is a complete blockage of one of the bundle branches, it is referred to as a bundle branch block. Otherwise, it is referred to as an IVCD. For now, we'll use the more commonly used term, bundle branch block, and concentrate on recognizing the ECG signs that show up in all bundle branch blocks, but be aware that sometimes wide QRS complexes we will see are not formed by a complete block of one or more bundle branches. This concept will be covered in the 12-lead ECG book.

The most obvious characteristic is a widened QRS complex. Remember, each QRS represents the depolarization of both the right and left ventricles. With a bundle branch block (BBB), the two QRS complexes merge, but not completely. Because one begins before the other, they overlap. As in ventricular rhythms and premature ventricular complexes, the block in the bundle branch conduction causes one ventricle to depolarize before the other. However, the QRS is narrower than what we see in most ventricular

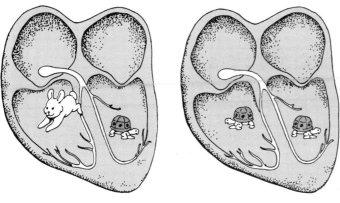

simultaneously rather than in sequence (Figs. 15–2B–C). In Figure 15–2B, the left ventricle has depolarized rapidly, followed by the right ventricle a bit more slowly. In fact, the right ventricle started depolarizing before the left ventricle had finished, but it took longer because it received the signal via the slow path. Still, the QRS is relatively narrow because both ventricles depolarized almost simultaneously.

Figure 15–2A shows normal conduction through the heart and the associated QRS complex. Figure 15–2B shows a QRS complex that resulted from a right bundle branch block. Although the QRS is wide, it isn't as wide as the QRS in the ventricular beat (see Fig. 15–2C) because the signal used the fast path to depolarize the left ventricle. The ventricle "fed" by the blocked bundle branch started depolarizing before the other ventricle had finished, shortening the total depolarization time. Figure 15–2C shows a QRS resulting from a beat that originated in the right ventricle. The QRS is very wide and bizarre, and the direction of the T-wave is opposite that of the QRS. The right ventricle was depolarized via the slow path, and only when the process was nearly complete did the left ventricle even begin depolarization. This sequential depolarization of the left and right ventricles maximizes the QRS interval time.

rhythms because some of the fast path is used (the overhead speaker is working on one side of the room). The width of the QRS is proportional to the size of the block: the more ventricular tissue is normally "fed" by the blocked portion of the bundle branch system, the wider the QRS.

FAST, FASTER, FASTEST

Figure 15–2 graphically demonstrates what occurs in a patient with normal ventricular conduction, a generic BBB, and a ventricular rhythm. Figure 15–2A shows what happens when both ventricles depolarize normally. The QRS complex is narrow because the two events have occurred

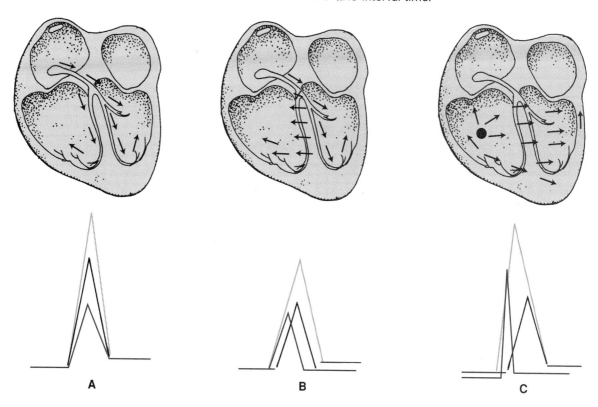

A   B   C

Fig. 15–2A–C Ventricular conduction and the resulting QRS complexes. A, In normal Bundle branch conduction, the QRS is ≤0.10 seconds. B, In a BBB, ventricular conduction is partly normal and partly delayed. The QRS is wider than normal but narrower than in a ventricular rhythm. C, In a ventricular rhythm, the right and left ventricles depolarize sequentially, producing a very wide QRS.

15-2 Racing Hearts

Imagine three pairs of runners at the starting line of a 100-meter race track. Each race will end only when both runners have crossed the finish line. In the first race (a normal rhythm), both runners start at the same time and run at about the same speed. In the second race (a bundle branch block), one runner is slow and the other fast. The slow runner starts just after the fast one, who stays a little ahead of him. In the third race (a ventricular rhythm), both runners are slow, but the first runner finishes most of the race before the late starter even begins.

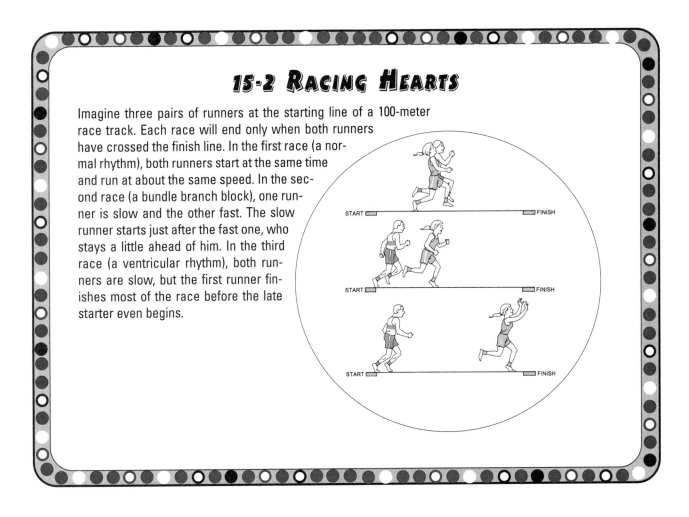

You can see how the use of the bundle branch pathways determines the formation of the QRS complex. A normally conducted beat (see Fig. 15–2A) has a narrow QRS because the left and right ventricles depolarize at nearly the same time. The QRS with the right bundle branch blocked (see Fig. 15–2B) is slightly wider because the left ventricle depolarized normally, while the right began depolarizing a little late and took a little longer because of the slower conduction pathway.

Remember, if depolarization is altered, so is repolarization. Therefore, a QRS complex with a bundle branch block will also have a different T-wave morphology. In fact, with a BBB, the direction of the T-wave is opposite the main direction of the QRS (especially the last portion of it). In normal conduction, the T-wave and most of the QRS should be in the same direction (Fig. 15–3).

So far, bundle branch block sounds a lot like a ventricular rhythm: a wide, bizarre QRS complex with a T-wave in the opposite direction. There are many subtle features that can help distinguish a BBB from a ventricular rhythm, but most need a 12-lead ECG. On a rhythm strip, aside from an occasional subtle difference in width, the QRSs in

ventricular beats and BBBs can look much alike. Rhythms with BBBs are occasionally mistaken for ventricular rhythms for this very reason. The key to differentiating them is to try to verify where the rhythm begins. To this end we can begin by looking at the P-waves.

POWER TO THE P-WAVE

Many rhythms can have P-waves. Even in atrial fibrillation, the occasional P-wave can turn up in an otherwise undulating baseline, and ventricular rhythms can have P-waves that are not associated with a QRS complex, especially in rhythms with third degree AV blocks.

The key to identifying a bundle branch block is to determine the relationship of the P-wave, if it's present, to the widened QRS complex. Suppose we have a rhythm with wide, bizarre QRSs and T-waves in the opposite direction. If there's a P-wave 0.16 seconds before every QRS, that strongly suggests (but doesn't guarantee) that the QRS was caused by the P-wave. If all of the QRSs are the same shape and if we can identify the P-waves that caused them, obviously the rhythm can't be ventricular. Why not? Because the signal started in the atria.

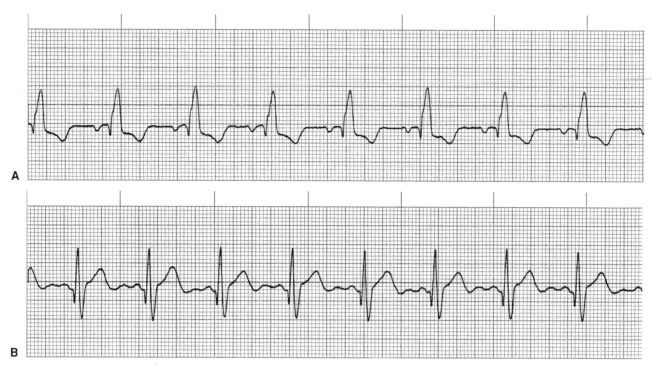

Fig. 15–3A–B In BBB rhythms, the direction of the T-wave, representing repolarization, is opposite that of the final portion of the QRS complex.

Tachycardias of the Fourth Kind

ORIGIN UNKNOWN

The three types of tachycardic rhythm we've discussed so far are atrial fibrillation and atrial flutter (Chapter 11), narrow-complex tachycardias apart from A-fib and atrial flutter (Chapters 10–12), and known ventricular tachycardia (Chapter 13). The fourth and final classification is *wide-complex tachycardia of unknown origin.*

All tachycardias with a QRS complex of more than 0.10 seconds are called *wide QRS complex tachycardias,* or *wide-complex tachycardias* for short. Interpreting these rhythms can give you a run for your money. It can be hard to distinguish between ventricular tachycardia and supraventricular tachycardia with a bundle branch block. You can usually pick out the P-waves fairly easily in a slower rhythm, but faster rhythms get tricky because P-waves may be hidden in the preceding QRS complex or T-wave (see Fig. 15–4). In tachycardic rhythms, checking other leads or getting a twelve-lead ECG may help to identify P-waves that are otherwise obscured.

Atrial fibrillation can accompany bundle branch block. Multifocal atrial tachycardia with a BBB is less common, but it does show up. In A-fib there are no P-waves to identify; in MAT the P-waves can be difficult to see. If the atrial rate is very rapid, nearer 600 bpm than 350 bpm,

you may not even be able to pick out the characteristic wavy baseline of A-fib.

PULLING A RABBIT OUT OF THE ECG

Wide-complex tachycardias are tricky to interpret. Here's a hint: look for the rabbit ears. Not the ones on the bunny or even the TV, but the ones on the ECG strip. Notice how the top of the QRS complex is notched and has two peaks—that's a rabbit ear pattern. Figure 15–5 shows some examples of QRS complexes with rabbit ears.

Rabbit ears can occur in both V-tach and SVT with a BBB. In some leads, the appearance of the rabbit ears can help us differentiate between these two possible

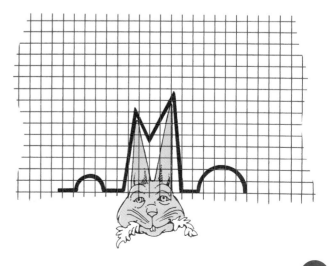

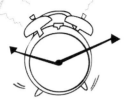

15-3 FIRST LOOK FOR V-TACH

You're looking at a tachycardic rhythm and you're not sure if it's ventricular or a bundle branch block. A key point to remember about ventricular tachycardia is that more than 75% of V-tach is regular. If BBB occurs in rhythms such as A-fib or MAT, even with the rapid ventricular rate, it's usually obvious that the rhythm is irregularly irregular. This method isn't foolproof, but it works in many cases.

Also, compare the QRS complexes with the patient's "normal" QRSs. For example, suppose the patient's normal rhythm is A-fib with a BBB and the heart rate suddenly increases to 200 bpm or more. Look at the QRS. If it's the same shape as it was before the tachycardia started, the rhythm is probably supraventricular tachycardia with a BBB. (This method works with all tachycardias.)

If you really can't differentiate between V-tach and supraventricular tachycardia with a BBB, you should assume that you're dealing with V-tach. Usually this rhythm is more dangerous and less well tolerated than SVT with a BBB; in addition, it's also more commonly found. Also, some medications used to treat SVT with a BBB, such as verapamil, can cause serious problems if administered to a patient with V-tach.

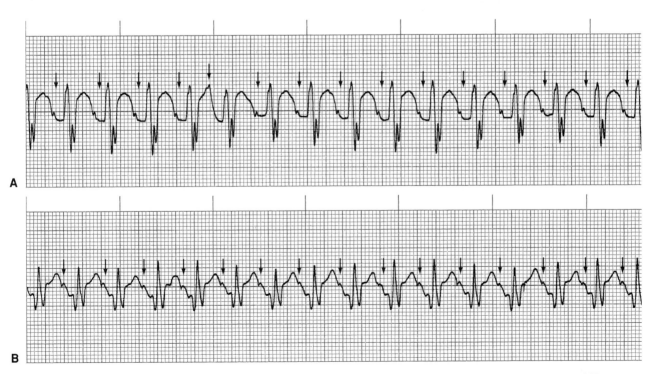

Fig. 15-4A–B Supraventricular tachycardia with a bundle branch block. Arrows indicate the P-waves preceding each wide QRS.

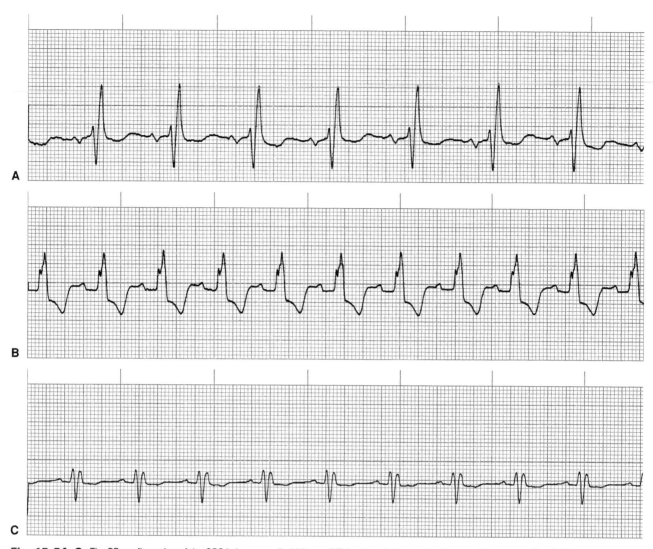

Fig. 15–5A–C The RR configuration of the QRS is known as "rabbit ears." This shape indicates that the ventricles are not depolarizing together.

origins for the widened QRS complex. If you're monitoring lead V_1 and the first rabbit ear is taller than the second, the pattern is suggestive of V-tach (Fig. 15–6A). However, if the first rabbit ear is shorter, we have a less-conclusive sign for SVT with a BBB (Fig. 15–6B–C).

DOES THE QRS STAY IN SHAPE?

If a rhythm strip or twelve-lead ECG was obtained before the wide-complex tachycardia developed, it may help you differentiate between the two types of rhythms. If the patient had a documented bundle branch block before developing a wide-complex tachycardia, you'll be able to compare the earlier QRS complexes with the present ones.

Figure 15–7A shows an example of sinus rhythm with a bundle branch block. Figure 15–7B, recorded later, shows a regular wide-complex tachycardia in the same patient. There are clearly no identifiable P-waves in the second strip, but notice that the QRS complex hasn't

changed shape. Remember, if any two waves of the same type are the same shape, they originated in the same place and followed the same path. In the first strip, the relationship between the P-wave and the QRS tells us that the rhythm is supraventricular, with the QRS originating in the AV node. Therefore, the second rhythm must also be supraventricular: the QRS is the same as in the first strip, so we know that it also originated in the AV node.

Do the Valsalva

BACK TO THE ROCK PILE

There's another piece to the tachycardic jigsaw puzzle, and it can come in handy once you know where it fits in.

Several locations in your body have pressure sensors that help to regulate your cardiovascular system. These sensors are located in the carotid arteries in your neck, the aortic arch in your chest, and, believe it or not, the arteries

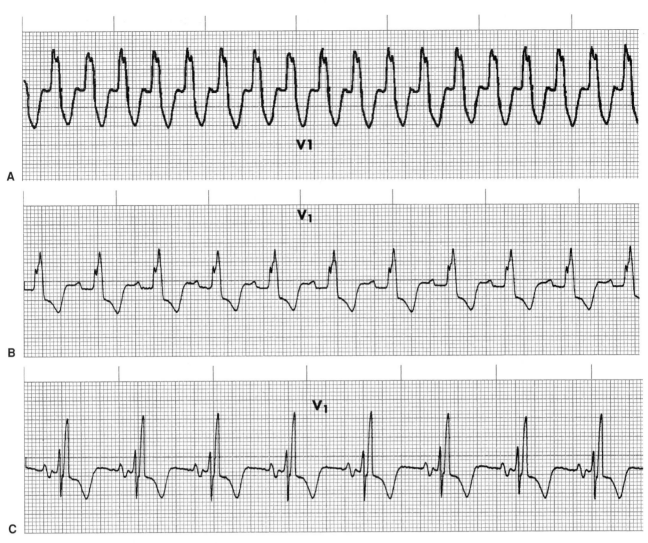

Fig. 15-6A–C A, Rabbit ears, with the first peak of the QRS higher than the second in lead V₁, suggest ventricular tachycardia. B and C, If the second ear is taller than the first in lead V₁, the rabbit ears give a less-conclusive indication of SVT with a BBB.

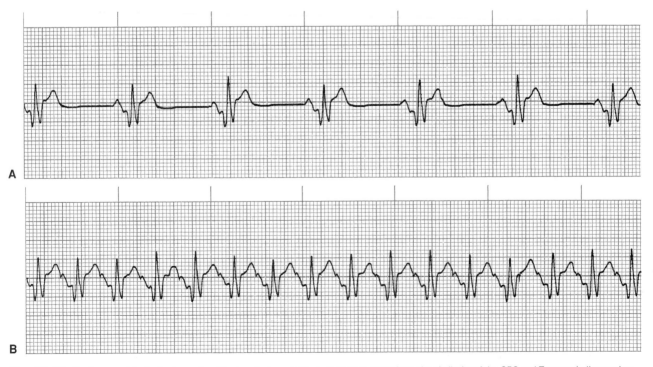

Fig. 15-7A–B Supraventricular tachycardia with a bundle branch block. In these two tracings, the similarity of the QRS and T-waves indicates that ventricular depolarization originated in the same location. In A, ventricular depolarization began in the AV node; therefore, we can safely assume the same about B.

in your rectum. The job of these sensors is to monitor the blood pressure in these locations and give feedback to the brain, which then can adjust your heart rate.

If you have a low blood pressure in any of these locations, some areas of your body may not be getting enough blood flow. As you know, blood pressure can fall if cardiac output is reduced. If the sensors sound a low blood pressure alarm, the brain increases the heart rate by sending signals that cause the sinus node to discharge more quickly and increase conduction speed through the AV node. Cardiac output increases—remember our rock-moving exercise in Chapter 1? Increased cardiac output increases blood flow to, and blood pressure in, the area of the low-pressure sensor, correcting the problem.

The opposite also works. If any of these sensors detects too high a blood pressure, it sends a warning to the brain, which decides that cardiac output is too high. The brain then sends a signal to the sinus node to discharge more slowly and decreases conduction through the AV node. Slowing the heart rate decreases cardiac output, correcting the high-pressure situation.

If the heart rate is too fast, we may be able to manipulate the pressure sensors to slow it down temporarily.

Once the heart rate has slowed sufficiently, we can identify any existing P-waves. We can learn something else, too: because most of this protective mechanism is felt by the sinus and AV nodes, a significant slowdown indicates strongly that the rhythm is supraventricular. If the rhythm originated in the ventricles, the sinus and AV nodes usually have no effect on the heart rate.

CONTENTS UNDER PRESSURE

We can activate the pressure sensors in several ways. One method, fortunately rarely used, was to submerge the patient's face in ice water. In a patient with coronary artery disease, this method could be dangerous because the patient could aspirate water into the lungs and the increase in adrenaline release can increase the oxygen demand of the heart, causing chest pain or worse. Also, you would not have a happy patient! A more current and merciful method is *carotid massage*. This should be performed only by a physician and only if the patient shows no evidence of carotid artery disease.

How can a non-physician bedside health-care practitioner activate the pressure sensors? Have the patient perform the Valsalva maneuver. There are two safe ways

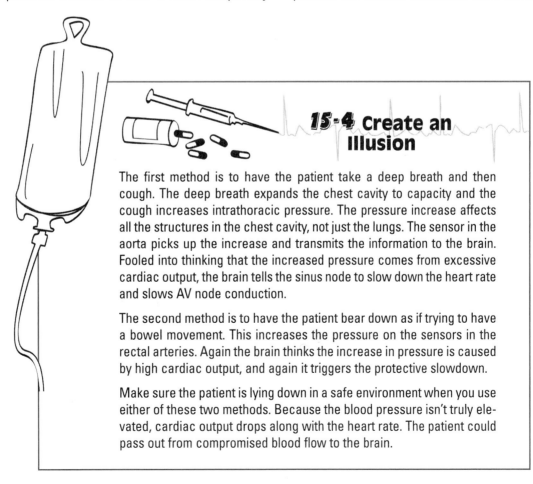

15-4 Create an Illusion

The first method is to have the patient take a deep breath and then cough. The deep breath expands the chest cavity to capacity and the cough increases intrathoracic pressure. The pressure increase affects all the structures in the chest cavity, not just the lungs. The sensor in the aorta picks up the increase and transmits the information to the brain. Fooled into thinking that the increased pressure comes from excessive cardiac output, the brain tells the sinus node to slow down the heart rate and slows AV node conduction.

The second method is to have the patient bear down as if trying to have a bowel movement. This increases the pressure on the sensors in the rectal arteries. Again the brain thinks the increase in pressure is caused by high cardiac output, and again it triggers the protective slowdown.

Make sure the patient is lying down in a safe environment when you use either of these two methods. Because the blood pressure isn't truly elevated, cardiac output drops along with the heart rate. The patient could pass out from compromised blood flow to the brain.

to do this. Neither method is foolproof—not all SVT rhythms will slow down, and some cases of V-tach will.

QRS Complexes in Accord

Whenever you have a wide-complex tachycardia in a stable patient, obtaining a 12-lead ECG should be a priority. Sometimes that's the only way to differentiate this starting point of these types of rhythms. Several algorithms, some better than others and none of them perfect, are used to differentiate supraventricular tachycardia with a bundle branch block from ventricular tachycardia. Every one of these methods relies on the multiple ECG leads.

Discussion of these algorithms is beyond the scope of this text. However, one unusual feature of the 12-lead ECG is so strongly suggestive of V-tach that I've decided to include it. Say hello to *precordial ventricular concordance*. In Chapter 4 we used the term "precordial" to describe the chest leads V_1 through V_6. "Concordance" means that all the precordial leads have the same deflection—that is, V_1 through V_6 all have completely positive or completely negative QRS complexes. Normally the deflection of the QRS is mostly negative in V_1. The positive portion increases until, by V_3 or V_4, the QRS is more

positive than negative, and finally by V_6 it's predominantly positive.

When all the V leads are completely positive or completely negative and all six of them are in the same direction, you've got positive ventricular concordance (even if the QRSs are all negatively deflected). More than 90% of wide-complex tachycardias with positive ventricular concordance turn out to be V-tach. However, the converse isn't true: a lack of concordance does not suggest SVT with a BBB.

Table 15–1 lists ECG features that suggest one type of rhythm over the other. These guidelines aren't perfect; however, the more features favor one rhythm over another, the more likely you are to make a correct diagnosis.

If It's Yellow, Waddles, and Quacks, It's Probably V-Tach

Sometimes it just isn't possible to differentiate wide-complex tachycardias using the bedside ECG. A more invasive method, called an *electrophysiology study* (EP study for short), maps the heart's electrical signals from inside the heart. The details are outside the scope of this book.

It's important to understand bundle branch blocks, their associated tachycardias, and how you can differentiate these rhythms by using some features of the surface ECG.

Table 15–1 Ventricular tachycardia or supraventricular tachycardia with bundle branch block?

Supraventricular Tachycardia with Bundle Branch Block	Ventricular Tachycardia
QRS ≤0.14 seconds	QRS ≥0.16 seconds
Decreased heart rate with Valsalva maneuver	Positive precordial ventricular concordance
P-Waves associated with QRSs	Regular P-waves that do not correspond to QRSs
QRS shape unchanged with increased heart rate	QRS shape changed with increased heart rate
Rabbit ears in V_1, with second peak taller than first peak	Rabbit ears in V_1, with first peak taller than second peak

But it's just as important to remember that most regular wide-complex tachycardias are V-tach, especially if the patient's QRS complex has changed shape significantly.

If you can't differentiate SVT with a BBB from V-tach using the information in this chapter, you still need to treat the patient. Treatment focuses on V-tach first, and you shouldn't try SVT treatments until you've eliminated that first possibility. If treatment still doesn't work, you should revert to treating the rhythm as V-tach. The key to treatment decisions is your assessment of how the rhythm affects the patient.

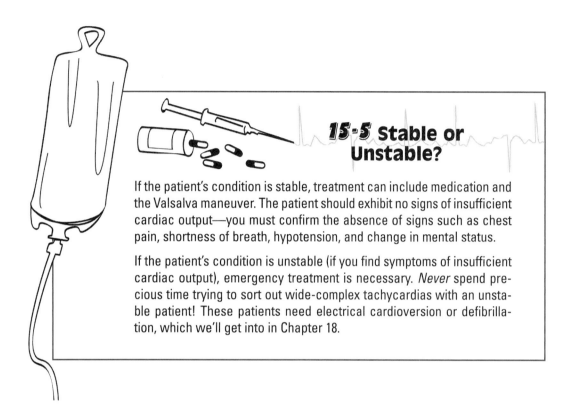

15-5 Stable or Unstable?

If the patient's condition is stable, treatment can include medication and the Valsalva maneuver. The patient should exhibit no signs of insufficient cardiac output—you must confirm the absence of signs such as chest pain, shortness of breath, hypotension, and change in mental status.

If the patient's condition is unstable (if you find symptoms of insufficient cardiac output), emergency treatment is necessary. *Never* spend precious time trying to sort out wide-complex tachycardias with an unstable patient! These patients need electrical cardioversion or defibrillation, which we'll get into in Chapter 18.

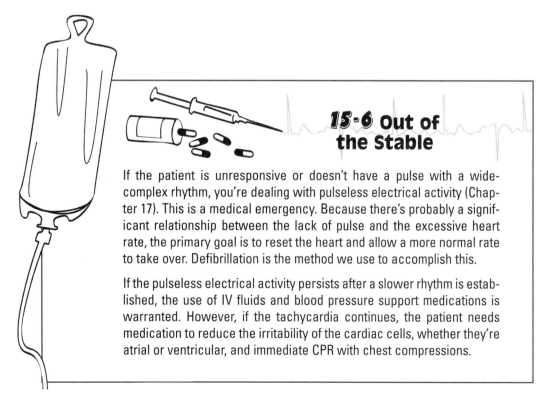

15-6 Out of the Stable

If the patient is unresponsive or doesn't have a pulse with a wide-complex rhythm, you're dealing with pulseless electrical activity (Chapter 17). This is a medical emergency. Because there's probably a significant relationship between the lack of pulse and the excessive heart rate, the primary goal is to reset the heart and allow a more normal rate to take over. Defibrillation is the method we use to accomplish this.

If the pulseless electrical activity persists after a slower rhythm is established, the use of IV fluids and blood pressure support medications is warranted. However, if the tachycardia continues, the patient needs medication to reduce the irritability of the cardiac cells, whether they're atrial or ventricular, and immediate CPR with chest compressions.

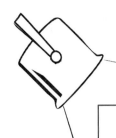

NOW YOU KNOW

A bundle branch block occurs when the signal transmitted from the AV node is unable to follow the normal paths through the bundle branches.

In rhythms with bundle branch blocks, the QRS complex and T-wave resemble those in a ventricular rhythm: wide, bizarre QRS complexes, and T-waves in the opposite direction from most of the QRS.

Bundle branch blocks by themselves are not dangerous and have little effect on cardiac output. They can complicate rhythm interpretation, causing delayed or incorrect treatment.

It's important to differentiate supraventricular tachycardia with a bundle branch block from ventricular tachycardia.

Treatment protocols are different for V-tach than for SVT with a BBB.

Treating V-tach with verapamil and similar drugs can be deadly.

When in doubt, or if the patient's condition is unstable, wide-complex tachycardia should be treated first as V-tach.

If a wide-complex tachycardia doesn't respond to treatment for V-tach, SVT medications should be used. If the rhythm persists, additional V-tach therapy should be resumed.

Test Yourself

1. What is a bundle branch block?
   _____

2. List three ECG features that point to ventricular tachycardia. _____

3. List three ECG features that point to supraventricular tachycardia with a bundle branch block. _____

4. What drug should never be given to a patient with ventricular tachycardia and why not?
   _____

5. How do you treat a patient with a wide-complex tachycardia when you can't differentiate between SVT with a BBB and V-tach?

6. In the following five strips, identify the rhythm as V-tach or SVT with a BBB. Note the feature or features that support your choice.

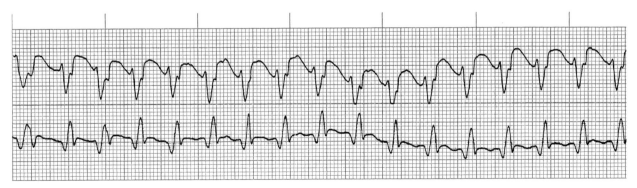

15–1

Regularity: _____ Heart rate: _____ PR interval: _____

P-waves: _____ QRS complex: _____

Interpretation: _____

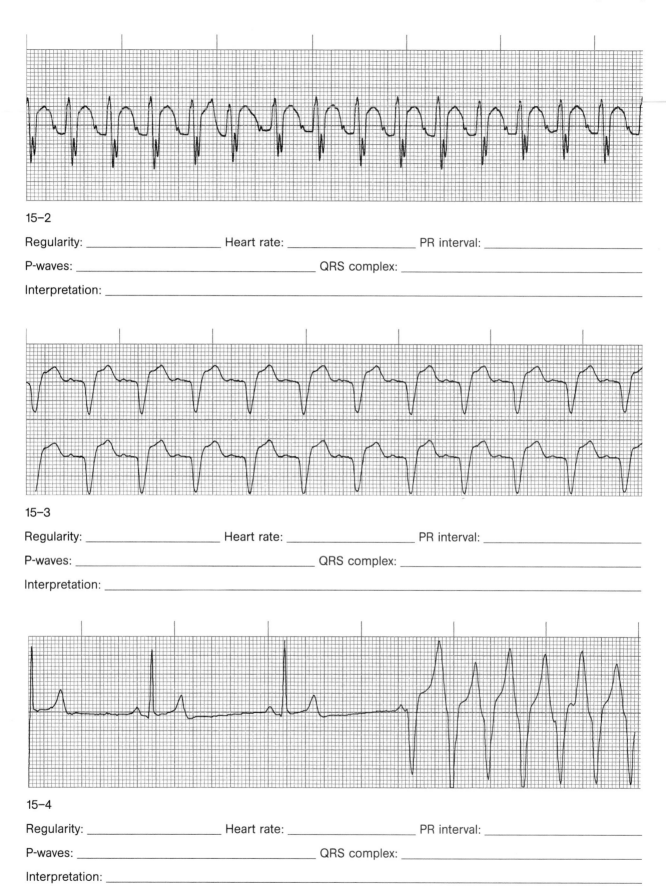

15–2

Regularity: _____ Heart rate: _____ PR interval: _____

P-waves: _____ QRS complex: _____

Interpretation: _____

15–3

Regularity: _____ Heart rate: _____ PR interval: _____

P-waves: _____ QRS complex: _____

Interpretation: _____

15–4

Regularity: _____ Heart rate: _____ PR interval: _____

P-waves: _____ QRS complex: _____

Interpretation: _____

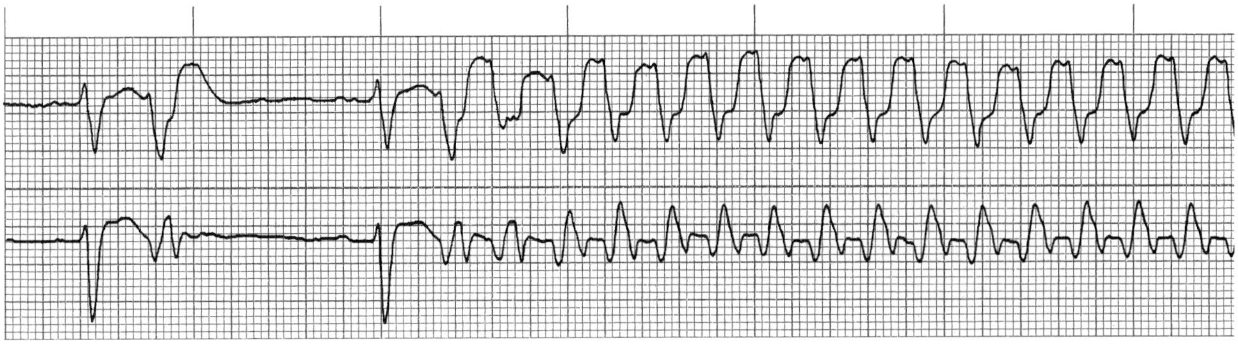

15–5

Regularity: _____ Heart rate: _____ PR interval: _____

P-waves: _____ QRS complex: _____

Interpretation: _____

7. Identify the rhythm in the following 10 strips:

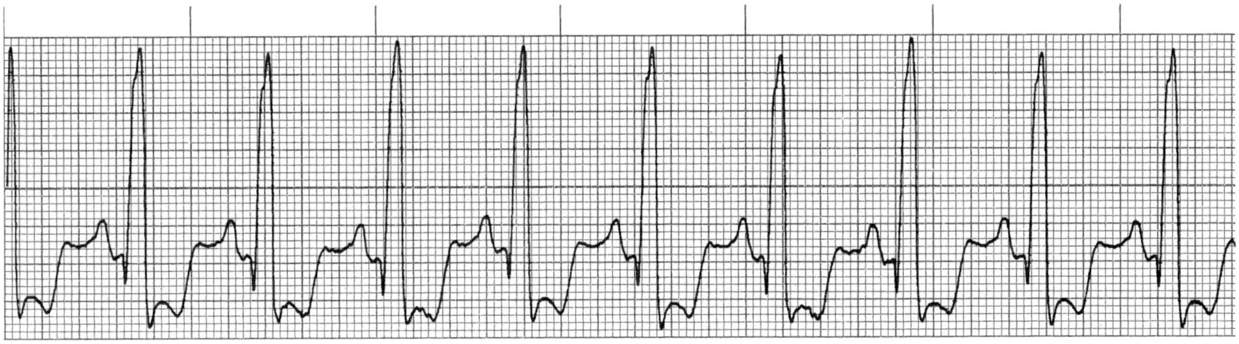

15–6

Regularity: _____ Heart rate: _____ PR interval: _____

P-waves: _____ QRS complex: _____

Interpretation: _____

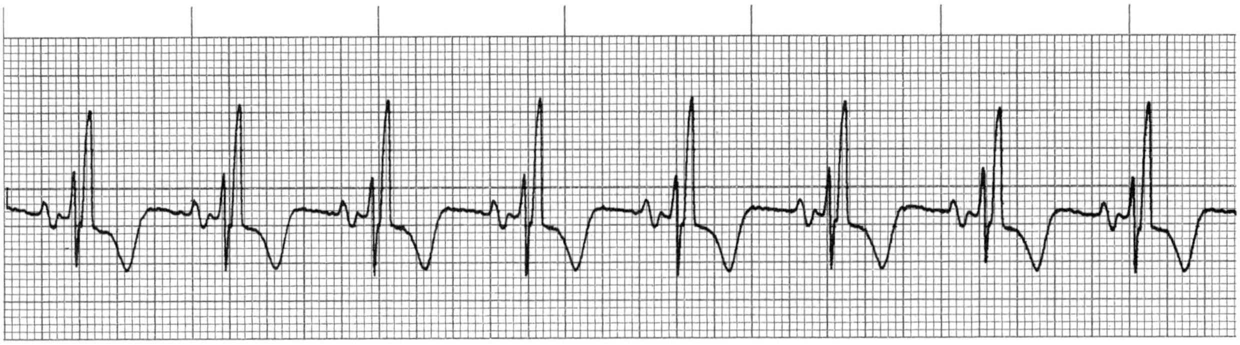

15–7

Regularity: _____ Heart rate: _____ PR interval: _____

P-waves: _____ QRS complex: _____

Interpretation: _____

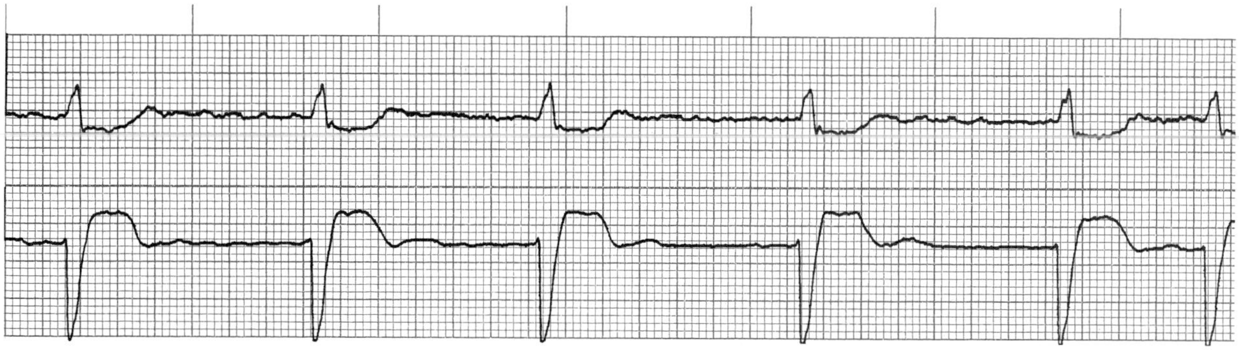

15-8

Regularity: _____ Heart rate: _____ PR interval: _____

P-waves: _____ QRS complex: _____

Interpretation: _____

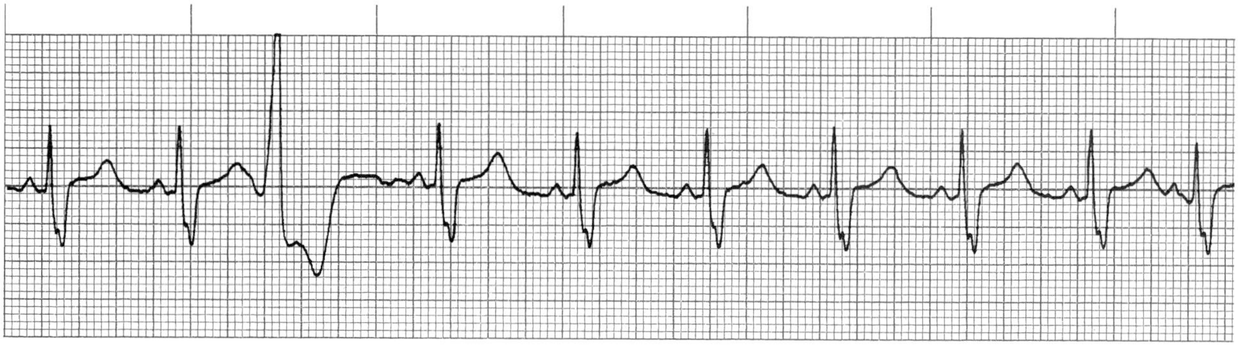

15-9

Regularity: _____ Heart rate: _____ PR interval: _____

P-waves: _____ QRS complex: _____

Interpretation: _____

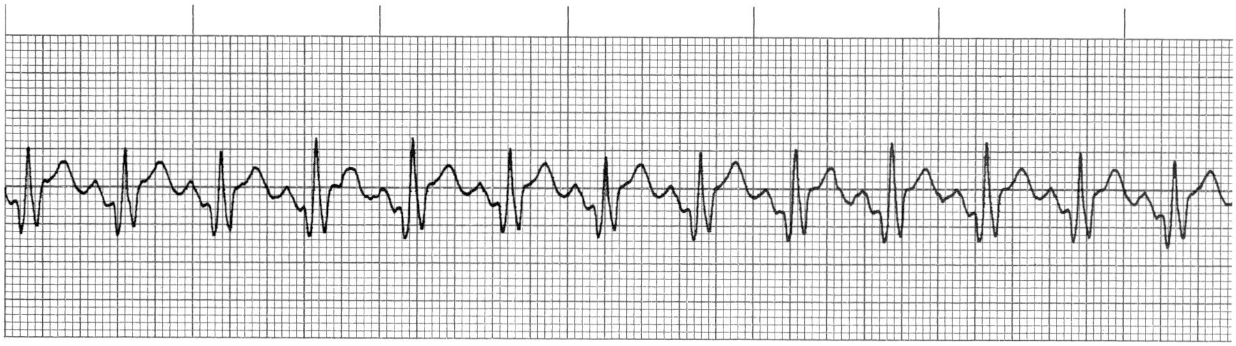

15-10

Regularity: _____ Heart rate: _____ PR interval: _____

P-waves: _____ QRS complex: _____

Interpretation: _____

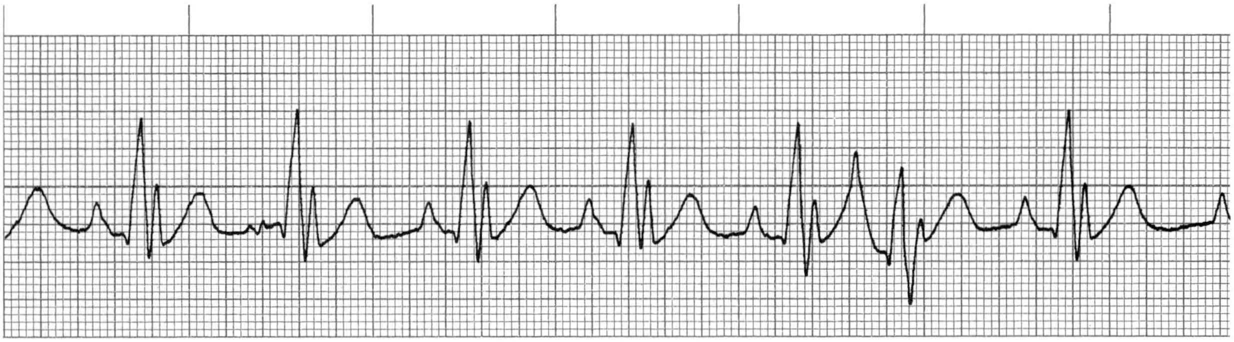

15–11

Regularity: _____ Heart rate: _____ PR interval: _____

P-waves: _____ QRS complex: _____

Interpretation: _____

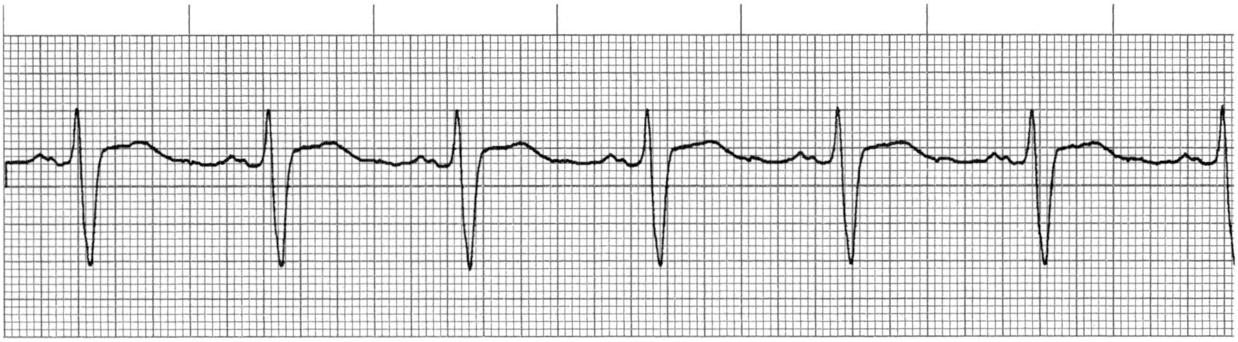

15–12

Regularity: _____ Heart rate: _____ PR interval: _____

P-waves: _____ QRS complex: _____

Interpretation: _____

II

MCL 1

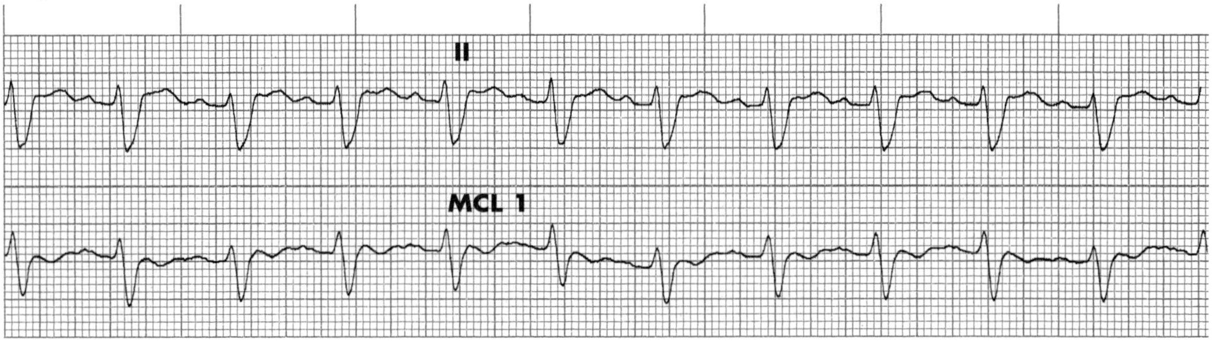

15–13

Regularity: _____ Heart rate: _____ PR interval: _____

P-waves: _____ QRS complex: _____

Interpretation: _____

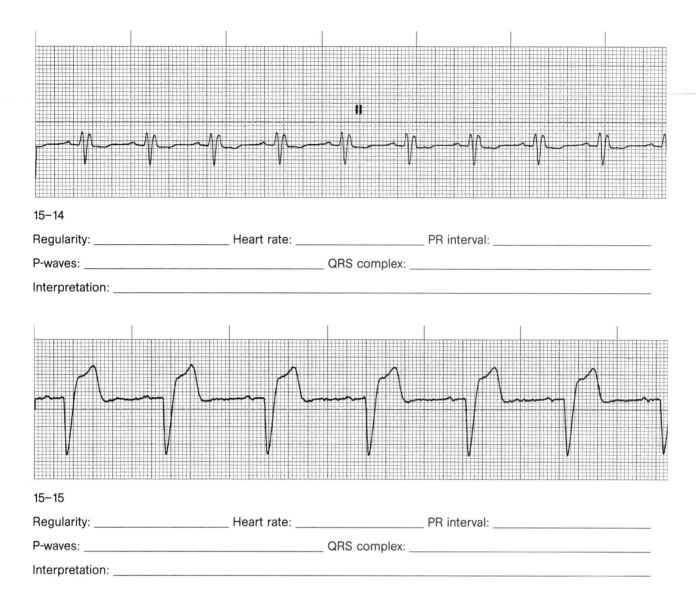

15–14

Regularity: _____ Heart rate: _____ PR interval: _____

P-waves: _____ QRS complex: _____

Interpretation: _____

15–15

Regularity: _____ Heart rate: _____ PR interval: _____

P-waves: _____ QRS complex: _____

Interpretation: _____

SECTION
5

Taking Advanced Lessons

Pacemakers: Keeping the Heart from Early Retirement

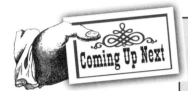

Coming Up Next

○ What is a pacemaker?

○ Why would a patient need a pacemaker?

○ Are there different types of pacemakers?

○ What is the NBG code and what is it used for?

○ Why should a pacemaker sense electrical activity?

○ What are the most common pacemaker modes?

○ How do pacemakers calculate heart rate?

An Electronic Superhero

We've already learned that the heart is an incredibly complex machine. However, experience tells us that no machine is perfect. Sometimes the heart takes a break; sometimes it tries to retire and stops altogether. When the heart slacks off or quits, the natural pacemakers aren't doing a sufficient job. The reasons for the failure vary but can include coronary artery disease, side effects of medication or disease, and aftereffects of cardiac surgery or myocardial infarction. There are many others. Whatever the origin, the end result is the same—inadequate cardiac output caused by a severe decrease in the heart rate.

The sinus node, atrial tissue, AV node, and ventricular tissue are all susceptible to failure. Although any one of them can generate a heart rhythm, that rhythm won't necessarily meet the body's needs. Sometimes the controlling pacemaker discharges too slowly or stops altogether. When that happens, if help doesn't arrive, the insufficient oxygen delivery causes organ failure and eventual death. But wait—it's a bird, it's a plane, no, it's an electronic pacemaker, appearing in the upper chest to save the day!

Would Somebody Help Me Here?

All the heart needs to do its job is a stimulus—any stimulus—to step up and start the process by depolarizing. It doesn't matter whether that stimulus comes from inside or outside the heart.

If an electrical void occurs in the heart, an artificial electronic pacemaker can fill it. An electronic pacemaker is a small computerized device that generates a repeating signal and delivers it to the heart via one or more wires that terminate in the cardiac tissue. These wires are known as *leads,* although the term is unrelated to the one used for ECG

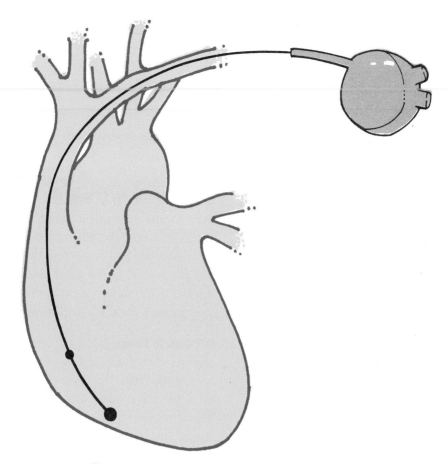

Fig. 16–1 A typical permanent pacemaker and its lead wires.

rhythm interpretation. Once the signal reaches the heart, it depolarizes the cardiac tissue at the contact point. After that the signal behaves just like a natural stimulus coming from that point. It spreads out in all directions, and eventually the heart depolarizes just as if it had generated its own signal. Figure 16–1 shows a pacemaker with its leads.

If this were all you needed to know about artificial pacemakers, we wouldn't dedicate an entire chapter to the subject. However, pacemakers are complicated, so we need to do some more exploring.

Initially pacemakers were used to maintain a minimum heart rate for patients with symptomatic bradycardia, whatever the point of origin. If the patient had a rhythm that was too fast, a pacemaker couldn't help. All that has changed. Today's pacemakers can deliver shocks, slow tachycardic rhythms by overdrive pacing, and even adjust their rates to the physiological needs of the patient. To keep things simple, we'll discuss only the type of pacemaker used in bradycardic rhythms.

Types of Pacemakers

TWO BASIC FLAVORS

Entire books have been written about pacemakers, which are evolving into more complex machines every day. This chapter will give you the basic facts you'll need to recognize pacemaker rhythms and identify the more common malfunctions.

All pacemakers generate rhythms the same way: they deliver electrical energy to the cardiac tissue. There's more than one way to accomplish that. Like flavors of ice cream, many different pacemaker categories exist, but someone with basic ECG interpretation skills is most likely to encounter two kinds: temporary and permanent. These two are the chocolate and vanilla of the pacemaker world.

From the Outside In One common type of temporary pacemaker is the *transcutaneous* pacemaker. As the name suggests, transcutaneous (trans-"through"; cutaneous-"skin") pacemakers are applied to the skin. This type uses more energy than any other because it must conduct its electrical signal through the skin, bones, and muscles of the chest and still deliver enough power to depolarize the heart. The energy used to depolarize cardiac tissue can also depolarize the muscles of the thorax, causing discomfort or outright pain. To conserve energy and avoid pain, we use transcutaneous pacemakers only as a stopgap measure in an emergency. Transcutaneous pacemakers are externally located but attach to a lead wire that enters the heart through a vein. They, along with epicardial pacemakers, behave similarly to internal pacemakers but are not permanent, long-term solutions.

Other types of temporary pacemaker are *transthoracic,* or *epicardial,* (epi-"upon") and *transesophageal.* These are uncommon in the basic ECG milieu, and we won't cover them here.

All on the Inside The other flavor is the *permanent,* or *internal,* pacemaker. In this type, the wires and the energy source, including all computerized parts, are placed inside the patient. These pacemakers need lower energy levels to achieve depolarization because the energy is delivered directly to the cardiac tissue.

This simplified discussion gives you what you need to understand basic pacemaker function. Although this chapter will focus on the interpretation of ECG rhythms generated by permanent pacemakers, most of the material can also apply to transcutaneous and other temporary pacemakers.

Decoding the Code

A GROUP OF LETTERS

Pacemakers are usually coded by a group of letters that describes the settings and capabilities of the machine. The **N**orth **A**merican **S**ociety of **P**acing and **E**lectrophysiology (NASPE) and the **B**ritish **P**acing **G**roup (BPG) devised a code known as the NBG (**N**ASPE and **B**PG **G**eneric) code for this purpose. There are other ways to describe pacemaker function, but this code is the easiest to understand and the most commonly used in clinical circles.

Although the code originally consisted of five letters, the first three are often the only ones used, particularly in older pacemakers. These three letters can provide all the information you'll need if the pacemaker has been inserted to treat symptomatic bradycardia.

WHAT THE LETTERS MEAN

Locating the Leads
The first letter of the code tells us in which chamber the lead wires are located and, therefore, which chamber or

chambers can be paced. There are four choices: A for *atrium,* V for *ventricle,* D for *dual* (both atrium and ventricle), and O for *none.* Now, I can see the confused look on your face as you say, "None? How can a pacemaker be designed to pace *no* chambers?" Well, stop worrying. The O designation is a temporary mode used by physicians and company representatives to assess pacemaker function, not to generate a rhythm.

A pacemaker can only deliver a stimulus to, or *pace,* a chamber if one of its lead wires is attached to tissue in that chamber. In a dual-chamber device, a pacing lead is attached in both the atrium *and* the ventricle. Each lead can serve two purposes: first, to deliver the signal from the pacemaker to the heart, and second, to act as an internal ECG monitor, sensing the heart's natural rhythm to determine when the pacemaker should take over.

It Helps to Listen
The pacemaker should listen for the natural electrical signals of the heart. Here's where the second letter comes in. If the pacemaker can sense electrical activity from inside the heart, this letter tells us which chambers it can sense. This entry in the NBG code, just like the first letter, can be A for *atrium,* V for *ventricle,* D for *dual* (both atrium and ventricle), or O for *none.*

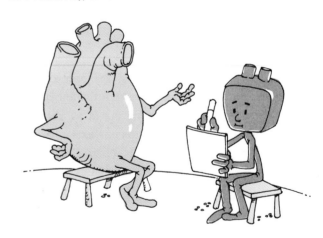

Keeping in Synch
The third letter describes what the pacemaker does when it senses a naturally occurring stimulus, that is, a naturally formed P-wave or QRS complex. We have four choices for this letter, too, but the choices are slightly different: I for *inhibited,* T for *triggered,* D for *dual* (both inhibited and triggered), and O for *none.*

Inhibition means that the pacemaker does not deliver a stimulus when it's already sensed one for that chamber. Inhibition usually acts on the chamber that has been sensed: if the pacemaker detects an atrial stimulus, its

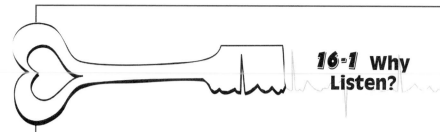

16-1 Why Listen?

We monitor the heart's electrical activity because we don't want to interfere with the natural rhythm. We don't want to take over if the heart is doing a sufficient job, only if it's not going fast enough. By "listening" for the patient's natural electrical activity, the *synchronous pacemaker* knows whether or not to deliver a stimulus. If the lead senses a stimulus from the chamber or chambers it's monitoring, only then does the third letter come into play.

complex without any atrial depolarization, would you want the pacemaker to depolarize the atria immediately after that? Probably not! Therefore the PVC, although sensed in the ventricle, can inhibit the pacemaker from generating an atrial impulse.

Triggering allows us to maximize the heart's natural function. If an atrial contraction isn't followed by a ventricular contraction, the heart has just wasted energy and cardiac output suffers. However, if the pacemaker fires, supplying the ventricular contraction that hasn't occurred naturally, then the day is saved.

atrial pacing ability is inhibited, and if it detects a ventricular stimulus, its ventricular pacing is inhibited. However, a natural beat sensed in one chamber can sometimes inhibit the pacemaker from pacing the other chamber. For example, if a patient had a premature ventricular

Here's where triggering comes in. Some pacemakers can sense atrial activity and wait for ventricular activity to follow. If it doesn't follow within a programmed time frame the pacemaker can be triggered to fire, preserving the normal atrioventricular coordination and thus atrial kick.

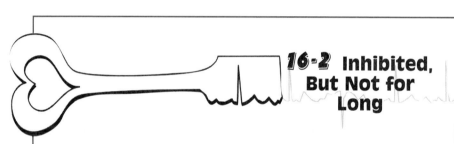

16-2 Inhibited, But Not for Long

It's important to note that inhibition is temporary. It lasts only for a fraction of a second or until the next beat is sensed. Its purpose is to give the advantage to naturally occurring beats and minimize competition between the natural heart rhythm and the pacemaker.

If the third letter is O, the pacemaker is in asynchronous mode because, even if it does sense the natural stimulus, it does nothing about it and goes on pacing the heart merrily, ignoring the sensed information.

16-3 GO CLEAN YOUR ROOM!

Think back to when you were a child and your parents told you to clean your room. Were you like me? I got chastised every Saturday, sent to my room, and told not to come out until it was clean. My banishment was as predictable as the sun rising in the east. However, if I had motivation, such as a baseball game I didn't want to miss, I'd clean my room during the week and keep it clean until Friday. (This didn't happen often.) When Saturday came, I wouldn't be hounded about my room because it was already clean. Why tell me to clean a clean room?

The same principle applies to demand pacemakers: they discharge only when they need to. What purpose would it serve to deliver a pacemaker beat if the patient's own heart had already done the job?

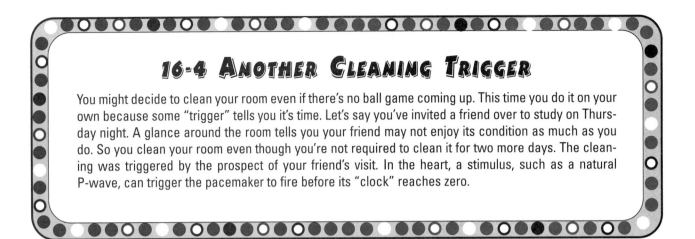

16-4 ANOTHER CLEANING TRIGGER

You might decide to clean your room even if there's no ball game coming up. This time you do it on your own because some "trigger" tells you it's time. Let's say you've invited a friend over to study on Thursday night. A glance around the room tells you your friend may not enjoy its condition as much as you do. So you clean your room even though you're not required to clean it for two more days. The cleaning was triggered by the prospect of your friend's visit. In the heart, a stimulus, such as a natural P-wave, can trigger the pacemaker to fire before its "clock" reaches zero.

Lead by Example

UNREAL MODES

Now that we have our three-letter code, let's try out some combinations and see what they mean to the heart's conduction system. With four possible letters for each of the three positions in the NBG code, there are 64 possible combinations; however, not all of them describe practical pacemaker modes. For instance, a pacemaker shouldn't be programmed as a VOT. Such a pacemaker would pace the ventricles (V) but wouldn't sense any stimuli (O). How can a pacemaker be triggered (T) if it can't sense anything?

Because the pacemaker lead doesn't lie in the sinus node or the AV node, the P-waves and QRS complexes will necessarily vary from "normal." For example, a pacemaker rhythm QRS is usually negatively deflected in lead II. This happens because the pacemaker wire is commonly embedded at the bottom of the ventricle, far from the AV node, the normal beginning point for ventricular depolarization (Fig. 16–3). In Figure 16–2B, the QRSs in ventricular paced beats look like a PVC or a bundle branch block—wide and bizarre, with the T-wave in the opposite direction—while the natural QRSs are narrow, as you might expect.

DOWN-TO-EARTH MODES

We can create many illusory letter combinations, and some other combinations are possible but are rarely if ever used. For simplicity we'll stick to some of the more common pacemaker modes and allow you to see the NBG code in action.

VOO This mode paces only the ventricles (Fig. 16–4). Because it doesn't sense any chamber, it may compete with the heart's natural pacemaker. This mode is called *competitive*, or *asynchronous*, pacing. In this mode, the pacemaker discharges at its programmed rate regardless of the patient's natural rhythm. The VOO setting was the only mode available in the early history of pacemakers, but now it's rarely used. This method of pacing a heart can be very dangerous. For more on what can happen, read Chapter 18.

VVI This mode paces only the ventricles, but the pacemaker senses

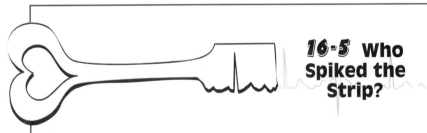

16-5 Who Spiked the Strip?

When the pacemaker depolarizes, it sends an electrical stimulus to the heart. This stimulus, like all electrical signals, is picked up by the ECG monitor. On the strip the stimulus appears as a short line, called a *pacemaker spike,* or *pacer spike,* immediately before the waveform it generates—P-wave, QRS complex, or both. The location of the spike, of course, depends on which chamber the pacemaker has stimulated. Figure 16–2 shows two ECG tracings with pacemaker spikes; one pacemaker has stimulated the atrial tissue (Fig. 16–2A) and the other the ventricular tissue (Fig. 16–2B).

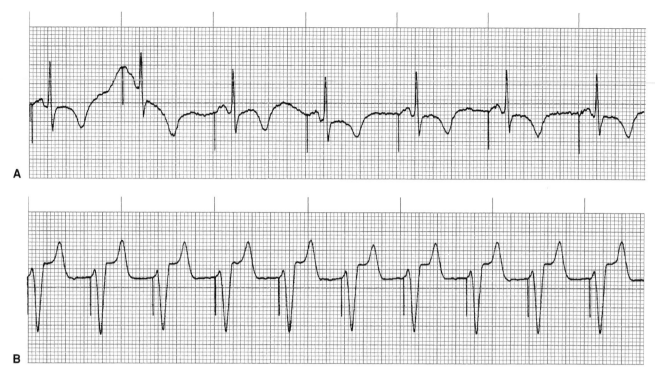

Fig. 16–2A–B Two ECG strips showing paced rhythms. A, In a rhythm with atrial pacing, the pacemaker spike occurs just before the P-wave. B, In a rhythm with ventricular pacing, the pacemaker spike occurs just before the QRS complex.

what's going on in the heart (Fig. 16–5). If it detects a stimulus in the ventricles, it's inhibited from discharging, whether the stimulus is a normal QRS complex from the AV node, a QRS from a PVC, or a QRS from a ventricular rhythm such as V-tach. No matter what ventricular activity it senses, the pacemaker is inhibited from discharging

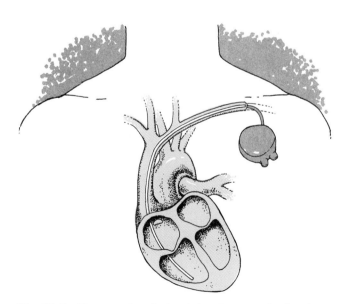

Fig. 16–3 The pacemaker wire travels from the pacemaker (here in the left chest wall) through blood vessels to the heart, where it attaches inside the right ventricle. The location shown is common, but precise location can vary.

and holds off until it's needed. This mode is known as *demand pacing* because the pacemaker discharges only when the heart is not doing its job. As I mentioned earlier, pacemakers that can coordinate their activity with the patient's intrinsic rhythm are collectively termed *synchronous pacemakers,* but the term is rarely used in clinical practice.

AAI Also a demand pacing mode, AAI paces the atria (Fig. 16–6). If the pacemaker senses a natural P-wave, it will not deliver a stimulus. With atrial pacing, it's critical to ensure that the AV node is working properly. If the pacemaker delivers a signal to the atria but the signal is blocked on its way to the ventricles, ventricular asystole and death can result.

DDD This mode paces both the atria and the ventricles (Fig. 16–7). It also monitors both of them for natural signals. If it senses an atrial or ventricular signal, it inhibits the corresponding pacemaker impulse. However, because the second letter is D (dual), this mode can also trigger. If the pacemaker senses a natural atrial signal, it waits for a ventricular signal to follow close behind. If no signal comes after the preprogrammed interval, the pacemaker will be triggered to deliver a ventricular stimulus. This pacemaker mode can masquerade as other modes. We'll talk more about it in the next section.

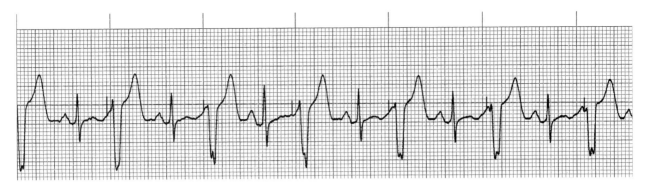

Fig. 16–4   An ECG strip generated by a pacemaker in VOO mode. The pacemaker is firing at a set rate of 60 bpm (five large boxes between paced beats), but the patient's natural sinus rhythm is much faster. Close examination reveals the clear beginnings of P-waves just before the pacemaker QRS complexes (arrows).

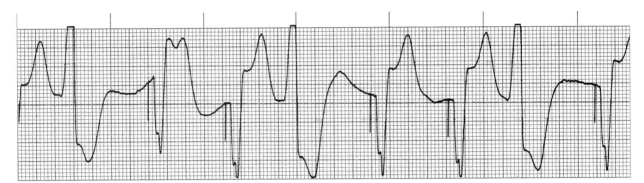

Fig. 16–5   An ECG strip generated by a pacemaker in VVI mode. Beginning with the first beat, every third beat is natural (no pacemaker spike and the QRS complex is in the opposite direction). The other beats are all pacemaker generated (a pacemaker spike at the beginning of the QRS complex). There are 21 small boxes between consecutive paced beats and about the same number between when the pacemaker sensed the natural and the next paced beat. The pacemaker has sensed the natural beat and has delayed firing.

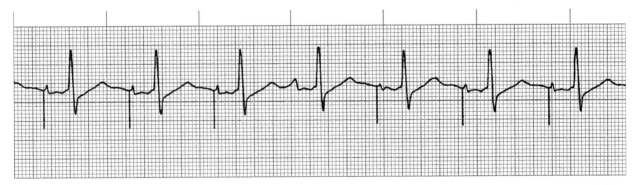

Fig. 16–6   An ECG strip generated by a pacemaker in AAI mode. The fourth P-wave is shaped differently from the others and is not preceded by a pacemaker spike. The pacemaker has sensed the natural P-wave and has delayed firing.

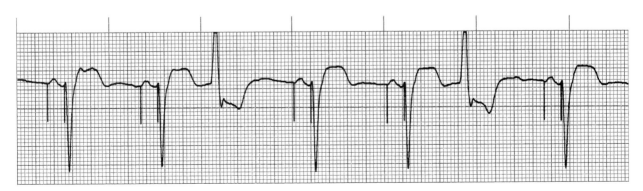

Fig. 16–7   An ECG strip generated by a pacemaker in DDD mode. Every third beat is a natural complex, which delays the pacemaker stimulus. Two pacemaker spikes show that the pacemaker has delivered a stimulus to both the atria and the ventricles.

DUAL-CHAMBER PACEMAKERS

Four different PQRST waveforms (Fig. 16–8) are possible with DDD pacemakers. If both the atria and the ventricles are paced (Fig. 16–8A), the waveform is easy to spot: it contains both an atrial and a ventricular pacemaker spike.

If only the atria are paced (Fig. 16–8B), the waveform looks like the one produced by a single-chamber atrial pacemaker: atrial spikes appear, but the QRS complexes are conducted normally. If only the ventricles are paced (Fig. 16–8C), the result is the same as from a single-chamber

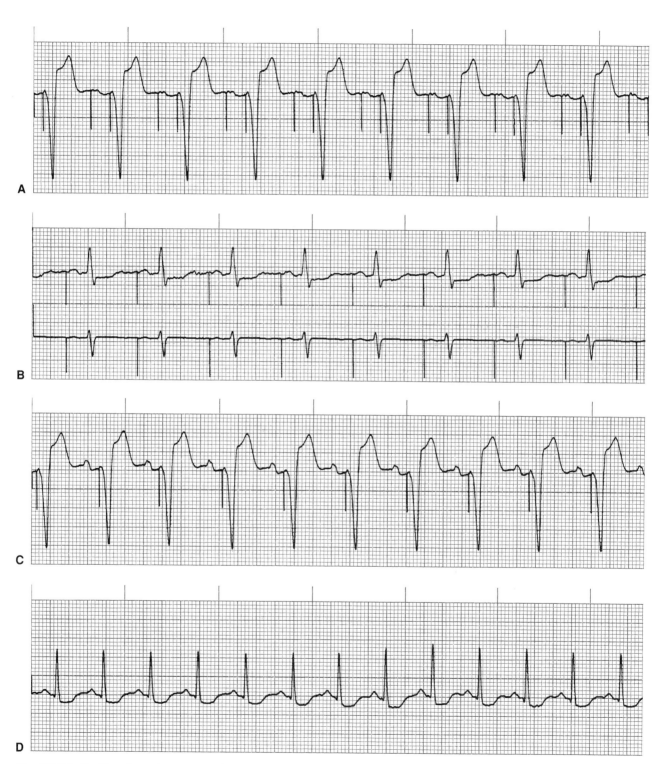

Fig. 16–8A–D These four strips were recorded at different times from the same patient with a DDD pacemaker. A, Both chambers are being paced. B, Only the atria are being paced. The signal is carried naturally through the AV node to the ventricles. C, Only the ventricles are being paced. The QRS complex is wide and bizarre and is preceded by a pacemaker spike and a P-wave. D, There are no pacemaker spikes; the rhythm is intrinsic. The pacemaker is not needed because the patient's heart rate is faster than the programmed minimum the pacemaker is inhibited.

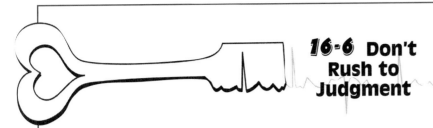

16-6 Don't Rush to Judgment

It's rare for one ECG strip to show all four of the possible dual pacemaker tracings described above. More commonly, one type of pacing (ventricular, for instance) will dominate for a while, change to another form (such as atrial or dual chamber), and then change back to the original. It's important to look at more than one strip before deciding that a single-chamber pacemaker produced the waveforms. In fact, you may not be able to properly identify the NBG code from the ECG strip at all. So it's better to simply describe which type of pacing you see. Figure 16–9 shows an ECG tracing from a dual-chamber pacemaker. The beginning of the strip shows only ventricular pacing, but the second half shows both atrial and ventricular pacing.

ventricular pacemaker: P-waves occur naturally, but the pacemaker runs the ventricles. Finally, if both the P-waves and the QRSs are natural (Fig. 16–8D), the heart's intrinsic rate must be higher than the set minimum rate for the pacemaker; therefore, the pacemaker hasn't been alerted to deliver an impulse.

Dual-chamber pacemakers don't discriminate among sinus P-waves, atrial P-waves, or atrial impulses triggered by the pacemaker. Whenever the atrial lead senses an electrical signal, the pacemaker expects a natural QRS complex to follow shortly. If the lead doesn't sense a QRS within a preprogrammed time frame, it triggers a ventricular pacemaker impulse. This impulse maximizes atrial kick by preserving the proper timing (the PR interval) between the atrial and ventricular contractions. Because of that advantage, the DDD mode is one of the most popular pacemaker settings. However, it shouldn't be used in certain situations, which we'll discuss later here and in Chapter 18.

Finally, there's one caveat to keep in mind. If the atrial rate is too high, the pacemaker may ignore some of the atrial contractions, just as the AV node would. Atrial fibrillation, for instance, produces more than 350 atrial impulses per minute, and clearly the pacemaker shouldn't generate a QRS complex for each of them. Instead, it waits a certain length of time (determined by the preprogrammed maximum heart rate) before responding to another atrial signal. In Figure 16–11, after the second QRS (which is natural), the pacemaker began responding to too many F-waves raising the heart rate significantly. The pacemaker ignored some of these flutter waves because it would have had to discharge faster than its programmed maximum rate, in this case 100 bpm.

Think Like a Pacemaker

KEEPING UP THE PACE

Internal pacemakers have come a long way since the first fully implantable pacemaker was used in the 1960s. Today's pacemakers can be programmed and reprogrammed. Some advanced pacemakers can even adjust their programs to the needs of the patient; they can change their discharge rate, vary the PR interval, and even terminate dangerous tachycardias by discharging at phenomenal rates!

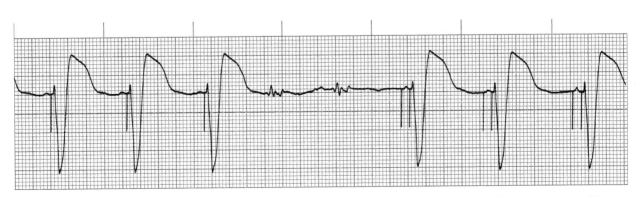

Fig. 16–9 This rhythm changes from single- to dual-chamber pacing. The first beats are single-chamber beats with ventricular pacing. Then they are two natural complexes. The last are dual-chamber beats.

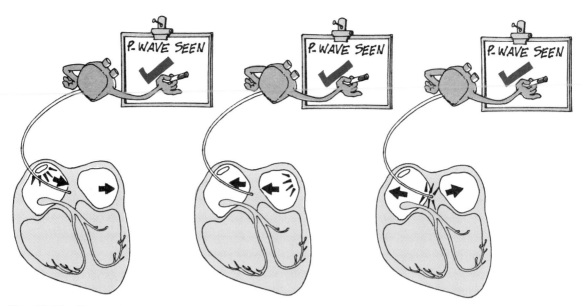

Fig. 16–10 No matter how the atrial signal is generated, if it reaches the pacemaker wire, it inhibits the pacemaker from generating an atrial impulse. It may also trigger a ventricular impulse if one does not occur soon after the pacemaker senses the P-wave.

As I mentioned earlier, we'll keep it simple in this chapter. We're concentrating on the type of pacemaker that corrects bradycardic rhythms by maintaining a programmed minimum heart rate. We can't understand these pacemakers until we understand how they determine whether or not to deliver an impulse.

AN INTERNAL CLOCK

How would you determine a patient's heart rate? At the bedside, you can simply check the pulse and count the number of beats in 1 minute, or listen to the patient's chest with a stethoscope and count the heart sounds. At the monitor, you can determine heart rate (but not pulse) by counting the number of QRS complexes in 1 minute. These methods work well for humans, but pacemakers need more precision.

A pacemaker doesn't bother calculating the number of beats per minute. To calculate heart rate, it determines the amount of time elapsed since the last beat. You already know this technique—it's the small-box method, in which we count the number of small boxes (0.04 seconds each) between consecutive QRS complexes. Well, the pacemaker is much more precise. It doesn't bother with calipers; it simply starts an internal clock when it discharges or senses an impulse and stops the clock at the next impulse. The impulses can be natural or paced, P-waves or QRSs—that depends on the pacemaker mode.

Programmed with a heart rate, the pacemaker transforms this rate into a time interval between consecutive beats. It does this by dividing the programmed heart rate into 60,000, the number of milliseconds in 1 minute. (1 millisecond is 0.001 seconds. There are 40 ms in one

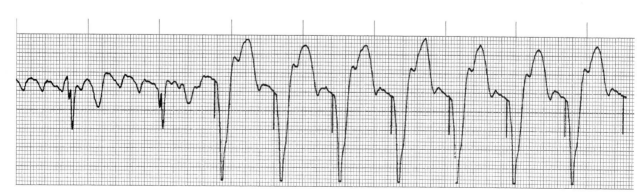

Fig. 16–11 Atrial flutter with triggered ventricular pacing. The pacemaker has ignored many of the flutter waves to keep the heart rate below the preprogrammed maximum of 100 bpm, demonstrated by the consecutive paced beats.

small box on the six second ECG strip!) Having decided how many milliseconds should occur between complexes in a regular rhythm, the pacemaker delivers a stimulus if that interval passes without a detectable complex.

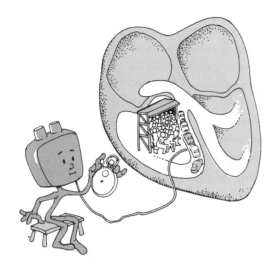

MORE MATH AGAIN

Pacemakers are programmed with a minimum as well as a maximum heart rate. If the minimum rate is set to 60 bpm, there should be no more than 60,000 ÷ 60, or 1000, milliseconds (1 second) between beats. When the pacemaker senses or delivers an impulse, the clock starts ticking. If the pacemaker senses another impulse before 1000 ms have passed, it resets the clock to zero and doesn't deliver a stimulus. If 1000 ms pass and the pacemaker doesn't sense a natural impulse, it delivers a stimulus and resets the clock to zero. Remember, though, if a natural stimulus triggers the pacemaker, it may fire faster—up to the maximum heart rate.

The story is the same, but the numbers are a bit different, if our pacemaker has a minimum rate set at 75 bpm. In that scenario the time interval between beats should be no more than 60,000 ÷ 75, or 800, ms. If the heart rate is increased 80, the pacemaker will wait 750 ms. In either case, when the time limit is reached and the pacemaker stimulus is finally delivered, the clock is reset to zero.

16-7 WATERING THE LAWN

Imagine that you water your lawn once every 7 days to keep the grass from dying. Every Saturday morning like clockwork, the automatic sprinklers deliver the water your lawn needs to survive. Now imagine a week when it pours rain on Thursday afternoon. Do you need to water your lawn on Saturday? No.

As a matter of fact, because excess watering can encourage disease and damage the lawn, it probably wouldn't be a good idea.

So you skip your normal Saturday watering. But then what? Your lawn needs to be watered every seven days, so waiting until next Saturday is also a bad idea. Therefore, if it doesn't rain by Thursday you should water that day. But if it rains before Thursday, you should adjust your watering schedule again. This method ensures that your lawn gets watered at least once a week regardless of the weather, just as our pacemaker ensures a beat at least every second but allows for more if it's needed.

SUN	MON	TUES	WED	THUR	FRI	SAT
						1
2	3	4	5	6	7	8
9	10	11	12	13	14	15
16	17	18	19	20	21	22
23	24	25	26	27	28	29
30	31					

The reliance on time intervals rather than beats per minute is an important safety feature. Suppose that your patient's ventricular pacemaker is set at 60 bpm and that it determines heart rate by sensing the total number of beats in 1 minute. If the patient has a 30-second run of atrial tachycardia at a rate of 120 followed by a 30-second pause, the total number of beats in 1 minute comes to 60, but the patient has gone an entire half minute with no cardiac output!

Suppose the same patient's pacemaker senses the time interval between beats. In this case, the natural rhythm (atrial tachycardia at 120 bpm) will run the heart for the first 30 seconds, generating 60 beats. The pacemaker will run the heart for the next 30 seconds, generating an additional 30 beats (one every 1000 ms during the pause), for a total of 90 bpm. That guarantees at least one beat per second and a much better outcome for the patient! For both our sake and the patient's, it's a good thing the pacemaker does the math; all it needs from us is the minimum heart rate.

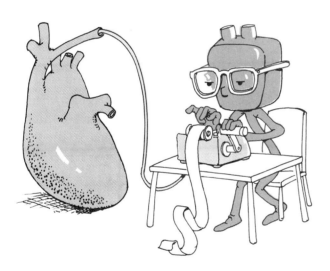

By the way, asynchronous pacemakers use an internal clock but don't sense the natural electrical activity of the heart. Therefore, the only way to reset the clock is for the pacemaker to deliver the stimulus.

THE SENSITIVE SIDE OF PACEMAKERS

The body is full of electrical signals, which drive nerves and muscles as well as the heart. To sense the heart's natural rhythms, a pacemaker must differentiate heart signals from all the extraneous non-heart noise in and around the body. The pacemaker uses its *sensitivity setting* to sort out the signals.

The sensitivity setting simply tells the pacemaker how much energy a signal needs to be designated a beat. If the pacemaker senses a lower energy level, it ignores the signal, even if the signal is a real heartbeat.

Sensitivity is programmed in demand pacemakers and can be individualized in both external and internal pacemakers. For our purposes, it's important just to understand the concept of sensitivity, not to know how to adjust it or what actual numbers are involved.

Recognizing Trouble

THE BASIC FOUR

Now that we've covered the basics of how pacemakers function, let's go on to see how they malfunction.

Many problems can occur with pacemakers. The four basic ones, which you must be able to recognize easily, are failure to fire, failure to capture, undersensing, and oversensing. Each type of malfunction has specific characteristics that define it on the ECG tracing. We'll go over these characteristics and their possible causes and potential treatments.

FAILURE TO FIRE

Failure to fire, or *failure to pace,* is probably the easiest malfunction to identify. Figure 16–12 shows an example; notice the absence of pacemaker spikes. The patient has a ventricular pacemaker with a minimum heart rate set at 60 bpm. Therefore, if the pacemaker doesn't sense a natural beat 1000 ms (five large boxes) after the last beat, it should fire. Look at what happens after the third QRS complex: the natural heartbeats stop, but no pacing occurs. The pacemaker should have fired but failed to do so.

The pacemaker can fail to fire for many reasons. The battery may be depleted, the lead wire may be broken or dislodged, or the pacemaker may be improperly programmed. Whatever the cause, it's important to assess the impact on the patient.

FAILURE TO CAPTURE

Capture occurs when the pacemaker delivers a stimulus that depolarizes an entire chamber causing a P-wave or QRS complex on the ECG, ideally generating a contraction. A dislodged or broken lead wire may deliver some,

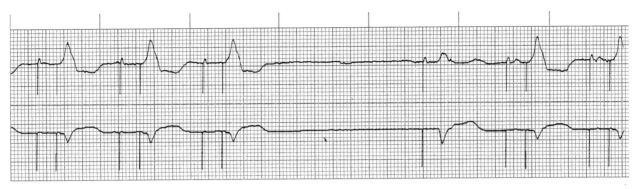

Fig. 16–12 Failure to fire. The pacemaker is set for a minimum heart rate of 71 bpm as calculated from the first three beats, which are paced. Then there is a pause. After 21 small boxes there should be a pacer spike, but there isn't .

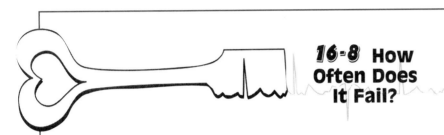

16-8 How Often Does It Fail?

If the pacemaker fails only once in a while, cardiac output will probably not change very much and the patient will suffer no ill effects. However, repeated or consecutive occurrences can decrease cardiac output significantly, with resulting chest pain, shortness of breath, nausea, and hypotension if the failures occur frequently enough.

but not all, of the needed energy. Sometimes scar tissue can develop at the point where the pacemaker wire attaches to the heart (scar tissue conducts electricity less effectively than regular cardiac tissue does). Failure to capture produces pacemaker spikes on the ECG as shown in Figure 16–13; that's how you distinguish it from failure to fire. The pacemaker stimulus is delivered, but the patient's heart doesn't depolarize.

Failure to capture can have a chemical basis, such as medication or an electrolyte imbalance. Many antiarrhythmic medications change the characteristics of the myocardial cell wall, making the cells less receptive to the pacemaker stimulus. The relative lack or abundance of electrolytes can stall the signal by affecting its ability to propagate from cell to cell.

UNDERSENSING

Undersensing (failure to sense; non-sensing) means that the pacemaker isn't responding to natural stimuli. This malfunction, shown in Figure 16–14, can be identified by a pacemaker spike that occurs too close to the previous beat. Notice the pace-

maker spike in the fifth QRS complex. This patient had a single-chamber ventricular pacemaker set at 75 bpm (you can measure out the pacemaker spikes on the strip). If the pacemaker had been sensing correctly, it would have been reset by this QRS complex, and the next spike would not have occurred for 800 milliseconds. Another pacemaker spike occurs too close to the seventh QRS complex.

Undersensing can cause a serious problem for the patient. One of its potential consequences is R-on-T phenomenon, which we'll discuss in depth in Chapter 18.

OVERSENSING

Picking Up the Wrong Signals

In *oversensing*, either the T-wave or some noncardiac electrical signal resets the pacemaker inappropriately, increasing the amount of time before the next discharge. Sometimes the large T-waves found in hyperkalemia or acute myocardial infarction can be intense enough to meet the sensitivity threshold. If so, the total heart rate will decrease because of the increased time interval between QRS complexes. The pacemaker can be adjusted, but some adjustments can cause more serious problems than the ones they correct.

Compared with other pacemaker malfunctions, oversensing is relatively benign. Pacemaker discharge is usually delayed for just a short time; the heart rate may dip slightly below minimum, but it can be corrected easily by a change in sensitivity or an increase in the programmed pacemaker rate.

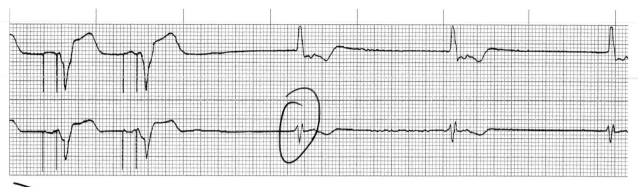

Fig. 16-13 Failure to capture. The first pacemaker spike is not immediately followed by a QRS as the next two are. The remaining pacemaker spikes don't capture as evidenced by the lack of QRS complexes. In the later beats, the pacemaker fires (note the spikes) but fails to capture (note the lack of QRSs).

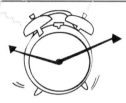

16-9 RESTORE THE HEART RATE

In both failure to fire and failure to capture, rapid assessment is essential. If the pacemaker isn't firing or capturing and the decreased cardiac output is causing symptoms, treatment is directed at restoring an adequate heart rate. This may prove difficult. Why? Because we're dealing with a permanent pacemaker. Patients with pacemakers may have impaired cardiac function or conduction and therefore often don't respond to the typical bradycardia medications given to increase heart rate. In addition, they may be taking medications that artificially decrease the heart rate, such as beta blockers or calcium channel blockers. The pacemaker provides a minimum heart rate as a safety net, so failure to fire can put such a patient in danger. Therefore, the intervention most likely to succeed is an external temporary pacemaker. Many defibrillators can also function as pacemakers. You should find out whether they're available at your facility before you need to use them.

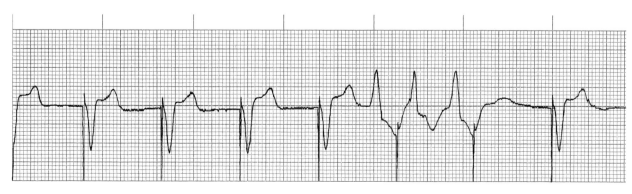

Fig. 16-14 Undersensing. Pacemaker spikes occur despite valid QRS complexes from a short run of PVCs. Undersensing of PVCs is fairly common.

Oversensing is easy to understand if you have an example to look at. Consider the ECG strip in Figure 16–15. This patient had a demand pacemaker with a minimum heart rate set at 75 bpm. With that setting, the pacemaker waits 800 ms (20 small boxes) after the last sensed event before it will discharge. Normally that event is a QRS complex. When the pacemaker senses a QRS, it resets its internal clock to zero and starts watching for the next event that meets the programmed sensitivity criteria. But if the next sensed event is a extra large T-wave, the pacemaker clock is again reset to zero, increasing the time between beats.

If the T-wave occurs two large boxes after the QRS complex, the pacemaker timer is reset twice: once at the beginning of the QRS and once during the T-wave. This pacemaker is sensing the T-wave as a QRS and delaying its impulse inappropriately. The time interval before the next delivered impulse increases to 1200 ms (800 ms programmed + 400 ms [two large boxes] delay for the T-wave), which corresponds to a heart rate of 50 bpm. The heart rate has been reduced by one third, a potential catastrophe for a cardiac patient, especially one dependent on a pacemaker to maintain an adequate heart rate.

Oversensing can also be caused by large *myopotentials* (electrical signals generated by muscle movements). These signals are usually too small for the pacemaker to pick up, and the pacemaker has shields and filters that minimize this type of problem. However, when a large muscle mass is involved, the pacemaker may sense the signals because of their sheer magnitude. Both shivering and seizures, which involve most of the muscles of the body, can bring on this effect. Like the ECG monitor, the pacemaker has algorithms to account for muscle movements (Chapter 17 has more on this subject), but these algorithms are not foolproof.

Bring in the Interrogator

Oversensing can be hard to identify; a dying battery or an inappropriately programmed minimum rate can also slow down the pacemaker. To be sure you're dealing with oversensing, you must know the pacemaker's minimum heart rate setting. The patient may not be able to give you this information—confusion can accompany a marked drop in cardiac output, or the patient may not know the rate to begin with. Without the proper information, you may need to have a company representative come out to "interrogate" the pacemaker and determine its settings.

Figure 16–16 gives examples of the four pacemaker malfunctions just described, shown side by side to help you compare them.

I Can Name that Pacemaker in Four Beats

CHALLENGE YOUR DESCRIPTIVE POWERS

When it comes to naming rhythms, a pacemaker can complicate matters. Identifying a pacemaker rhythm is usually easy because the spikes stick out like a sore thumb, but naming the rhythm can be tricky. We've demonstrated that we can't always determine the pacemaker mode with a single strip or even many strips.

So how do we name the rhythms? We usually refer to the chamber or chambers being paced. A rhythm can be *atrial paced, ventricular paced,* or *dual-chamber paced,* also called simply *AV paced.*

Pacemaker rhythms are often secondary, which means that the patient has at least one other rhythm. In

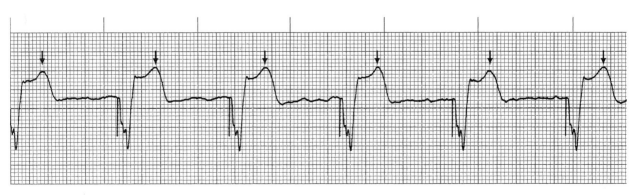

Fig. 16–15   Oversensing. This pacemaker is programmed for a minimum heart rate of 75 bpm, with 800 ms between beats. Because it senses the large T-wave (arrow) as a QRS complex, it resets its internal clock, artificially delaying the paced beat for a total interval of 1200 ms. However, the time between the T-wave and the next beat is the programmed 800 ms.

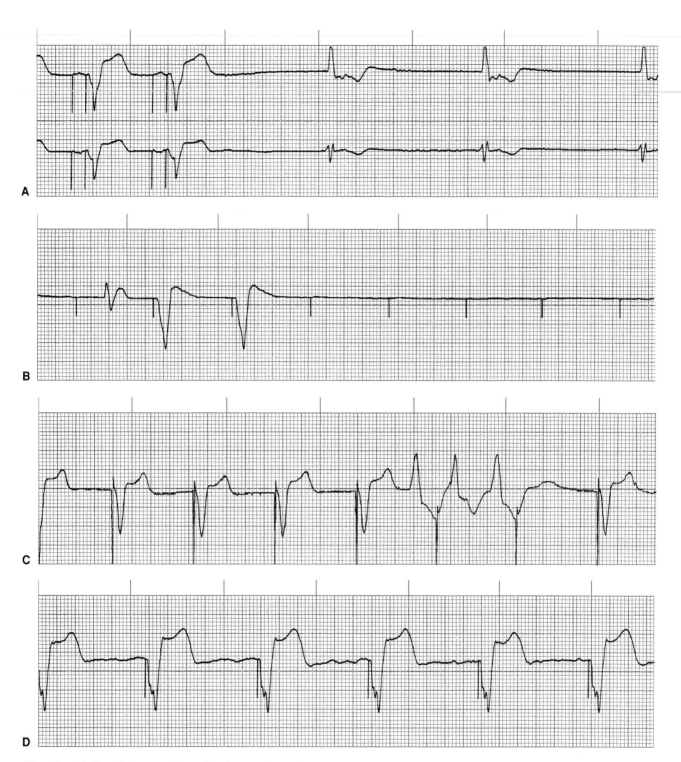

Fig. 16–16A–D All the pacemaker malfunctions are shown side by side for easy comparison. A, Failure to fire. B, Failure to capture. C, Undersensing. D, Oversensing.

Figure 16–17, although the QRS complexes are generated by the pacemaker, all the P-waves are the patient's own. How do we describe this rhythm? As with premature beats, we note the tissue that sets the heart rate (in this case the sinus node) and then add the modifier (in this case ventricular pacing). Also, we usually indicate how often the modifier occurs: for example, sinus rhythm with frequent PACs. For pacemaker rhythms, we can use the adjectives "frequent," "occasional," and "rare." These terms are used often, but we can describe "frequent" and "occasional" more precisely in terms of percentage.

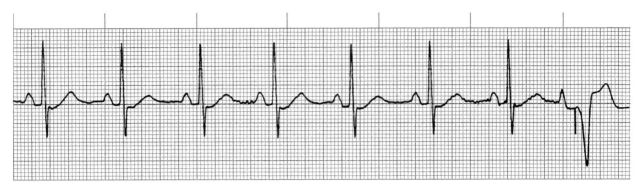

Fig. 16–17 Sinus rhythm with PACs. All the P-waves and QRS complexes are intrinsic, except the last QRS complex which is generated by the pacemaker. The irregularity of the rhythm is not caused by the pacemaker but occurs because the eighth P-wave is premature. The pacemaker senses the P-wave but doesn't sense a QRS following it, so it generates one.

I believe in using percentages to describe pacemaker-generated rhythms, although this information isn't required. You can use the 6-second strip to help you calculate. First, count the number of paced beats in the strip; next, divide that number by the total number of beats. Alternatively, you can count the number of paced beats in a group of 10 beats and simply add a zero. If all the beats are paced, the percentage is 100.

Let's get back to Figure 16–17. We're looking at a sinus rhythm with 100% ventricular pacing. This description tells us that the P-waves originated in the sinus node, at a rate between 60 and 100 bpm, and that all the QRSs were generated by the pacemaker.

In Figure 16–18, all of the P-waves are pacemaker generated but the rest of the conduction is normal. Because the pacemaker generates the P-waves and therefore the heart rate, we'd describe this rhythm as 100% atrial pacing, indicating that all the P-waves are generated by the pacemaker in the atrium. (We don't need a modifier to explain the QRS complexes because they're generated naturally; in fact, the absence of a modifier implies that they are.) Figure 16–19, which shows abnormal bundle branch conduction, is

described as 100% atrial pacing with BBB. In both of these strips, all conduction is assumed to be normal unless an abnormality is mentioned specifically. Figure 16–20 is described as 100% AV pacing. This term indicates that both the P-waves and the QRSs are pacemaker generated.

KEEP THE BATTERY JUICED

Figure 16–21 demonstrates one way to indicate the approximate percentage of pacemaker-generated beats in combination rhythms. Counting the number of paced beats (four) in 6 seconds of this strip, dividing by the total number of beats (seven), and rounding to the nearest 10%, we get about 60% paced beats. Therefore, the rhythm would be sinus rhythm with 60% ventricular pacing.

There's more than one reason to keep track of percentages. A significant increase or decrease in the frequency of paced beats can indicate a change in the patient's condition. Also, the more frequently a pacemaker generates the rhythm, the sooner its batteries become depleted, so knowing the percentage of paced beats can give you an idea of how much battery juice the patient is using.

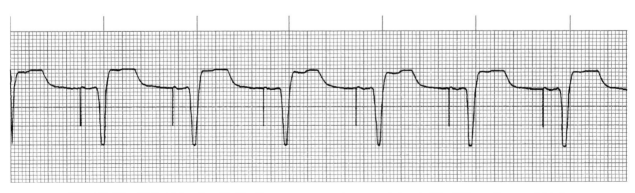

Fig. 16–18 100% atrial pacing. All of the P-waves are pacemaker generated, and all the QRS complexes are intrinsic.

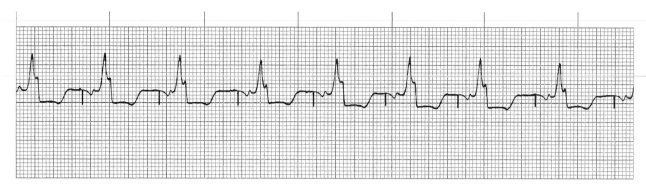

Fig. 16–19 100% atrial pacing with bundle branch block. All of the P-waves are pacemaker generated, and all of the QRS complexes are intrinsic. A wide QRS and a T-wave in the opposite direction indicate a BBB.

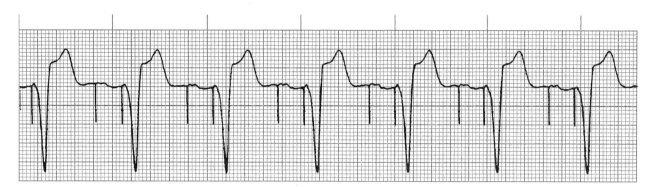

Fig. 16–20 100% AV pacing. All of the P-waves and all of the QRS complexes are pacemaker generated.

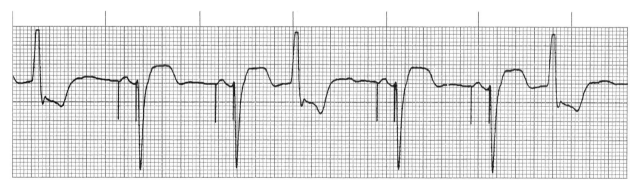

Fig. 16–21 In the first 6 seconds of this strip, four of the seven beats are paced, so the rhythm is 57% paced. Because this figure is only an estimate, we can round it to 60% paced beats. Therefore, the rhythm is sinus rhythm with 60% ventricular pacing.

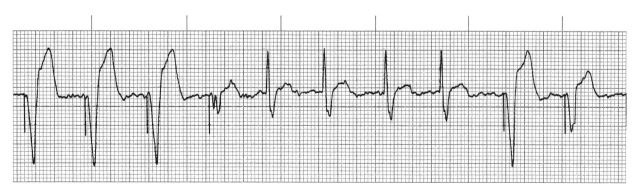

Fig. 16–22 Atrial fibrillation with 60% ventricular pacing. In the first 10 beats of this strip, about 60% are pacemaker generated.

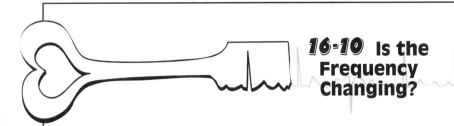

16-10 Is the Frequency Changing?

Noting the relative frequency of paced beats can help you identify changes in the patient's ECG. If the relative number of paced beats is increasing, something could be suppressing the patient's natural rhythm; causes might include myocardial infarction, medication, and hypoxia. A decreasing percentage of paced beats could indicate that the heart is getting more irritable and needs intervention. On the other hand, the patient's condition might just be improving. You won't know either way until you investigate.

ANOTHER CRACK AT PERCENTAGES

Here's another simple way to approximate percentage. Just count the number of paced beats in 10 consecutive beats and multiply by 10. For example, in Figure 16–22, some QRS complexes are pacemaker generated and some are natural. Counting, we find six paced beats out of the 10 beats on the strip. We'd describe this rhythm as atrial fibrillation with 60% ventricular pacing.

If we find significant stretches with no paced beats, we can substitute "rare" for the percentage figure, as in "sinus rhythm with rare ventricular paced beats."

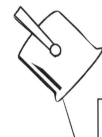

Now You Know

An electronic pacemaker is a device that can help to maintain a minimum heart rate.

A pacemaker may be needed if the cardiac conduction system fails to maintain an adequate output despite medication or other conservative treatments.

Pacemakers can be simply classified as internal or external; permanent or temporary.

The NBG code allows a simple description of pacemaker mode. Common pacemaker modes are DDD, VVI, and AAI. Many others are possible.

A pacemaker can be triggered or inhibited according to its programming and to the patient's condition and needs.

A pacemakers can be programmed to sense the patient's natural beats, minimizing potentially dangerous competition.

Asynchronous pacemakers compete with the patient's natural heartbeats and are therefore dangerous.

Demand pacemakers don't compete with the patient's natural rhythm but supplement it.

Pacemakers calculate heart rate by a method similar to the small-box method. They measure the intervals between two consecutive beats and convert those intervals into a heart rate.

Test Yourself

1. Why are transcutaneous pacemakers used only as a stopgap measure? _____

2. The pacemaker's electrical discharge should show up on the ECG strip as a small _____.

3. Describe how a VVI pacemaker functions.
   _____
   _____

4. What condition precludes the use of an AAI pacemaker? _____ Why?
   _____
   _____

5. Why are asynchronous pacemakers less popular than they used to be? _____
   _____

6. Why is pacemaker inhibition an important feature? _____
   _____
   _____

7. Why is triggering an important pacemaker feature? _____
   _____
   _____

8. How do you calculate the percentage of heartbeats generated by the pacemaker?
   _____
   _____

9. Where is the ventricular lead located in most permanent pacemakers?
   _____
   _____

10. Match the pacemaker malfunctions with their identifying features:

    _b_ A. Failure to fire   a. Paced beats consistently occurring late

    _c_ B. Failure to capture   b. A long interval with no natural or paced beats.

    _d_ C. Undersensing   c. Pacemaker spikes occurring when expected with no PQRST following

    _a_ D. Oversensing   d. Pacemaker spikes occurring too close to the previous beat.

11. Identify the rhythms in the following 25 strips involving pacemakers and identify any malfunctions:

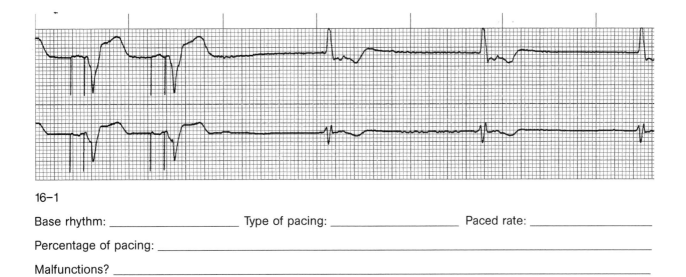

16–1

Base rhythm: _____ Type of pacing: _____ Paced rate: _____

Percentage of pacing: _____

Malfunctions? _____

Interpretation: _____

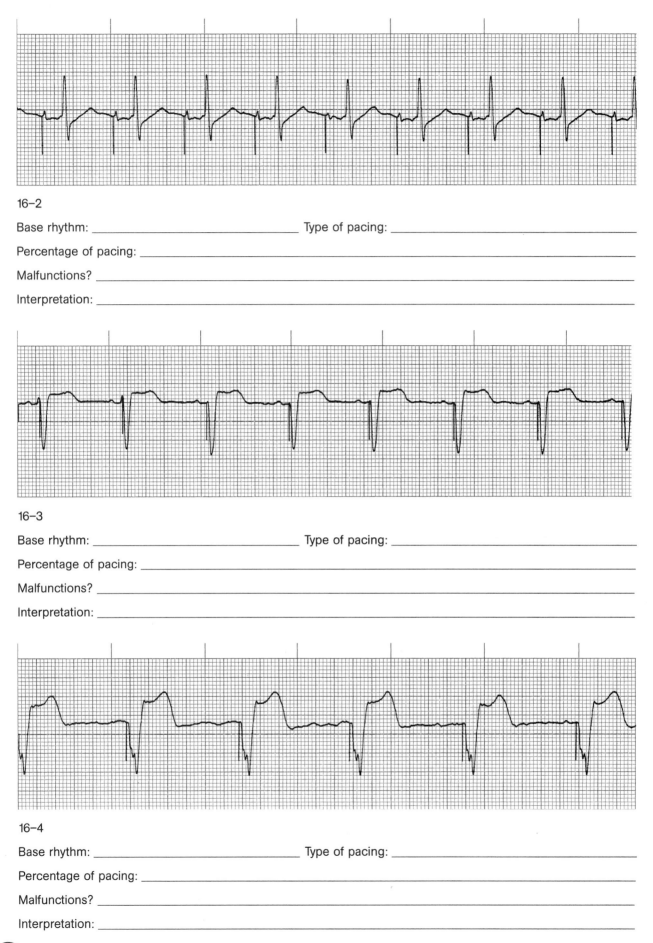

16–2

Base rhythm: _____ Type of pacing: _____

Percentage of pacing: _____

Malfunctions? _____

Interpretation: _____

16–3

Base rhythm: _____ Type of pacing: _____

Percentage of pacing: _____

Malfunctions? _____

Interpretation: _____

16–4

Base rhythm: _____ Type of pacing: _____

Percentage of pacing: _____

Malfunctions? _____

Interpretation: _____

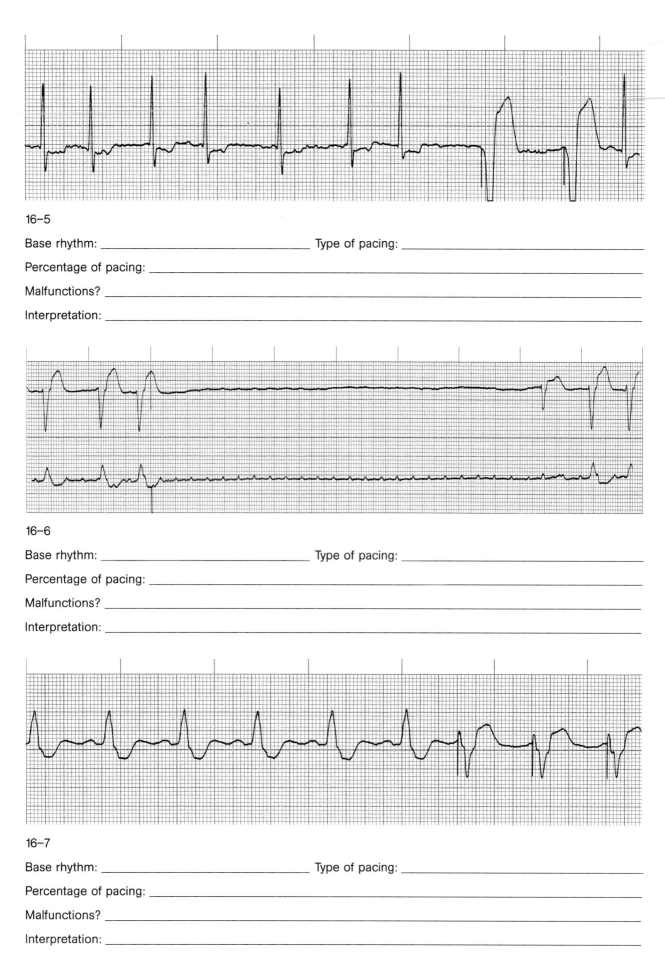

16–5

Base rhythm: _____ Type of pacing: _____

Percentage of pacing: _____

Malfunctions? _____

Interpretation: _____

16–6

Base rhythm: _____ Type of pacing: _____

Percentage of pacing: _____

Malfunctions? _____

Interpretation: _____

16–7

Base rhythm: _____ Type of pacing: _____

Percentage of pacing: _____

Malfunctions? _____

Interpretation: _____

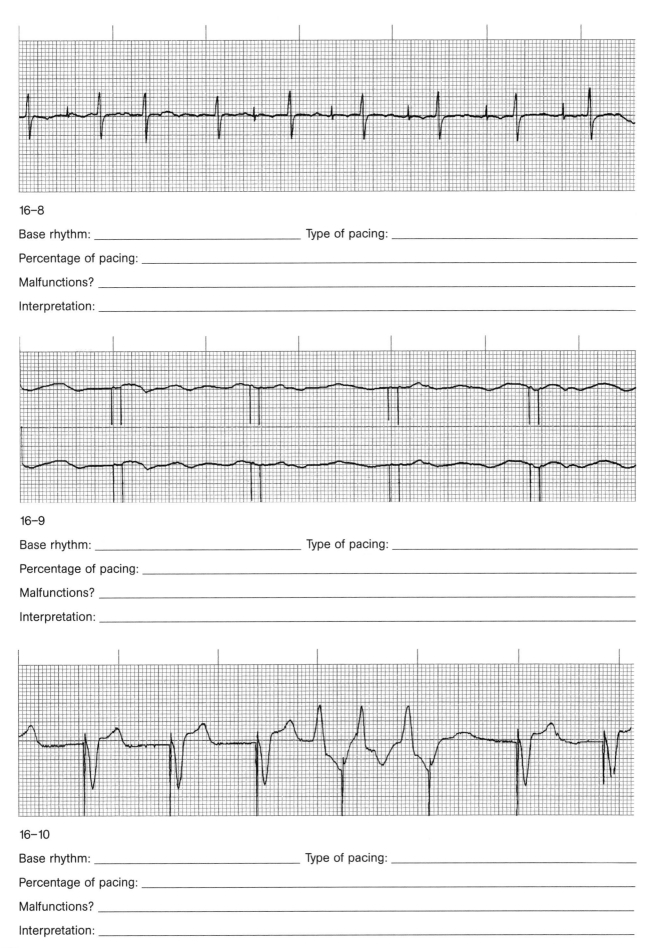

16–8

Base rhythm: _____ Type of pacing: _____

Percentage of pacing: _____

Malfunctions? _____

Interpretation: _____

16–9

Base rhythm: _____ Type of pacing: _____

Percentage of pacing: _____

Malfunctions? _____

Interpretation: _____

16–10

Base rhythm: _____ Type of pacing: _____

Percentage of pacing: _____

Malfunctions? _____

Interpretation: _____

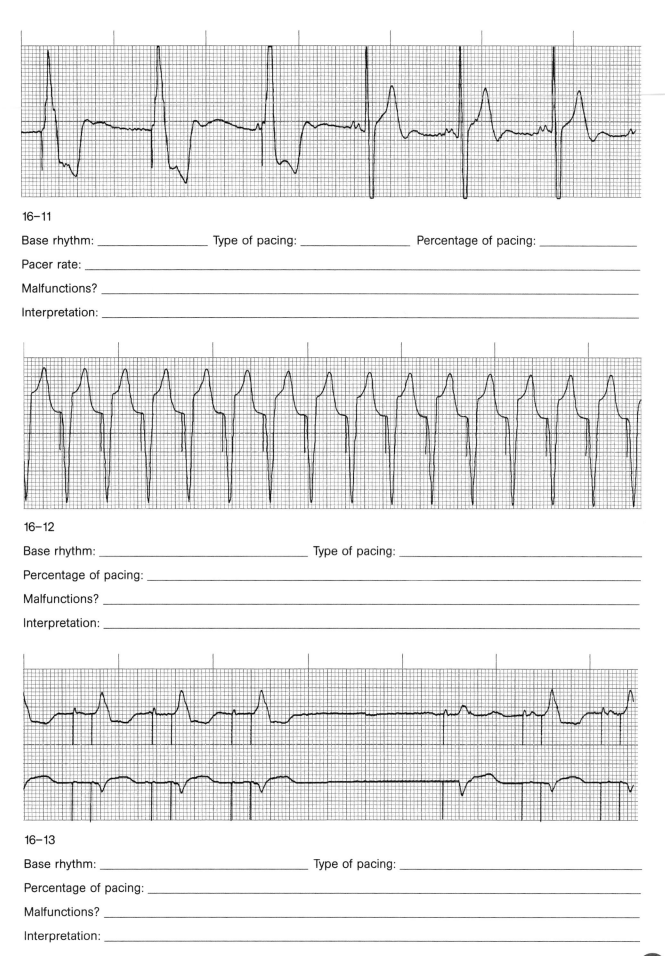

16–11

Base rhythm: _____ Type of pacing: _____ Percentage of pacing: _____

Pacer rate: _____

Malfunctions? _____

Interpretation: _____

16–12

Base rhythm: _____ Type of pacing: _____

Percentage of pacing: _____

Malfunctions? _____

Interpretation: _____

16–13

Base rhythm: _____ Type of pacing: _____

Percentage of pacing: _____

Malfunctions? _____

Interpretation: _____

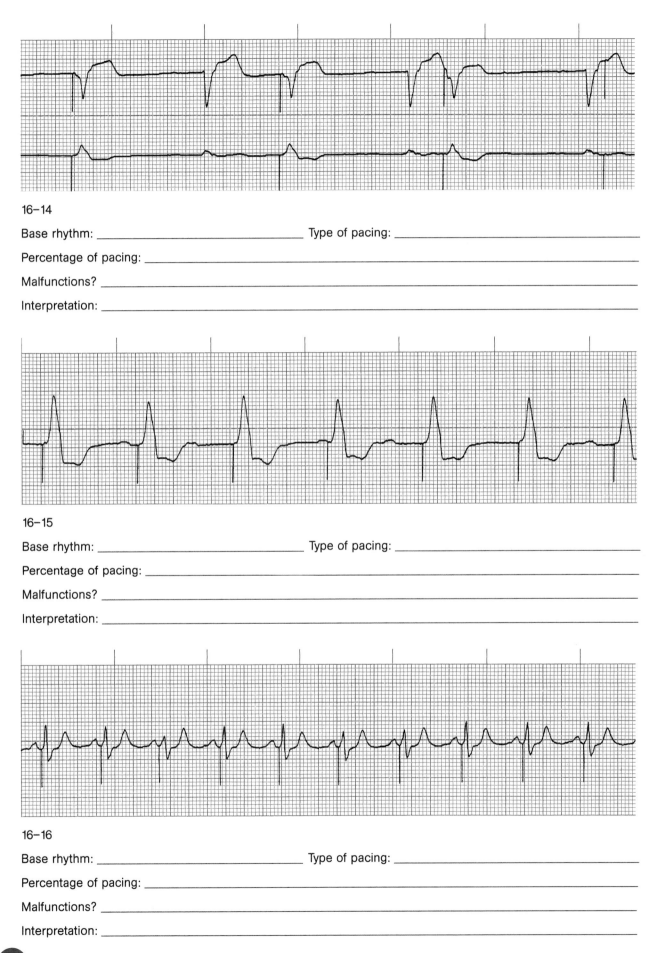

16-14

Base rhythm: _____ Type of pacing: _____

Percentage of pacing: _____

Malfunctions? _____

Interpretation: _____

16-15

Base rhythm: _____ Type of pacing: _____

Percentage of pacing: _____

Malfunctions? _____

Interpretation: _____

16-16

Base rhythm: _____ Type of pacing: _____

Percentage of pacing: _____

Malfunctions? _____

Interpretation: _____

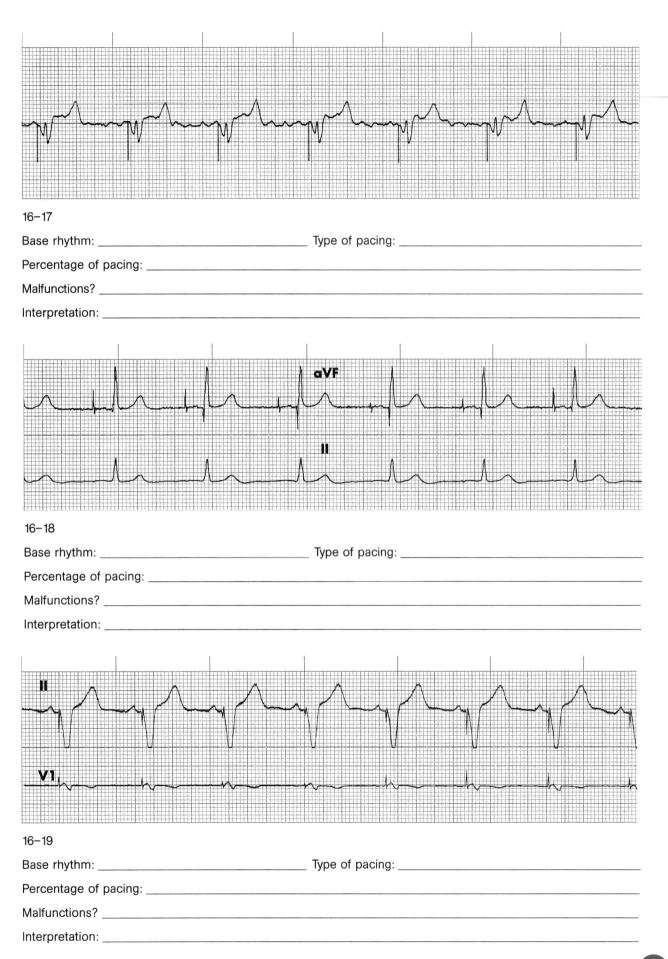

16–17

Base rhythm: _____ Type of pacing: _____

Percentage of pacing: _____

Malfunctions? _____

Interpretation: _____

aVF

II

16–18

Base rhythm: _____ Type of pacing: _____

Percentage of pacing: _____

Malfunctions? _____

Interpretation: _____

II

V1

16–19

Base rhythm: _____ Type of pacing: _____

Percentage of pacing: _____

Malfunctions? _____

Interpretation: _____

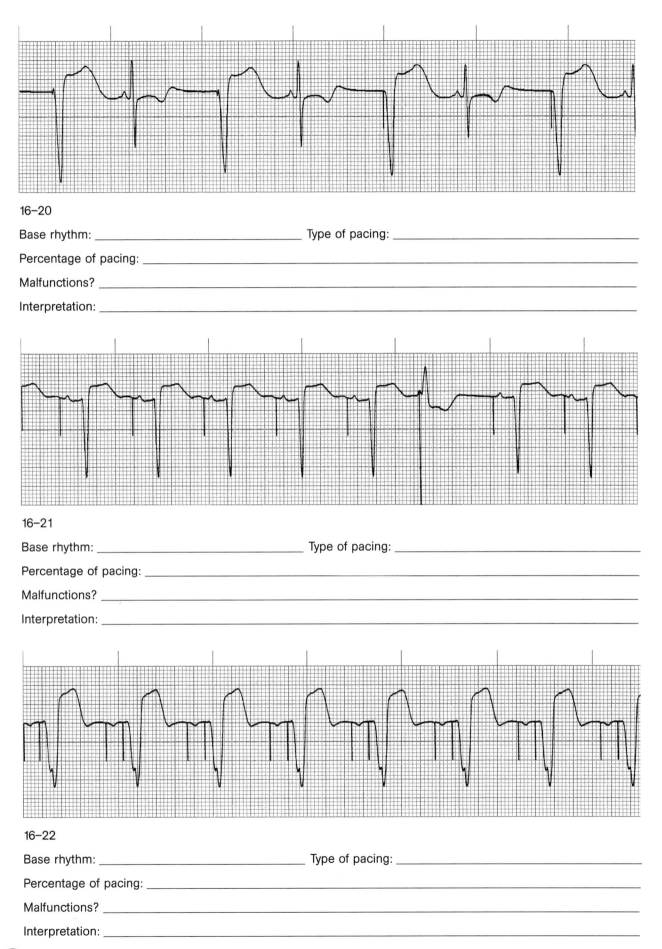

16–20

Base rhythm: _____ Type of pacing: _____

Percentage of pacing: _____

Malfunctions? _____

Interpretation: _____

16–21

Base rhythm: _____ Type of pacing: _____

Percentage of pacing: _____

Malfunctions? _____

Interpretation: _____

16–22

Base rhythm: _____ Type of pacing: _____

Percentage of pacing: _____

Malfunctions? _____

Interpretation: _____

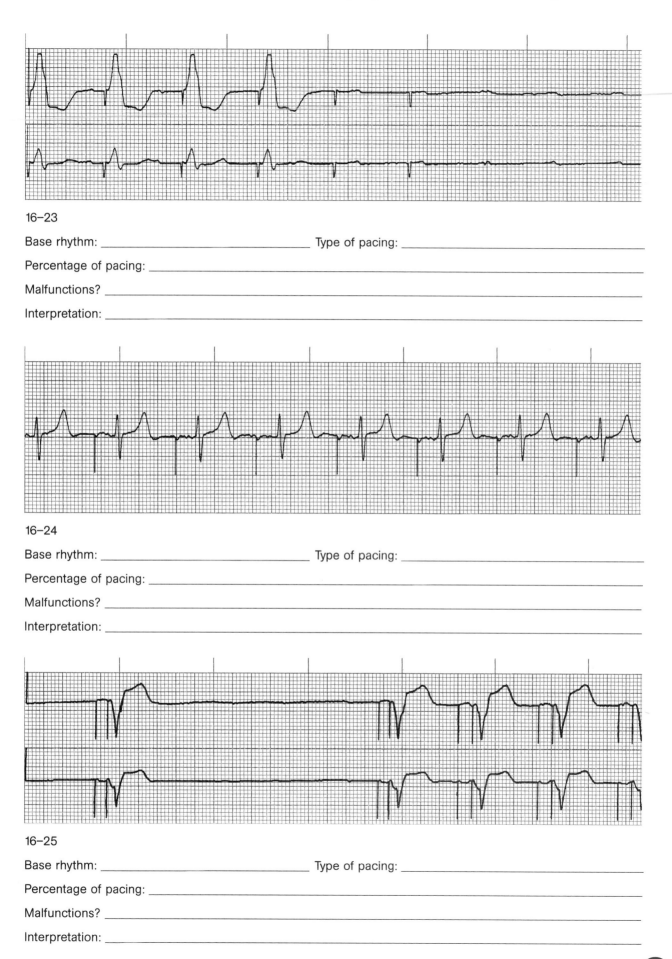

16–23

Base rhythm: _____ Type of pacing: _____

Percentage of pacing: _____

Malfunctions? _____

Interpretation: _____

16–24

Base rhythm: _____ Type of pacing: _____

Percentage of pacing: _____

Malfunctions? _____

Interpretation: _____

16–25

Base rhythm: _____ Type of pacing: _____

Percentage of pacing: _____

Malfunctions? _____

Interpretation: _____

Some Artifacts Aren't Rare or Valuable

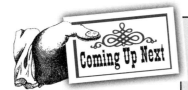

Coming Up Next

○ What is artifact?

○ How can electrical appliances affect the ECG monitor?

○ Why does artifact occur?

○ Which three elements of the ECG acquisition process can cause artifact?

○ What causes of artifact originate with the patient and how can you eliminate them?

○ Why can changing a patch or monitoring a different lead affect the amount of artifact?

○ How can a patient have a normal ECG rhythm but not have a pulse?

Snow in Your House

Has it ever happened to you? You're sitting at home watching a beach scene on TV when suddenly the beach scene is covered in snow! If your TV is like mine, one swift hit on the side will melt the snow fast. Or an adjustment to the cable (in earlier days, the rabbit-ear antennae) does the trick. If any of this sounds familiar, you've experienced *artifact.*

Taber's Cyclopedic Medical Dictionary defines "artifact" as "the appearance of a spurious signal not consistent with results expected from the signal being studied." An ECG artifact is defined loosely as anything that shows up on the ECG tracing and is not generated by the heart's electrical conduction system. This interference can vary in origin and impact. There are several common types of artifact. For each type, we'll discuss key features, what rhythms it can mimic, and how to correct it. Artifact has three basic sources: the patient, an external influence, and the ECG equipment.

In real life, artifact is everywhere, TV snow and radio static being among the most common examples. If you like, poor communication between partners is a kind of artifact. The key is that something interferes with the signal

we're trying to receive. When it snows on TV, the cable may be broken or improperly connected to the back of the set. Radio static can come from signal blockage, as when you drive through a tunnel or under strong electrical power lines. When partners miscommunicate, the signal gets through but is misinterpreted because of emotion, fatigue, or distraction.

Everyday, real-life artifacts can interfere with the reception and interpretation of ECG signals. Remember Chapter 4, where we learned that ECG patches receive their electrical signals from all directions? Like the TV and radio, the electrodes can pick up all kinds of electrical signals, not just the ones we want them to. The ECG patch can't decide which signals really come from the heart and which are spurious.

Check Your Patient

LARGE-MUSCLE ARTIFACT

Patients can cause three common types of artifact. The first is *large-muscle artifact,* also known as *somatic (body-related) artifact*, such as tremors. It occurs when

17-1 WEED OUT THE STATIC

Like the uncomprehending partner, the ECG monitor processes every signal it receives. With some effort, even a disgruntled person can usually separate the message from the static. In the ECG monitor, the computer uses algorithms to weed through all of the extra information and "decide" which signals to transform into the tracing we'll interpret. However, just like people, computers are imperfect, so extraneous signals often get through so strongly that they completely scramble the ECG tracing. It's our job to recognize the artifact and not misinterpret it as a dysrhythmia.

large amounts of muscle tissue are stimulated. If the lead we're monitoring has a patch in close proximity to the muscle movement, we can get this type of artifact.

Figure 17–1 shows what havoc simply using a toothbrush can cause. In a right-handed patient, the rapid motion produces lots of electrical activity over the RA lead as the arm and chest muscles move the hand up and down. If the patient is monitored in lead I or lead II, the strip may show many waves that resemble QRS complexes—the electrical activity from the muscles overpowers the small amount coming from the heart. This "rhythm," commonly known as "toothbrush tachycardia," can also occur with chills, muscle spasms, or a rapid tap with a finger on the lead.

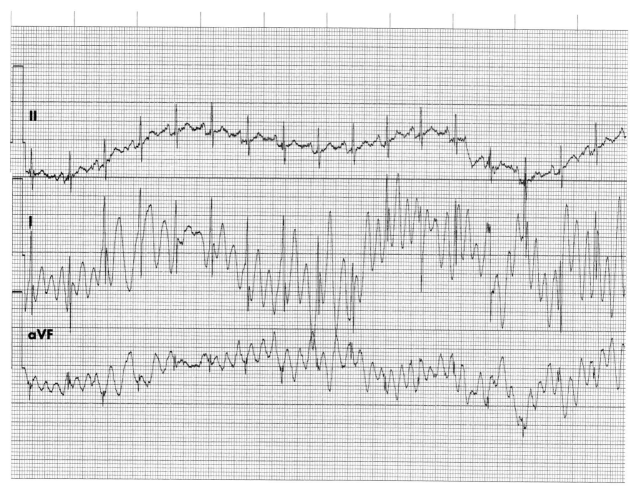

Fig. 17–1 Sinus rhythm with somatic artifact, sometimes called "toothbrush tachycardia." This tracing shows how large-muscle movement near a patch can affect a recording of sinus rhythm. The tracing can easily be mistaken for V-tach, but the true QRSs (arrows) are identifiable with close attention.

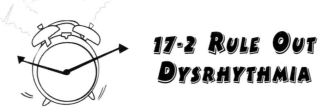

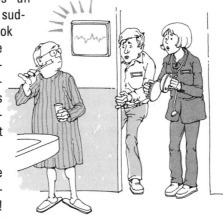

17-2 RULE OUT DYSRHYTHMIA

When the computer sounds an alarm, it may be reacting to the sudden onslaught of spikes that look like QRS complexes, or the patient may really have ventricular tachycardia. If the computer announces a dangerous dysrhythmia, how can we distinguish a toothbrush artifact from a case of V-tach?

The first step, which should be obvious, but is often overlooked: check your patient! When you're in doubt, immediate assessment is critical. If the problem isn't artifact but a dangerous rhythm, the patient needs immediate treatment. Measure the patient's vital signs, such as heart rate, blood pressure, and oxygen saturation, and do a thorough assessment. If you're dealing with artifact, you're still at bedside to correct the problem.

If the patient isn't in danger, check the ECG tracing. In large-muscle artifact, we often see normal QRS complexes sticking out from the top and bottom of the tracing. If the true rhythm is regular, we can look for a real QRS and then try to march out the others. Look back at Figure 17–1; In the top tracing the P-waves and QRS complexes are easy to identify. Look below the QRS complexes in that tracing and

you can see the QRS complexes in the lower two strips. That can help you to see sharp points that interrupt the toothbrush tachycardia. These are the true QRSs sticking their heads up out of the artifact. Although you won't always be able to see them, their presence is a strong indicator of artifact. Figure 17–2 shows another artifact strip. This time the true QRSs are irregular; see if you can identify them.

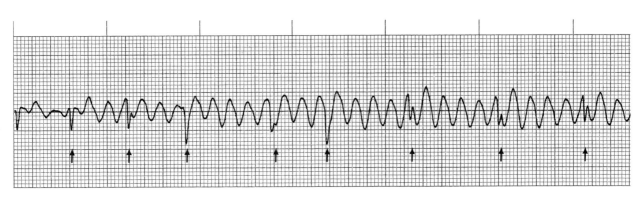

Fig. 17–2 Atrial fibrillation with somatic artifact, mimicking V-tach. The irregularity of the true rhythm may make it hard to identify the QRSs (arrows) on the tracing. Patient assessment, including palpation for a pulse, can easily distinguish this rhythm from V-tach.

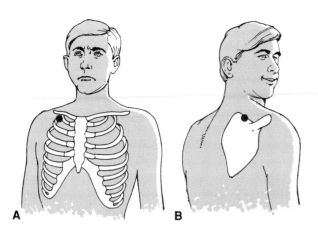

Fig. 17–3a–b The "cure" for somatic artifact is to relocate the affected patches to areas that have less electrical activity. Here the patches are moved from the large pectoralis muscles of the chest (a) to the much smaller and less frequently used muscles of the upper back (b). The tracing becomes much easier to read, although it may change slightly because the patches have been moved.

The approach to large-muscle artifact is to stop muscle stimulation under the patches for the monitored lead. You may be able to do this by changing to a lead that doesn't rely so heavily on that patch. However, because each patch is used to evaluate multiple leads, this approach may not work. Also, you may have a reason to monitor that particular lead: the patient may have a history of myocardial infarction, or you may need to observe P-waves.

A second approach is to move the patch away from the offending muscle group. If the RA lead is the problem, moving it from the anterior chest to the upper portion of the posterior chest, as shown in Figure 17–3, may solve the problem, or at least minimize it. Be careful—any deviation of lead placement from the assigned locations can introduce small changes in the ECG tracing. The lead has changed its perspective, so you're monitoring a different vector. Any alternative lead placement should be recorded in the nurse's notes and on the strip if the difference is significant. Otherwise someone might misinterpret the new ECG waveform as a change in patient condition instead of a change in patch location.

Look back at Figure 17–2. This patient had tremors in her left arm. Her hand would lift slightly off the patch, and the base of her hand would then tap the patch gently in a rapidly repeating cycle. The treatment for the resulting "tachycardia" was to simply move the patient's hand off the LL lead. Too bad all tachycardias aren't so easily treated.

BASELINE SWAY

Another common patient-generated artifact is *baseline sway,* in which the whole rhythm rises from the normal baseline. This artifact has many possible causes. Lotion, sweat, or body oil may come between the patient and the electrode, altering the conduction of the electrical signal between the patient's skin and the patch. This kind of interference is the easiest to correct. Simply remove the offending patch, clean the skin with an alcohol swab, dry it thoroughly, and apply a new patch. The area may need light shaving to improve contact.

Another cause of baseline sway is breathing. Breathing depends on large groups of muscles working in a rhythmic pattern. When muscles below the patch contract, the signal is added to the ECG tracing and raises the rhythm

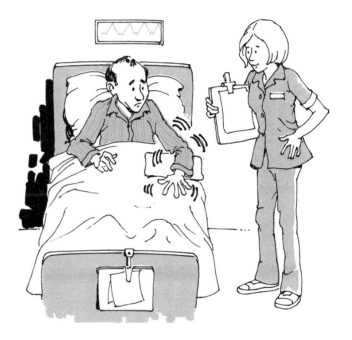

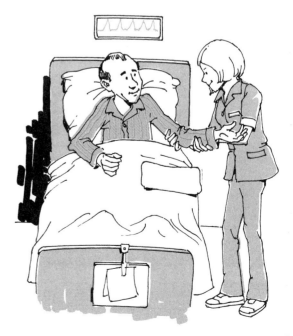

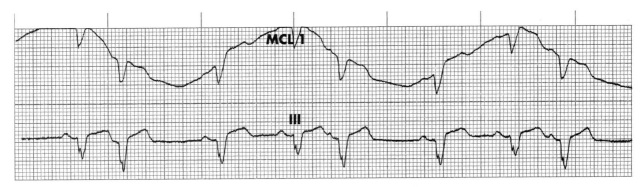

Fig. 17–4 The top tracing shows respiratory artifact caused by the chest patch in lead MCL₁. The bottom tracing, which doesn't rely on the chest patch, is normal. This patient's respiratory rate, about 23 per minute, can be determined from the distance between the peaks or valleys of the baseline sway. Changing the location of the chest lead to the MCL position may also correct the artifact.

from the baseline. When the same muscles relax, the tracing returns whence it came. This artifact usually does nothing but irritate the person watching the monitor. The slow, rhythmic up-and-down undulations, which reflect the patient's respiratory rate, usually don't affect rhythm interpretation and are generally restricted to certain leads (Fig. 17–4). They just make it a little harder to take measurements and may set off some monitor alarms repeatedly.

In some patients, electrode placement and lead selection can correct baseline sway. It may help to make sure that the lower patches don't rest on the diaphragm

(about the base of the ribcage). Also, men tend to be abdominal breathers—the abdomen rises and falls to assist with chest expansion. As a result, the abdomen moves in and out from front to back, rather than from side to side. Therefore, moving the lower patches (LL and RL) to the sides, not the front, of the abdomen (Fig. 17–5) can help to diminish or even eliminate this type of artifact.

PULSELESS ELECTRICAL ACTIVITY

A patient may have an underlying rhythm and still need cardiopulmonary resuscitation (CPR) or some other

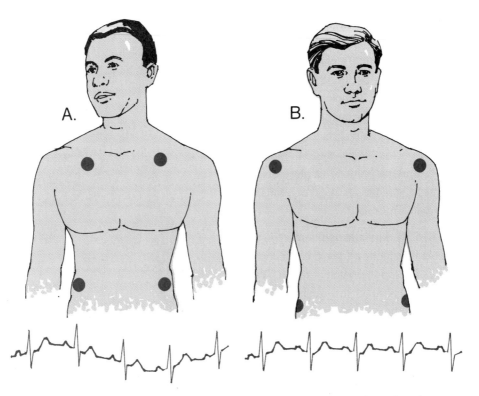

Fig. 17–5A–B Respiratory baseline sway. A, The affected patches should be moved away from the areas of respiratory muscle movement. B, The lower two patches have been moved away from the diaphragm.

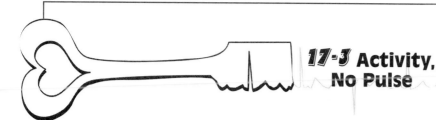

17-3 Activity, No Pulse

A patient with PEA can have any rhythm, from junctional bradycardia to sinus rhythm to ventricular tachycardia. Simply, PEA is any rhythm that doesn't generate a pulse. It can be caused by insufficient cardiac output or by a heart muscle that can't contract because of an electrolyte disturbance such as hypokalemia, hyperkalemia, or hypocalcemia. Remember, the wrong concentration of electrolytes can prevent the shift across the cell membrane that causes the muscle to contract.

Pulseless electrical activity isn't really a rhythm interpretation. Even so, it's important to understand the concept that a normal-looking ECG strip doesn't necessarily guarantee a pulse.

drastic intervention. The rhythm may be bradycardic and too slow to sustain life. On the other hand, it may look normal but not generate a pulse. This second situation, called *pulseless electrical activity* (PEA), is life threatening.

In PEA, the patient's rhythm may look like a perfectly normal sinus rhythm in the 80s, but the patient may be dead. This phenomenon used to be called *electrical-mechanical dissociation* ("EMD" in clinical settings), which implied that the electrical signals in the heart were not causing mechanical contraction. That term isn't necessarily accurate. The heart may be contracting, but its condition may prevent it from filling properly with blood or

from ejecting all of the blood it receives. Therefore, "pulseless electrical activity" is a better description of what's happening—the patient has electrical activity with no palpable pulse.

Other causes of PEA include tension pneumothorax, in which air leaks into the chest cavity, and pericardial tamponade, in which the sac around the heart fills with excessive fluid. Both conditions can put excessive pressure on the heart. The pressure weakens contractions and can minimize the amount of blood returning to the heart, decreasing cardiac output until a pulse is no longer detectable. Severe internal bleeding from a ruptured aortic aneurysm can also cause PEA by decreasing the amount of blood returning to the heart. Other culprits are pulmonary embolism, which blocks ejection of blood from the right ventricle, and myocardial infarction, which minimizes ventricular contraction. (The MATCHx5ED mnemonic that was covered in Chapter 13 when we discussed the common causes of asystole also works for PEA.)

Treatment of PEA is aimed at identifying and removing the cause. It's important to realize the limits of the ECG: it gives us an "electrical" heart rate, but the only way to check for a "physical" heart rate—in other words, a pulse—is to assess the actual patient! That means you can't go up to the person watching the monitors and ask for your patient's pulse.

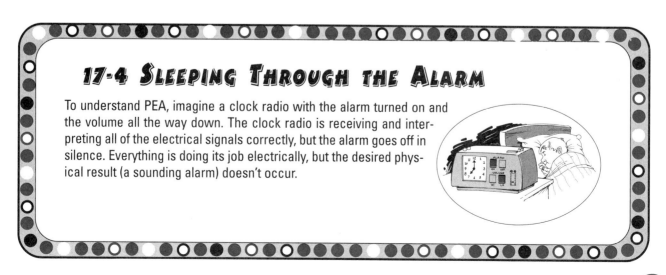

17-4 Sleeping Through the Alarm

To understand PEA, imagine a clock radio with the alarm turned on and the volume all the way down. The clock radio is receiving and interpreting all of the electrical signals correctly, but the alarm goes off in silence. Everything is doing its job electrically, but the desired physical result (a sounding alarm) doesn't occur.

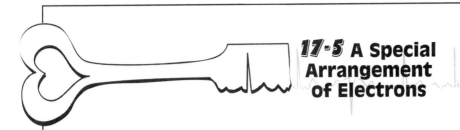

17-5 A Special Arrangement of Electrons

Magnets are electrical devices that arrange their electrons in a specific pattern. All electrical currents, including those in the body, generate magnetic fields. That's why we have positive and negative leads and why batteries have a positive and a negative end. Even wires that conduct electricity, like the wires connecting the ECG patches to the monitor, generate small magnetic fields as electricity courses through them.

The ECG monitor picks up tiny changes in the electrical field of the chest and interprets them as the tracing. Anything that can generate a magnetic field, such as a magnet or an electrical appliance, can alter the electrical signal we're trying to monitor.

Under the Influence

60-CYCLE INTERFERENCE...

The electricity that comes from the walls is known as *alternating current.* That means its polarity varies from positive to negative in a repeated, rapid pattern. It usually changes at a speed of 60 hertz, which has nothing to do with the car rental company. "Hertz" means "cycles per second," or the number of times in 1 second that the polarity changes from positive to negative and back. That's where we get the name for this type of artifact—*60-cycle interference.*

... AND HOW IT INTERFERES

We commonly find 60-cycle interference when outlets or electrical equipment (IV pumps, tube feeding pumps, electric razors) aren't properly grounded or when the insulation covering a wire has even a small break. If there's no obvious problem with the equipment, the wall outlet may be providing faulty grounding. Whatever the reason, the electricity traveling through the cord "leaks." When the electrical cord is close to or wrapped around the ECG wires or cables, the result is the type of tracing you see in Figure 17–6. This rhythm is regular but has a wavy baseline. A wavy baseline raises the suspicion of atrial fibrillation, but A-fib should be irregularly irregular. The baseline also looks thick, being much darker than the rest of the tracing. Normally, even in A-fib, the baseline is much thinner.

If you look closely at Figure 17–6, you can barely make out 12 or so little "P-waves" in every large box. Extrapolating out, we can calculate about 60 of these little P-waves every second (five large boxes per second × 12 P-waves per large box). Each P-wave represents a cycle in the electricity feeding the offending device. Of course, these P-waves are 60-cycle imposters, but they're frequently mistaken for the real thing.

Compare the first two strips in Figure 17–7. The first shows atrial fibrillation, with the irregularly irregular QRS complexes that help us identify it; the second shows sinus rhythm with 60-cycle interference. Notice the regularity of the QRSs in Figure 17–7b. It's possible for 60-cycle interference to occur in any rhythm, including atrial fibrillation and sinus rhythm with PACs. In Figure 17–7c, the artifact is only present in one lead. Look carefully for the P-waves before each QRS; they frequently show up in lead II despite the 60-cycle interference. That's because the artifact is small enough and regular enough that the large P-waves in this lead are usually visible.

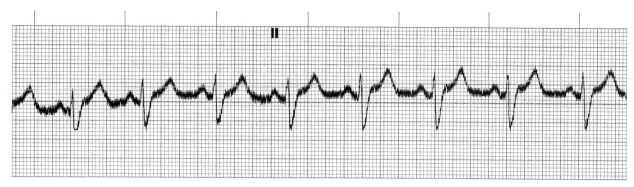

Fig. 17-6 A sinus rhythm tracing with 60-cycle interference. The baseline looks thick and fuzzy. The QRS is frequently not affected because of its greater height. Because 60-cycle interference has a continuous, consistent effect, the underlying rhythm can often be identified.

You may want to run a clean strip to post in the patient's medical record or to check for rhythm changes if they're suspected. You can usually eliminate 60-cycle interference by moving the offending electrical equipment as far from the ECG wires and cables as possible. If not, unplugging any equipment that can run on batteries may do the trick. Either way, the biomedical engineering department should be notified so they can investigate the cause of the

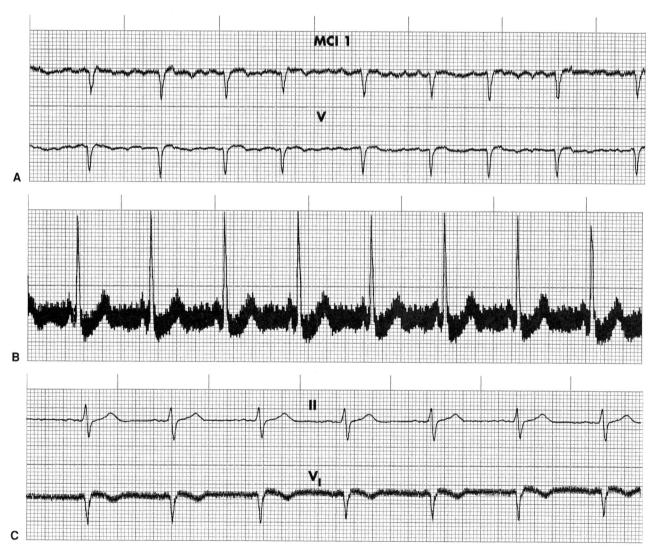

Fig. 17-7A-C Three common rhythms with 60-cycle interference. Because the artifact blurs the baseline, these rhythms can be easily misinterpreted. A, Atrial fibrillation. The artifact in the top tracing conceals the wavy baseline, removing a key feature of the rhythm. The wavy baseline is more easily seen in the bottom tracing. B, Sinus rhythm with 60-cycle interference. The P-waves are nearly obscured. C, Sinus rhythm. The artifact nearly obscures the typically smaller P-waves in lead V_I, making the rhythm appear to be junctional but the P-waves are clearly visible in lead II.

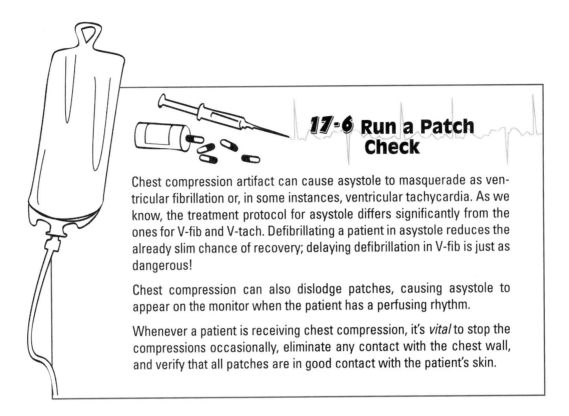

17-6 Run a Patch Check

Chest compression artifact can cause asystole to masquerade as ventricular fibrillation or, in some instances, ventricular tachycardia. As we know, the treatment protocol for asystole differs significantly from the ones for V-fib and V-tach. Defibrillating a patient in asystole reduces the already slim chance of recovery; delaying defibrillation in V-fib is just as dangerous!

Chest compression can also dislodge patches, causing asystole to appear on the monitor when the patient has a perfusing rhythm.

Whenever a patient is receiving chest compression, it's *vital* to stop the compressions occasionally, eliminate any contact with the chest wall, and verify that all patches are in good contact with the patient's skin.

interference. Leaking current from a broken wire, or improperly grounded electrical outlets or equipment can put patients at risk for electrical shock.

CARDIAC COMPRESSION

Chest compressions can cause artifact in a patient receiving CPR. The rhythm has a rounded waveform that corresponds to the compressions (Fig. 17–8). The rate should be around 100 bpm, the American Heart Association's recommended rate of chest compressions in an adult patient. If cardiac compression is the cause of the rhythm, the rounded undulations should resolve after compression stops. In an actual resuscitation, the practitioner can stop compressions for a few seconds and watch the monitor to determine whether the patient is producing an ECG tracing. In the absence of a life-sustaining rhythm, the chest compressions should continue.

The Ghost in the Machine

Sometimes artifact can come from the last place you'd think of—the ECG equipment itself. Like the other types of artifact, it usually declares itself by producing a characteristic tracing.

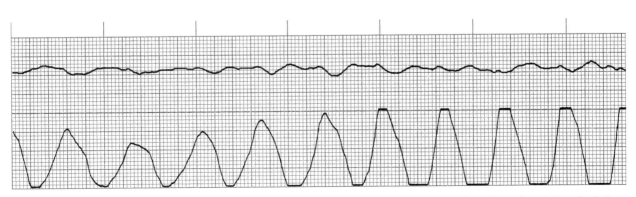

Fig. 17–8 Chest compression artifact, occurring at a rate slightly slower than 100 bpm. In the top tracing, the artifact is less obvious; the rhythm appears to be V-fib, although the actual rhythm is asystole.

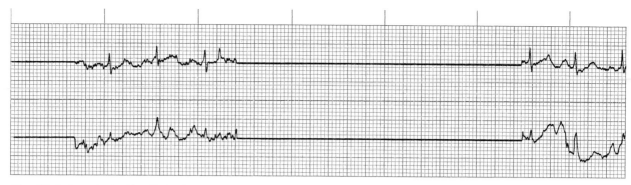

Fig. 17-9 Loose lead artifact. Notice the erratic nature of the tracing. When patch contact is good, the rhythm appears normal. When contact is poor, the deflections vary wildly. When the pads briefly lose all contact, the tracing becomes a flat line indicating that the equipment is not receiving any electrical signals.

LOOSE LEADS SINK STRIPS

In my experience, the most common type of ECG equipment artifact is caused by loose leads. Although we call it "loose lead artifact," it's really the individual patches that get loose. In Chapter 4 we discussed some characteristics of the electrodes. Remember the silver chloride gel that conducts the electrical signal to the ECG cables? This gel is a good conductor, but it tends to dry out over time. Influenced by conditions such as room humidity and skin moisture, patches can dry out in as little as 1 day.

Figure 17-9 is an example of loose lead artifact. You'll notice periods in which the tracing is normal, followed by sudden, wildly varying deflections interspersed with completely flat, straight lines. The flat lines represent periods when the patch is disconnected and completely unable to conduct.

It's not unusual for loose lead artifact to shift the tracing from a normal rhythm to a perfectly flat line and return it quickly back to normal. The flat, nonconducted periods, if present, are usually preceded and followed by wildly flailing waveforms.

Sometimes, if the silver chloride gel is drying out, you can get loose lead artifact even if all the patches are firmly in place. Another suspect is a broken wire. Loose lead artifact can mimic a short period of asystole, although a sudden change to asystole and back to a normal rhythm just doesn't occur.

You may be able to spot a broken lead wire by looking at the cables; however, sometimes the wire inside the cable can be broken without obvious external damage. Artifact caused by a broken wire can look just like loose lead artifact and should be suspected if all other causes have been eliminated.

GOOD ARTIFACT. . .

As I said earlier in this chapter, computer algorithms can be used to weed out extraneous signals. For instance, cable TV boxes use algorithms to remove the snowy artifact when their signals get scrambled. We already know that the wrong signals get through sometimes, but these algorithms have another trick up their sleeve: they can remove signals that should get through. The resulting distortion can throw off your interpretation of the rhythm. Most commonly, this type of artifact occurs in patients who have pacemaker rhythms, discussed in Chapter 16.

The algorithms are designed to remove high-frequency signals. These signals, which are large and very short, don't usually occur naturally in the heart. But they're exactly the type of signal that a pacemaker delivers: a large, short burst of electricity, meant to initiate a rhythm in the heart chamber being paced. When the algorithm identifies this kind of signal as artifact, we call it *pacemaker artifact*.

Most ECG monitoring equipment has a special setting to identify pacemaker artifact. Usually a button can activate the *pacemaker mode* to alert the monitor if the patient has a pacemaker. Armed with this information, the computer purposely lets the high-frequency artifact get through. Any time you see a regular rhythm that looks ventricular, turn on the monitor's pacemaker mode to check for pacemaker spikes. Doing this may save you some embarrassment—not all pacemakers are externally visible, and not all patients are able to tell you that they have one.

Compare the two strips in Figure 17-10. These two tracings were taken from the same patient 1 minute apart. Although the QRS complexes are identical, only the first strip shows pacemaker artifact; the second was taken with the pacemaker mode turned off.

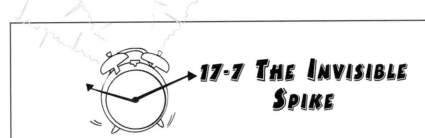

17-7 THE INVISIBLE SPIKE

The telltale spike that identifies a pacemaker rhythm may actually be removed by the very equipment that's supposed to pick it up! In this case, a pacemaker-generated rhythm, which tells us that the pacemaker is functioning, can masquerade as a ventricular rhythm, which might indicate trouble.

. . .GONE BAD

Although pacemaker artifact helps to identify pacemaker rhythms, it can have its down side. As the old saying goes, "If some is good, more is not always better!" That's especially true with pacemaker artifact. When the pacemaker mode is in use, the monitor lets through all high-frequency artifact within a particular range. As Figure 17–11 shows, that can wreak havoc on the strip. You can see the underlying rhythm, but are all those spikes really from the pacemaker? If so, too many can indicate a dangerous situation in which the pacemaker is definitely malfunctioning. As you recall from Chapter 16, it would be both failing to sense and failing to capture. Are *any* of them from the pacemaker? It can be hard to tell.

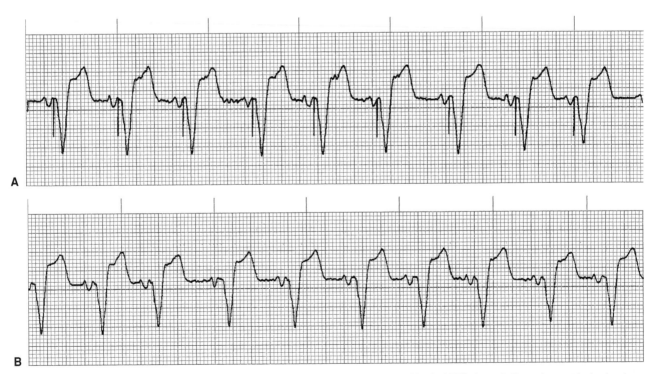

Fig. 17–10A–B Pacemaker artifact. Both strips come from the same patient 1 minute apart. Identical QRS shapes indicate that ventricular depolarization started at the same location in both strips. A, The pacemaker mode is turned on, producing a typical pacemaker spike. B, The pacemaker mode is turned off. The rhythm looks identical to A except for the absence of the pacemaker spike.

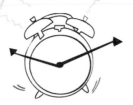

17-8 TURN OFF THE SETTING

To verify that the pacemaker is working, turn off the ECG pacemaker mode, at least temporarily. Eliminating the source of the artifact usually eliminates the extra pacemaker spikes. A few extra spikes may remain, and it's important to take care in determining whether they come from the pacemaker or from intermittent artifact. You can find this out by monitoring other leads. Frequently the extra spikes won't appear in other leads because the artifact causing a false pacemaker spike exists in only specific leads.

If you measure from one spike to the next in Figure 17–11, you'll find pacemaker rates ranging from about 100 bpm (between the two normally paced beats) up to more than 1500 bpm (the two closest spikes are less than one small box apart). No pacemaker is programmed to discharge at such high rates, so this raises our suspicion immediately.

Figure 17–11 also has an erratic baseline, probably from somatic artifact. All of the extra spikes come from short movements of a muscle mass. These could reflect anything from fine tremors in Parkinson's, to chills, to sudden or rhythmic movements such as raising a hand and waving. In fact, anything that can cause artifact can create extra pacemaker spikes. The underlying pacemaker rhythm, is probably normal.

Know What You're Dealing With

It's essential to distinguish artifact from true dysrhythmias. In some instances, the rhythm may behave like a malfunctioning pacemaker, and at other times it may behave like ventricular tachycardia or even asystole. The wrong interpretation can easily lead to inappropriate treatment.

A quick, thorough check of the ECG monitoring system is usually sufficient to identify and correct artifact. Changing or relocating patches, replacing broken wires, unplugging or moving equipment, monitoring other leads, or alerting the monitor to expect a certain artifact—all of these precautions take just a few minutes and can open the way to identifying true dysrhythmias.

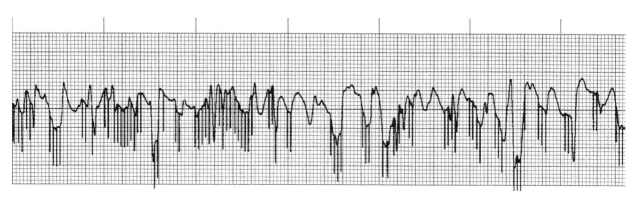

Fig. 17–11 Pacemaker artifact. Both the number and the spacing of the pacemaker spikes suggest a malfunction, but the rhythm looks normal when the pacemaker mode is turned off. Such large, erratic spikes are almost always caused by an artifact other than pacemaker failure.

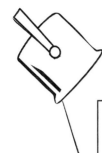

Now You Know

The term "artifact" refers to electrical signals that don't come from the heart and that interfere with proper ECG rhythm interpretation.

Artifact can occur naturally, as from muscle movements, or artificially, as from electrical appliances or chest compressions.

Sixty-cycle interference can make the baseline appear thick and wavy.

Sometimes changing a single patch or monitoring a different lead can undo the influence of artifact.

The ECG patches pick up all electrical activity from all sources that reach the patches.

Pulseless electrical activity (PEA) is not a rhythm but a symptom of a condition in which the heart can't function adequately.

Causes of PEA can include massive internal bleeding, tension pneumothorax, pericardial tamponade, pulmonary embolism, significant electrolyte disturbances, and myocardial infarction.

Pulseless electrical activity is life threatening, and treatment is directed at identifying and removing the cause.

Test Yourself

1. Baseline sway caused by breathing may be corrected by _____ some ECG patches.

2. During resuscitation, it's important to periodically _____ chest compressions because the artifact they generate may interfere with rhythm identification.

3. _____ can be caused by any electrical device that leaks current, or is improperly grounded.

4. In which rhythms can pulseless electrical activity occur? _____

5. List at least three possible causes of PEA.
   _____

6. Artifact can occur because the ECG patches transmit _____ electrical signals that reach them; not just those from the heart's electrical system.

7. Some rhythm strips do not have artifact because the monitoring equipment has built-in _____ to filter the electrical signals received from the ECG patches.

8. It's impossible to obtain a patient's _____ from the ECG monitor.

9. Identify which of the following 20 strips have artifact and the probable cause for the artifacts:

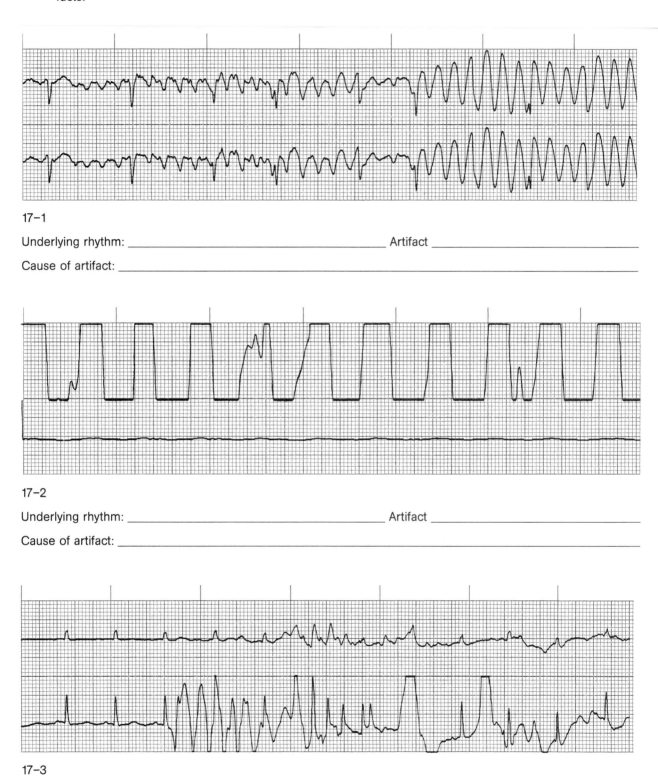

17–1

Underlying rhythm: _____ Artifact _____

Cause of artifact: _____

17–2

Underlying rhythm: _____ Artifact _____

Cause of artifact: _____

17–3

Underlying rhythm: _____ Artifact _____

Cause of artifact: _____

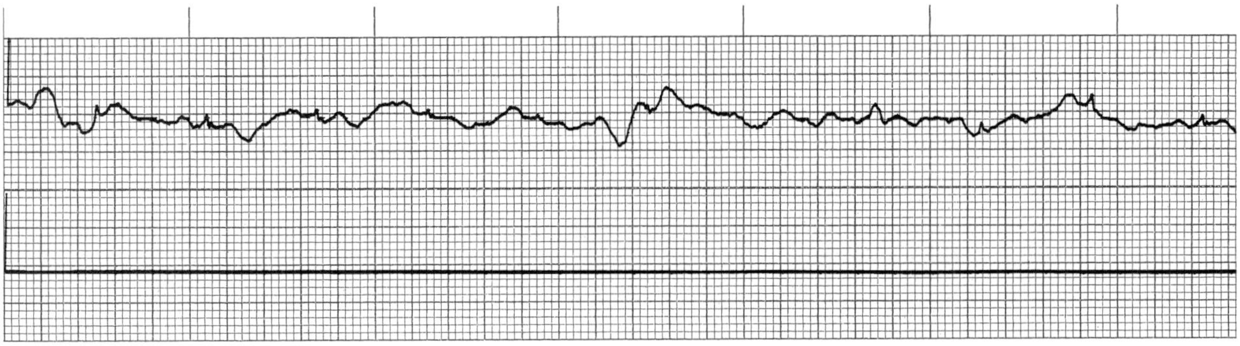

17–4

Underlying rhythm: _____ Artifact _____

Cause of artifact: _____

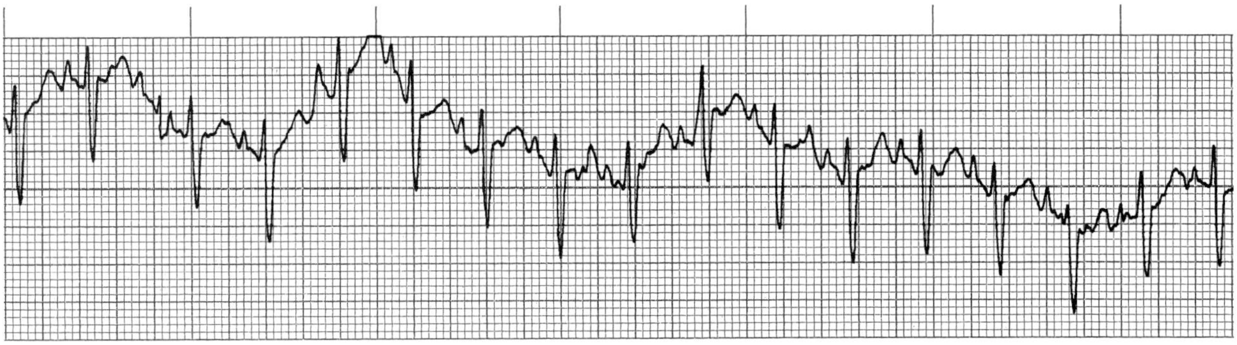

17–5

Underlying rhythm: _____ Artifact _____

Cause of artifact: _____

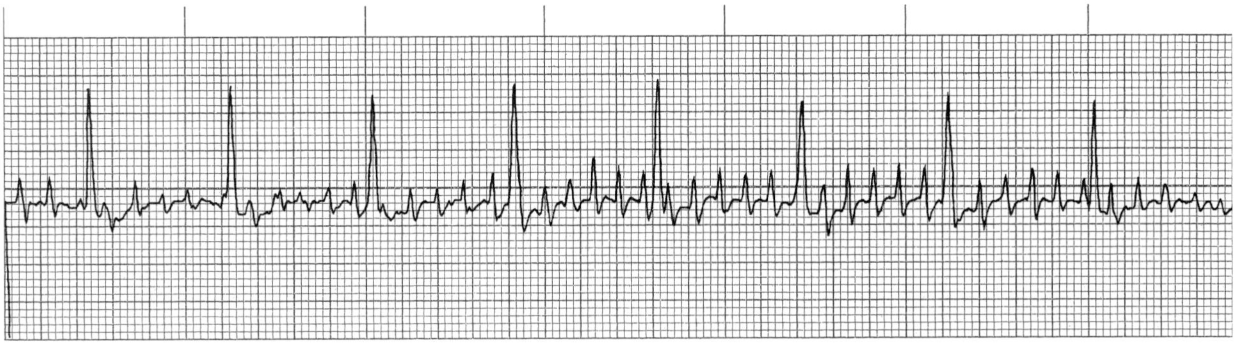

17–6

Underlying rhythm: _____ Artifact _____

Cause of artifact: _____

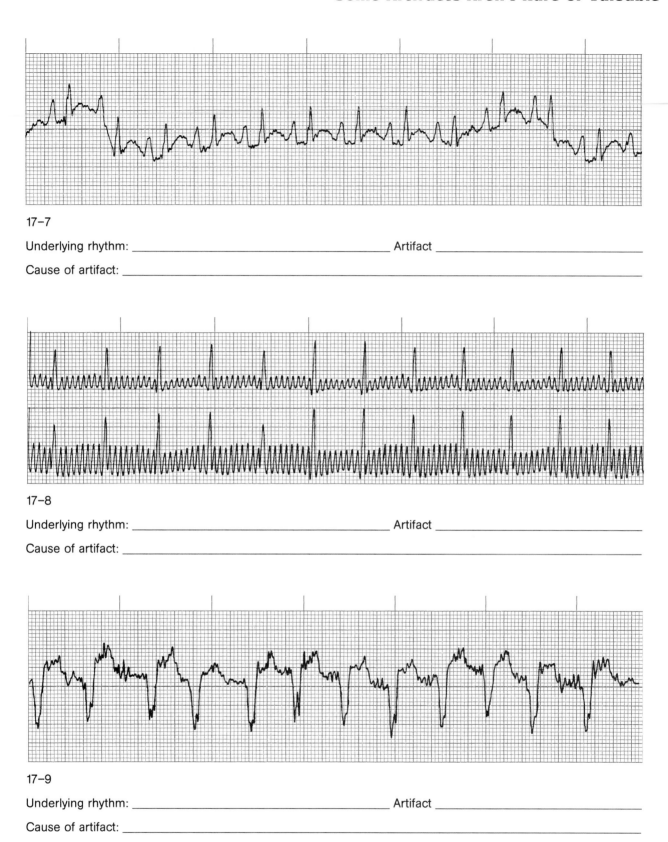

17–7

Underlying rhythm: _____ Artifact _____

Cause of artifact: _____

17–8

Underlying rhythm: _____ Artifact _____

Cause of artifact: _____

17–9

Underlying rhythm: _____ Artifact _____

Cause of artifact: _____

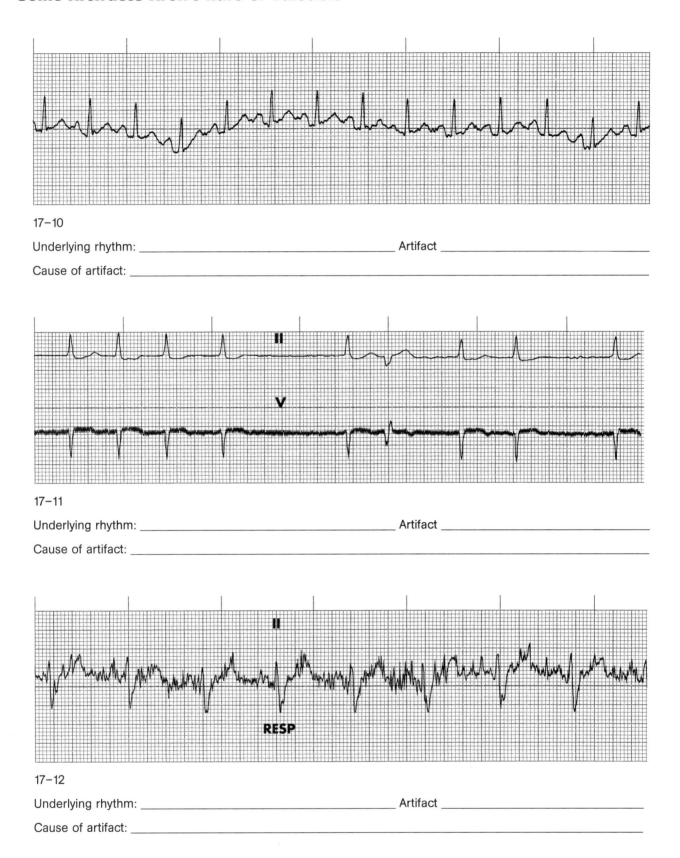

17-10

Underlying rhythm: _____ Artifact _____

Cause of artifact: _____

17-11

Underlying rhythm: _____ Artifact _____

Cause of artifact: _____

17-12

Underlying rhythm: _____ Artifact _____

Cause of artifact: _____

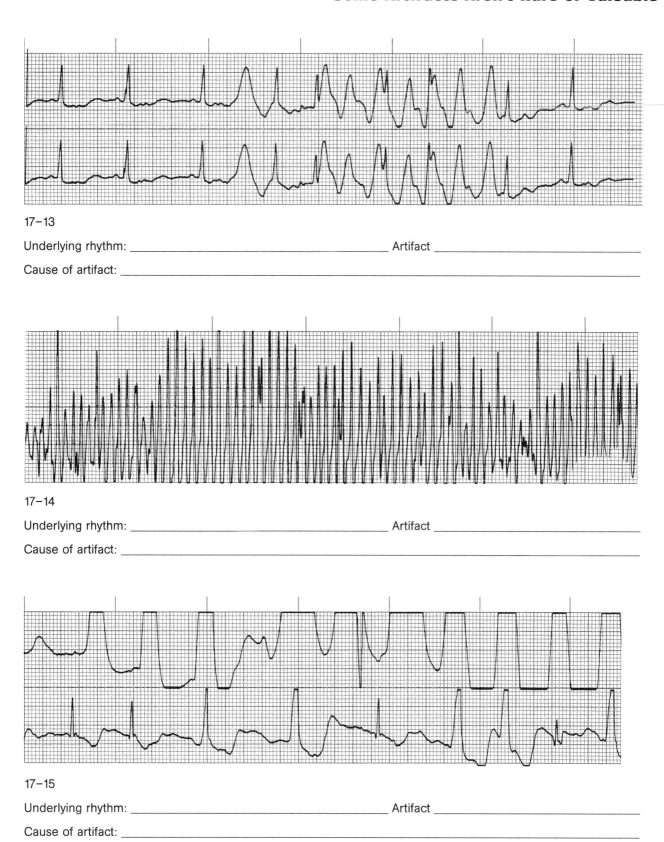

17–13

Underlying rhythm: _____ Artifact _____

Cause of artifact: _____

17–14

Underlying rhythm: _____ Artifact _____

Cause of artifact: _____

17–15

Underlying rhythm: _____ Artifact _____

Cause of artifact: _____

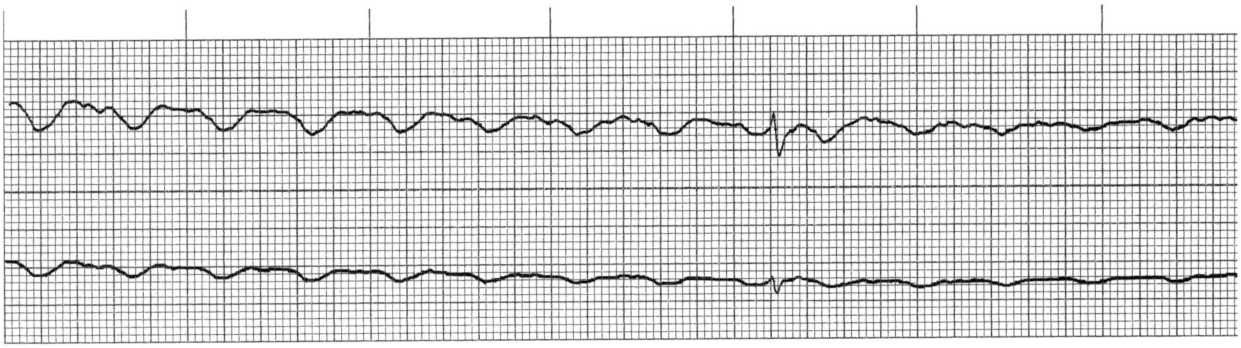

Some Artifacts Aren't Rare or Valuable

17–16

Underlying rhythm: _____ Artifact _____

Cause of artifact: _____

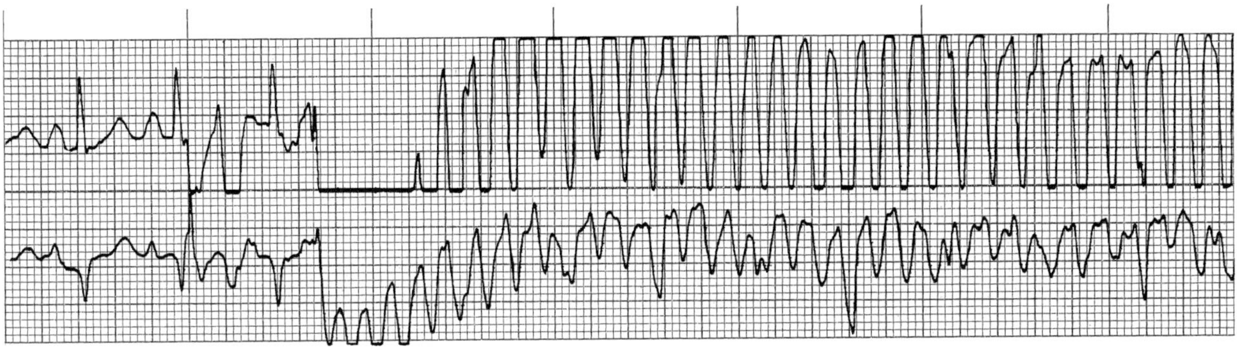

17–17

Underlying rhythm: _____ Artifact _____

Cause of artifact: _____

MCL₁

III

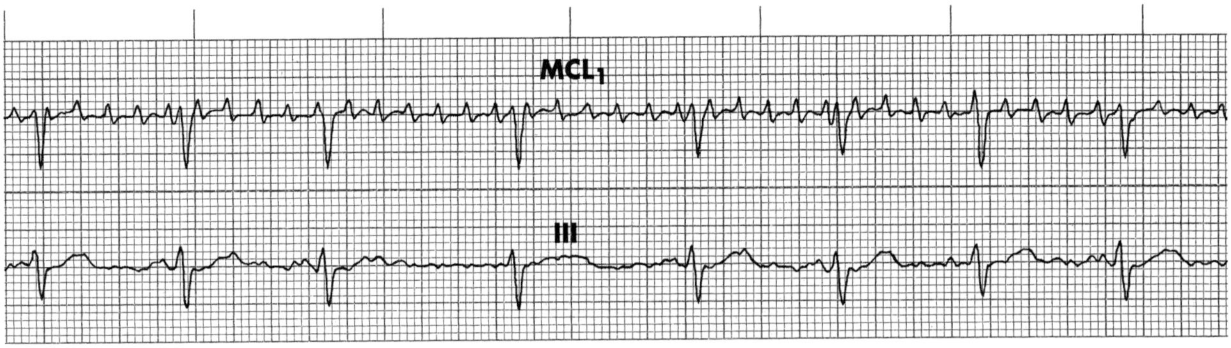

17–18

Underlying rhythm: _____ Artifact _____

Cause of artifact: _____

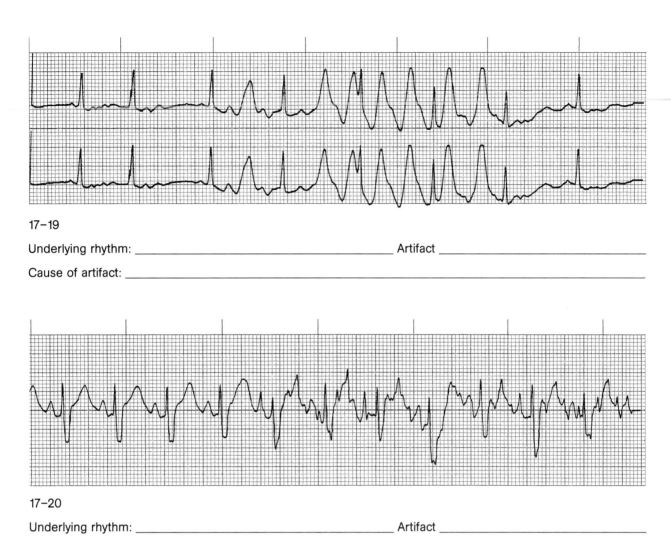

17–19

Underlying rhythm: _____ Artifact _____

Cause of artifact: _____

17–20

Underlying rhythm: _____ Artifact _____

Cause of artifact: _____

Timing Really

Is Everything

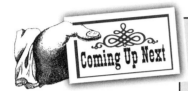

Coming Up Next

○ What is the QT interval and what does it contain?

○ Why do we need to worry about the QT interval?

○ How do we know if the QT interval is normal?

○ What is the difference between the absolute and relative refractory periods?

○ What is R on T phenomenon and why is it important?

○ What are fusion beats, pseudo-fusion beats, and pseudo–pseudo-fusion beats?

○ What are cardioversion and defibrillation, and how do they differ?

What's a QT Interval?

The title of this chapter shouldn't come as a great surprise when you consider that everything we've discussed so far has been about timing. From atrial kick to atrial fibrillation, from electronic pacemaker sensing to natural depolarization, from AV blocks to bundle branch blocks—timing crops up everywhere we look.

This chapter covers a mixed bag of topics, all timing related and indirectly related to rhythm interpretation. The first topic is the QT interval. We touched on this just briefly in Chapter 5, but now we'll cover it in more detail. An abnormal QT interval doesn't change our rhythm interpretation. However, it can determine how we treat that rhythm and can help us assess a patient's risk for developing ventricular tachycardia, ventricular fibrillation, or some other dangerous dysrhythmia.

The QT interval contains the QRS complex, the ST segment, and the T-wave. The QRS represents the depolarization of the ventricles, and the T-wave represents their repolarization. We won't need the ST segment for this chapter; its role in rhythm interpretation will become clear in Chapter 19.

For all intents and purposes, the QT interval measures how long the ventricles take to depolarize and repolarize. That seems simple enough. Why is this part of the tracing so important?

Measuring the QT Interval

A RULE OF THUMB

The QT interval is as simple to measure as the PR interval; it begins at the beginning of the QRS complex and ends at the end of the T-wave. Figure 18–1 shows a QT measurement. Unlike the normal ranges for PR intervals and QRS complex durations, the range for QT intervals isn't set. That's because they vary with the heart rate and depend on the length of time since the last beat. For QT intervals, normality is relative.

In our discussion of the AV node back in Chapter 6, I said that the AV node can repolarize more quickly when the heart rate is faster. Well, the same rule applies here; the ventricular tissue repolarizes more quickly at a faster heart rate.

Here's a good rule of thumb: if the QT interval is near normal, the T-wave should end before the halfway point between two consecutive QRS complexes. Compare the two strips in Figure 18–2. In the first strip, the T-wave ends well before the midpoint; in the second strip, which shows an abnormally long QT interval, the T-wave passes the midpoint.

There's a generally accepted formula for estimating whether a QT interval is normal: $QTc = QT / \sqrt{\text{previous RR}}$ interval. The value is *a corrected QT interval* (thus the "c" in "QTc"). Not that the QT interval was incorrect to begin

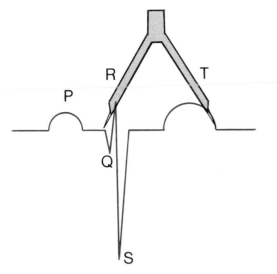

Fig. 18–1 The QT interval is measured from the beginning of the QRS complex to the end of the T-wave and represents one complete depolarization-repolarization cycle for the ventricles.

with: the term is misleading. It means that the measured QT interval has been adjusted for the given heart rate. A normal value for the QTc is 440 msec (0.44 sec) or less.

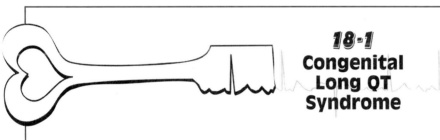

18-1
Congenital Long QT Syndrome

Some people are born with a cardiac anomaly known as _congenital long QT syndrome._ These patients will always have a longer-than-normal QT interval, which increases their risk for sudden cardiac death from V-tach or V-fib. Because it lacks symptoms, a long QT interval is often discovered incidentally when a patient goes for a physical exam that includes a 12-lead ECG.

THIS IS YOUR QT ON DRUGS

A normal QT interval changes from beat to beat, but should never varies outside the normal range for any given heart rate. However, treatment for a dysrhythmia can cause the QT interval to wander out of bounds.

Some cardiac medications, specifically the class IA drugs, can increase the QT interval. Two commonly used medications of this type are quinidine and procainamide. They can be used for a wide variety of dysrhythmias from atrial fibrillation to premature ventricular contractions. However, it's especially important to monitor a patient taking either of these medications,

especially when they're initially prescribed or given intravenously. They can throw off the QT interval pretty quickly and send it out of the normal range. If it wanders too far outside the normal range, the offending medication must be reduced or even discontinued.

If a patient receives cardiac monitoring while taking a class IA drug, it's important to measure the QT interval and, if possible, compare it with the QT measured during the previous visit. If the QT has increased 50% from baseline, the medication is discontinued. An overdose of these medications can cause severe symptoms, cardiac and otherwise.

Too Long a Rest

R ON T PHENOMENON

If the ventricles contract when they're supposed to, why do we care how long they take to recuperate? As the chapter title suggests, it's a question of timing. If the ventricles take too long to repolarize, the lag may interfere with the next depolarization and therefore with the QRS complex.

If the ventricles begin to depolarize before they finish repolarizing, you could be dealing with an _R on T phenomenon._ To understand this term, look at Figure 18–3. You can see that the QRS complex (often referred to as simply the R-wave) falls on top of the T-wave. Remember, the T-wave represents ventricular _re_polarization, and the QRS (R-wave) represents ventricular _de_polarization. If these two events happen simultaneously, they occur at the same point on the ECG tracing.

If the QRS complex falls on top of the QRS, why do we use the term "R on T"? What happened to Q and S? If you remember, back when we learned to measure heart rate, you learned the term "R to R interval." The same principle is operating here. We use the R-wave as the simplest reference point because it's the most common and most prominent feature of the QRS complex.

How dangerous is R on T phenomenon? That depends on two things: which part of the ventricles produced the interfering QRS complex and, more importantly, how much ventricular tissue has been repolarized and is ready

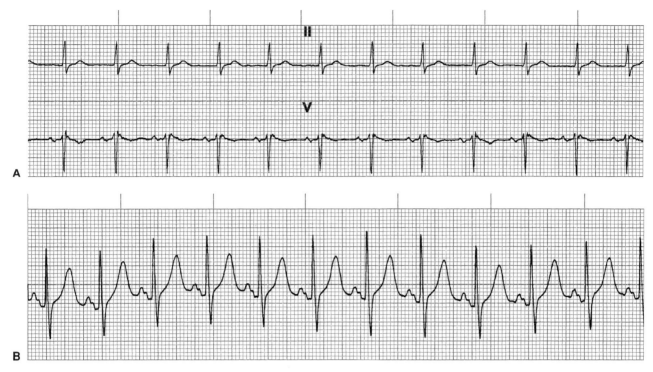

Fig. 18–2A–B Despite identical heart rates, the QT intervals vary. A, The R to R interval is 0.58 seconds, and the QT interval is only 0.26 seconds, less than half the R to R interval. B, The R to R interval is 0.58 seconds as in A, but the QT interval is 0.36 seconds, more than half the R to R interval.

to take part in the QRS. In the worst case, a chaotic rhythm such as torsade de pointes, multifocal V-tach, or V-fib can occur.

THE RELATIVITY OF READINESS

Refusing to Budge

The T-wave represents ventricular repolarization. Its distance from the QRS complex determines the length of the QT interval. If only one ventricular cell is repolarized, the chance of an R on T situation causing a problem is small, but if a sufficient number of ventricular cells are ready to discharge again, the risk is higher. Enter the *refractory period*.

When a heart cell or group of cells is completely depolarized, it's *absolutely refractory* to another signal. Regardless of how hard we try, or how intense an electrical signal reaches that cell or cell group, depolarization is impossible. A cell or cell group is *relatively refractory* if it's capable of depolarizing given a sufficiently strong signal. This situation usually occurs during repolarization, when the sodium, potassium, and calcium are returning to their starting positions.

The division between the absolute and relative refractory periods occurs near the middle of the T-wave (Fig. 18–4). Because there's no magical line visible, we approximate the division for convenience. This approximation helps us understand the R on T concept.

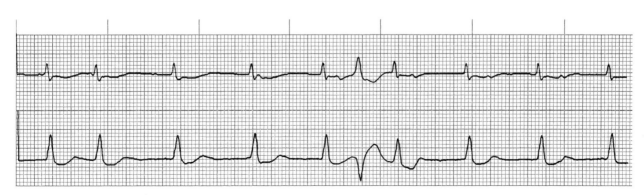

Fig. 18–3 The 6th QRS complex is premature and falls on the T-wave. The bottom tracing shows this event more clearly. In the T-wave after the 5th beat, the QRS falls on the downward portion of the T-wave, a dangerous place. Comparison with the previous T-waves shows the difference.

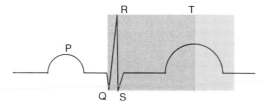

Fig. 18–4 The absolute refractory period encompasses the QRS complex and about the first half of the T-wave. The relative refractory period encompasses the remainder of the T-wave and sometimes a portion of variable length immediately after it.

Suppose a new ventricular stimulus comes during the absolute refractory period. If that happens, the ventricular tissue can't sustain the depolarization and therefore won't produce a QRS complex. We covered a similar concept in the chapter on AV blocks: if the AV node receives a signal before it's ready to transmit one, no signal gets through and the QRS can't occur. In an R on T situation, it's the ventricular tissue that isn't ready, but the patient still ends up without a QRS.

Following a Crooked Path

Figure 18–5 shows what can happen when a stimulus occurs in the ventricles during the relative refractory period, past the middle of the T-wave. A point in the ventricles begins to depolarize when only a few cells have repolarized. Those are the only cells that can respond to the signal. By the time they depolarize, the other cells have repolarized.

Now the signal can follow only the newly repolarized paths. When this new path depolarizes, the old path repolarizes, creating an unstable cyclical path through the ventricles. Because fragments of ventricular tissue contract out of sync instead of the entire ventricle's contracting at once, the patient is left with ineffective contractions. This situation can quickly deteriorate into V-tach or V-fib.

Pacemakers and the QT Interval

AN ILL-TIMED SPIKE

Artificial pacemakers can cause a variation of R on T phenomenon by failing to sense the patient's natural QRS complexes. If the pacemaker stimulates the ventricles, the spike represents the beginning of the QRS complex, the "R" of "R on T." If the pacemaker fails to sense the natural QRS, the pacemaker will not be inhibited and will continue to wait. After its programmed interval has passed, the pacemaker discharges, delivering a stimulus to the ventricles.

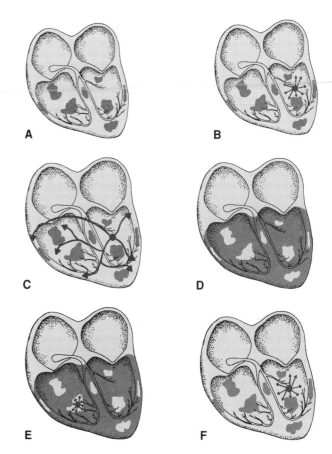

Fig. 18–5A–F A, The ventricles are partially repolarized (pink areas) until the end of the T-wave. B, A point in the ventricles begins to depolarize before repolarization is complete. C, The signal can travel only to the repolarized cells. D, By the time the repolarized cells depolarize (dark areas), other cells have repolarized (white areas). E, The signal can travel down only the repolarized paths. F, When the new path depolarizes, the old path repolarizes. The resulting path is unstable and causes ineffective contractions.

If the stimulus falls on the T-wave during the absolute refractory period, the ECG tracing will show only the pacemaker spike. No matter how intense a stimulus they receive, the ventricles can't respond and therefore can't produce a QRS. If the stimulus is delivered during the relative refractory period, it may depolarize part of the ventricles, causing a dysfunctional depolarization wave to propagate through partially prepared tissue. Finally, if the stimulus is delivered after the T-wave is complete, the risk for trouble is much lower because now the signal can depolarize the entire ventricle the way it's supposed to. However, the relative refractory period may extend for a few small boxes after the apparent end of the T-wave, so you may not be out of the woods when you think you are.

While we're on the topic of improper timing, let's find out what happens when pacemaker spikes interfere with other parts of the ECG tracing.

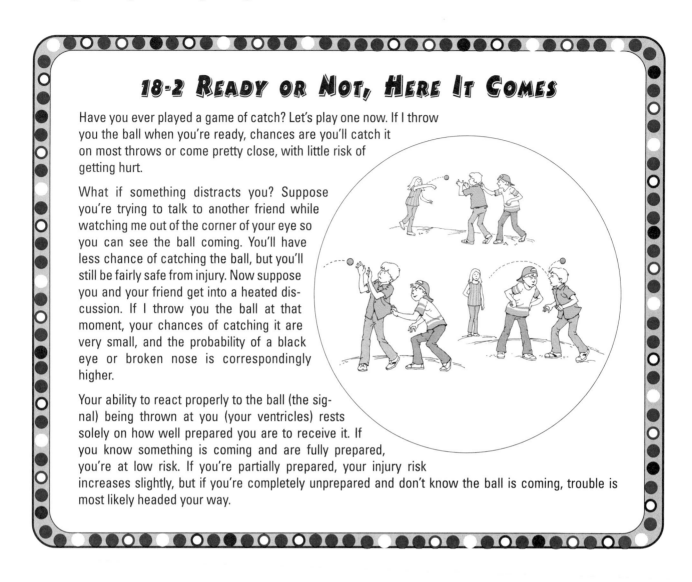

18-2 Ready or Not, Here It Comes

Have you ever played a game of catch? Let's play one now. If I throw you the ball when you're ready, chances are you'll catch it on most throws or come pretty close, with little risk of getting hurt.

What if something distracts you? Suppose you're trying to talk to another friend while watching me out of the corner of your eye so you can see the ball coming. You'll have less chance of catching the ball, but you'll still be fairly safe from injury. Now suppose you and your friend get into a heated discussion. If I throw you the ball at that moment, your chances of catching it are very small, and the probability of a black eye or broken nose is correspondingly higher.

Your ability to react properly to the ball (the signal) being thrown at you (your ventricles) rests solely on how well prepared you are to receive it. If you know something is coming and are fully prepared, you're at low risk. If you're partially prepared, your injury risk increases slightly, but if you're completely unprepared and don't know the ball is coming, trouble is most likely headed your way.

FUSION BEATS

Pacemaker leads usually aren't inserted along the normal conduction pathway. For instance, most ventricular pacemaker leads are placed at the bottom of the right ventricle. Figure 18–6 shows what happens if the pacemaker begins to fire just as a natural signal begins traveling from the AV node down the bundle branches. Remember, when the signal travels through the bundle branches, it generates no waveform on the ECG tracing. Therefore, the first deflection we can see is the pacemaker spike at the beginning of the QRS complex.

However, because some of the signal has taken the fast track down the bundle branches, it depolarizes most of the ventricular tissue. Therefore, the QRS complex will represent a *fusion* of a normal pacemaker-induced QRS and a natural one. The QRS will be a hybrid, with some characteristics of each type. Because part of the ventricular tissue is depolarized via the fast track, the QRS will be narrower than the one the pacemaker normally produces, but wider than a purely natural QRS.

Figure 18–7 shows an example of fusion beats. The first QRS complex is pacemaker generated. The second is stimulated mostly by the bundle branches and strongly resembles the natural QRS size and shape. The fifth and sixth QRSs are completely natural, stimulated only by the bundle branches. All the other QRSs represent fusion beats of one kind or another. The variation among the fusion beats is caused by the relative contributions of the bundle branch and pacemaker stimuli.

Many people are concerned that fusion beats represent a failure to sense, but the pacemaker never gets the opportunity to fail. That's because the signal from the AV node doesn't reach the ventricular sensor before the pacemaker delivers the stimulus. There simply isn't anything for the pacemaker to sense.

Fusion beats occur normally and are benign. Because the entire ventricle is ready to receive a stimulus, the pacemaker can't cause the problems that come from a signal delivery during the vulnerable period of the T-wave.

18-3 Waiting at a Red Light

You stop at a red light because, as a safe driver, you understand the importance of obeying traffic signals. You're eager to get going again, but you can be patient—up to a point. Traffic light tolerance varies with each person and each situation, but if the light takes longer than *you* think it should, you start getting irritated. Finally, convinced the light will stay red forever, you can't take it anymore. With a quick look left and right, you plunge into the intersection.

You'll probably escape with no consequences, or you may have a near miss with another car. However, you could end up in an accident, colliding in the middle of the intersection with a car that has the green light.

If the ventricles take too long to repolarize, they may begin to depolarize again before the process is complete. Like the impatient driver, one QRS complex can just miss the other or can crash into it with serious consequences, including death.

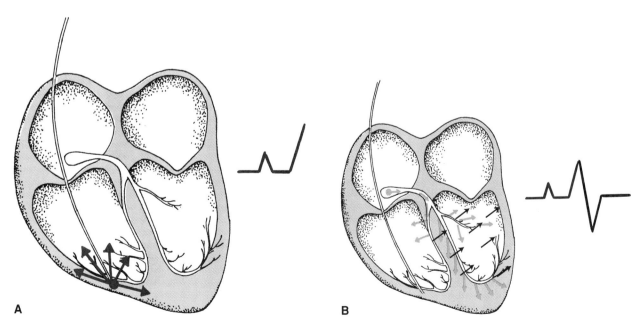

Fig. 18–6A–B Depolarization from AV node and pacemaker stimuli. A, The pacemaker depolarizes and begins to generate a QRS complex on the ECG tracing, but the bundle branches do not generate any tracing. B, The pacemaker depolarization continues to generate a QRS, but now the natural stimulus has left the bundle branches and is depolarizing ventricular tissue. The natural stimulus adds to the pacemaker QRS tracing and generates a fusion beat.

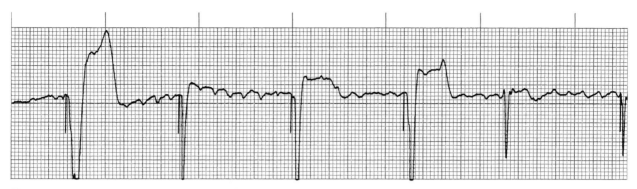

Fig. 18–7 Pacemaker rhythm with fusion beats. A QRS complex predominantly from a pacemaker stimulus resembles a typical pacemaker QRS; one generated mostly by the bundle branches resembles a natural QRS. Here the first QRS is completely pacemaker generated. Beats 2–4 are fusion beats, whereas the fifth is caused by normal AV mode – Bundle Branch conduction.

PSEUDO-FUSION BEATS

If the natural signal arrives at the pacemaker site just as the pacemaker begins to deliver its stimulus, we have a *pseudo-fusion beat.* In this scenario, the pacemaker contributes nothing to the QRS complex, but its discharge creates a pacemaker spike at the beginning of the QRS. The QRS itself looks completely normal, unlike the one produced by a fusion beat. In this case, the ventricles have depolarized completely from the natural stimulus.

Figure 18–8 shows two examples of pseudo-fusion beats; look at the second and fourth QRS complexes of Figure 18–8A. The QRS appears perfectly normal except for the pacemaker spike protruding from the beginning of it. Figure 18–8B has two pseudo-fusion beats, the first and fourth QRSs. They appear identical to the normal QRSs except for the spike immediately preceding them. Pseudo-fusion beats can occur with normal pacemaker function, as fusion beats can, and give no cause for alarm.

PSEUDO-PSEUDO-FUSION BEATS

I know—"When is this 'pseudo' thing going to end?" Well, there's one more pacemaker phenomenon that masquerades as a fusion or a pseudo-fusion beat. *Pseudo–pseudo-fusion beats* aren't routinely discussed, but they reflect a timing problem and can cause confusion about what the heart is really doing.

These pretenders can occur only in dual-chamber pacemakers. Atrial and ventricular pacemaker spikes can

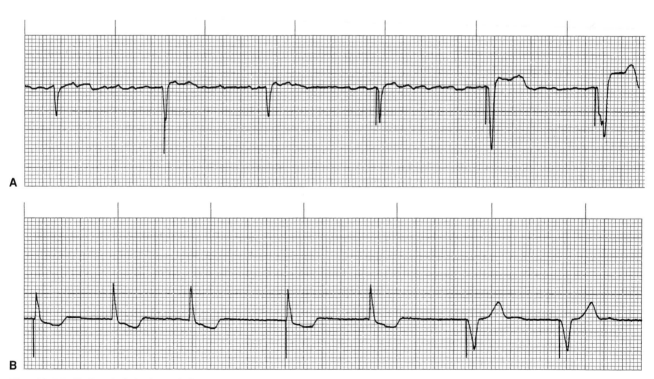

Fig. 18–8A–B Pseudo-fusion beats. A, The 3rd and 5th beats are pseudo-fusion beats. Despite the pacemaker spikes, which occur as expected, the QRSs appear identical to the patient's normal ones. B, The 1st and 4th beats are pseudo-fusion beats.

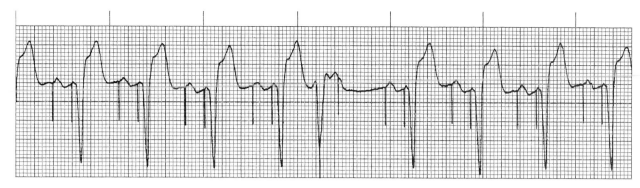

Fig. 18–9 The 5th beat in this strip, which shows a dual-chamber pacemaker, is a pseudo–pseudo-fusion beat. Notice the two pacemaker spikes, one on the bottom of the QRS and the other in the T-wave. The 1st pacemaker spike is from the atrial wire and therefore can't affect the QRS.

look identical. Therefore, if an atrial pacemaker spike occurs at the beginning of a QRS complex, we may mistake it for a ventricular spike and call it a pseudo-fusion beat (the atrial spike wouldn't actually distort the QRS because it doesn't occur in the ventricles). Figure 18–9 shows a pseudo–pseudo-fusion beat. In the fifth beat, the atrial pacemaker spike occurs at the bottom of the QRS. The other spike is the ventricular one, which falls on the T-wave.

When an atrial pacemaker spike falls on the T-wave, there's no risk for an R on T phenomenon, even if the spike occurs during the relative refractory period. Why not? The pacemaker is attempting to depolarize the atrial tissue, not the ventricular tissue. Unless the signal is in the ventricles, it can't depolarize them to any degree.

Shocking News on the QT

DEFIBRILLATION OR CARDIOVERSION?

It's important to monitor the QT interval because the longer it is, the higher the risk for an R on T situation. We've already seen that the R on T stimulus can occur naturally, as a PVC, or artificially, as a pacemaker-generated signal. There's one more way for an inappropriate stimulus to strike the T-wave—through an electrical shock given to convert a dangerous rhythm. Such a shock can be delivered in two ways, which we've touched on in earlier chapters. The difference is a matter of timing.

The shock takes one of two forms: *synchronized cardioversion* and *defibrillation* (unsynchronized cardioversion).

Either way, the signal is generally delivered through paddles or through gel pads applied to the chest wall but may be delivered from an internal device (Fig. 18–10). Paddles must be placed on a conducting gel before being used. Pads already contain the gel and adhere to the chest wall, allowing hands-free delivery of the shock. As with electrodes, the gel improves conduction and decreases the risk for electrical burns. The paddles and pads work the same way as the ECG patches do, but the stimulus goes the other way: it's delivered *to* the patient instead of being received *from* the patient.

In both methods, the idea boils down to "resetting" the heart. Figure 18–11 shows an example of what the shock looks like on the ECG strip. Notice the large deflections that go all the way to the top of the paper and then all the way down to the bottom. The defibrillator that delivers the shock will usually print out the energy level on the strip, as well as a marker indicating where the shock was

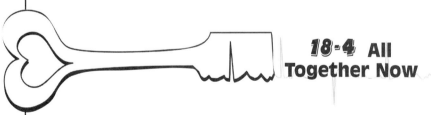

18-4 All Together Now

Remember, the fastest pacemaker wins. If an alternate pacemaker site has become irritable, it will discharge faster than the higher pacemakers—the sinus node, atria, and junctional tissue. Tachycardic rhythms can also reflect a circular path in the AV node, ventricular tissue, or other areas, and this cycle can outpace the natural pacemakers' intrinsic rates.

When the heart receives the cardioversion stimulus, all cells that are not in the absolute refractory period will depolarize in response to the intense signal. The hope is that once all the heart's cells get into sync by being depolarized at the same time, the sinus node will retake control and return the patient to a sinus rhythm.

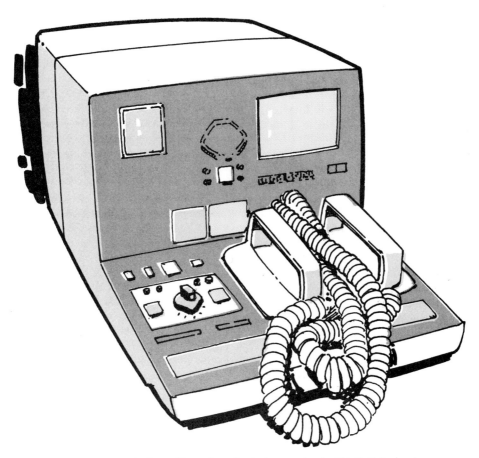

Fig. 18–10 Equipment typically used in cardioversion, both unsynchronized (defibrillation) and synchronized.

delivered. Figure 18–11 shows the shock as a small lightning bolt near the bottom of the strip.

DEFIBRILLATION: NO TIME TO LOSE

The difference between the two methods comes down to the medical credo "first, do no harm." Defibrillation, designed to deliver a shock to a fibrillating (quivering) heart, is used when the heart is unable to pump any blood—that is, when the patient is basically dead. Therefore, time is of the essence. The American Heart Association states clearly in its Advanced Cardiac Life Support algorithms that in an adult patient with V-fib or pulseless V-tach, defibrillation should not be delayed for *any* reason except chest compressions. Studies have shown up to a 90% decrease in survival rates for such patients when defibrillation was delayed by a mere 8 minutes, even when proper CPR had been performed.

Defibrillation shocks the heart with a large amount of energy over a very short period. The shock may occur in any part of the cardiac cycle (thus, the term "unsynchronized"),

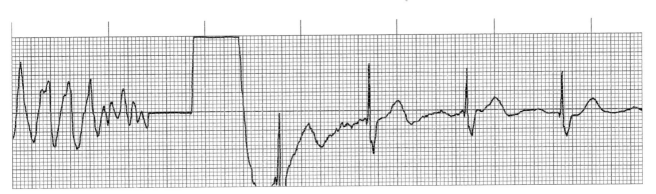

Fig. 18–11 Defibrillation artifact. The initial rhythm is V-fib, and the shock is delivered as indicated by the small lightning bolt at the bottom of the strip. The method, energy, and resistance are all listed on the bottom margin of the strip.

including the relative refractory period. But, since the heart isn't functioning and delay can mean failure, we don't care about anything except delivering the shock. The only timing concern can be summed up in one word—*now!*

CARDIOVERSION: A SYNCHRONIZED SHOCK

Cardioversion, also called *synchronized cardioversion* or *synchronized electrical cardioversion*, is a little more discriminating. In this method of shock delivery, the stimulus is timed to coincide with the R-wave to eliminate the possibility of R on T phenomenon.

To perform cardioversion, you must activate the "sync" mode on a capable defibrillator. The monitor on the defibrillator begins identifying the R-wave and tagging it with a special marker that appears on, above, or below it on the strip (Fig. 18–12). The marker can be a small square, a dot, a triangle, or any other symbol. This is the monitor's way of saying, "Here's the R-wave; I can see it clearly." When

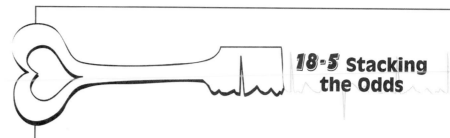

18-5 Stacking the Odds

If a pacemaker spike occurs in the QRS complex, it's much less likely to disrupt ventricular depolarization than a spike that comes during the relative refractory period. In theory, the same principle applies to electrical shocks, but it isn't foolproof. In practice, we may run into trouble because we're delivering so much energy through a poorly conducting medium (the skin) to a heart that's already behaving abnormally enough to need drastic intervention. A timed shock delivery won't necessarily prevent the patient's rhythm from deteriorating into V-fib, pulseless V-tach, or asystole; it simply reduces the chance.

you press the buttons to deliver the shock, the stimulus is delayed briefly (usually a fraction of a second) until the monitor senses an R-wave. Only then does it deliver the shock.

Cardioversion can begin with energy levels of 25 to 100 J. The energy levels increase until a more stable rhythm is restored or the maximum energy level (360 J) is reached. Medication is often used as an adjunct in cardioversion. It

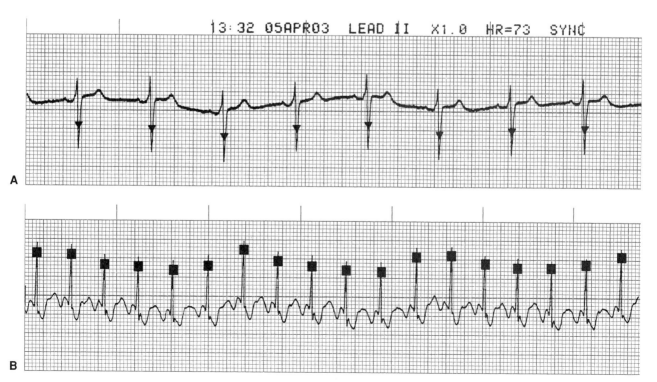

Fig. 18–12A–B Two different types of markers for identifying the QRS in synchronized cardioversion mode.

can decrease the irritability of all the competitor sites, maximizing the probability that the sinus node will regain control.

Cardioversion may be used in both stable and unstable situations, but the patient must have a rhythm and a pulse. If the patient's condition deteriorates, and the monitor is not able to recognize the R-wave for any reason, such as artifact, mechanical failure, or a sudden loss of rhythm, the machine should be taken out of synch mode and put into defibrillation mode immediately. In cardioversion, the shock may never be delivered if the monitor can't see the R-wave.

A powerful electrical shock may be the only intervention that will reset the heart. The longer it takes to deliver the shock, the less chance it has to succeed. Remember, timing is everything.

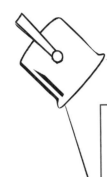

Now You Know

The QT interval consists of the QRS complex, the ST segment, and the T-wave.

The QT interval measures how long the ventricles take to depolarize and repolarize.

If the QRS complex takes too long to do its job, another QRS can occur before the ventricle is completely depolarized.

The QT interval does not have a set normal range like the PR interval or the QRS complex. Instead, it varies with the heart rate according to the formula $QTc = $ measured $QT/ \sqrt{\text{previous RR interval}}$.

In a normal QT interval, the T-wave should be completed before the midpoint between two QRS complexes.

The absolute refractory period lasts from the beginning of the QRS complex to about the middle of the T-wave. The relative refractory period lasts from about the middle to the end of the T-wave.

R on T phenomenon occurs when the R-wave comes before the ventricular tissue is completely repolarized (before the T-wave ends).

Fusion beats occur when both a pacemaker spike and a natural stimulus partly depolarize the ventricles.

A pseudo-fusion beat occurs when a pacemaker spike precedes a natural QRS complex but doesn't change it. The pacemaker spike location gives the false impression that the spike influenced the QRS.

A pseudo–pseudo-fusion beat occurs only with dual-chamber pacemakers. It looks just like a pseudo-fusion beat, but the pacemaker spike occurs in the atria, not the ventricles.

Cardioversion is the delivery of an electrical shock to convert a dangerous rhythm. The shock is timed to minimize the possibility of an R on T phenomenon.

Defibrillation is the delivery of an electrical shock that isn't coordinated with the ECG. It's usually reserved for V-fib, pulseless V-tach, equally dangerous pulseless rhythms, and situations in which synchronized cardioversion is impossible or delay would be hazardous.

Test Yourself

1. The T-wave should end before the _____ point between two consecutive QRS complexes.

2. The normal values for QT intervals vary according to _____.

3. During the _____, no stimulus, no matter how large, can initiate another QRS complex.

4. The _____ refractory period begins approximately at the _____ of the T-wave and ends at the end of the T-wave.

5. In _____, which are benign, QRS complexes are formed by two different locations initiating ventricular depolarization at the same time.

6. _____ may cause ventricular fibrillation because a new stimulus tries to depolarize the ventricles before they are fully ready.

7. Identify the pacemaker timing anomalies in the following eight strips:

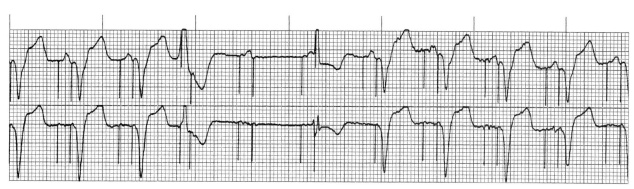

18–1

Answer: _____ .

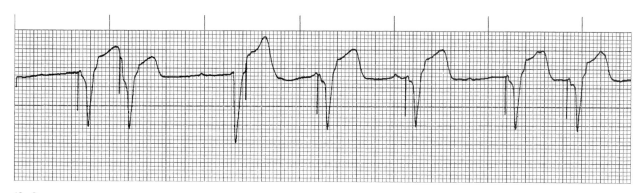

18–2

Answer: _____ .

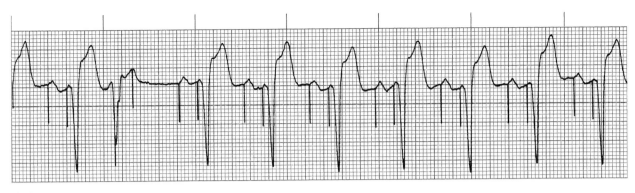

18–3

Answer: _____.

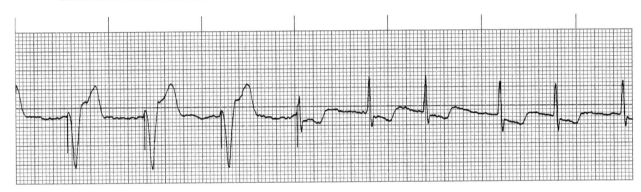

18–4

Answer: _____.

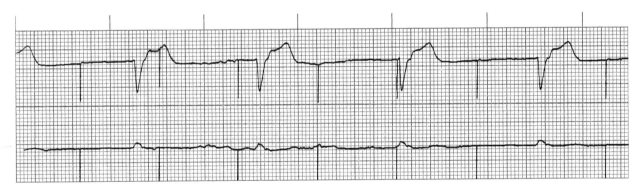

18–5

Answer: _____.

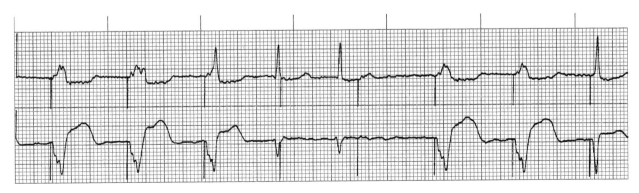

18–6

Answer: _____.

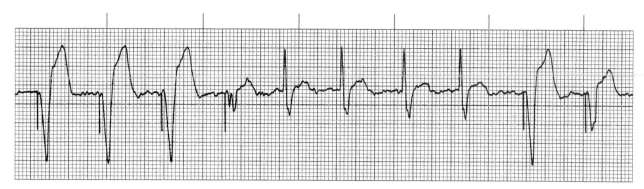

18-7

Answer: _____.

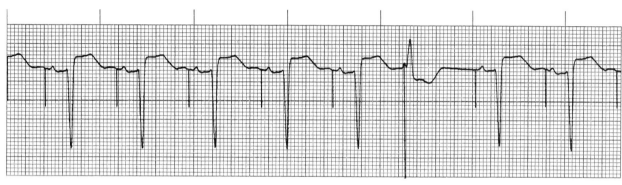

18-8

Answer: _____.

Are There Really Three I's in MI?

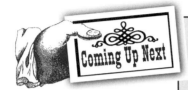

Coming Up Next

- ○ What are ischemia, injury, and infarction in relation to the coronary arteries?
- ○ What is arteriosclerosis and why is it bad?
- ○ What areas of the heart are supplied by which coronary arteries?
- ○ What can the ST segment and T-wave tell us about the heart's blood supply?
- ○ Why don't we see Q-waves more often?
- ○ What is the widow maker and how did it get its notorious name?
- ○ How long does it take for most of the damaged cells to die after a heart attack starts?
- ○ What does the saying "time is muscle" mean?

Shifting Focus

YOU'VE ACCOMPLISHED A LOT

Congratulations; you've come a long way. You can identify the more common dysrhythmias, recognize their expected signs and symptoms, and suggest basic treatment options. You have nearly all the tools for rhythm interpretation that you need, so your basic ECG training is almost complete. However, you need to learn one more feature of ECG interpretation. It has nothing to do with rhythm identification per se, but it's so important that I'm devoting this entire chapter to it.

Up until now, we've focused on the heart's electrical system to explain the dysrhythmias that can result from inadequate blood flow to different parts of the heart, among other causes. But certain other changes can alert us to poor coronary artery perfusion, and we need to understand them to round out our discussion of ECG interpretation.

The rhythm strip can help identify problems with the heart's plumbing system, as well as its electrical system. It's critically important to catch this kind of trouble because it affects the delivery of blood to cardiac tissue and this can cause any of the dysrhythmias covered in this book. This chapter will teach you to identify the clues that warn you

when parts of the heart stop receiving adequate blood flow and, more specifically, which vessels are likely involved.

MANY NAMES, ONE PROBLEM

You know it by many names: Coronary. Heart attack. Myocardial infarction and its ubiquitous abbreviation, MI. Whatever the name, a complete blockage in a coronary artery causes cardiac cell death, and you'd better believe that's serious.

Ischemia, injury, and *infarction* are three stages that cardiac tissue goes through when a complete blockage occurs in a coronary artery. The chapter title refers to these three stages and the associated changes in the ECG waveform. We'll discuss each stage in a little while, but first let's visit the arteries.

An Advanced Lesson in Plumbing

A NEW LOOK AT THE ARTERIES

Remember how the heart gets its blood supply? We introduced this topic in Chapter 1 but didn't go into great detail. Now it's time for a closer look.

Table 19-1 Which arteries supply which areas?

Coronary Artery	Areas Supplied
Left anterior descending	Right bundle branch Intraventricular septum (anterior) Ventricles, anterior walls Left ventricle, lateral wall (anterior) Left ventricle, anterior fascicle
Right coronary	Sinus node (55%*) AV node (90%) Right atrium Intraventricular septum (posterior) Left ventricle, posterior fascicle Right ventricle
Left circumflex	Sinus node (45%) AV node (10%) Left atrium Left ventricle, lateral wall (posterior) Left ventricle, inferior wall Left ventricle, posterior fascicle
*Percentage refers to occurrence in the population.	

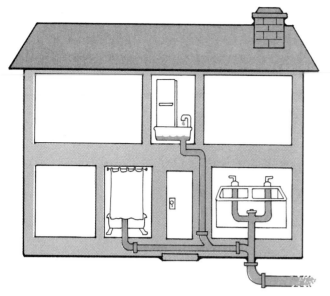

Fig. 19-1 The heart's coronary arteries are like pipes in your house; they direct life-giving fluid to the areas that need it.

The heart muscle receives its blood from the two coronary arteries that branch off from the base of the aorta. The coronary arteries supply the heart with enough blood to achieve more than 1 billion beats in an average lifetime while removing the metabolic wastes generated by these same beats. Think of the plumbing in your home: it supplies life-giving water and removes the waste we generate by living.

Each coronary artery delivers blood to specific areas of the heart. For the most part we can generalize about which arteries supply which areas, although some individual variation occurs (Table 19–1).

LEFT, RIGHT, LEFT

The left main coronary artery plays a more important role in the heart than the right coronary artery. Although both are vital to a properly functioning heart, complete blockage in the left main coronary artery is so serious that it's often called "the widow maker." This morbid name was chosen because most patients with 100% blockage of this vessel die without immediate intervention. After a couple of centimeters, the left main coronary artery branches into the left anterior descending and left circumflex arteries, which supply many areas, including most of the left ventricle.

Left Anterior Descending Artery The left anterior descending artery (LAD) feeds a large amount of the cardiac muscle mass. It delivers blood to the anterior walls of the left and right ventricles, as well as the anterolateral wall of the left ventricle and the anterior two thirds of the intraventricular septum. It also supplies the right bundle branch and the anterior left fascicle. The heart's ability to pump blood to the body can decrease dramatically if blood flow to these areas is compromised.

Right Coronary Artery The right coronary artery (RCA) supplies certain higher pacemakers: the sinus node in about 55% of people, the AV node in about 90%, and the right atrium. The RCA also feeds the posterior third of the intraventricular septum, most of the right ventricle, and the posterior left fascicle.

Left Circumflex Artery The final major branch of the coronary artery system is the left circumflex artery (LCx). It supplies the sinus node in about 45% of people, the AV node in about 10%, and the left atrium. In addition, it supplies the posterior lateral wall and part of the inferior wall of the left ventricle. It also supplies the posterior left fascicle (this fascicle is supplied by two different coronary arteries and is therefore least likely to become blocked).

The Three I's

ISCHEMIA: HOLDING BACK THE BLOOD

What's Blocking the Way?

The word *ischemia* comes from Greek and literally means "to restrain the blood." Clinically, ischemia is a lack of

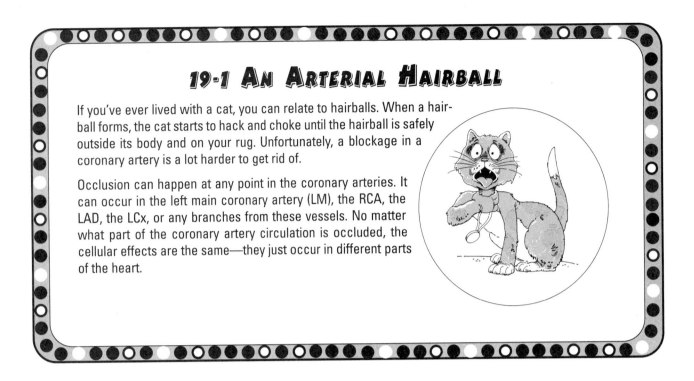

19-1 An Arterial Hairball

If you've ever lived with a cat, you can relate to hairballs. When a hairball forms, the cat starts to hack and choke until the hairball is safely outside its body and on your rug. Unfortunately, a blockage in a coronary artery is a lot harder to get rid of.

Occlusion can happen at any point in the coronary arteries. It can occur in the left main coronary artery (LM), the RCA, the LAD, the LCx, or any branches from these vessels. No matter what part of the coronary artery circulation is occluded, the cellular effects are the same—they just occur in different parts of the heart.

sufficient blood flow to tissue—any tissue. In the heart, this lack of blood flow can come from many causes, including low blood pressure, significant bleeding anywhere in the body, or a blockage, or *occlusion,* of one of the coronary arteries.

Coronary artery blockages come from two related disorders: arteriosclerosis and atherosclerosis. *Arteriosclerosis,* also known as "hardening of the arteries," decreases the ability of the blood vessels to respond to changes in the heart's need for blood.

Atherosclerosis, a form of arteriosclerosis, comes from the Greek terms *athērē,* meaning "sludge" or "gruel," and *sklērōsis,* meaning "hardness." Atherosclerosis comes from a buildup of plaques, or lesions. Plaques narrow the blood vessel, making it more difficult for blood to pass through. These lesions can result from deposition of cholesterol on the inside of the vessels. Our knowledge of what triggers cholesterol deposition is constantly expanding but includes high levels of LDL ("bad") cholesterol, low levels of HDL ("good") cholesterol, diabetes, cigarette smoking, and, more recently, inflammation. (The cholesterol abbreviations stand for "low-density lipoprotein" and "high-density lipoprotein.")

So what's the difference between arteriosclerosis and its offshoot, atherosclerosis? Arteriosclerosis is a more general term. In this condition, plaques may be present or absent. If they're absent, the hardening of the arteries may be caused by high blood pressure. In atherosclerosis, plaques are always present.

Angina Pectoris

Arteriosclerosis limits blood flow to the areas supplied by diseased coronary arteries. The decrease in blood flow can be partial or complete. If the decreased flow is both partial and temporary, the result is a type of ischemia called *angina pectoris,* or simply *angina.*

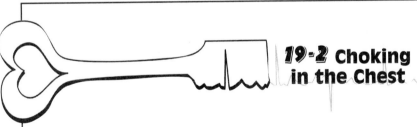

19-2 Choking in the Chest

The term *angina* comes from a Greek word meaning "to choke." Although there are many types of angina, the word nearly always refers to angina pectoris—the "choking" is occurring in the pectoral area, or chest.

Angina falls into two general categories: stable and unstable. In stable angina, chest pain is triggered predictably by an increase in the heart's demand for oxygen, as with exercise or emotional stress, and goes away with rest or elimination of the trigger.

Unstable angina (often abbreviated USA) is known for its unpredictability. Even without a trigger, the capacity of the coronary arteries is compromised suddenly and without warning. Unstable angina can occur at any time, even during sleep, when the heart's oxygen demands are normally at their lowest.

INJURY: SOMETHING ISN'T RIGHT

Everyone knows the word *injury*. But, as with all ubiquitous words, its original meaning has become skewed. It may surprise you to learn that the word comes from the Latin *injurius,* meaning "not right." Although vague, this sense of the word describes what happens in the heart during a myocardial infarction. If ischemia continues long enough, chemical derangement worsens to the point where cellular damage and dysfunction begins. Cell membranes become unstable, and metabolic processes begin to go haywire. However, prompt treatment can restore the damaged area to normal, just as it can repair a twisted ankle or broken bone.

Inadequate blood flow has some serious consequences. It decreases the delivery of glucose and oxygen and the removal of metabolic byproducts such as water and carbon dioxide. Oxygen, glucose, and the correct pH are all needed to control the flow of calcium, sodium, potassium, and magnesium ions across the cell membrane. The loss of oxygen and glucose causes metabolic changes, and the buildup of waste products alters chemical reactions because of changes in acidity. Many changes occur, but the end result is that the cells become dysfunctional. Their ability to depolarize is affected severely, but the first evident change is in the repolarization. We'll talk more about this later.

INFARCTION: JUST STUFF IT IN

No Oxygen, No Energy

Infarction comes from a Latin word meaning "to stuff." The material blocking the artery is stuffed, or crammed, into the vessel lumen and is unable to move forward or allow blood to pass around it. When an infarction occurs, no blood is flowing to the area of the heart served by the diseased vessel.

In a complete occlusion, no blood is getting past the blockage, so the parts of the heart fed by that vessel are starved of oxygen and glucose. The hypoxic cells start to

become dysfunctional. Remember, it takes energy to move the electrical signal through the heart and a lot of energy to return a cell to its resting state.

Time Is Muscle

Although prevention is an important goal in cardiac disease, it's impossible to eliminate heart attacks, especially since we're still learning how heart disease occurs. As long as people go on having heart attacks, early recognition will remain vital.

The longer the blockage persists, the more heart muscle is damaged. The patient has the best chance when the blockage is recognized within the first 6 hours. That's why early recognition is so important. After more than 6 hours, a large percentage of the hypoxic muscle will have died. At that point, the risks of treatment with angioplasty or thrombolytics may outweigh the potential amount of tissue salvaged, so treatment becomes more conservative. By 12 hours, tissue death is nearly complete.

That's "Conical," Not "Comical"

In two dimensions, as on the surface of the heart, the damage appears to be triangular (Fig. 19–2). Although we're most accustomed to seeing the heart in two dimensions—most of the artwork in this book is drawn that way—the heart is really a three-dimensional object. If you're looking at a drawing of the ventricles, for instance, you need to remember that the ventricular walls have depth as well as width. The blood supply from the coronary arteries is also three dimensional: the arteries branch out along the surface in a triangle, but they also penetrate into the thick ventricular walls. Therefore, in myocardial infarctions, the damaged area radiates outward in a cone shape, with the point of blockage at the tip of the cone (Fig. 19–2).

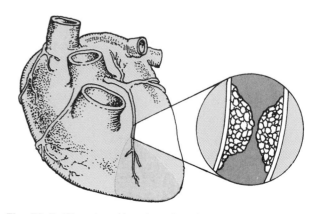

Fig. 19–2 When viewed from the surface of the heart, the damage from a blocked coronary artery appears triangular.

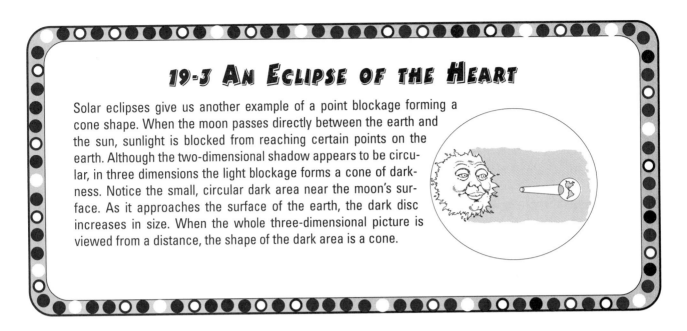

19-3 AN ECLIPSE OF THE HEART

Solar eclipses give us another example of a point blockage forming a cone shape. When the moon passes directly between the earth and the sun, sunlight is blocked from reaching certain points on the earth. Although the two-dimensional shadow appears to be circular, in three dimensions the light blockage forms a cone of darkness. Notice the small, circular dark area near the moon's surface. As it approaches the surface of the earth, the dark disc increases in size. When the whole three-dimensional picture is viewed from a distance, the shape of the dark area is a cone.

The Sensitive T-Wave

THE LAST TWO PIECES

In previous chapters you learned about various waves, complexes, and intervals. You practiced locating and measuring the most clinically significant features, and you learned the criteria for distinguishing normal waveforms from abnormal ones. Each part of the total ECG waveform has given us a different piece of information about the heart and its electrical system. The P-wave shows atrial activity, the PR interval tells us about AV node functionality, and the QRS complex reports on ventricular depolarization. Even the QT interval plays a role, showing us how quickly the ventricles get ready for the next QRS. However, to evaluate the heart's plumbing system completely, we need to discuss two more pieces of the ECG waveform: the ST segment and the T-wave.

As I mentioned earlier, lack of oxygen can affect depolarization, but the first change occurs during repolarization and alters the T-wave. The T-wave can change in response to either decreased blood flow or a complete blockage of a coronary artery. T-waves can become either inverted or hyperacute (we'll meet both these terms in

a little while). Initially at least, the QRS complexes will remain normal because depolarization hasn't been affected yet.

Normal T-waves should be less than one third the height of the associated QRS complex, and, as we know from Chapter 15, they should also be in the same direction as the end portion of the QRS. Any T-wave changes should be taken in the context of patient symptoms. Although electrolyte imbalances can also alter the shape,

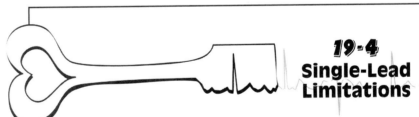

19-4 Single-Lead Limitations

Heart attacks can happen anywhere in the heart: the front, the back, the side, you name it. Trouble is, each lead views only one aspect of the heart, so single-lead monitoring is limited both in scope and accuracy. Lead II, for example, monitors the inferior portion of the heart. If a patient were having an MI in the side of the heart, we'd miss it completely. Remember, each lead is like a camera: it images only the part of the heart that the positive electrode points toward.

Therefore, to monitor more areas of the heart for damage, not just dysrhythmias, we need more leads. It's time to reintroduce the 12-lead ECG. In the following sections you'll see that we need this many leads to ensure that heart attacks are diagnosed accurately. We'll return to this topic in a little while.

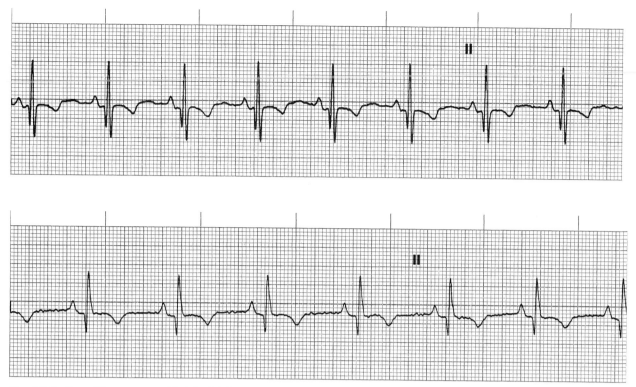

Fig. 19–3 Normal T-waves are upright in leads I, II, III, V$_3$–V$_6$, aVL, and aVF. Inverted T-waves with a QRS complex of normal width, as shown here, frequently indicate ischemia.

size, and direction of the T-wave, a patient with cardiac symptoms such as chest pain and hypotension is probably showing the effects of altered coronary artery blood flow.

WHEN IT TURNS UPSIDE DOWN

The term *inverted* refers to T-waves that are negatively deflected, as in Figure 19–3. Normally the T-wave is upright in leads I, II, III, V$_3$ through V$_6$, aVF, and aVL. Remember, T-waves may be inverted even if ischemia is not present; this form shows up in ventricular rhythms, bundle branch blocks, and ventricular paced beats. In these situations it's difficult, if not impossible, to diagnose coronary artery blockages. T-waves are also normally inverted in lead aVR, which is not used in determining MI location or in any rhythm interpretation.

Inverted T-waves usually indicate that ischemia is occurring. Inversion may be an early warning of an MI, but more commonly, it simply indicates that a particular area of the heart isn't getting the oxygen it needs to work at the level that's being demanded. Inversion can reflect any condition that causes ischemia: significant blood loss, stable angina with increased activity, unstable angina at rest, low blood pressure, respiratory distress—the list goes on and on.

HYPERACUTE DOESN'T MEAN "REALLY CUTE"

A *hyperacute*, or *peaked*, T-wave is narrower than usual, pointed, symmetrical, and, most important, much taller than normal. In fact, it can rival the QRS complex in size (Fig. 19–4). These alarming T-waves are associated with acute blockage of a coronary artery. Hyperacute T-waves can have other causes, such as electrolyte disturbances.

Hyperacute T-waves usually warn us that myocardial cell injury is beginning. After they appear, ST segment elevation usually begins.

STRANGE ST STATES

Normally the ST segment should stay at the baseline. In other words, the TP, PR, and ST segments should all be on the same level as in Figure 19–5. If the ST segment is not at baseline, we have a phenomenon called *ST segment deviation*.

If the ST segment is deviated above the baseline, it's *elevated;* if deviated below the baseline, it's *depressed*. Both elevation and depression can indicate occlusion of a coronary artery. Although the ST segment can change for many reasons including use of medications such as

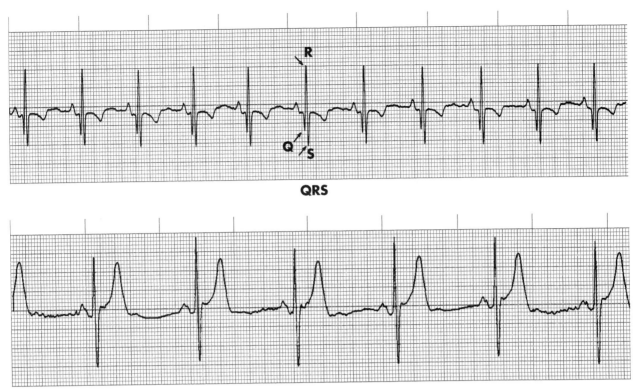

Fig. 19–4 Normal T-waves are rounded and much smaller than the QRS complex. T-waves that are narrow, tall, and peaked may indicate dysfunctional myocardial cells and possibly an impending MI. An MI was diagnosed 20 minutes after this strip was run.

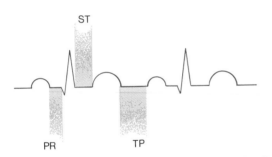

Fig. 19–5 The TP, PR, and ST segments all should be on the baseline because they represent no measurable cardiac electrical activity. If electrical activity occurs during one of these segments, something is wrong.

digoxin, acute changes are usually related to coronary artery occlusion and need further assessment, such as a 12-lead ECG and laboratory tests, to rule out an MI.

Now let's discuss what causes these changes in the ST segment and T-wave.

The Rise and Fall of the ST Segment

SUBTLE BUT SIGNIFICANT

Changes in the ST segment and the T-wave can be subtle, especially in the initial stages of an MI or in a "small heart attack," in which the blockage occurs in a small, distal branch of a coronary artery.

During ischemia, the ST segment may initially become depressed, as in Figure 19–6A–B. The T-wave may be inverted, as in Figure 19–6A, or may be normal, as in Figure 19–6B. In an MI, however, the initial changes occur in the T-wave, which may become hyperacute or, less commonly, inverted. Changes in the ST segment usually follow these changes in the T-wave.

The ST segment reveals injury within minutes to hours of a blockage, becoming elevated as in Figure 19–7. Elevation of the ST segment can occur for other reasons, including some acute conditions. One of these is *pericarditis,* an inflammation of the sac around the heart.

THE ECG COMES FIRST

Although we've covered rhythm interpretation from the perspective of just one or two monitoring leads, we need the 12-lead ECG to identify an MI. However, a single- or dual-lead ECG strip frequently offers clues that something is "not right," which should prompt the practitioner to obtain a 12-lead ECG. But even that isn't infallible.

We have a wealth of tests available for detecting myocardial infarction. Some are invasive—lab tests and coronary angiography, for example. Noninvasive methods include echocardiography and stress tests. But the initial test, the one that usually precedes all the others, is the

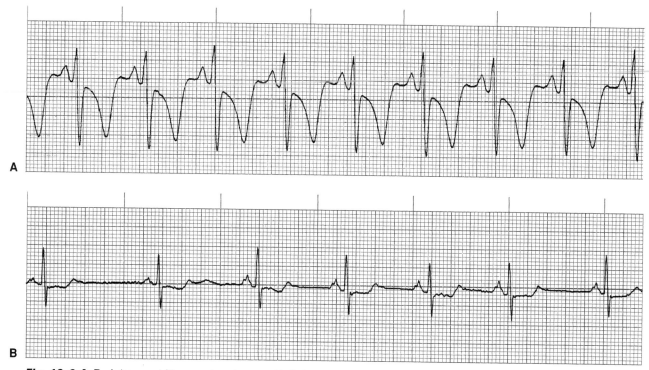

Fig. 19–6 A–B A depressed ST segment can be caused by ischemia or by some common cardiac drugs. If new, it should be investigated.

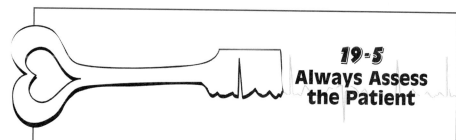

19-5
Always Assess the Patient

All of this ECG mumbo-jumbo is great. We can diagnose many diseases and disorders, even some noncardiac problems, with the help of the 12-lead ECG. However, notice the word "help." The ECG is far from perfect, and that's why it's important to assess the patient. A "normal" ECG can mask an acute MI, just as a patient with significant ST segment elevation can prove to have nothing wrong. Does the patient have chest pain, shortness of breath, nausea, or an impending sense of doom? If none of these findings are present, we need to think hard before diagnosing an MI from ECG changes alone. Remember to treat the patient, not the monitor!

12-lead ECG. Although it's a good first-line intervention, because it can be performed in minutes with immediate results, it identifies only 40% to 60% of acute MIs. Therefore, you should be able to recognize the ECG changes that suggest any kind of heart damage.

Sometimes changes that look significant on the patient's monitor strip disappear in the same lead during a 12-lead ECG. Because the 12-lead ECG is a brief snapshot of the heart's electrical activity, not a long movie, we can process the signals in greater detail to get more precise information. However, when monitoring one or two leads continuously, we use different filtering algorithms to speed the processing. These different filtering effects can sometimes distort single- or dual-lead tracings. That's why we refer to these tracings as "rhythm strips": because the strips are used to interpret rhythms, not to diagnose conditions.

The rhythm strip and the 12-lead ECG differ in one other important way—detail. We don't need the exact size of the P-wave or the precise deviation of the ST segment to interpret the patient's rhythm. We can expedite signal processing and show 5, 10, 20, or more patients on one nursing station monitor by filtering out signals that aren't relevant to rhythm interpretation. The range of frequencies accepted by the ECG monitor for rhythm strips is 0.5 to 30 MHz, which gives a generally clear picture of the P-wave, QRS complex, and T-wave. This picture is known as a "monitor-quality" ECG tracing.

19-6 A SMILE OR A FROWN?

Not all ST segment elevations are created equal. Some deviate up and then remain level before returning to baseline. Others turn down, not returning to baseline, and back up again; we call these *concave elevations*. They usually indicate early repolarization and are considered benign, so we don't worry about them. Another type of elevation turns up and then backs down. These *convex elevations* are the ones we do worry about because this shape usually indicates an MI. You can remember the difference by thinking of the concave elevation as a smile and the convex elevation as a frown.

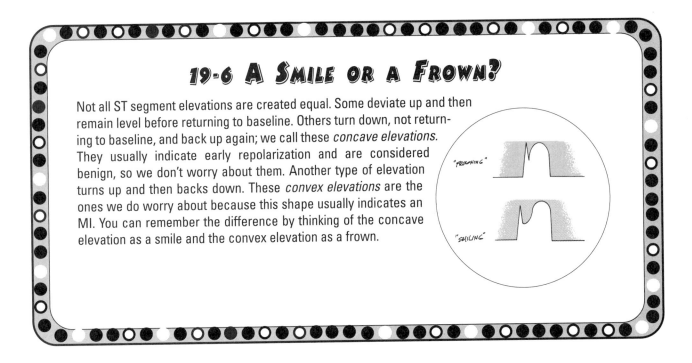

A QUICK LOOK AT Q-WAVES

The 12-lead, on the other hand, accepts frequencies from 0.05 to 150 MHz. Almost all possible signals are accepted and interpreted. Much more intensive signal processing is needed to convert the larger frequency range into a tracing in only 10 seconds. In the case of a 12-lead ECG, we get 12 different tracings in those 10 seconds. Therefore, sometimes these changes may appear on a monitor strip, but will not appear on the 12-lead and vice versa.

If blood flow is not rapidly restored after the ST segment elevates, myocardial tissue begins to die. This tissue death can sometimes be seen on the ECG and frequently remains visible for the rest of the patient's life, in the form of a Q-wave.

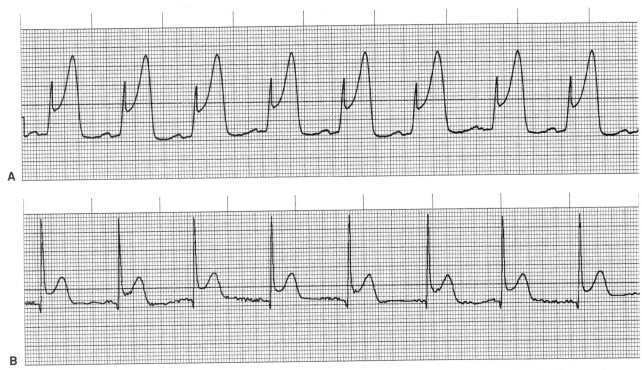

A

B

Fig. 19–7 A–B An elevated ST segment elevation may indicate myocardial injury. If the T-wave begins above the baseline, the ST segment is considered elevated even if the actual segment is not seen.

19-7 CAMERA ANGLES

Imagine that you're getting your picture taken. Do you have some feature you aren't happy with—a bald spot on the back of your head or a scar on your cheek, maybe? If you don't want that in the picture, all you have to do is turn your head to conceal the offending part. However, if I take 12 pictures, all from different angles, the chances increase dramatically that I will capture that feature on film.

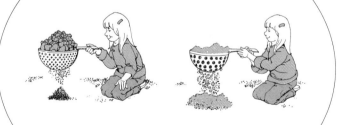

The ability to see any ECG change, whether it's caused by ischemia, injury, or infarction, depends on which leads you monitor. The positive ECG patch is the key to determining what part of the heart you're looking at. Now think of the positive patch as a camera.

If you aim that camera toward the negative patch in any lead and snap a picture, you'll see only a portion of the heart's muscle and related electrical conduction system. If the damage isn't happening in view of that camera, you won't be able to see it.

19-8 PLAYING IN THE SAND

Remember playing with a strainer as a child? You may have used one at the beach to sift away the sand and find shells. If the holes in the strainer were very small, then only the grains of sand would get through and the rest of the contents would be trapped in the strainer.

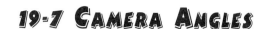

Now make the holes bigger. What happens? Not only sand, but larger material, such as shell fragments or maybe even small pebbles, can get through. Because so much more gets through the strainer, your pile of sand and debris increases much more quickly.

The same thing happens with a 12-lead: the greater frequency range allows more signals to get through the larger "strainer holes" of the monitor, giving us more signals to interpret.

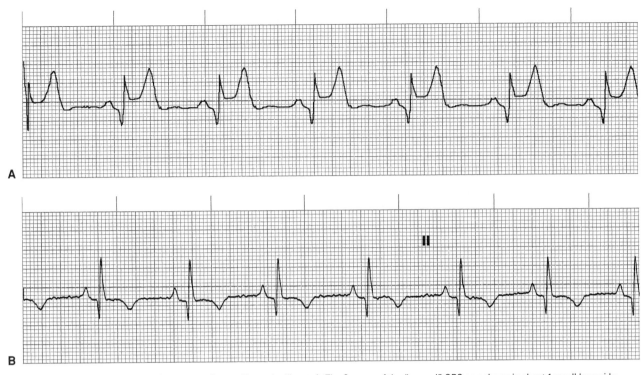

Fig. 19-8 A-B The Q-waves in these two strips qualify as significant. A, The Q-wave of the "normal" QRS complexes is about 1 small box wide. B, The Q-wave is wide and is nearly one third the height of the entire QRS.

We've seen Q-waves before in many of the tracings we've studied, but if you look back, you'll notice that most of them are small and barely worth mentioning. For a Q-wave to indicate myocardial tissue *necrosis* (from a Greek word meaning "death"), it must have certain characteristics.

First, its size must be "significant." To be considered significantly large, a Q-wave must be wider than one small box (0.04 seconds), more than one third (some experts say 25%) the height of the total QRS complex, or both (Fig. 19-8A-B). Larger, or more significant, Q-waves usually indicate larger areas of necrotic tissue. The Q-wave can indicate that the patient had an MI but not when. It may

have happened a day or two ago or more than decade ago. Once the tissue dies, it can't tell us anything other than that it's dead.

Second, Q-waves should not appear in any lead except aVR, which isn't involved in our MI determination, and V_1. Occasionally a nonsignificant Q-wave turns up in lead III. It's common for lead V_1 to show a large QS complex, but V_2, which also looks at the intraventricular septum, should not have a Q-wave. We'll learn more about leads V_1 and V_2 in a later section.

Other issues can confound the significance of the Q-wave (Fig. 19-9). It isn't as reliable in bundle branch blocks,

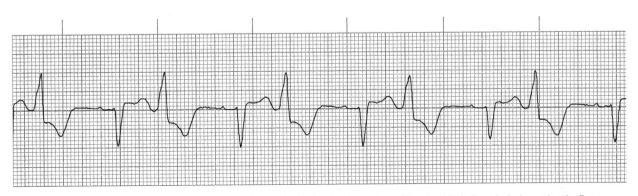

Fig. 19-9 At first glance, there appears to be a large Q-wave, indicating that the patient suffered an MI. A closer look shows that the first deflection is a small r-wave, making the large negative deflection an S-wave.

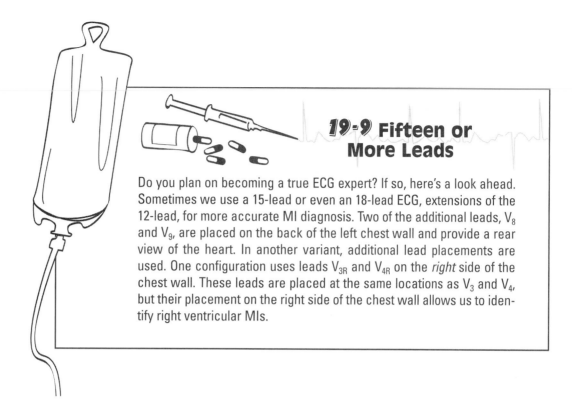

19-9 Fifteen or More Leads

Do you plan on becoming a true ECG expert? If so, here's a look ahead. Sometimes we use a 15-lead or even an 18-lead ECG, extensions of the 12-lead, for more accurate MI diagnosis. Two of the additional leads, V_8 and V_9, are placed on the back of the left chest wall and provide a rear view of the heart. In another variant, additional lead placements are used. One configuration uses leads V_{3R} and V_{4R} on the *right* side of the chest wall. These leads are placed at the same locations as V_3 and V_4, but their placement on the right side of the chest wall allows us to identify right ventricular MIs.

pacemaker rhythms, or ventricular rhythms. In these rhythms, the depolarization of the ventricles is altered and Q-waves are not as specific as they would be in other circumstances.

WHERE ARE THE Q-WAVES

ECGs that generate ST-segment elevation and Q-waves are known as STEMI (ST-segment Elevation Myocardial Infarction), or Q-wave MIs. But, not all myocardial infarctions produce significant Q-waves. Some do not even generate the typical ST segment elevation. When the ECG misses the heart attack, we can turn to the laboratory to diagnose myocardial damage with "cardiac markers". Cardiac markers, such as troponin-I, or CPK-MB will never miss an acute MI because these chemicals are released whenever any cardiac tissue dies. The 12-lead, or the 15 (or more)-lead, ECG only focuses on specific areas of the heart. If the area of damaged myocardium is small and not being watched by one of the leads, then we will not see the damage occurring. If there is ST-segment elevation, there will usually be a Q-wave. Therefore, heart attacks that do not produce ST-segment elevation are known as NSTEMIs (Non ST-segment Elevation Myocardial Infarctions) or non Q-wave MIs.

These types of heart attacks, recognized by laboratory values and not ECG changes, can occur more than 50% of the time. Therefore, if a patient presents with signs and symptoms of an acute myocardial infarction, he may be having an MI even with a normal 12-lead ECG! Treat the patient, not the monitor!

RECIPROCAL CHANGES

When a myocardial infarction occurs in one location, the ST segment becomes elevated in the leads facing the necrotic tissue. However, in the leads that view the damaged tissue from a different angle, the ECG changes are reversed. The elevated ST segment becomes depressed and the Q-waves, if they're present, shift above the baseline to become tall R-waves. These "opposite view" changes are collectively called *reciprocal changes*.

We can take advantage of reciprocal changes to identify a posterior wall MI by using leads V_1 and V_2, which view the opposite area—the anterior intraventricular septum. Because the heart is tilted and slightly rotated in the chest, this area lies directly in front of the posterior wall of the left ventricle. The 12-lead ECG doesn't monitor leads that view the heart from the back, so we rely on V_1 and V_2 to show the reciprocal changes that indicate an MI in progress. Because V_1 and V_2 normally show small R-waves or none at all, the presence of tall R-waves may reflect reciprocal changes caused by a posterior wall MI. Also, since the T-waves in these leads are usually upright, ST-segment elevation, the opposite of ST-elevation, and deep T-wave inversion, the opposite of hyperacute T-waves, can also indicate a posterior wall MI.

Are There *Really* Three I's in MI?

Reciprocal changes not only indicate posterior wall MIs but also help confirm that an MI has caused the ST segment elevation in other leads. Although reciprocal changes don't appear in all MIs, their presence underscores the presumptive MI diagnosis.

Table 19–2 sums up what we've learned about ST segment elevation. Table 19–3 brings together all the MI diagnostic information we've covered in this chapter. Remember, though, that rhythm strips may suggest ST segment changes, but only a 12-lead can confirm those changes.

WHERE DO WE SEE IT?

The evidence for myocardial infarction on the 12-lead ECG presents itself in the leads that look at the area. Not all the leads need to show the changes, but at least two leads looking at the same part of the heart (referred to as contiguous leads) must show changes. If only one lead does you can not diagnose an MI. It may be an anomaly or a lead placement error.

Treating Myocardial Infarctions

THREE BASIC APPROACHES

Acute myocardial infarction treatment is too complex for us to discuss in depth. However, it's important to get a basic, general understanding of the techniques involved. As you know, acute MI treatment is a race against time. Because arterial blockage starves the heart tissue, more cells are dying every minute. There are three basic ways to return blood flow to the starving tissue: thrombolytics, angioplasty, and surgery.

CLOT BUSTERS

Thrombolytics are chemicals that dissolve blood clots. (The Greek prefix *thrombo-* refers to blood clots; *-lytic* comes from a word meaning "dissolution.") Thrombolytics can reopen some blocked coronary arteries, particularly if the blockage is a blood clot. However, some blockages have

Table 19–2 Characteristics of ST segment elevation

Diagnosis	Key Features	Clinical Significance
Pericarditis	Usually present in many leads. No reciprocal changes noted.	Can occur after MI or with infection. May be life threatening.
Early repolarization	Concave elevations ("smiles") usually ≤2 mm. No reciprocal changes noted.	Benign; often found in healthy males aged 13–29 years.
Myocardial infarction	Convex elevations ("frowns") in two or more contiguous leads. Reciprocal changes present.	Life-threatening condition

Table 19–3 Diagnostic criteria for myocardial infarction

Location of Infarction	Primary Changes (ECG Lead)	Reciprocal Changes (ECG Lead)	Artery Involved	Associated Complications	Comments
Anterior	V_1–V_4	II, III, aVF	LAD	3° AVB with ventricular escape rhythm Bradycardia New BBBs	Poor prognosis
Lateral	I, aVL, V_5, V_6		LCx	Ventricular aneurysm	Fair prognosis
Inferior	II, III, aVF	V_2–V_4	RCA	3° AVB with junctional escape rhythm	Fair prognosis
Septal	V_1, V_2	V_8, V_9	LAD	Ventricular septal defect	Good prognosis
Posterior	V_8, V_9 (none on 12-lead ECG)	V_1, V_2	LCx or LAD	Lesser AV blocks	Good prognosis

19-10 A Backed-Up Sink

If you have a sink that won't drain, you're dealing with a blockage that needs to be removed. You can use any of three methods to drain your sink: dissolve the blockage chemically, remove it mechanically, or go around it. All three methods work, but each one presents different problems.

Chemical dissolution may not remove the whole blockage or may not address its cause (a roughened, damaged pipe lining). In either case, a new blockage is more likely to form than if the pipe were in perfect condition. If the blockage is caused by something the chemical can't dissolve, it will remain in place. Mechanical removal can damage the pipe lining, inviting future blockages, or may actually break the pipe and cause it to leak. Bypassing the blockage is costly and traumatic to the pipes, and the alteration in flow can increase the likelihood of a new blockage.

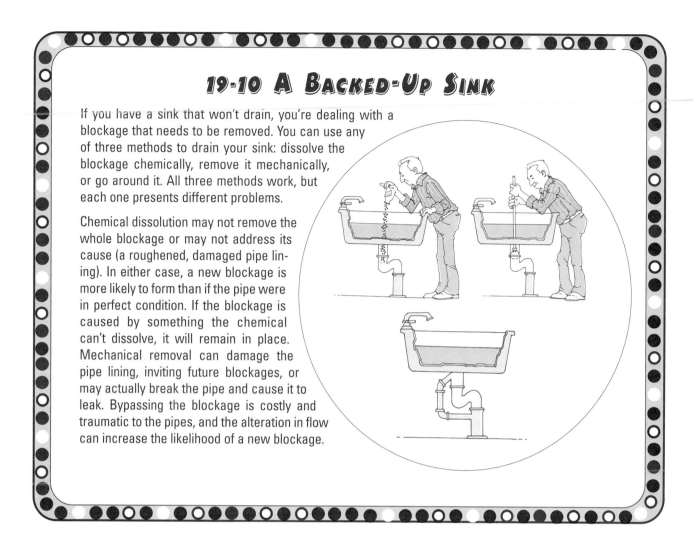

other causes, and thrombolytics won't touch them. In addition, thrombolytics can cause significant, even life-threatening, bleeding from other areas of the body, such as the brain and abdomen, and so should be used with caution.

ANGIOPLASTY

Here's a mouthful: *percutaneous* (through the skin) *transluminal* (through a space, the blood vessel) *coronary* (heart) *angioplasty* (shaping of a blood vessel). Thankfully, we fall back on the abbreviation PTCA. In this procedure, a catheter is fed into the diseased coronary artery from either a brachial or femoral artery and then into the narrowed portion of the vessel. Once the catheter reaches the blockage, a balloon is inflated under high pressure (measured in multiples of atmospheric pressure), squeezing the blockage against the vessel wall. The balloon is then deflated and removed, allowing blood to flow to the starving cells. Angioplasty, like thrombolytics, puts the patient at risk for bleeding. If

used incautiously, this method can rupture the coronary artery. Also, the plaque that originally blocked the artery may also travel further into it, causing an occlusion in a more distal portion of the same artery or one of its branches. If this kind of blockage occurs, the patient may need emergency open-heart surgery.

Frequently a device called a *stent* is used during a PTCA. The stent acts as a scaffolding to keep the vessel from reoccluding (Fig. 19–10). Drug-eluting stents can contain additional medications that inhibit clot formation, but patients are usually kept on additional medications for months after stent placement to keep clots from forming on the raw edges of the newly deformed plaque.

CABBAGE, ANYONE?

Coronary artery bypass graft (CABG) is frequently called "cabbage" because of the abbreviation. In this surgical procedure, a natural blood vessel such as a leg vein or small

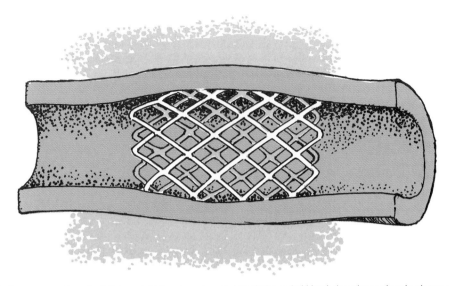

Fig. 19–10 A coronary artery stent. This metal tube-shaped scaffolding helps to hold back the atherosclerotic plaque after angioplasty.

chest artery or an artificial blood vessel such as a graft is used to deliver blood around the blockage. This surgery is serious and involves great risks, which include death during surgery, graft failure, arterial reocclusion, and wound infection. Still, it's the best treatment if the patient has multiple blockages or if the other two methods have failed.

THE SOONER THE BETTER

The key to successful MI treatment, of course, is recognition. Early identification means early treatment, minimized tissue death, and the maximum amount of retained cardiac function. Because many factors affect the outcome, the patient may need longer-term treatment to support cardiac function or to prevent recurrence.

We have just skimmed the surface of coronary artery disease and its relationship to ECG interpretation. But look how much you've learned. Now you can spot ECG changes that indicate blocked coronary arteries, identify the area of the heart and the possible blood vessels affected, and know which dysrhythmias to watch for. Congratulations again—you've made a great start.

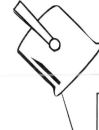

Now You Know

Ischemia means "to restrain the blood" and occurs when the coronary arteries can't meet the heart's need for oxygen.

Injury occurs when the lack of oxygen begins to affect the functioning of cardiac cells.

Infarction occurs when the cells are starved of oxygen for too long and begin to die.

Arteriosclerosis—hardening of the arteries—can be caused by either high blood pressure or atherosclerosis. Either type increases the risk for a heart attack.

The left anterior descending artery supplies the anterior walls of the left and right ventricles.

The left circumflex artery supplies the lateral wall of the left ventricle and the sinus node in about 50% of the population.

The right coronary artery supplies the sinus node in the other 50% of the population and the AV node in 90%.

The left main coronary artery supplies most of the left ventricle. It's called "the widow maker" because untreated blockage of this artery is fatal.

A depressed ST segment indicates coronary artery ischemia; an elevated ST segment indicates injury to cardiac cells.

The faster a heart attack is diagnosed and treated, the more muscle is saved.

Cardiac cells begin to die within minutes of a heart attack, but it takes more than 12 hours for most of them to die. Many cells can be saved in the first 6 hours.

The 12-lead ECG is important in MI diagnosis because it images different parts of the heart at the same time, allowing a more detailed picture.

Test Yourself

1. ST segment _____ can be a sign of ischemia in a cardiac patient.

2. ST segment _____ can be a sign of cardiac cell injury.

3. Early repolarization is a benign cause of _____.

4. The AV node receives its blood supply from the _____, in most patients.

5. Blockage of the left anterior descending artery is associated with which type of myocardial infarction? _____.

6. If a patient is having an acute inferior wall MI, which additional ECG lead should you check? Why? _____.

7. Identify the features associated with MIs in the following four strips:

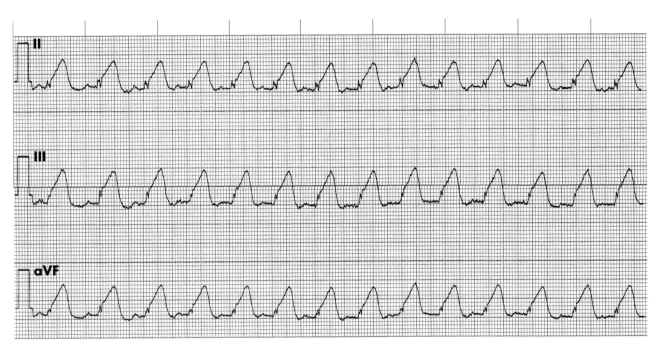

19–1

Diagnosis: _____

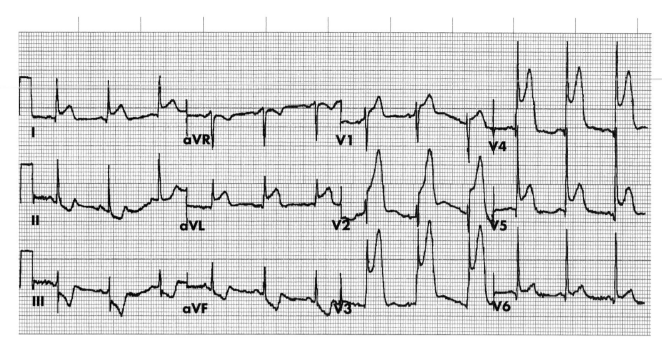

19–2

Diagnosis: _____

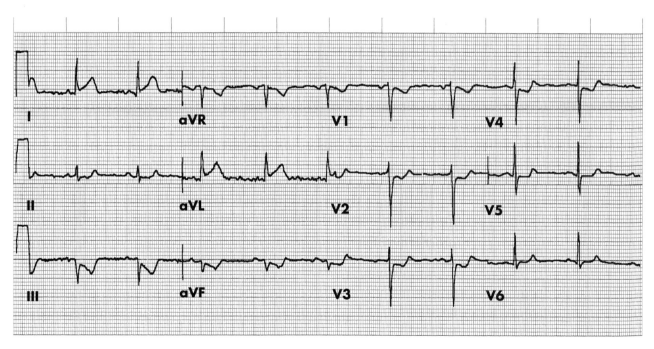

19–3

Diagnosis: _____

Are There *Really* Three I's in MI?

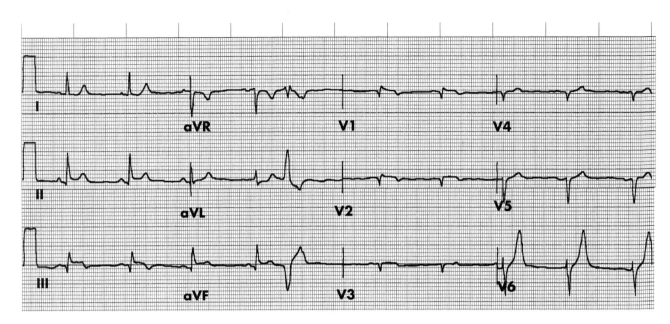

19–4

Diagnosis: _____

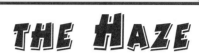

CUTTING THROUGH

THE HAZE

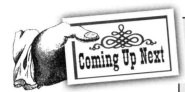

❍ What rhythms cause the most confusion?

❍ What are the key differences to help us keep them straight?

❍ What techniques can we use to differentiate ventricular tachycardia from toothbrush tachycardia?

❍ What rhythm is Wenckebach block commonly confused with? What are the consequences of this confusion?

❍ What else do we need to consider when interpreting an ECG strip?

Sorting Things Out

Now you can interpret common ECG dysrhythmias as well as identify patients likely suffering a life-threatening heart attack. If you think you've learned a lot, you're right, but some areas are probably still a little fuzzy. If you find yourself peering into the haze, you're most likely confused by a rhythm that can be easily mistaken for another. Let's take this final opportunity to review the most important areas of potential confusion.

Irregular Rhythms with P-Waves

Here's a trio of rhythms that cause a great deal of confusion. We've met them all: sinus arrhythmia, sinus rhythm with premature atrial contractions, and wandering atrial pacemaker. Each of these rhythms is irregular, each has a P-wave before every QRS complex, each has a different cause, and all are usually benign. Careful review of the strip can help you to pick out their differences and correctly name the strip.

SINUS ARRHYTHMIA

Sinus arrhythmia is usually related to respiration—significant changes in the heart rate depend on whether the patient is breathing in or breathing out. The key feature to distinguishing this rhythm is that all the P-waves are identical, as in Figure 20–1. The sinus node is in complete control of the rhythm, but the rate varies. This rhythm usually is a non-issue and is treated only if slowing of the heart rate causes symptoms of low cardiac output. These rare cases may require a pacemaker or a cardiac medication adjustment.

SINUS RHYTHM WITH PREMATURE ATRIAL CONTRACTIONS

In sinus rhythm with premature atrial contractions, the rhythm is regular except for the PACs. However, frequent

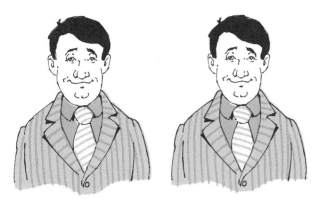

WANDERING ATRIAL PACEMAKER

In a wandering atrial pacemaker, control of the rhythm moves back and forth among the sinus node, the atria, and occasionally even the junctional tissue. This constant shift causes some irregularity because one single point isn't generating all the P-waves. The key difference distinguishing WAP from the two preceding rhythms is the presence of at least three different, and frequently more, P-waves in a 6-second strip (Fig. 20–3). This feature tells us that the rhythm has originated in at least three different points over a brief period—in other words, that it has wandered. Also, this rhythm can be more regular than either sinus arrhythmia or sinus rhythm with PACs because many atrial foci are willing to take control. If one focus isn't ready, there's always another in the wings waiting for a chance to "strut its stuff."

PACs can make it appear irregular. The key feature of this dysrhythmia is the different shape of the P-wave preceding some beats; this different waveform indicates that part of the rhythm didn't originate in the sinus node (Fig. 20–2). Also, the rate doesn't usually vary in a predictable up-and-down pattern as it does in sinus arrhythmia. The premature beats are usually caused by increased irritability, or automaticity, of the atrial tissue. Causes of PACs can include stimulants such as caffeine or cocaine, anxiety, and many other factors, which we discussed in Chapter 11. But PACs don't vary with respirations.

Table 20–1 sums up the information we've just covered.

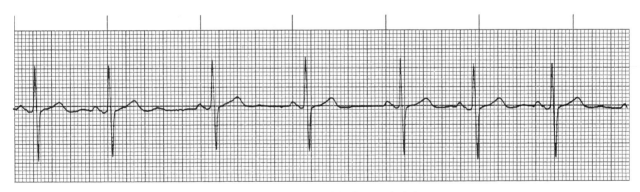

Fig. 20–1 Sinus arrhythmia. All the P-waves look the same.

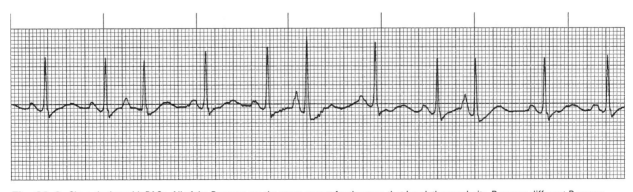

Fig. 20–2 Sinus rhythm with PACs. All of the P-waves are the same except for the ones that break the regularity. Because different P-waves mean different starting points and not all of the P-waves originate in the same place, the rhythm can't be purely sinus.

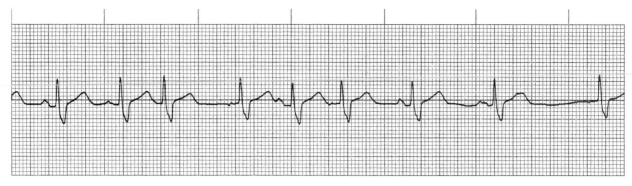

Fig. 20–3 Wandering atrial pacemaker. Several P-waves in a row started in a different location (they have different shapes) even if they were not premature.

Artifact or Ventricular Tachycardia?

Toothbrush tachycardia can put on a convincing show of ventricular tachycardia. Here's a statistic that may surprise you: as much as 10% of the treated episodes of V-tach are really artifact related and not truly V-tach. If a patient with artifact is treated for V-tach, the result can be fatal! Because misidentification can lead to a catastrophe, I'll re-emphasize some key points to help you differentiate these two rhythms.

ANY UNUSUAL FEATURES?

In any V-tach, even torsade de pointes, the QRS complexes usually have straight lines and sharp points associated with them (Fig. 20–4A). Artifact, however, may show points too frequently (Fig. 20–4B) or may show a few points disrupting an otherwise smooth tracing (Fig. 20–4C). The points may represent the artifact, as in Figure 20–4B, or the true QRSs, as in Figure 20–4C. The apparent QRSs (Fig. 20–4B) are caused by somatic artifact, but in toothbrush tachycardia (Fig. 20–4C) they're caused by external stimulation to the patches of the lead involved.

DOES IT START SLOWLY?

Rhythms with artifact can give themselves away by starting slowly. Look at the strip in Figure 20–5. Notice the oddly shaped waveforms between the patient's normal beats in the beginning of the strip—don't they look like QRS complexes? These odd QRSs increase in frequency until they dominate the rhythm. This occurrence, common in toothbrush tachycardia, can be caused by tremors in the patient's body. The tremors start out slowly and build up in a crescendo. When they slow down again, the process reverses—the odd QRSs may occur less frequently and the normal QRSs are increasingly visible.

A DIFFERENT POINT OF VIEW

Because toothbrush tachycardia can occur from repetitive contact with one ECG patch, a lead with a different positive patch may show the patient's QRS complexes more clearly (Fig. 20–6). When patients are monitored in multiple leads, all the leads frequently share the same positive patch. For example, in leads II, III, and aVF, the positive patch is the LL lead. If the patient's tremor affects the LL patch and therefore those three leads, the artifact may obscure the patient's normal QRSs, and

Table 20–1 Irregular rhythms with P-waves

Rhythm	Regularity	P-Waves	Comments
Sinus arrhythmia	Regularly irregular	All the same shape	Related to breathing
Sinus rhythm with PACs	"Regular except"	Different P-waves in premature beats	Increased atrial irritability
Wandering atrial pacemaker	Slightly or grossly irregular	At least three different P-waves in 6-second strip	Can be caused by increased atrial stretch

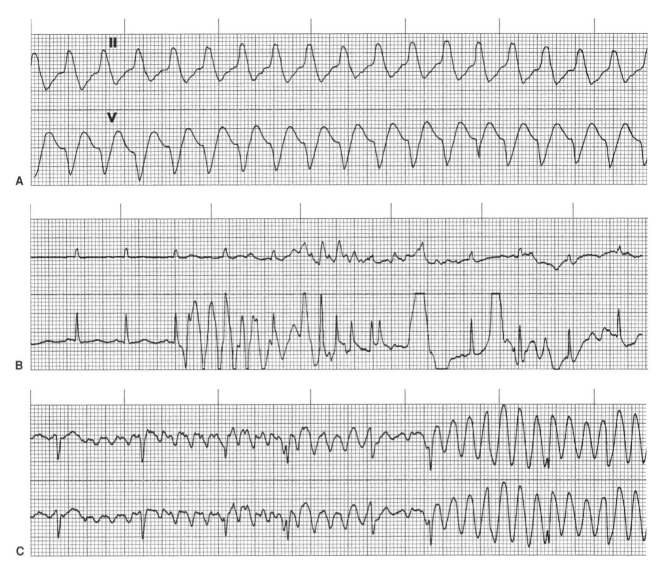

Fig. 20–4A–C Three ECG strips from the same patient. A, Genuine V-tach. B, Somatic artifact from the patient turning over in bed. C, Toothbrush tachycardia from left arm tremor.

rhythm interpretation will suffer. You can get a clearer tracing if you monitor the patient in lead I, which uses the LA lead as the positive patch. Then, although you may not get rid of the artifact, it won't be as large, and you may be able to uncover the mimic.

Absent P-Waves

Junctional rhythm and atrial fibrillation differ significantly, but each can masquerade as the other. We've learned that junctional tissue, in some unusual circumstances,

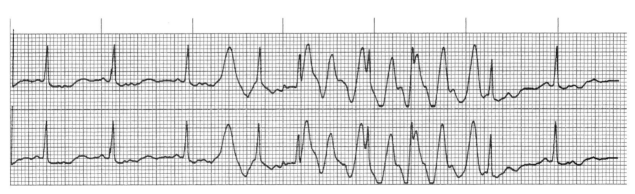

Fig. 20–5 Artifact, marked by a slow onset. Extended time of onset or termination, or both, are key clues that the rhythm is not V-tach.

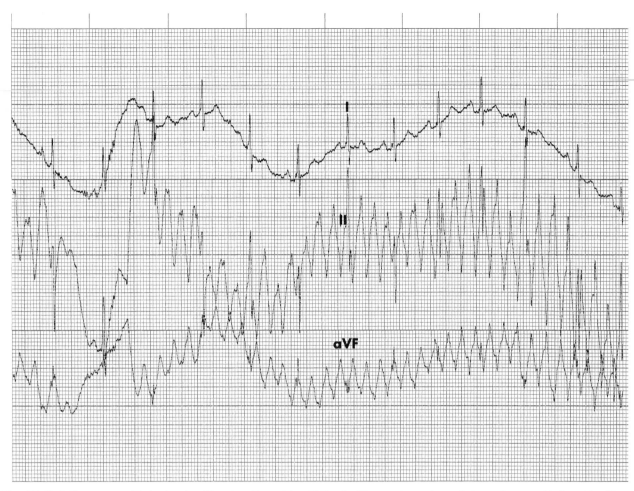

Fig. 20–6 Artifact generated by leads using different positive patches. Notice the difference in prominence between the top and bottom strips. The top tracing is lead I, which uses the LA patch as the positive; the bottom tracing, lead II, uses the LL patch. This tracing was generated while the author tapped rapidly on the LL patch. Despite the mild baseline sway artifact, the top strip clearly shows sinus rhythm, but the bottom tracing is impossible to interpret because of the artifact.

wrestles control from other potential pacemakers. When it does act as the pacemaker, it's generally regular because it's reliable (Fig. 20–7A). Now and then, a junctional rhythm can show slight irregularity. By contrast, in atrial fibrillation, the AV node has to transport atrial signals that vary in frequency and intensity, so the rhythm is grossly irregular (Fig. 20–7B).

Atrial fibrillation may have a fine, indistinct baseline in one lead, but the characteristic wavy baseline may be seen more clearly in an alternate lead. If artifact interferes with a junctional rhythm, the baseline can appear wavy and throw off the interpretation, so regularity is key.

As in any rhythm where artifact is getting in the way, you can try to eliminate the artifact by relocating patches in the affected lead, monitoring another lead, or administering ordered sedation if the artifact is caused by patient motion.

Blocking AV Block Errors

WENCKEBACH OR SINUS RHYTHM?

Wenckebach phenomenon can be confused with several other types of block. Sometimes the confusion is benign, as when Wenckebach is mistaken for sinus rhythm with blocked PACs. Sometimes, however, confusion can bring serious consequences—for example, when third-degree AV block is mistaken for Wenckebach.

REGULARITY IS KEY

The key to keeping our blocks straight is regularity. It's important to remember that AV blocks, particularly Wenckebach and third-degree block, generally have regular P-waves. The conduction problem is not in the sinus node but in the AV node. Therefore, the P-waves in Wenckebach (Fig. 20–8A) should march out. In sinus rhythm with blocked PACs (Fig. 20–8B), the rhythm

20-1 FAKE FIGHTING

You've all seen movies in which one person beats up another. As you know, the fight scenes are staged and often involve no contact between fists and faces. The secret lies in the camera angle. In the ECG tracing, the positive patch in a lead acts just like a camera; it allows you to see things from only one specific angle.

If you sneaked a peek at a fight scene from a different camera angle, you'd see punches whisking past the actor's nose as he feigns the impact of being hit. In ECG land, viewing a different camera angle (using a lead with a different positive patch) can sometimes reveal the deception.

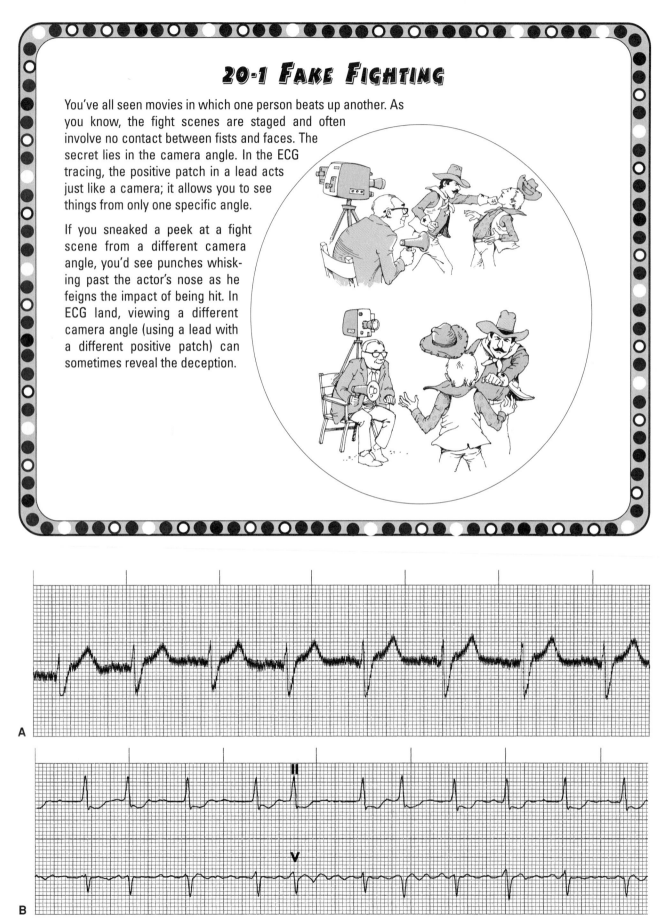

A

II

V

B

Fig. 20–7A–B A, Junctional rhythm with artifact obscuring the baseline is regular. B, True A-fib is irregularly irregular.

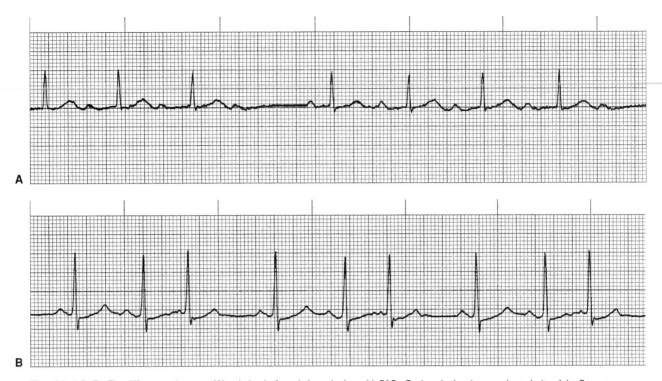

Fig. 20–8A–B The differences between Wenckebach, A, and sinus rhythm with PACs, B, show in the shape and regularity of the P-waves.

description tells us that the P-waves don't march out; they can't because the PACs are premature by definition.

Here's another clue: because all the P-waves in Wenckebach originate in the sinus node, they should all have the same shape—another difference from sinus rhythms with PACs. So, even though both rhythms occasionally show

P-waves without QRS complexes, you can differentiate them with close inspection and a few measurements.

WENCKEBACK OR THIRD-DEGREE?

If you're trying to differentiate third-degree AV block (Fig. 20–9) from Wenckebach, the P-waves won't help because

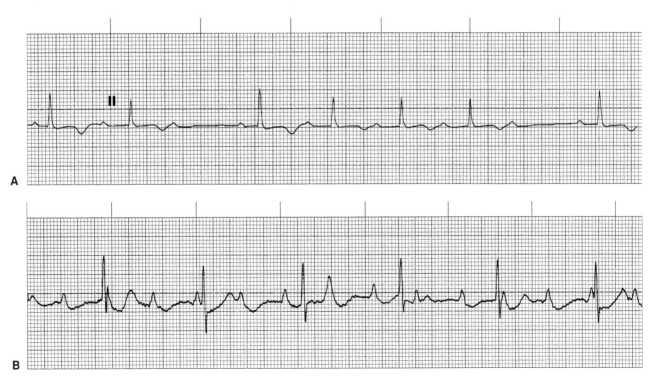

Fig. 20–9A–B The key difference between sinus rhythm with Wenckebach, A, and sinus rhythm with 3° AV block, B, shows in the QRS regularity.

Table 20–2 Is it Wenckebach or not?

Rhythm	Are P-waves regular?	P-Wave shapes	Are QRSs regular?
Wenckebach	Yes	All the same	No
Sinus rhythm with blocked PACs	No	Some different	No
3° AV Block	Yes	All the same	Yes

they march out and are all the same shape for both rhythms. Instead we look at the QRS complexes. In Wenckebach (Fig. 20–9A), the QRSs are irregular because the AV node sends some, but not all, of the atrial signals to the ventricles. Transport time varies for the signals that do get through, causing the PR intervals to be inconsistent. In third-degree AV block (Fig. 20–9B), the AV node doesn't conduct any signals at all. The PR interval changes in this rhythm because the atria and the ventricles are depolarizing independently. When this happens, a lower pacemaker, either the junctional or the ventricular tissue, steps in to control ventricular depolarization. Both lower pacemakers are known for their regularity, reflected in the QRS regularity. Therefore, even though the P-waves don't help us, the regular QRSs tell us what we need to know.

Table 20–2 summarizes our discussion of blocks.

Ventricular Fibrillation or Asystole?

It's easy to confuse ventricular fibrillation with asystole. The difference between these two rhythms is a matter of degree, and recognizing it is less a science than an art.

Both rhythms are lethal if untreated, but the treatments vary. In treating asystole you must discover and remove the cause; remember MATCH (× 5) ED from Chapter 13?

Electrical shocks are contraindicated because, if the heart is not generating any electrical signals, stunning it more will only suppress the return of natural pacemaker sites. In treating V-fib, you'd use electrical defibrillation without delay, possibly followed by antidysrrhythmic medications.

Asystole is defined as the absence of electrical activity, and therefore the ECG tracing should be essentially flat in all leads (Fig. 20–10). Fine V-fib may appear flat in some leads, but other leads clearly show a fine fibrillation baseline (Fig. 20–11). That's one reason why we have to verify asystole in more than one lead. Patient assessment may help us differentiate asystole from loose lead artifact, but we can't use it to distinguish asystole from V-fib—in both cases we're dealing with a patient who has no pulse and is essentially dead.

Antidisestablishmentarianism

We've seen combination rhythms before. That's what we get when one rhythm converts into another—for example, sinus rhythm converting into an ectopic atrial pacemaker rhythm. But, as you've learned, rhythm naming can get a lot more complex than that. You need to scour the entire rhythm strip for any and all elements before you can complete the naming process. Sometimes the name can be longer than the strip itself!

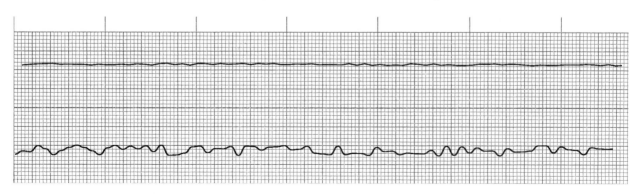

Fig. 20–10 Both leads on this strip show fine V-fib. The true rhythm shows in the top tracing; if you viewed only the bottom tracing, you might misidentify this rhythm as asystole.

20-2 TWO KINDS OF BLINDNESS

In V-fib and asystole, although neither rhythm shows coordinated activity, the treatments are vastly different. Think in terms of light and darkness. If you're in a totally dark room, you're effectively blinded. The same thing happens if a glaring light shines in your eyes. In one case you don't have enough light to see by; in the other you have an overwhelming excess. You can see in a dark room if light is added, but if the room is too bright already, adding more light only makes you see less. Decreased light will help you see in the bright room, but in the dark room it only deepens your blindness.

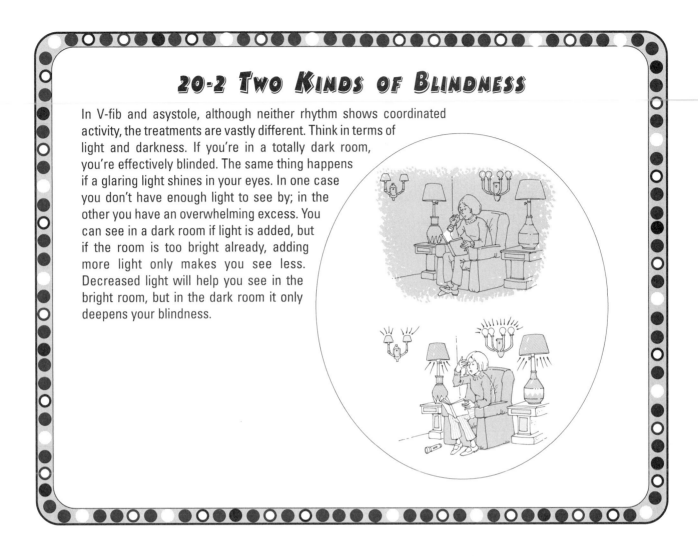

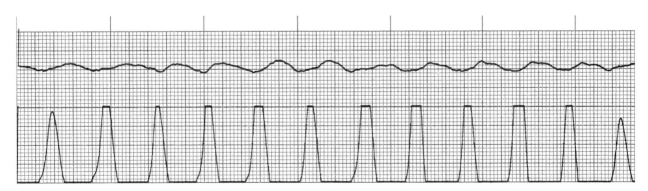

Fig. 20–11 This strip shows true asystole in two different leads, with chest compression artifact.

Figure 20–12 shows a complex rhythm strip. Here we have sinus rhythm with third-degree AV block and junctional escape rhythm bigeminal, unifocal PVCs. Whew, what a mouthful! But all the pieces are important. The sinus rhythm tells us that the sinus node is the fastest supraventricular pacemaker, which is good news. The third-degree AV block tells us that the AV node is not functioning adequately. The junctional escape rhythm tells us that the junctional node is responding to the AV node block by picking up the slack—more good news. The bigeminal PVCs show increased ventricular irritability, and that's bad news.

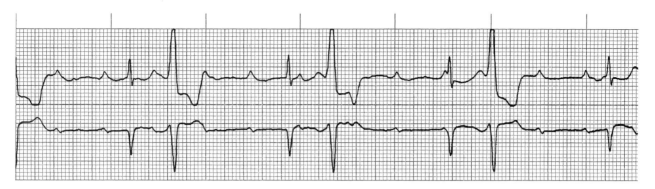

Fig. 20–12 Sinus rhythm with 3° AV block and junctional escape rhythm with bigeminal, unifocal PVCs. It is important to identify all parts of a rhythm.

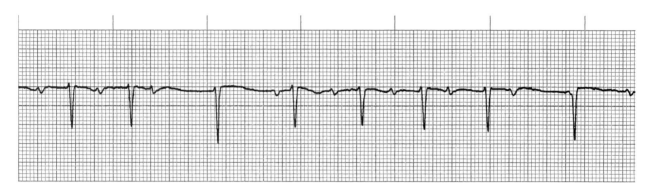

Fig. 20–13 The complete interpretation of this strip is sinus rhythm with 2° AV block type I (Wenckebach) with junctional escape beats. Notice that the 3rd QRS is later than it should be, and is not preceded by a P-wave.

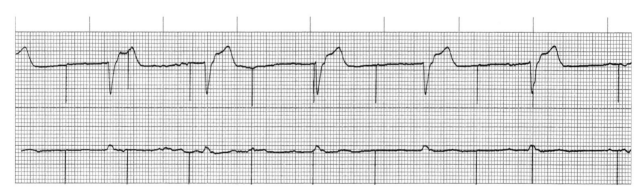

Fig. 20–14 The complete interpretation of this strip is accelerated idioventricular rhythm with pacer spikes (presumably ventricular) with failure to capture and failure to sense.

Incomplete rhythm naming won't necessarily cause problems. However, when you call a physician to report a rhythm change, it's important to provide as much information as possible. Figures 20–13 and 20–14 give additional examples of complex rhythms for you to practice with.

You'll find other potential areas of confusion in basic ECG interpretation, but we've covered the ones I run into most often when I teach. You now have an ECG interpretation library inside your head, and I hope this chapter has cleared some cobwebs from the shelves.

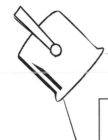

Now You Know

The following rhythms are easily confused:

Sinus arrhythmia, sinus rhythm with PACs, and wandering atrial pacemaker

Ventricular fibrillation and asystole

Toothbrush tachycardia and V-tach

Wenckebach phenomenon, sinus rhythm with blocked PACs, and third-degree AV block

If you find P-waves without QRS complexes, as in AV block, you should analyze P-wave and QRS regularity carefully.

If you can monitor multiple leads simultaneously, you should monitor leads with different positive patches to minimize the effect of artifact.

Incorrect rhythm interpretations include

Wandering atrial pacemaker mistaken for a benign sinus arrhythmia

V-fib mistaken for asystole, resulting in the wrong treatment

Third-AV block, a life-threatening dysrhythmia, mistaken for Wenckebach.

You must analyze all the complexes in a strip to make sure you've identified all the elements of the rhythm.

APPENDIX 1

Heart Rate Tables

Heart Rate Table I

Small boxes	Large boxes	Heart rate	Small boxes	Large boxes	Heart rate
1		1500	31		48
2		750	32		47
3		500	33		45
4		375	34		34
5	1	300	35	7	43
6		250	36		42
7		214	37		41
8		188	38		39
9		167	39		38
10	2	150	40	8	38
11		136	41		37
12		125	42		36
13		115	43		35
14		107	44		34
15	3	100	45	9	33
16		94	46		33
17		88	47		32
18		83	48		31
19		79	49		31
20	4	75	50	10	30
21		71	51		29
22		68	52		29
23		65	53		28
24		63	54		28
25	5	60	55	11	27
26		58	56		27
27		56	57		26
28		54	58		26
29		52	59		25
30	6	50	60	12	25

Heart Rate Table I

Small boxes	Large boxes	Heart rate	Small boxes	Large boxes	Heart rate
1		1500	31		48
2		750	32		47
3		500	33		45
4		375	34		34
5	1	300	35	7	43
6		250	36		42
7		214	37		41
8		188	38		39
9		167	39		38
10	2	150	40	8	38
11		136	41		37
12		125	42		36
13		115	43		35
14		107	44		34
15	3	100	45	9	33
16		94	46		33
17		88	47		32
18		83	48		31
19		79	49		31
20	4	75	50	10	30
21		71	51		29
22		68	52		29
23		65	53		28
24		63	54		28
25	5	60	55	11	27
26		58	56		27
27		56	57		26
28		54	58		26
29		52	59		25
30	6	50	60	12	25

APPENDIX 1

Heart Rate Tables

Heart Rate Table II

Heart rate	Large boxes	Small boxes	Heart rate	Large boxes	Small boxes
1500		31	48		1
750		32	47		2
500		33	45		3
375		34	44		4
300	1	35	43	7	5
250		36	42		6
214		37	41		7
188		38	39		8
167		39	38		9
150	2	40	38	8	10
136		41	37		11
125		42	36		12
115		43	35		13
107		44	34		14
100	3	45	33	9	15
94		46	33		16
88		47	32		17
83		48	31		18
79		49	31		19
75	4	50	30	10	20
71		51	29		21
68		52	29		22
65		53	28		23
63		54	28		24
60	5	55	27	11	25
58		56	27		26
56		57	26		27
54		58	26		28
52		59	25		29
50	6	60	25	12	30

Heart Rate Table II

Heart rate	Large boxes	Small boxes	Heart rate	Large boxes	Small boxes
1500		31	48		1
750		32	47		2
500		33	45		3
375		34	44		4
300	1	35	43	7	5
250		36	42		6
214		37	41		7
188		38	39		8
167		39	38		9
150	2	40	38	8	10
136		41	37		11
125		42	36		12
115		43	35		13
107		44	34		14
100	3	45	33	9	15
94		46	33		16
88		47	32		17
83		48	31		18
79		49	31		19
75	4	50	30	10	20
71		51	29		21
68		52	29		22
65		53	28		23
63		54	28		24
60	5	55	27	11	25
58		56	27		26
56		57	26		27
54		58	26		28
52		59	25		29
50	6	60	25	12	30

Post-Test Questions

#1

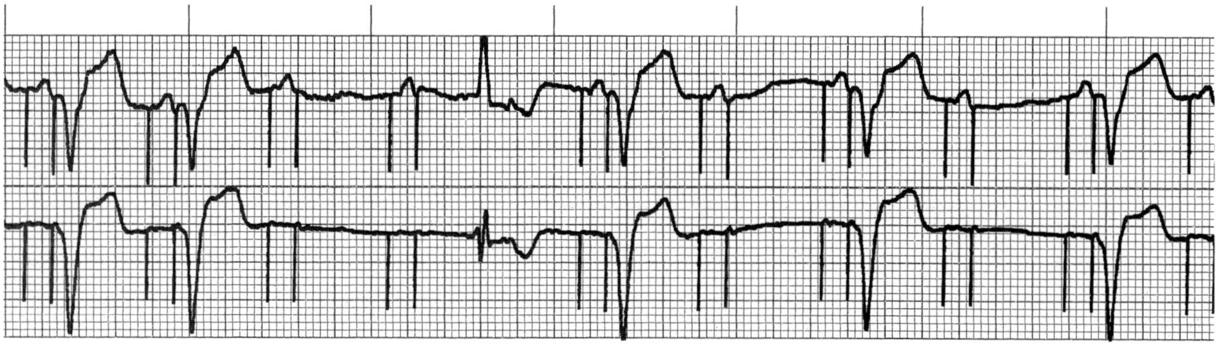

Regularity: _____ Heart rate: _____ PR interval: _____

P-waves: _____QRS complex: _____

Interpretation: _____

#2

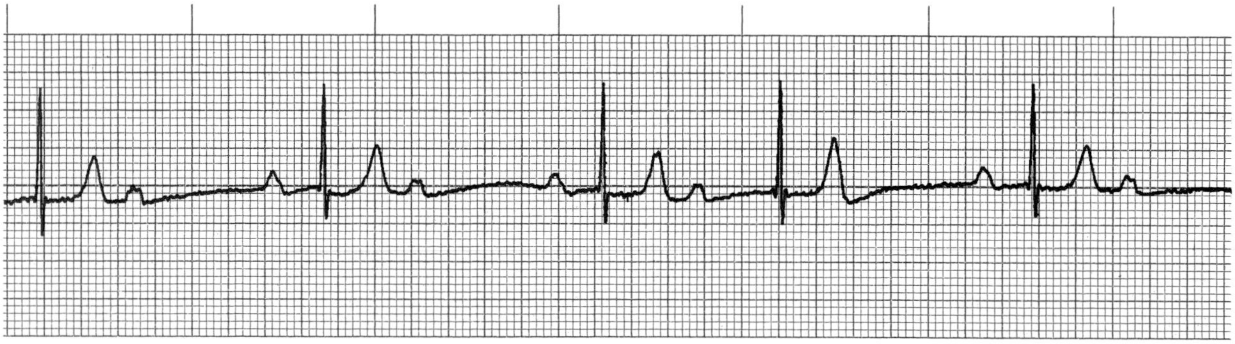

Regularity: _____ Heart rate: _____ PR interval: _____

P-waves: _____QRS complex: _____

Interpretation: _____

#3

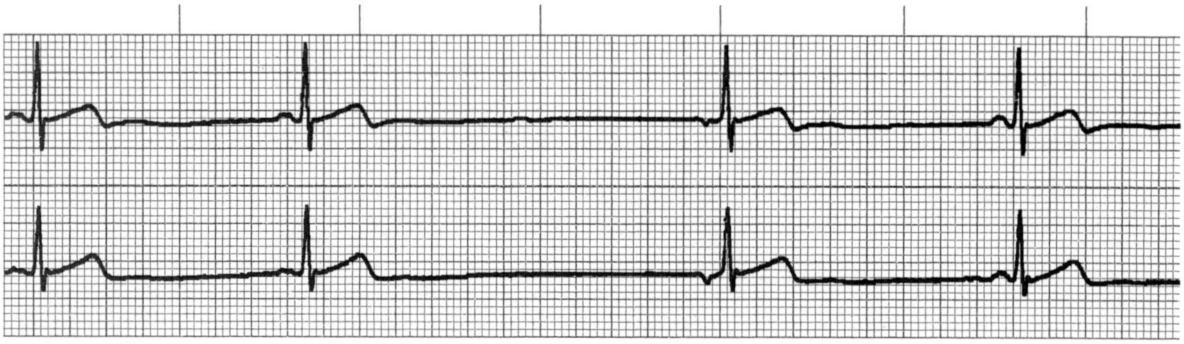

Regularity: _____ Heart rate: _____ PR interval: _____

P-waves: _____QRS complex: _____

Interpretation: _____

#4

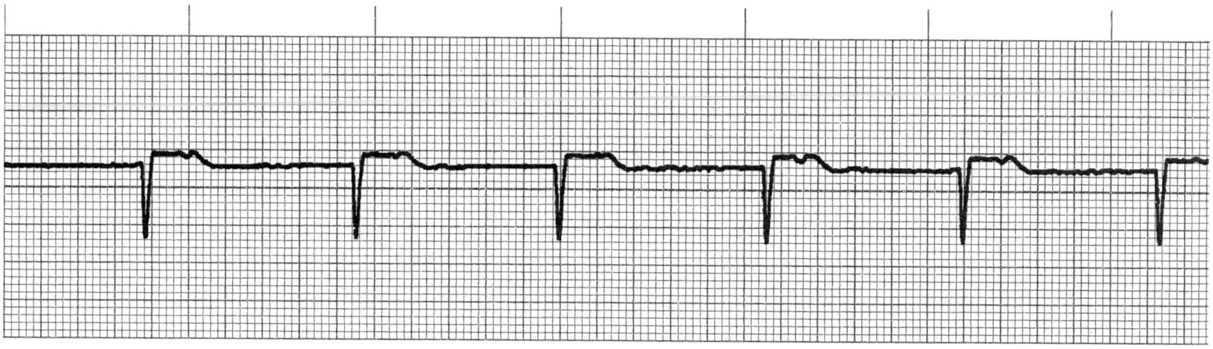

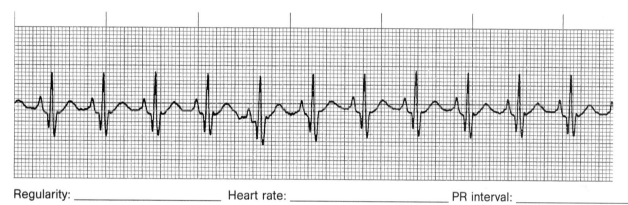

Regularity: _____ Heart rate: _____ PR interval: _____

P-waves: _____QRS complex: _____

Interpretation: _____

#5

Regularity: _____ Heart rate: _____ PR interval: _____

P-waves: _____QRS complex: _____

Interpretation: _____

#6

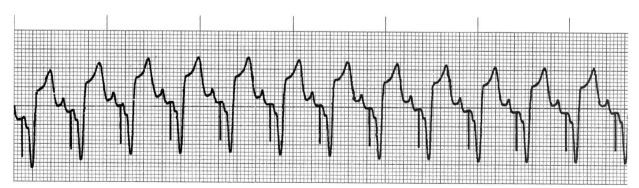

Regularity: _____ Heart rate: _____ PR interval: _____

P-waves: _____QRS complex: _____

Interpretation: _____

Post-Test Questions

#7

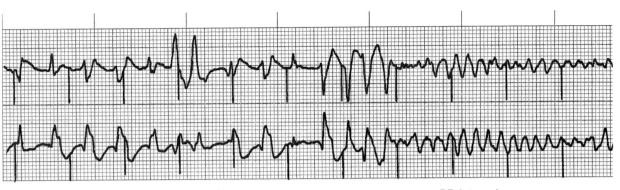

Regularity: _____ Heart rate: _____ PR interval: _____

P-waves: _____ QRS complex: _____

Interpretation: _____

#8

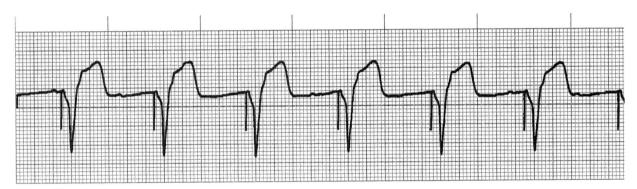

Regularity: _____ Heart rate: _____ PR interval: _____

P-waves: _____ QRS complex: _____

Interpretation: _____

#9

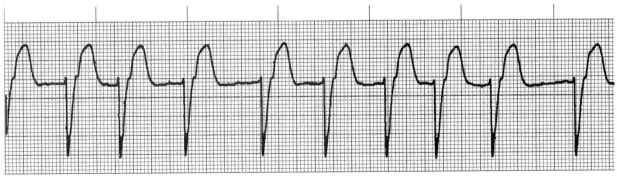

Regularity: _____ Heart rate: _____ PR interval: _____

P-waves: _____ QRS complex: _____

Interpretation: _____

#10

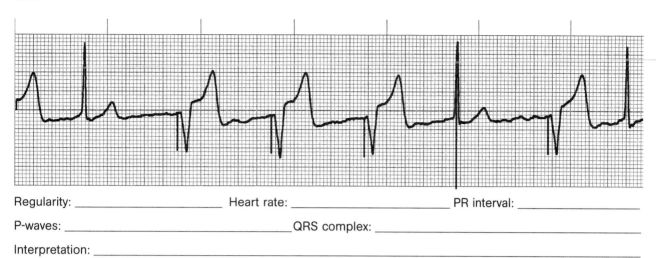

Regularity: _____ Heart rate: _____ PR interval: _____

P-waves: _____ QRS complex: _____

Interpretation: _____

#11

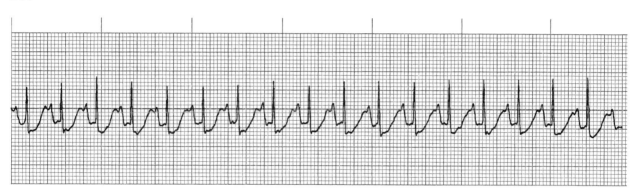

Regularity: _____ Heart rate: _____ PR interval: _____

P-waves: _____ QRS complex: _____

Interpretation: _____

#12

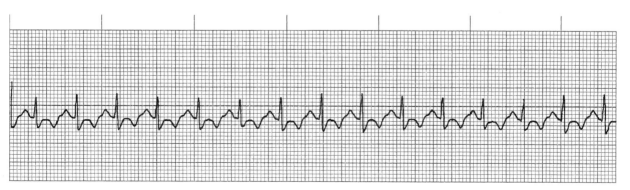

Regularity: _____ Heart rate: _____ PR interval: _____

P-waves: _____ QRS complex: _____

Interpretation: _____

Post-Test Questions

#13

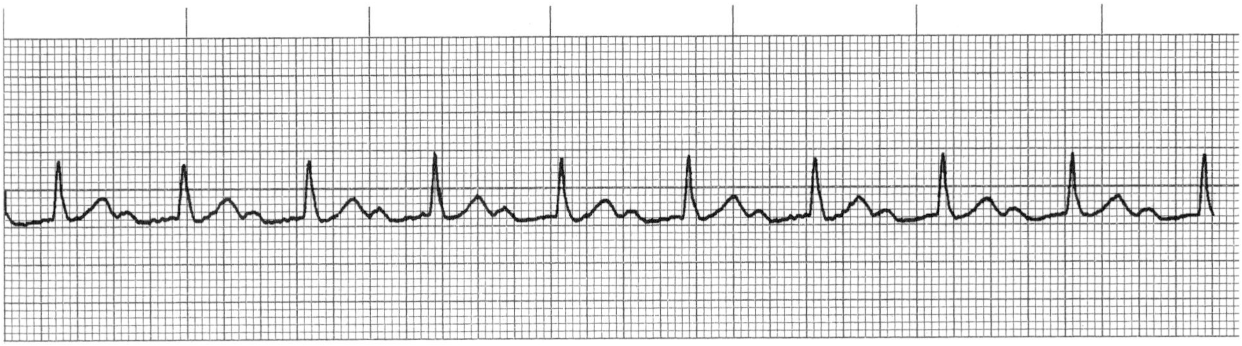

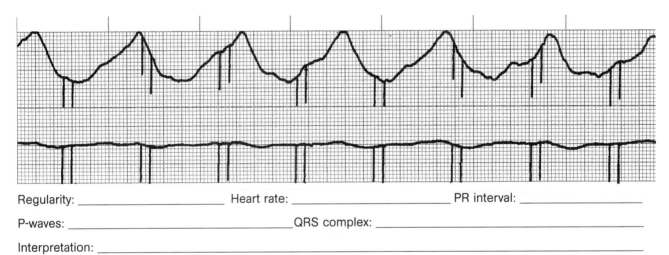

Regularity: _____ Heart rate: _____ PR interval: _____

P-waves: _____ QRS complex: _____

Interpretation: _____

#14

Regularity: _____ Heart rate: _____ PR interval: _____

P-waves: _____ QRS complex: _____

Interpretation: _____

#15

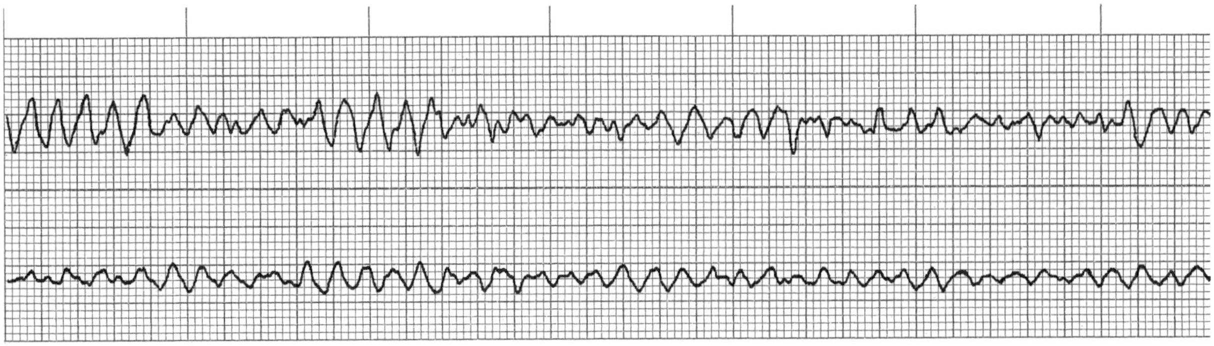

Regularity: _____ Heart rate: _____ PR interval: _____

P-waves: _____ QRS complex: _____

Interpretation: _____

#16

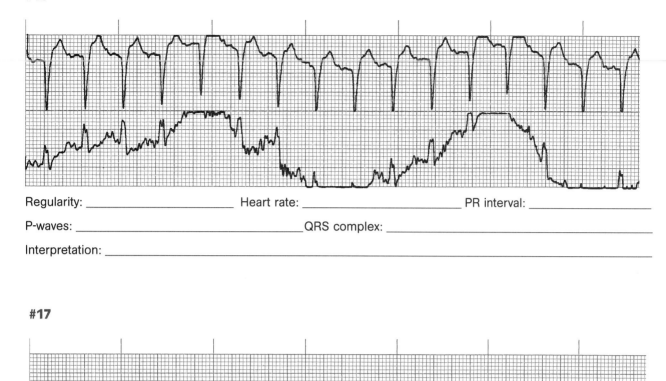

Regularity: _____ Heart rate: _____ PR interval: _____

P-waves: _____ QRS complex: _____

Interpretation: _____

#17

Regularity: _____ Heart rate: _____ PR interval: _____

P-waves: _____ QRS complex: _____

Interpretation: _____

#18

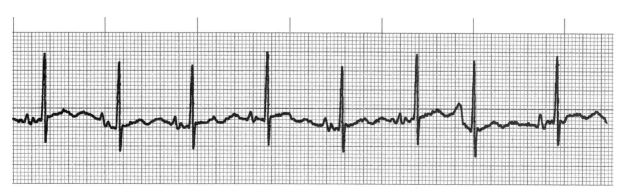

Regularity: _____ Heart rate: _____ PR interval: _____

P-waves: _____ QRS complex: _____

Interpretation: _____

#19

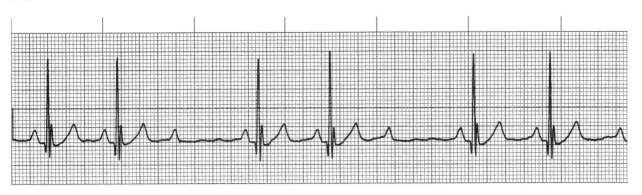

Regularity: _____ Heart rate: _____ PR interval: _____

P-waves: _____ QRS complex: _____

Interpretation: _____

#20

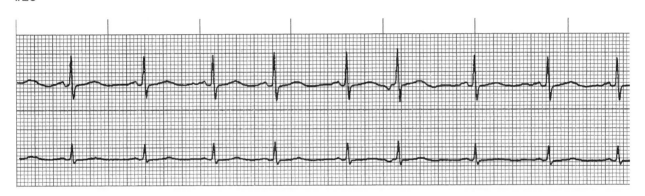

Regularity: _____ Heart rate: _____ PR interval: _____

P-waves: _____ QRS complex: _____

Interpretation: _____

#21

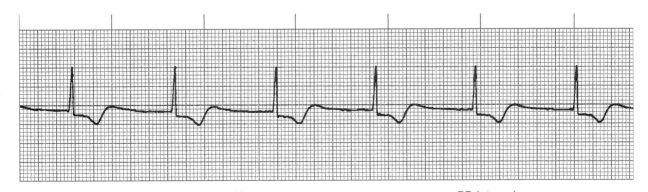

Regularity: _____ Heart rate: _____ PR interval: _____

P-waves: _____ QRS complex: _____

Interpretation: _____

#22

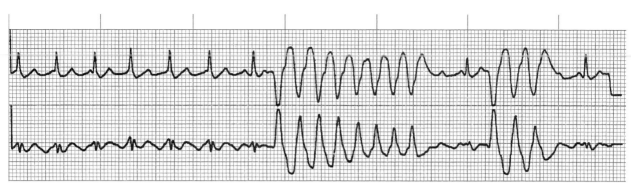

Regularity: _____ Heart rate: _____ PR interval: _____

P-waves: _____ QRS complex: _____

Interpretation: _____

#23

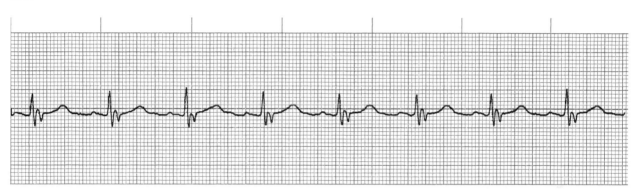

Regularity: _____ Heart rate: _____ PR interval: _____

P-waves: _____ QRS complex: _____

Interpretation: _____

#24

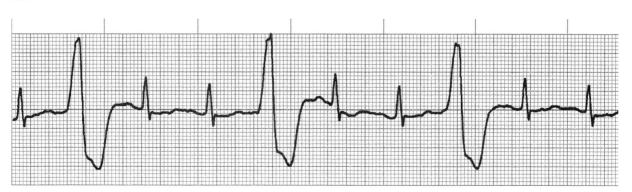

Regularity: _____ Heart rate: _____ PR interval: _____

P-waves: _____ QRS complex: _____

Interpretation: _____

#25

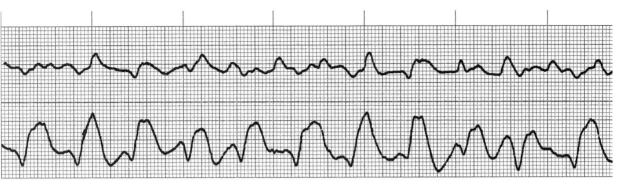

Regularity: _____ Heart rate: _____ PR interval: _____

P-waves: _____ QRS complex: _____

Interpretation: _____

#26

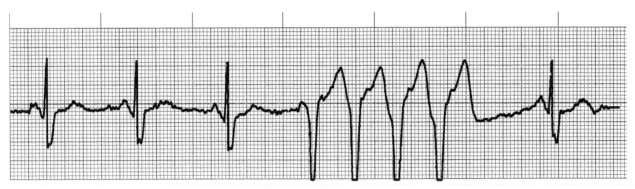

Regularity: _____ Heart rate: _____ PR interval: _____

P-waves: _____ QRS complex: _____

Interpretation: _____

#27

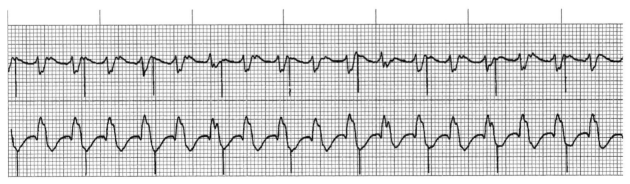

Regularity: _____ Heart rate: _____ PR interval: _____

P-waves: _____ QRS complex: _____

Interpretation: _____

#28

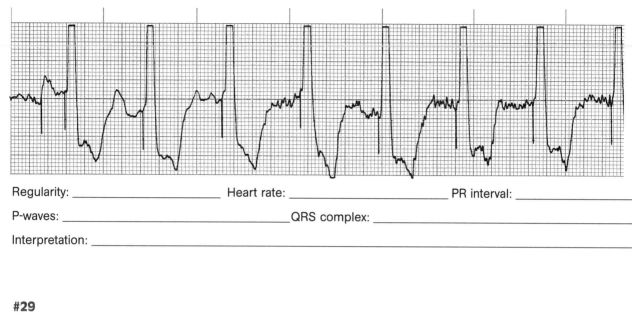

Regularity: _____ Heart rate: _____ PR interval: _____

P-waves: _____ QRS complex: _____

Interpretation: _____

#29

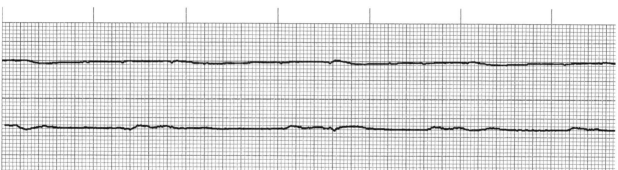

Regularity: _____ Heart rate: _____ PR interval: _____

P-waves: _____ QRS complex: _____

Interpretation: _____

#30

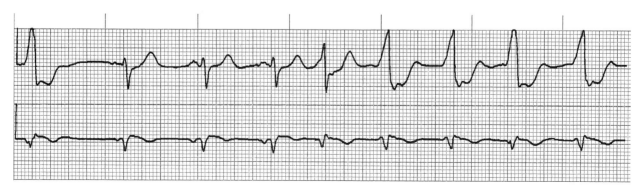

Regularity: _____ Heart rate: _____ PR interval: _____

P-waves: _____ QRS complex: _____

Interpretation: _____

#31

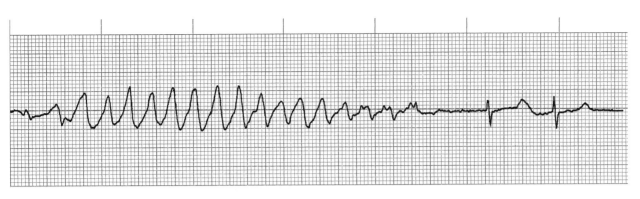

Regularity: _____ Heart rate: _____ PR interval: _____

P-waves: _____ QRS complex: _____

Interpretation: _____

#32

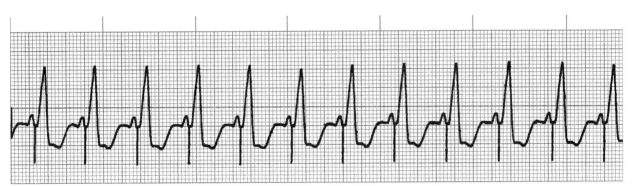

Regularity: _____ Heart rate: _____ PR interval: _____

P-waves: _____ QRS complex: _____

Interpretation: _____

#33

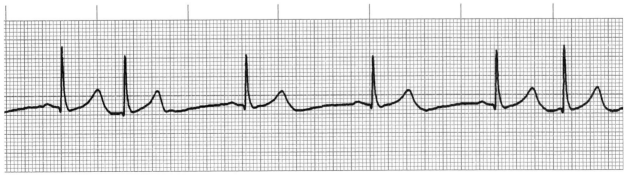

Regularity: _____ Heart rate: _____ PR interval: _____

P-waves: _____ QRS complex: _____

Interpretation: _____

#34

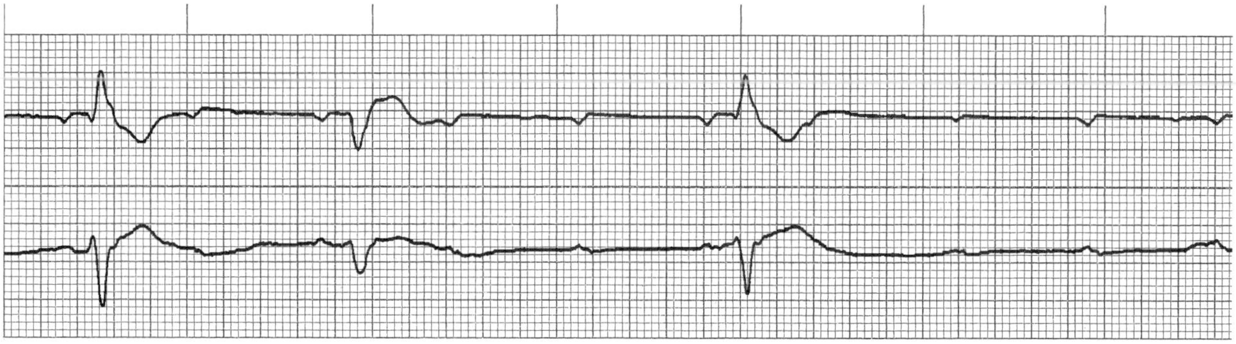

Regularity: _____ Heart rate: _____ PR interval: _____

P-waves: _____ QRS complex: _____

Interpretation: _____

#35

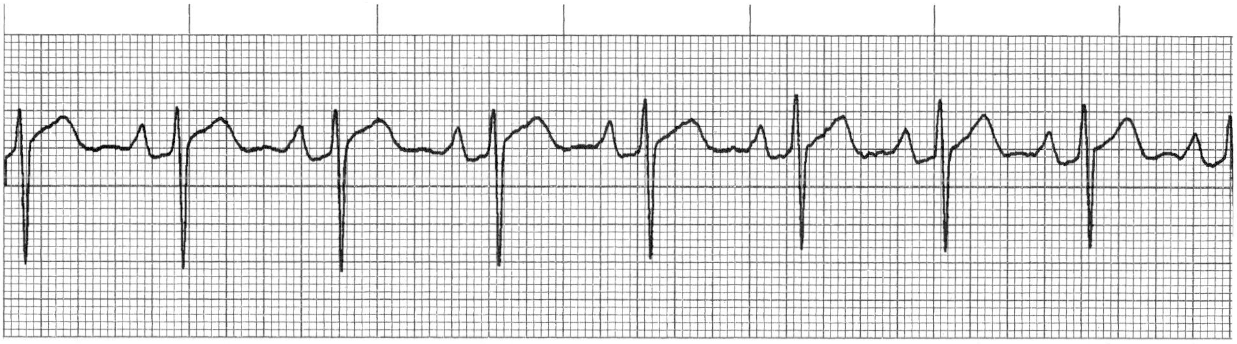

Regularity: _____ Heart rate: _____ PR interval: _____

P-waves: _____ QRS complex: _____

Interpretation: _____

#36

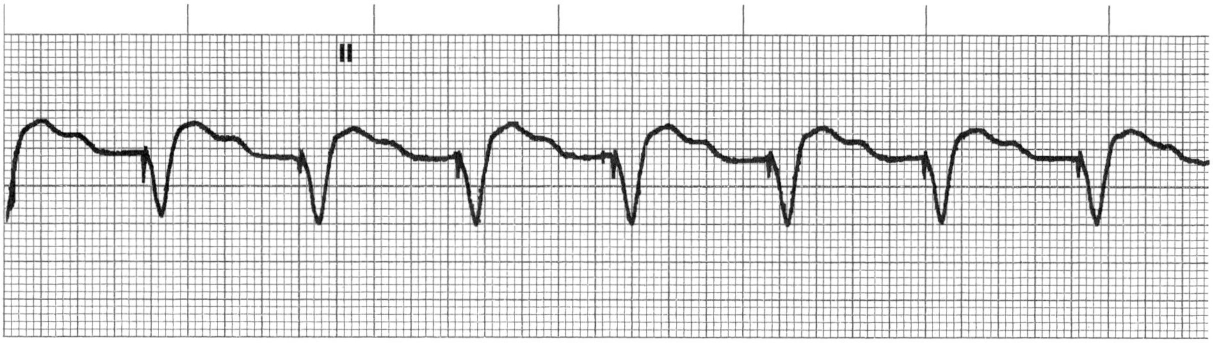

Regularity: _____ Heart rate: _____ PR interval: _____

P-waves: _____ QRS complex: _____

Interpretation: _____

#37

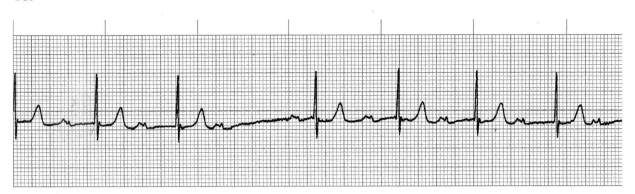

Regularity: _____ Heart rate: _____ PR interval: _____

P-waves: _____ QRS complex: _____

Interpretation: _____

#38

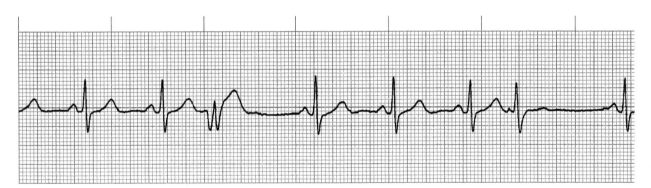

Regularity: _____ Heart rate: _____ PR interval: _____

P-waves: _____ QRS complex: _____

Interpretation: _____

#39

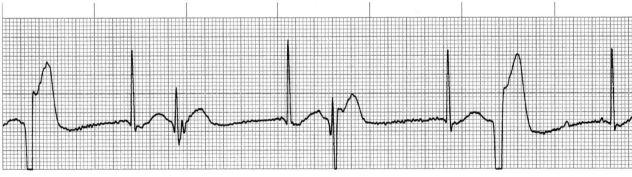

Regularity: _____ Heart rate: _____ PR interval: _____

P-waves: _____ QRS complex: _____

Interpretation: _____

#40

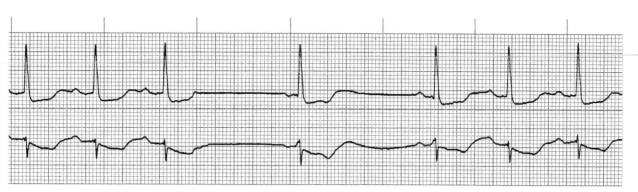

Regularity: _____ Heart rate: _____ PR interval: _____

P-waves: _____QRS complex: _____

Interpretation: _____

#41

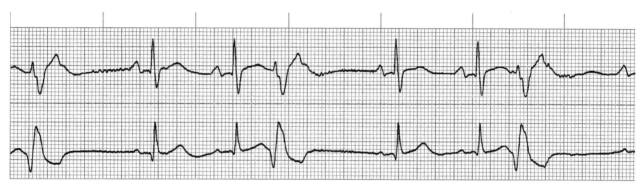

Regularity: _____ Heart rate: _____ PR interval: _____

P-waves: _____QRS complex: _____

Interpretation: _____

#42

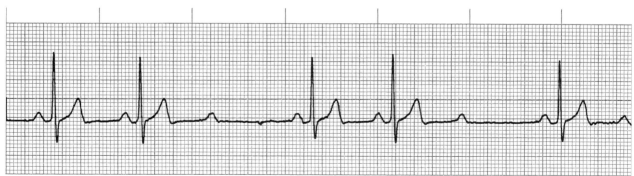

Regularity: _____ Heart rate: _____ PR interval: _____

P-waves: _____QRS complex: _____

Interpretation: _____

#43

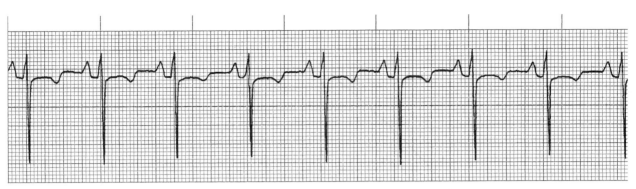

Regularity: _____ Heart rate: _____ PR interval: _____

P-waves: _____QRS complex: _____

Interpretation: _____

#44

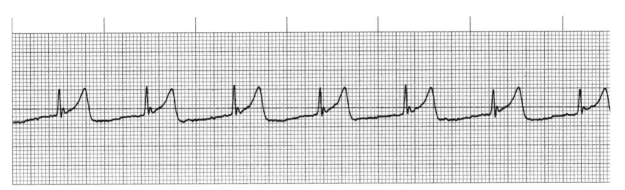

Regularity: _____ Heart rate: _____ PR interval: _____

P-waves: _____QRS complex: _____

Interpretation: _____

#45

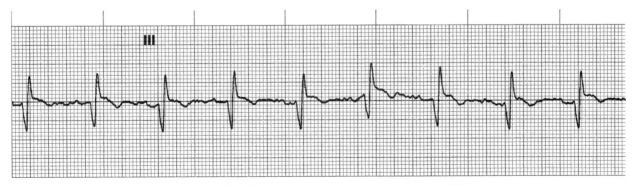

Regularity: _____ Heart rate: _____ PR interval: _____

P-waves: _____QRS complex: _____

Interpretation: _____

#46

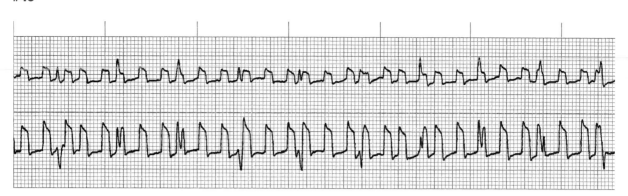

Regularity: _____ Heart rate: _____ PR interval: _____

P-waves: _____QRS complex: _____

Interpretation: _____

#47

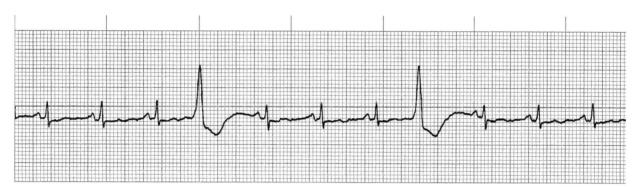

Regularity: _____ Heart rate: _____ PR interval: _____

P-waves: _____QRS complex: _____

Interpretation: _____

#48

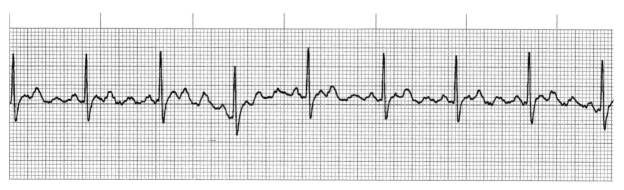

Regularity: _____ Heart rate: _____ PR interval: _____

P-waves: _____QRS complex: _____

Interpretation: _____

#49

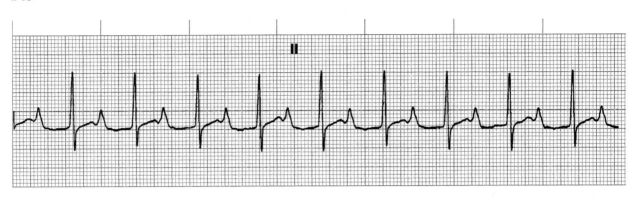

Regularity: _____ Heart rate: _____ PR interval: _____

P-waves: _____ QRS complex: _____

Interpretation: _____

#50

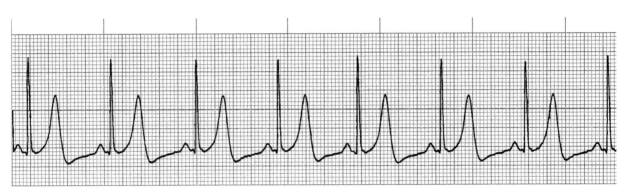

Regularity: _____ Heart rate: _____ PR interval: _____

P-waves: _____ QRS complex: _____

Interpretation: _____

#51

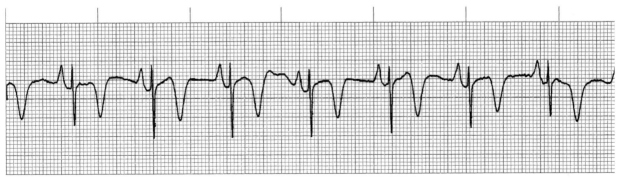

Regularity: _____ Heart rate: _____ PR interval: _____

P-waves: _____ QRS complex: _____

Interpretation: _____

#52

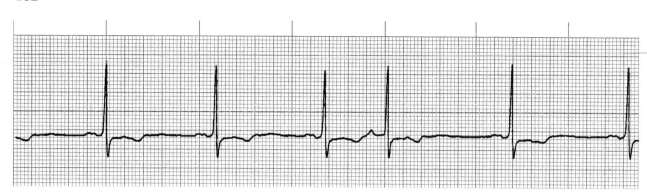

Regularity: _____ Heart rate: _____ PR interval: _____

P-waves: _____ QRS complex: _____

Interpretation: _____

#53

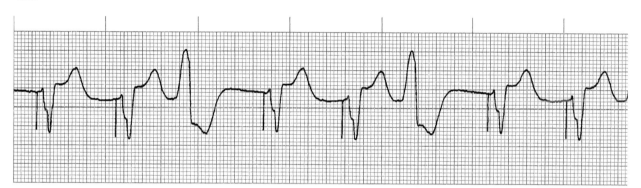

Regularity: _____ Heart rate: _____ PR interval: _____

P-waves: _____ QRS complex: _____

Interpretation: _____

#54

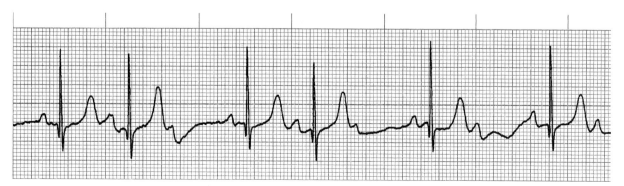

Regularity: _____ Heart rate: _____ PR interval: _____

P-waves: _____ QRS complex: _____

Interpretation: _____

#55

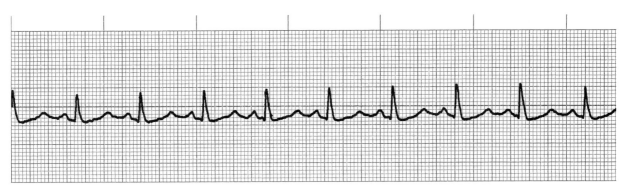

Regularity: _____ Heart rate: _____ PR interval: _____

P-waves: _____ QRS complex: _____

Interpretation: _____

#56

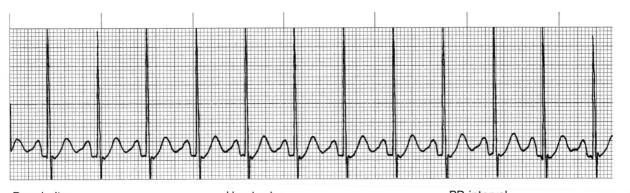

Regularity: _____ Heart rate: _____ PR interval: _____

P-waves: _____ QRS complex: _____

Interpretation: _____

#57

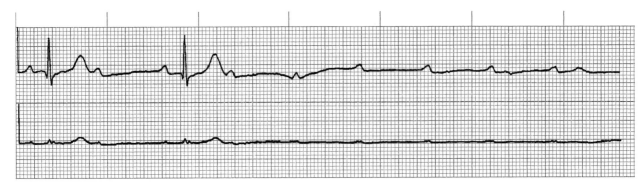

Regularity: _____ Heart rate: _____ PR interval: _____

P-waves: _____ QRS complex: _____

Interpretation: _____

#58

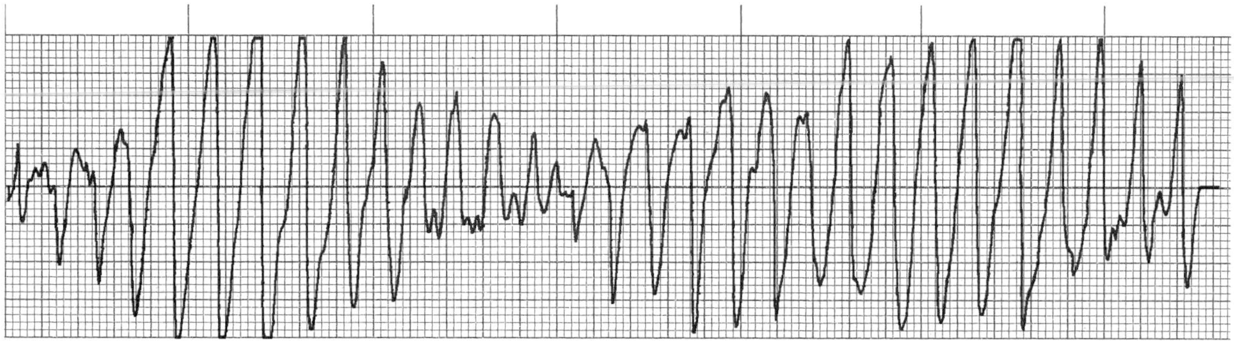

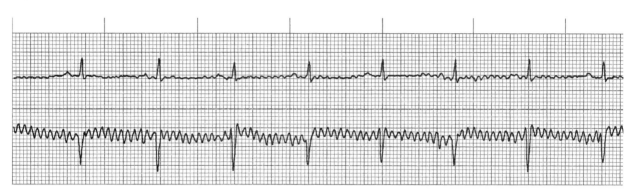

Regularity: _____ Heart rate: _____ PR interval: _____

P-waves: _____ QRS complex: _____

Interpretation: _____

#59

Regularity: _____ Heart rate: _____ PR interval: _____

P-waves: _____ QRS complex: _____

Interpretation: _____

#60

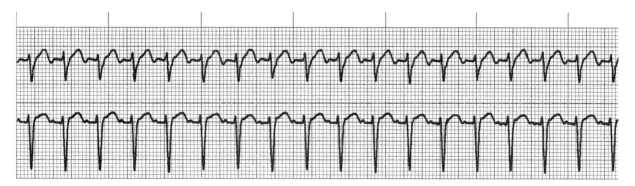

Regularity: _____ Heart rate: _____ PR interval: _____

P-waves: _____ QRS complex: _____

Interpretation: _____

#61

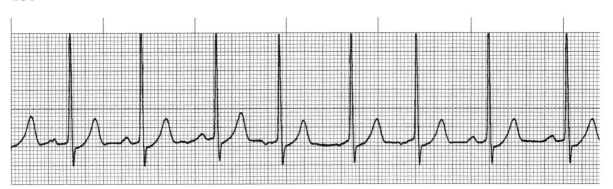

Regularity: _____ Heart rate: _____ PR interval: _____

P-waves: _____ QRS complex: _____

Interpretation: _____

#62

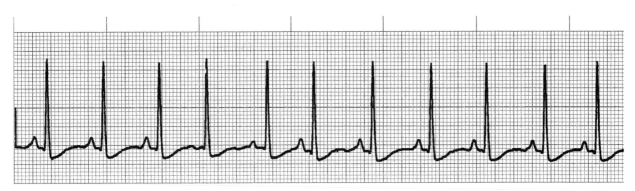

Regularity: _____ Heart rate: _____ PR interval: _____

P-waves: _____ QRS complex: _____

Interpretation: _____

#63

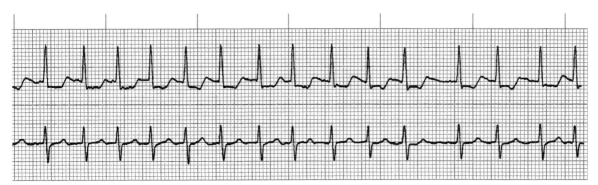

Regularity: _____ Heart rate: _____ PR interval: _____

P-waves: _____ QRS complex: _____

Interpretation: _____

#64

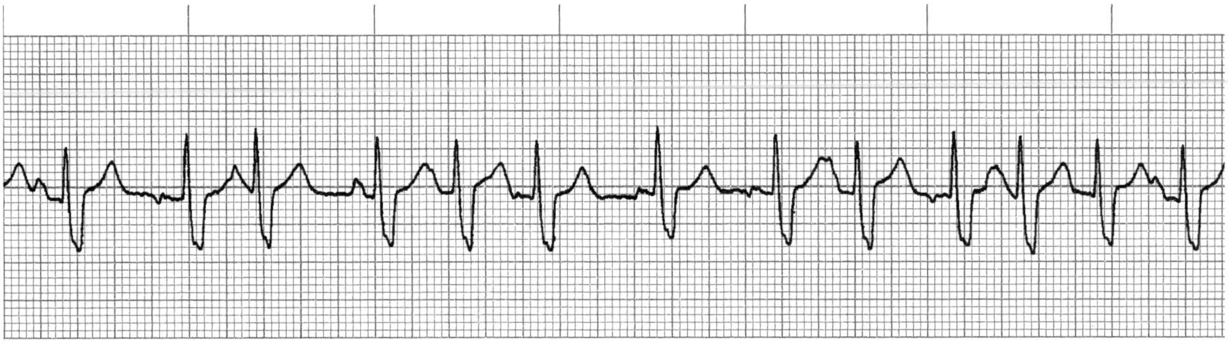

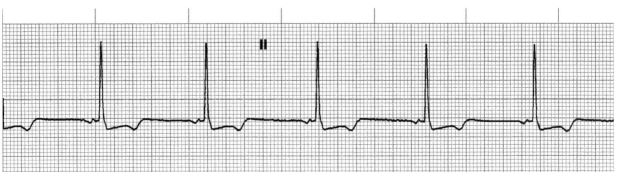

Regularity: _____ Heart rate: _____ PR interval: _____

P-waves: _____ QRS complex: _____

Interpretation: _____

#65

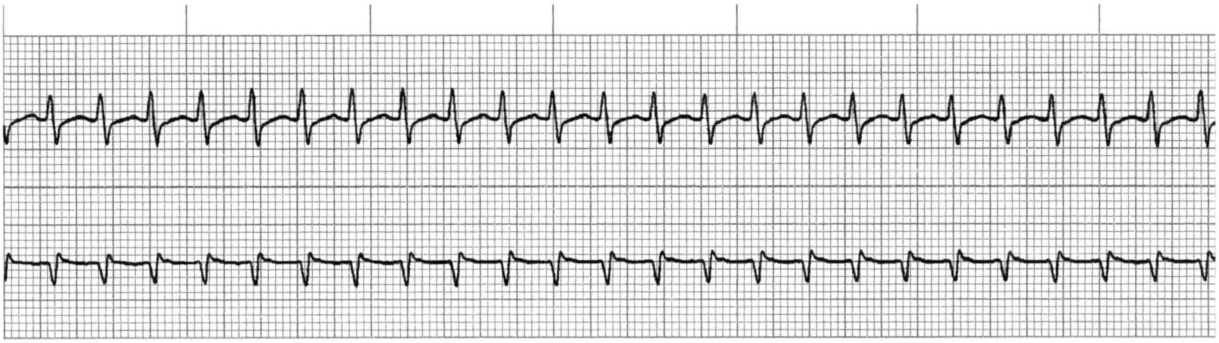

Regularity: _____ Heart rate: _____ PR interval: _____

P-waves: _____ QRS complex: _____

Interpretation: _____

#66

Regularity: _____ Heart rate: _____ PR interval: _____

P-waves: _____ QRS complex: _____

Interpretation: _____

#67

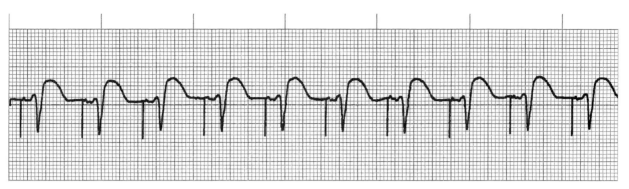

Regularity: _____ Heart rate: _____ PR interval: _____

P-waves: _____ QRS complex: _____

Interpretation: _____

#68

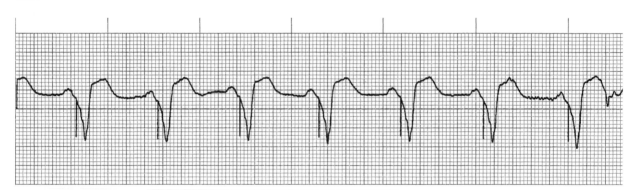

Regularity: _____ Heart rate: _____ PR interval: _____

P-waves: _____ QRS complex: _____

Interpretation: _____

#69

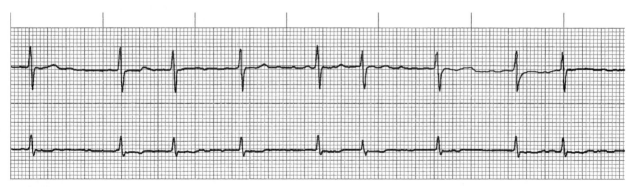

Regularity: _____ Heart rate: _____ PR interval: _____

P-waves: _____ QRS complex: _____

Interpretation: _____

#70

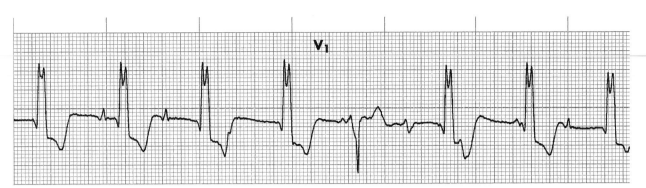

Regularity: _____ Heart rate: _____ PR interval: _____

P-waves: _____QRS complex: _____

Interpretation: _____

#71

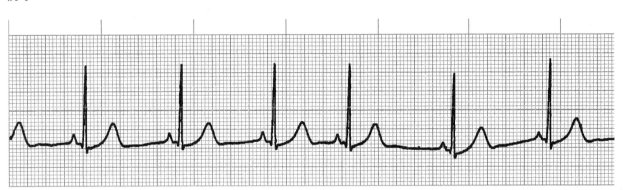

Regularity: _____ Heart rate: _____ PR interval: _____

P-waves: _____QRS complex: _____

Interpretation: _____

#72

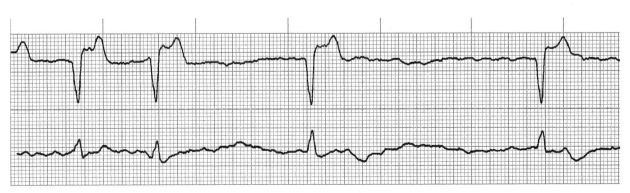

Regularity: _____ Heart rate: _____ PR interval: _____

P-waves: _____QRS complex: _____

Interpretation: _____

Post-Test Questions

#73

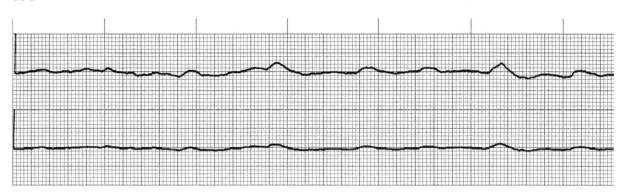

Regularity: _____ Heart rate: _____ PR interval: _____

P-waves: _____QRS complex: _____

Interpretation: _____

#74

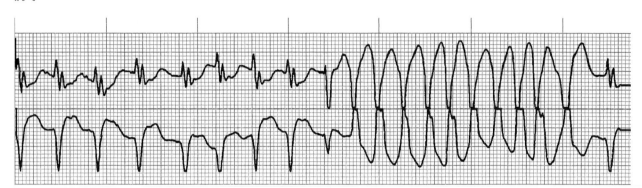

Regularity: _____ Heart rate: _____ PR interval: _____

P-waves: _____QRS complex: _____

Interpretation: _____

#75

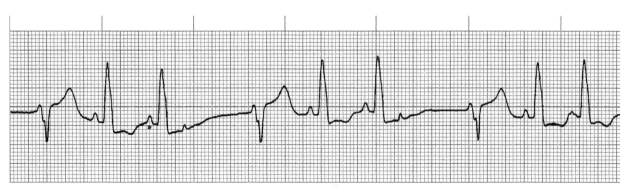

Regularity: _____ Heart rate: _____ PR interval: _____

P-waves: _____QRS complex: _____

Interpretation: _____

#76

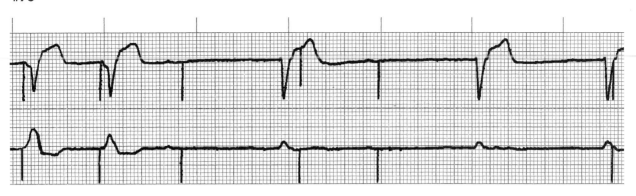

Regularity: _____ Heart rate: _____ PR interval: _____

P-waves: _____QRS complex: _____

Interpretation: _____

#77

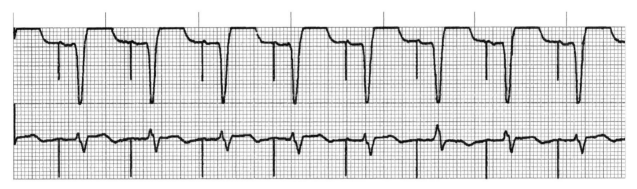

Regularity: _____ Heart rate: _____ PR interval: _____

P-waves: _____QRS complex: _____

Interpretation: _____

#78

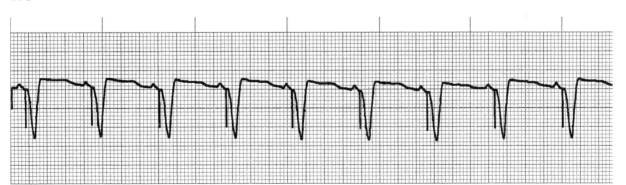

Regularity: _____ Heart rate: _____ PR interval: _____

P-waves: _____QRS complex: _____

Interpretation: _____

#79

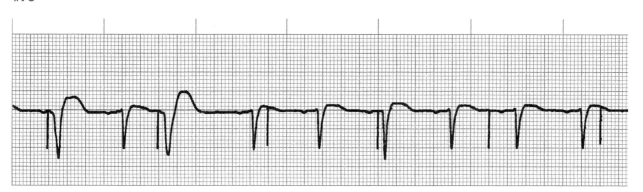

Regularity: _____ Heart rate: _____ PR interval: _____

P-waves: _____ QRS complex: _____

Interpretation: _____

#80

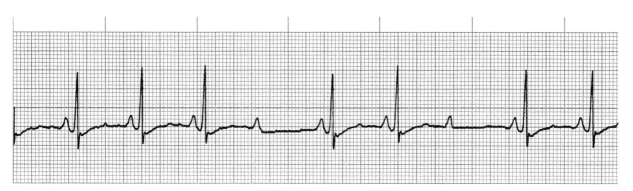

Regularity: _____ Heart rate: _____ PR interval: _____

P-waves: _____ QRS complex: _____

Interpretation: _____

#81

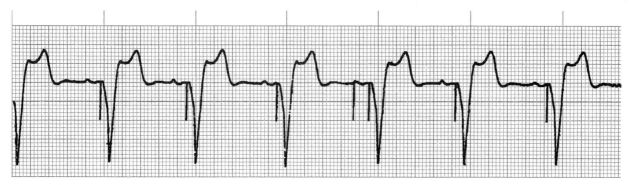

Regularity: _____ Heart rate: _____ PR interval: _____

P-waves: _____ QRS complex: _____

Interpretation: _____

#82

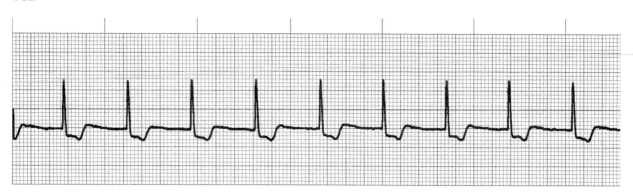

Regularity: _____ Heart rate: _____ PR interval: _____

P-waves: _____ QRS complex: _____

Interpretation: _____

#83

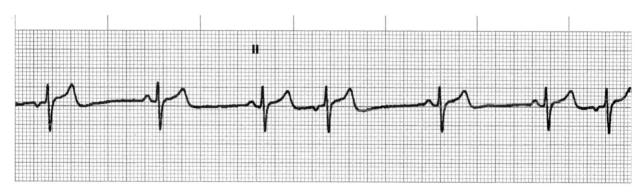

Regularity: _____ Heart rate: _____ PR interval: _____

P-waves: _____ QRS complex: _____

Interpretation: _____

#84

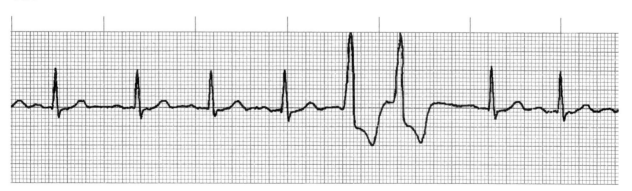

Regularity: _____ Heart rate: _____ PR interval: _____

P-waves: _____ QRS complex: _____

Interpretation: _____

Post-Test Questions

#85

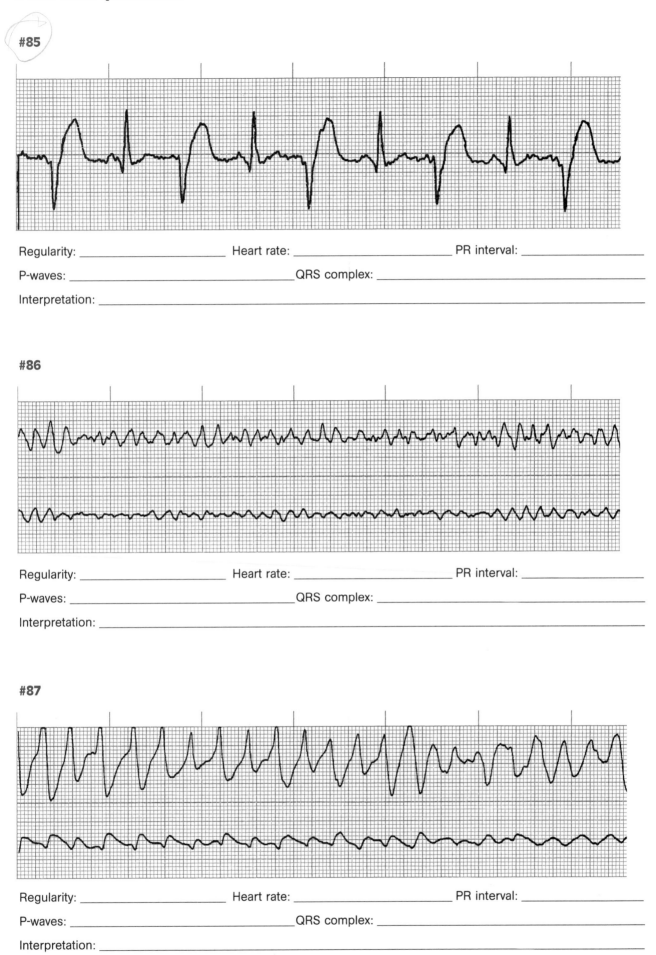

Regularity: _____ Heart rate: _____ PR interval: _____

P-waves: _____ QRS complex: _____

Interpretation: _____

#86

Regularity: _____ Heart rate: _____ PR interval: _____

P-waves: _____ QRS complex: _____

Interpretation: _____

#87

Regularity: _____ Heart rate: _____ PR interval: _____

P-waves: _____ QRS complex: _____

Interpretation: _____

#88

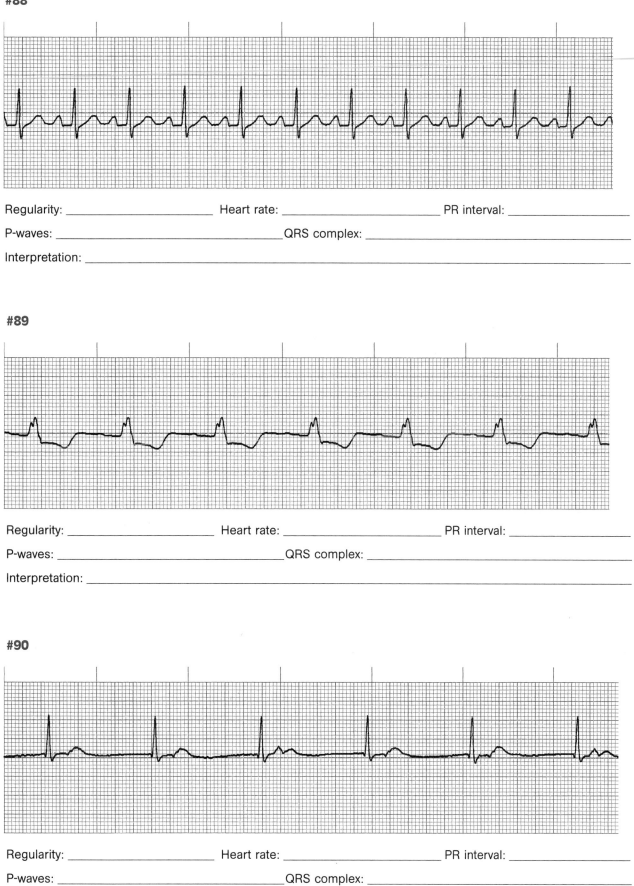

Regularity: _____ Heart rate: _____ PR interval: _____

P-waves: _____ QRS complex: _____

Interpretation: _____

#89

Regularity: _____ Heart rate: _____ PR interval: _____

P-waves: _____ QRS complex: _____

Interpretation: _____

#90

Regularity: _____ Heart rate: _____ PR interval: _____

P-waves: _____ QRS complex: _____

Interpretation: _____

Post-Test Questions

#91

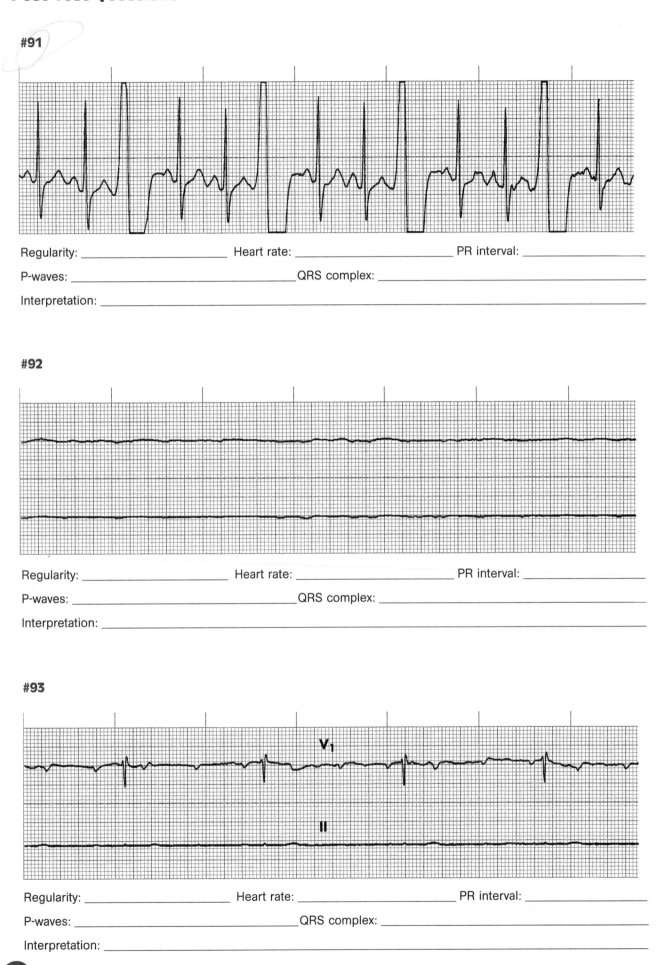

Regularity: _____ Heart rate: _____ PR interval: _____

P-waves: _____ QRS complex: _____

Interpretation: _____

#92

Regularity: _____ Heart rate: _____ PR interval: _____

P-waves: _____ QRS complex: _____

Interpretation: _____

#93

Regularity: _____ Heart rate: _____ PR interval: _____

P-waves: _____ QRS complex: _____

Interpretation: _____

#94

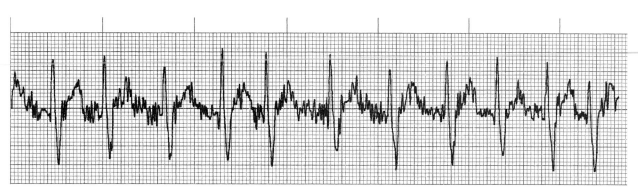

Regularity: _____ Heart rate: _____ PR interval: _____

P-waves: _____ QRS complex: _____

Interpretation: _____

#95

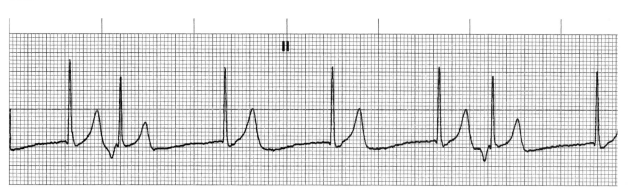

Regularity: _____ Heart rate: _____ PR interval: _____

P-waves: _____ QRS complex: _____

Interpretation: _____

#96

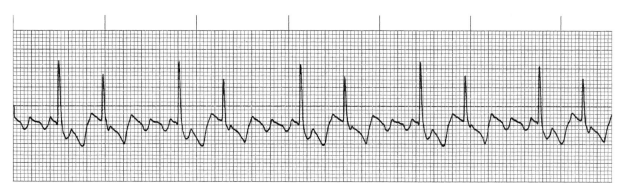

Regularity: _____ Heart rate: _____ PR interval: _____

P-waves: _____ QRS complex: _____

Interpretation: _____

Post-Test Questions

#97

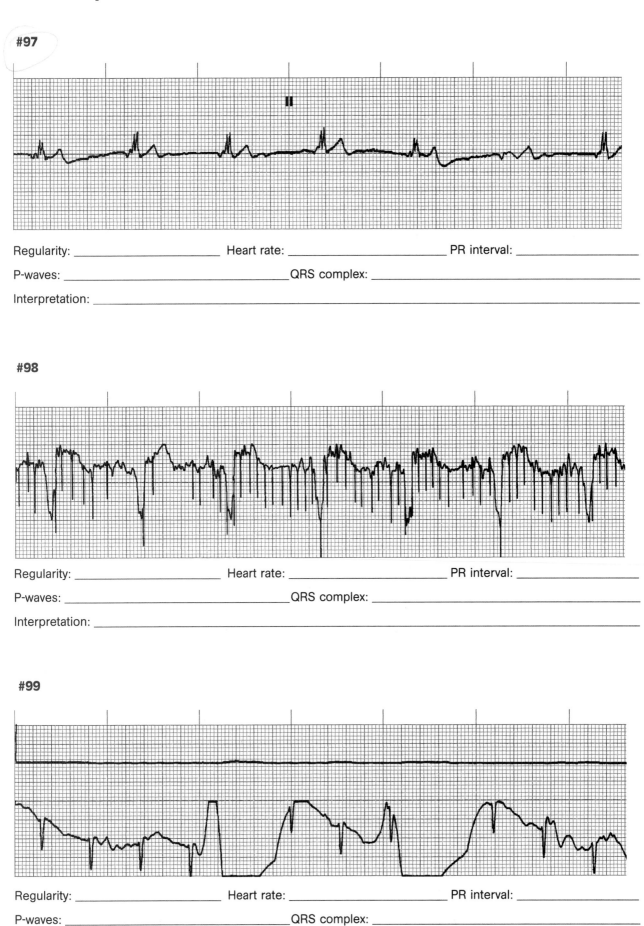

Regularity: _____ Heart rate: _____ PR interval: _____

P-waves: _____ QRS complex: _____

Interpretation: _____

#98

Regularity: _____ Heart rate: _____ PR interval: _____

P-waves: _____ QRS complex: _____

Interpretation: _____

#99

Regularity: _____ Heart rate: _____ PR interval: _____

P-waves: _____ QRS complex: _____

Interpretation: _____

#100

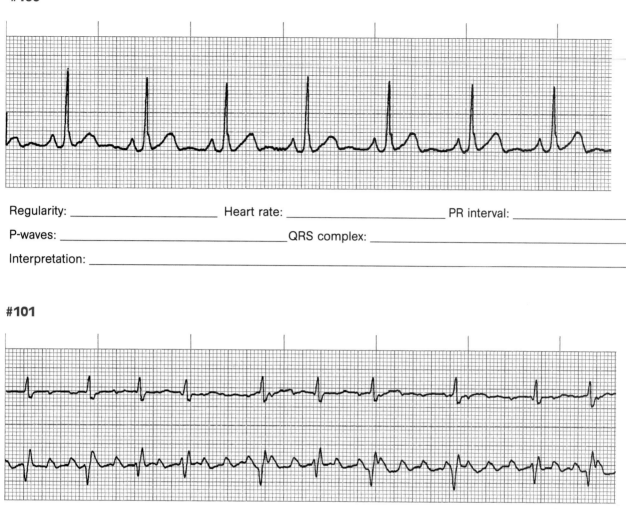

Regularity: _____ Heart rate: _____ PR interval: _____

P-waves: _____ QRS complex: _____

Interpretation: _____

#101

Regularity: _____ Heart rate: _____ PR interval: _____

P-waves: _____ QRS complex: _____

Interpretation: _____

#102

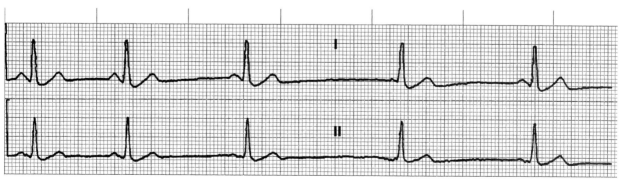

Regularity: _____ Heart rate: _____ PR interval: _____

P-waves: _____ QRS complex: _____

Interpretation: _____

#103

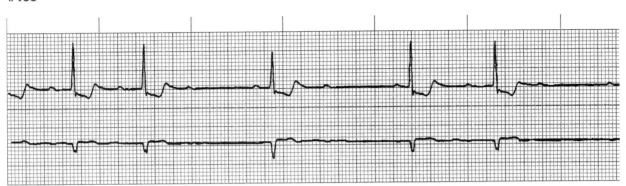

Regularity: _____ Heart rate: _____ PR interval: _____

P-waves: _____ QRS complex: _____

Interpretation: _____

#104

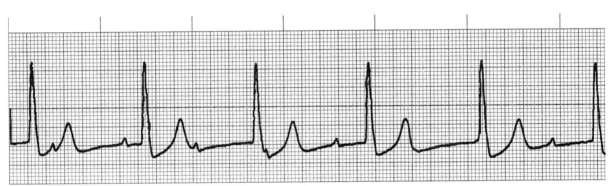

Regularity: _____ Heart rate: _____ PR interval: _____

P-waves: _____ QRS complex: _____

Interpretation: _____

#105

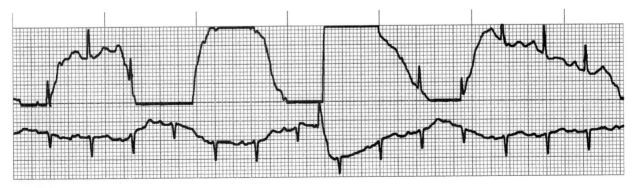

Regularity: _____ Heart rate: _____ PR interval: _____

P-waves: _____ QRS complex: _____

Interpretation: _____

#106

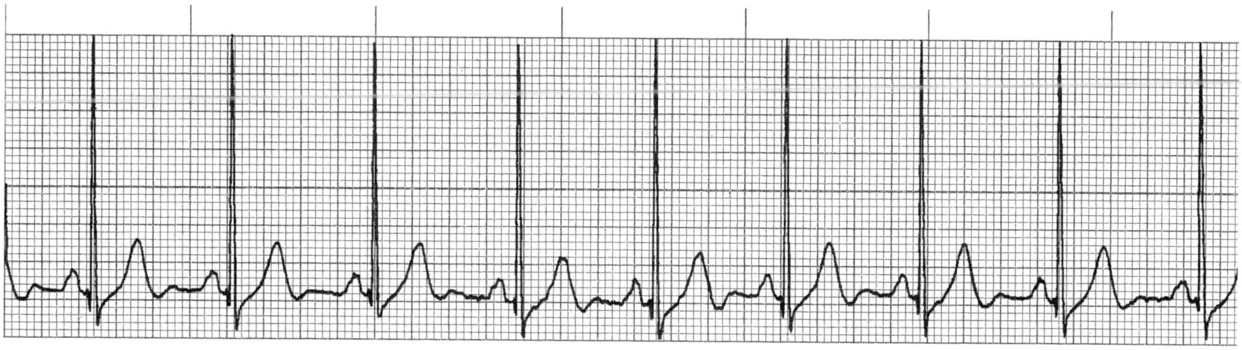

Regularity: _____ Heart rate: _____ PR interval: _____

P-waves: _____ QRS complex: _____

Interpretation: _____

#107

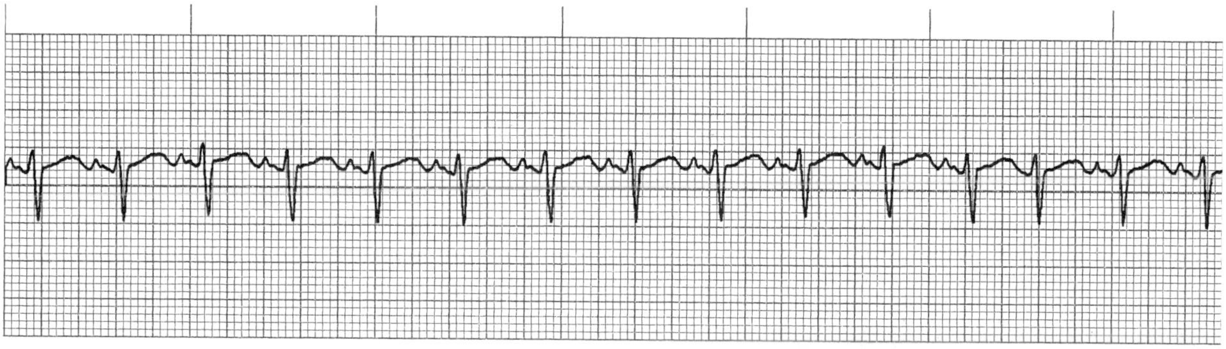

Regularity: _____ Heart rate: _____ PR interval: _____

P-waves: _____ QRS complex: _____

Interpretation: _____

#108

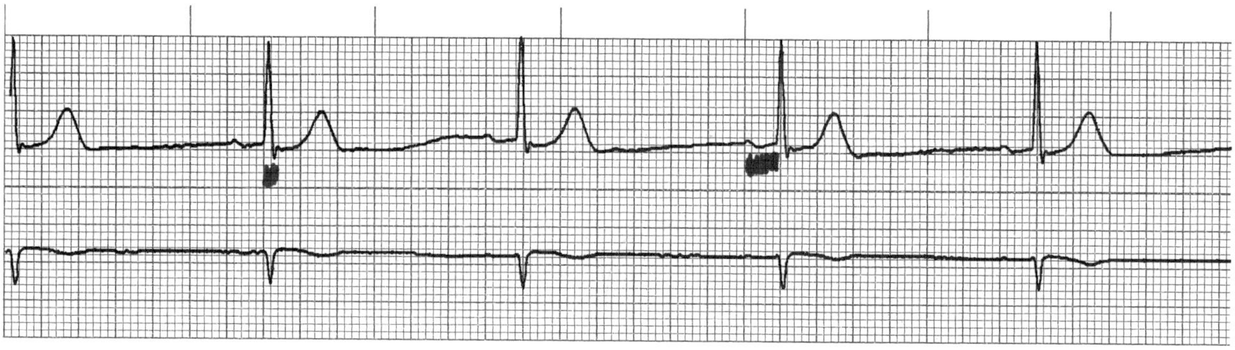

Regularity: _____ Heart rate: _____ PR interval: _____

P-waves: _____ QRS complex: _____

Interpretation: _____

Post-Test Questions

#109

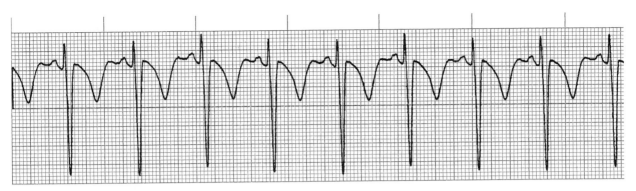

Regularity: _____ Heart rate: _____ PR interval: _____

P-waves: _____ QRS complex: _____

Interpretation: _____

#110

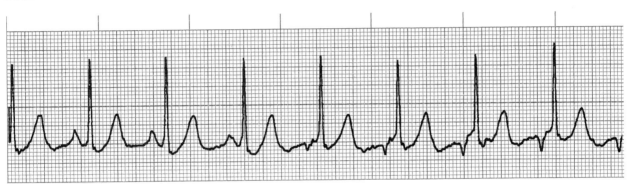

Regularity: _____ Heart rate: _____ PR interval: _____

P-waves: _____ QRS complex: _____

Interpretation: _____

#111

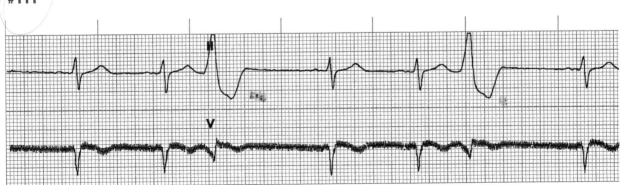

Regularity: _____ Heart rate: _____ PR interval: _____

P-waves: _____ QRS complex: _____

Interpretation: _____

#112

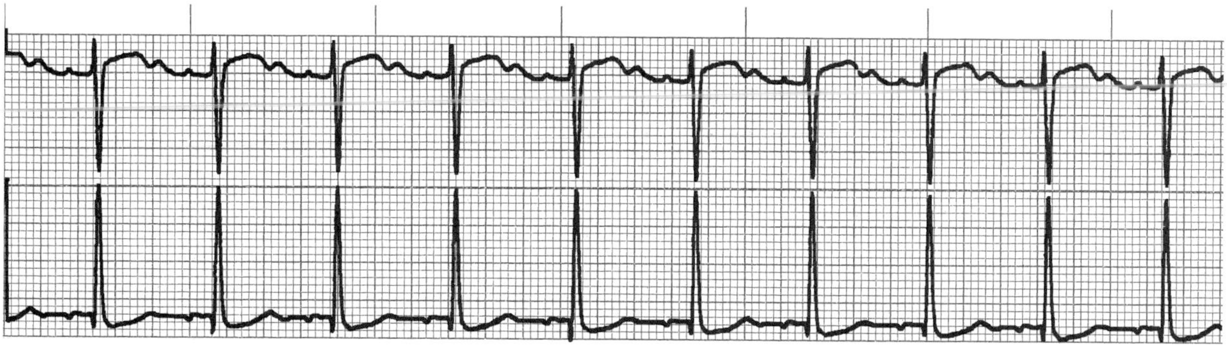

Regularity: _____ Heart rate: _____ PR interval: _____

P-waves: _____ QRS complex: _____

Interpretation: _____

#113

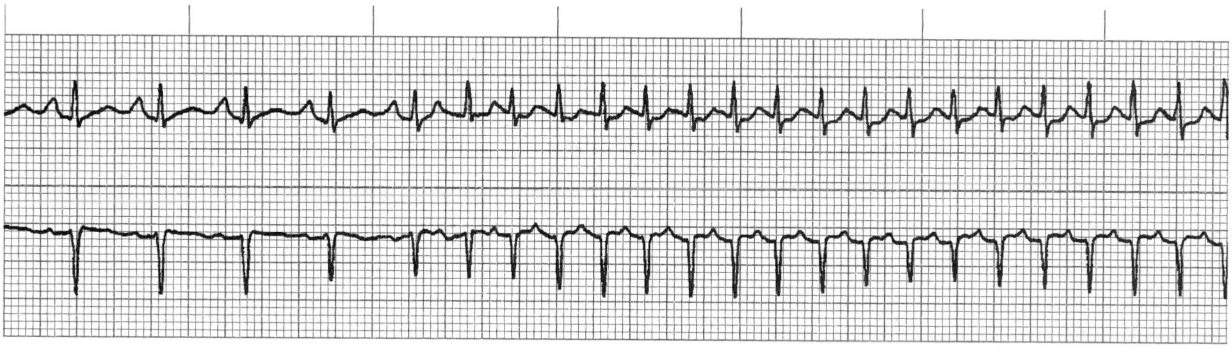

Regularity: _____ Heart rate: _____ PR interval: _____

P-waves: _____ QRS complex: _____

Interpretation: _____

#114

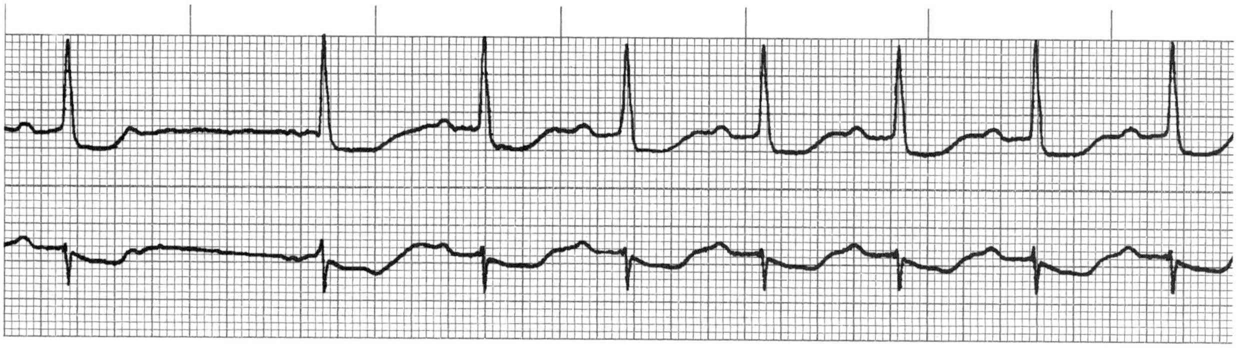

Regularity: _____ Heart rate: _____ PR interval: _____

P-waves: _____ QRS complex: _____

Interpretation: _____

#115

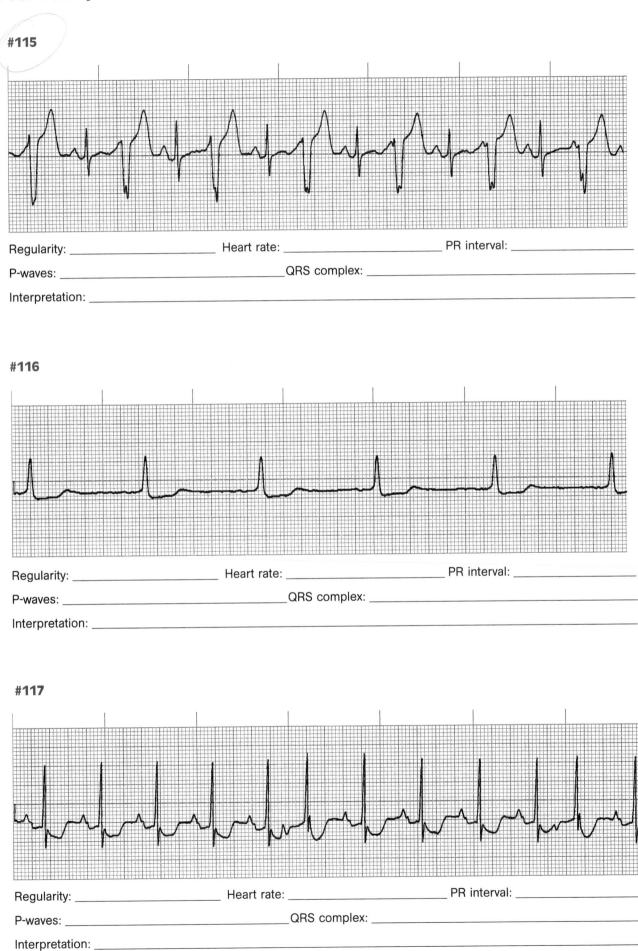

Regularity: _____ Heart rate: _____ PR interval: _____

P-waves: _____ QRS complex: _____

Interpretation: _____

#116

Regularity: _____ Heart rate: _____ PR interval: _____

P-waves: _____ QRS complex: _____

Interpretation: _____

#117

Regularity: _____ Heart rate: _____ PR interval: _____

P-waves: _____ QRS complex: _____

Interpretation: _____

#118

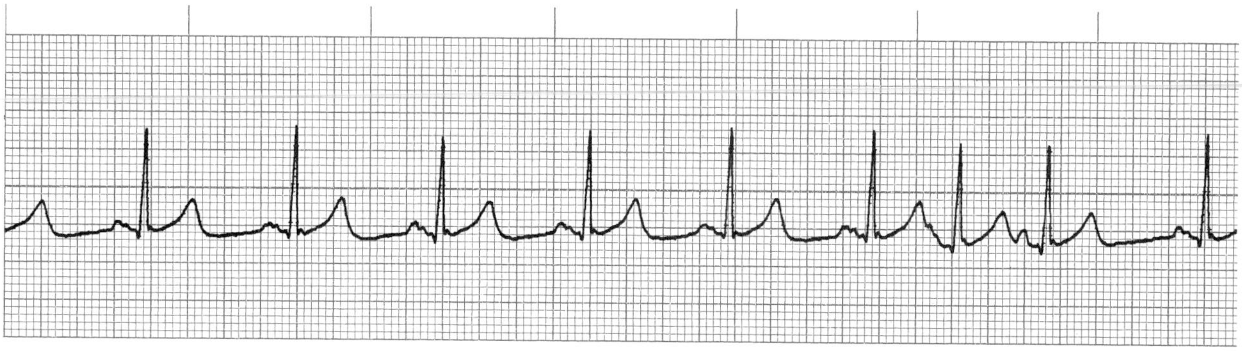

Regularity: _____ Heart rate: _____ PR interval: _____

P-waves: _____ QRS complex: _____

Interpretation: _____

#119

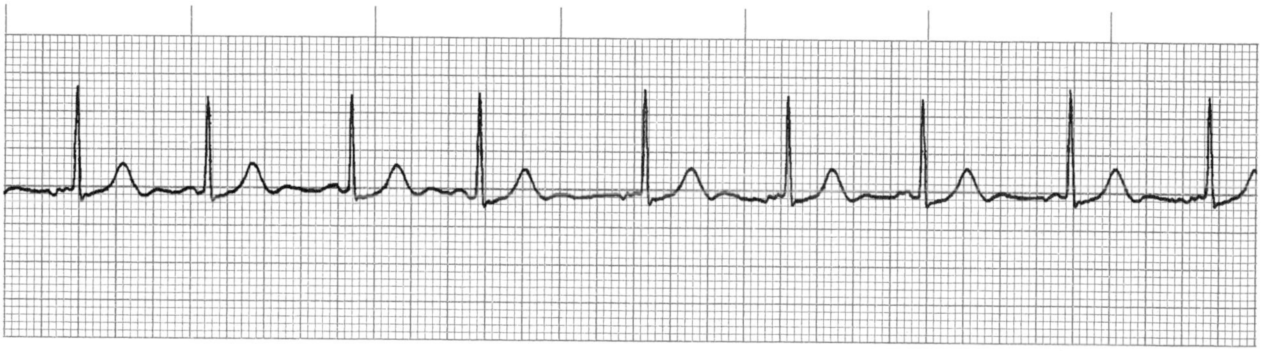

Regularity: _____ Heart rate: _____ PR interval: _____

P-waves: _____ QRS complex: _____

Interpretation: _____

#120

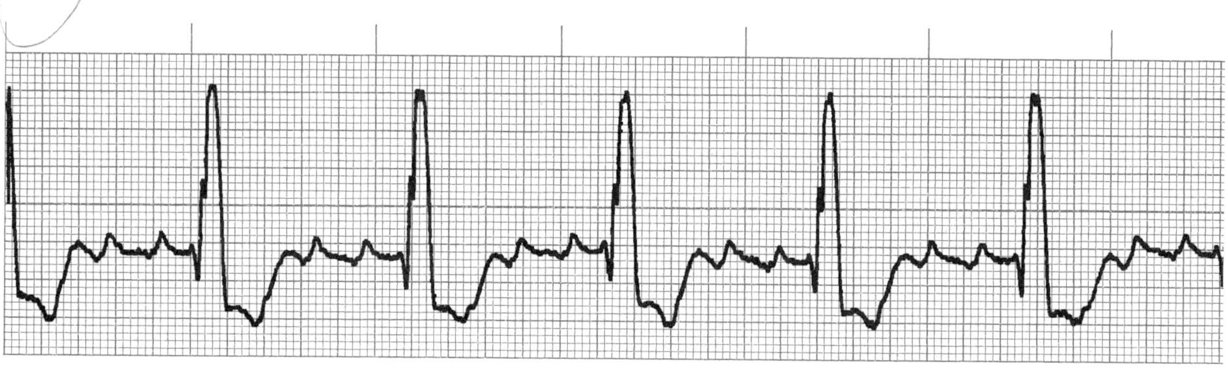

Regularity: _____ Heart rate: _____ PR interval: _____

P-waves: _____ QRS complex: _____

Interpretation: _____

Post-Test Questions

#121

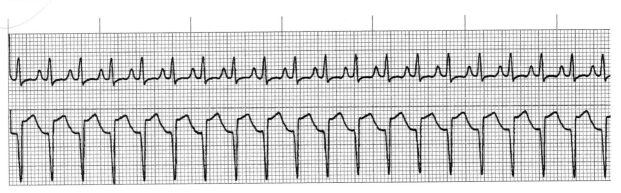

Regularity: _____ Heart rate: _____ PR interval: _____

P-waves: _____ QRS complex: _____

Interpretation: _____

#122

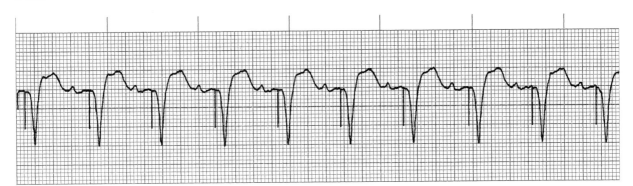

Regularity: _____ Heart rate: _____ PR interval: _____

P-waves: _____ QRS complex: _____

Interpretation: _____

#123

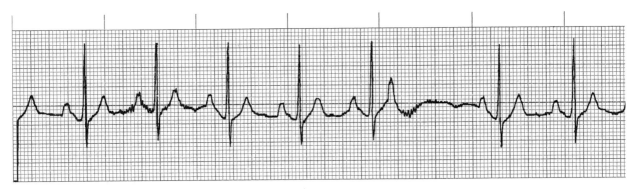

Regularity: _____ Heart rate: _____ PR interval: _____

P-waves: _____ QRS complex: _____

Interpretation: _____

#124

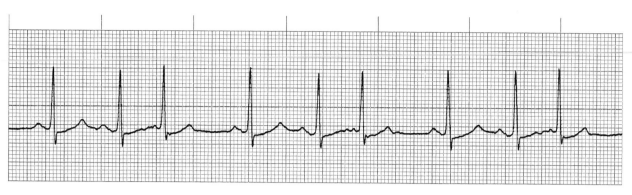

Regularity: _____ Heart rate: _____ PR interval: _____

P-waves: _____ QRS complex: _____

Interpretation: _____

#125

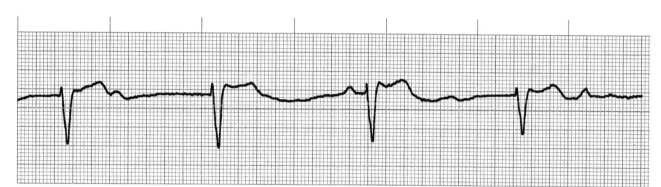

Regularity: _____ Heart rate: _____ PR interval: _____

P-waves: _____ QRS complex: _____

Interpretation: _____

#126

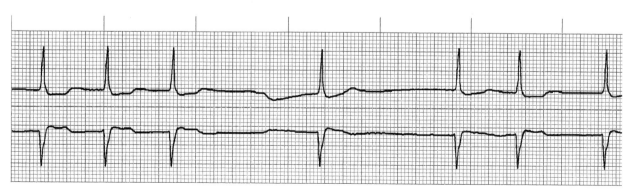

Regularity: _____ Heart rate: _____ PR interval: _____

P-waves: _____ QRS complex: _____

Interpretation: _____

#127

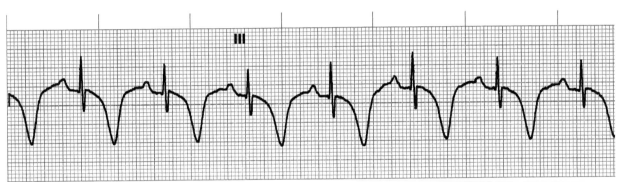

Regularity: _____ Heart rate: _____ PR interval: _____

P-waves: _____ QRS complex: _____

Interpretation: _____

#128

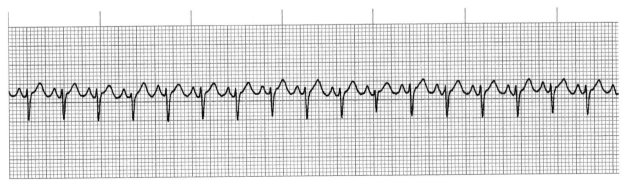

Regularity: _____ Heart rate: _____ PR interval: _____

P-waves: _____ QRS complex: _____

Interpretation: _____

#129

Regularity: _____ _____ Heart rate: _____ PR interval: _____

P-waves: _____ QRS complex: _____

Interpretation: _____

#130

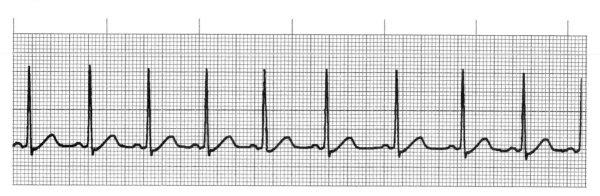

Regularity: _____ Heart rate: _____ PR interval: _____

P-waves: _____ QRS complex: _____

Interpretation: _____

#131

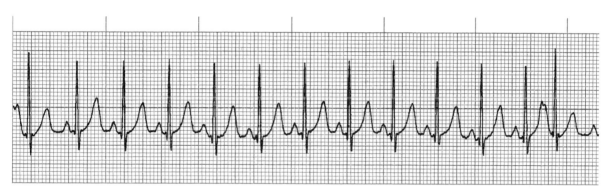

Regularity: _____ Heart rate: _____ PR interval: _____

P-waves: _____ QRS complex: _____

Interpretation: _____

#132

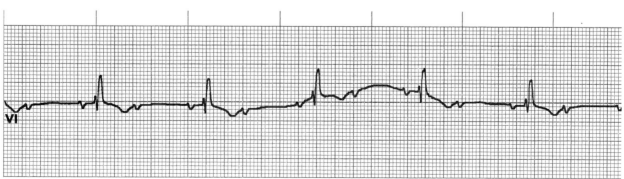

Regularity: _____ Heart rate: _____ PR interval: _____

P-waves: _____ QRS complex: _____

Interpretation: _____

Post-Test Questions

#133

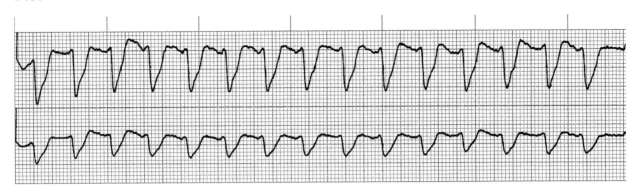

Regularity: _____ Heart rate: _____ PR interval: _____

P-waves: _____ QRS complex: _____

Interpretation: _____

#134

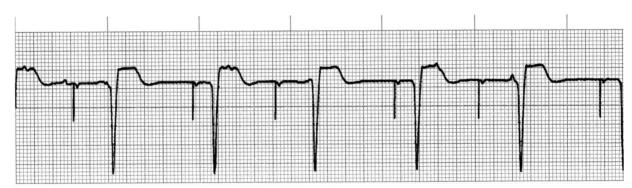

Regularity: _____ Heart rate: _____ PR interval: _____

P-waves: _____ QRS complex: _____

Interpretation: _____

#135

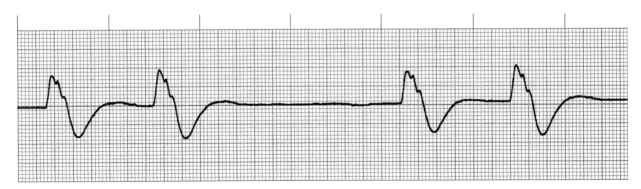

Regularity: _____ Heart rate: _____ PR interval: _____

P-waves: _____ QRS complex: _____

Interpretation: _____

#136

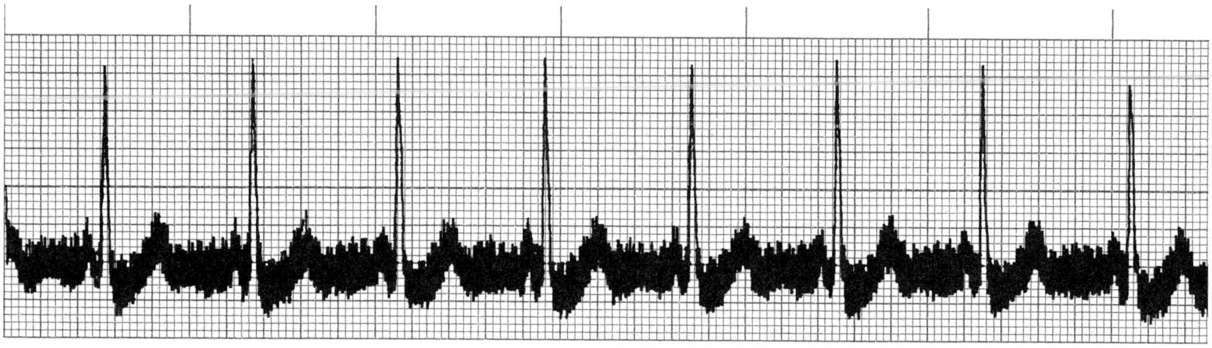

Regularity: _____ Heart rate: _____ PR interval: _____

P-waves: _____ QRS complex: _____

Interpretation: _____

#137

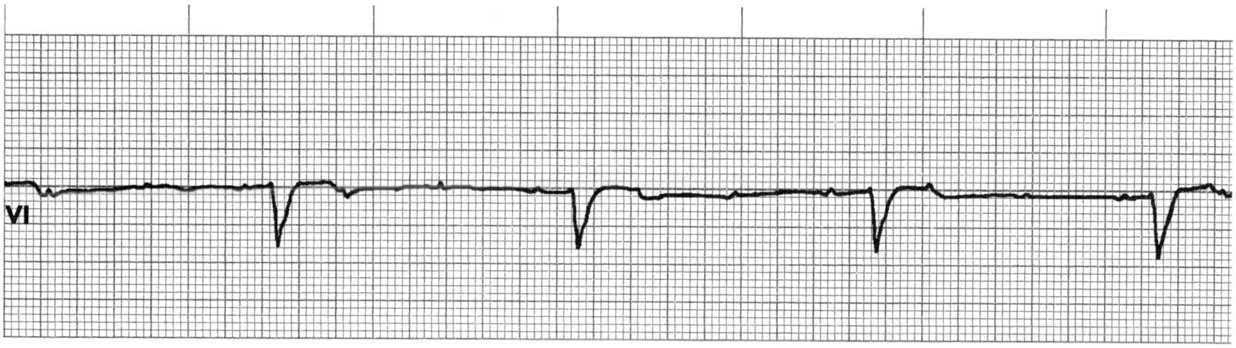

Regularity: _____ Heart rate: _____ PR interval: _____

P-waves: _____ QRS complex: _____

Interpretation: _____

#138

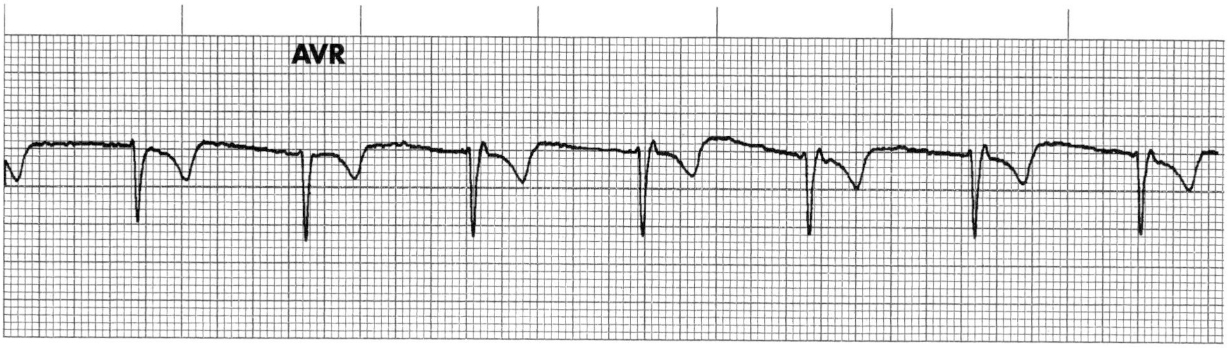

Regularity: _____ Heart rate: _____ PR interval: _____

P-waves: _____ QRS complex: _____

Interpretation: _____

#139

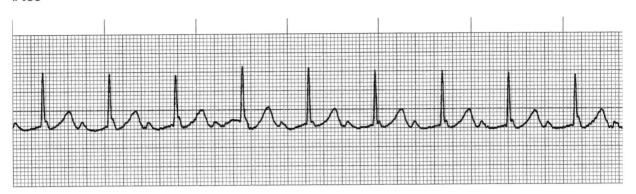

Regularity: _____ Heart rate: _____ PR interval: _____

P-waves: _____ QRS complex: _____

Interpretation: _____

#140

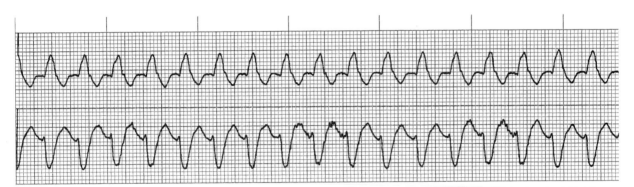

Regularity: _____ Heart rate: _____ PR interval: _____

P-waves: _____ QRS complex: _____

Interpretation: _____

#141

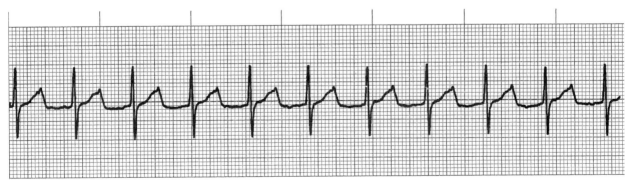

Regularity: _____ Heart rate: _____ PR interval: _____

P-waves: _____ QRS complex: _____

Interpretation: _____

#142

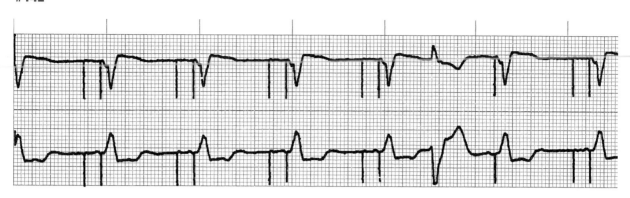

Regularity: _____ Heart rate: _____ PR interval: _____

P-waves: _____ QRS complex: _____

Interpretation: _____

#143

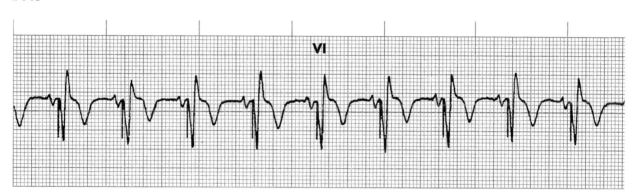

Regularity: _____ Heart rate: _____ PR interval: _____

P-waves: _____ QRS complex: _____

Interpretation: _____

#144

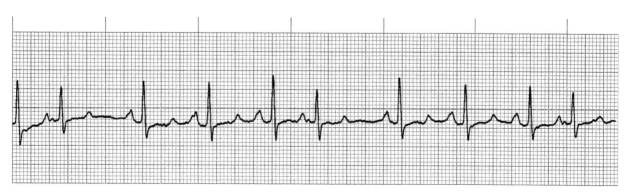

Regularity: _____ Heart rate: _____ PR interval: _____

P-waves: _____ QRS complex: _____

Interpretation: _____

#145

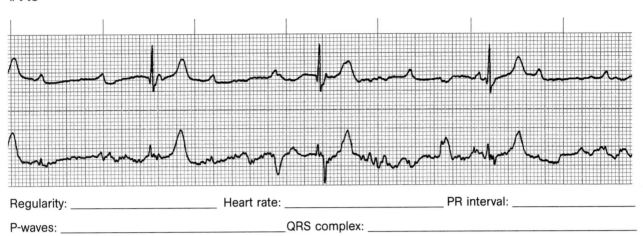

Regularity: _____ Heart rate: _____ PR interval: _____

P-waves: _____ QRS complex: _____

Interpretation: _____

#146

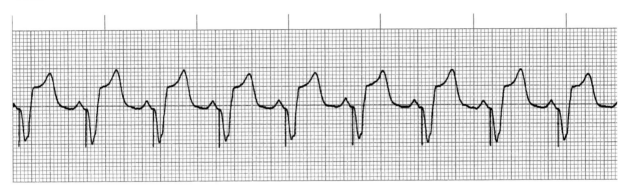

Regularity: _____ Heart rate: _____ PR interval: _____

P-waves: _____ QRS complex: _____

Interpretation: _____

#147

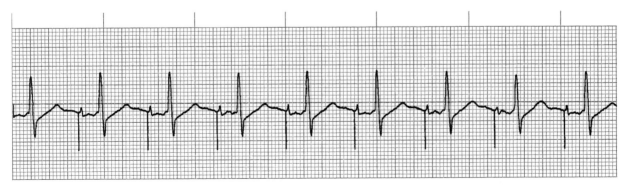

Regularity: _____ Heart rate: _____ PR interval: _____

P-waves: _____ QRS complex: _____

Interpretation: _____

#148

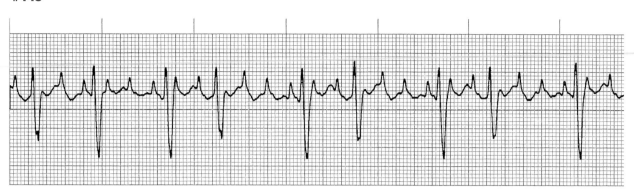

Regularity: _____ Heart rate: _____ PR interval: _____

P-waves: _____ QRS complex: _____

Interpretation: _____

#149

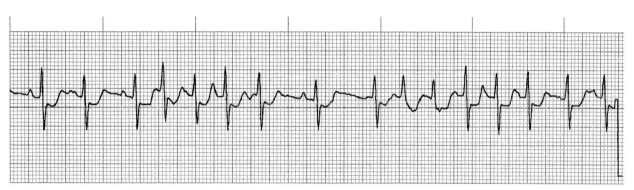

Regularity: _____ Heart rate: _____ PR interval: _____

P-waves: _____ QRS complex: _____

Interpretation: _____

#150

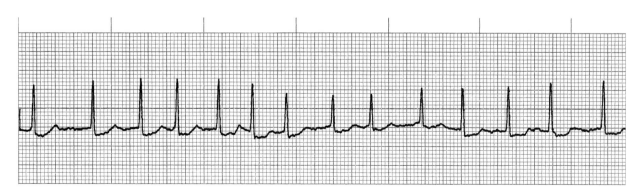

Regularity: _____ Heart rate: _____ PR interval: _____

P-waves: _____ QRS complex: _____

Interpretation: _____

Post-Test Questions

#151

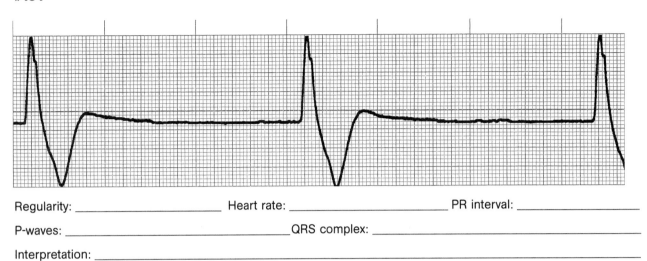

Regularity: _____ Heart rate: _____ PR interval: _____

P-waves: _____ QRS complex: _____

Interpretation: _____

#152

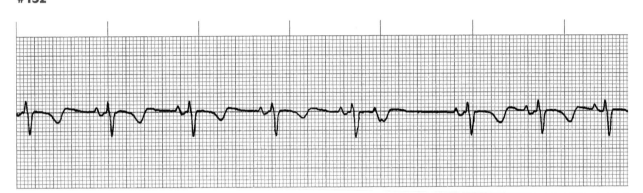

Regularity: _____ Heart rate: _____ PR interval: _____

P-waves: _____ QRS complex: _____

Interpretation: _____

#153

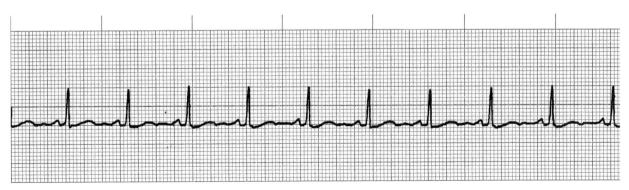

Regularity: _____ Heart rate: _____ PR interval: _____

P-waves: _____ QRS complex: _____

Interpretation: _____

#154

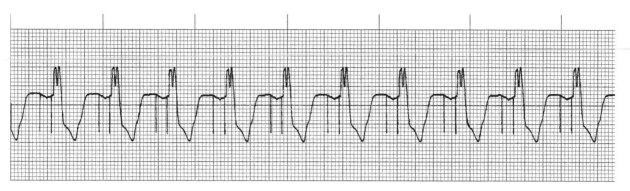

Regularity: _____ Heart rate: _____ PR interval: _____

P-waves: _____ QRS complex: _____

Interpretation: _____

#155

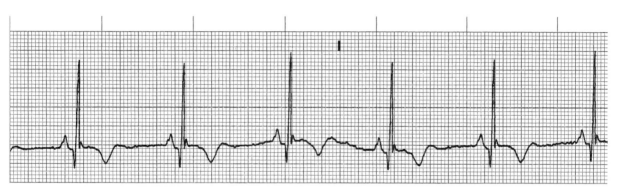

Regularity: _____ Heart rate: _____ PR interval: _____

P-waves: _____ QRS complex: _____

Interpretation: _____

#156

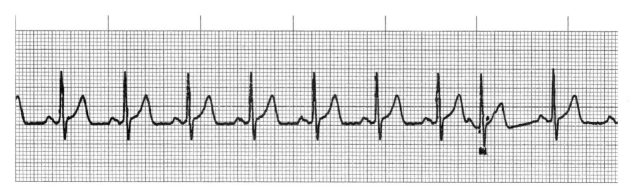

Regularity: _____ Heart rate: _____ PR interval: _____

P-waves: _____ QRS complex: _____

Interpretation: _____

#157

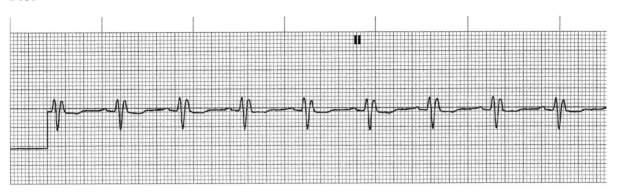

Regularity: _____ Heart rate: _____ PR interval: _____

P-waves: _____ QRS complex: _____

Interpretation: _____

#158

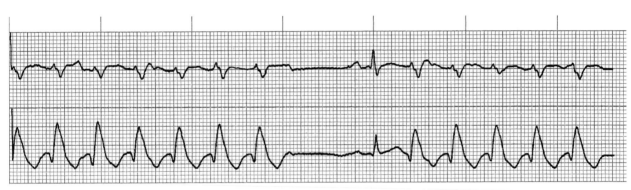

Regularity: _____ Heart rate: _____ PR interval: _____

P-waves: _____ QRS complex: _____

Interpretation: _____

#159

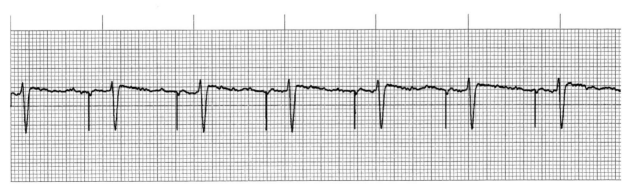

Regularity: _____ Heart rate: _____ PR interval: _____

P-waves: _____ QRS complex: _____

Interpretation: _____

#160

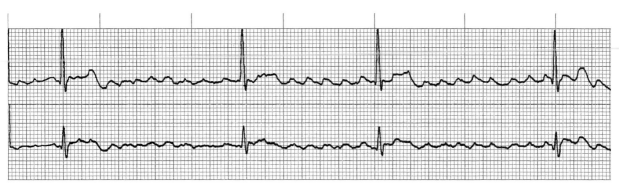

Regularity: _____ Heart rate: _____ PR interval: _____

P-waves: _____ QRS complex: _____

Interpretation: _____

#161

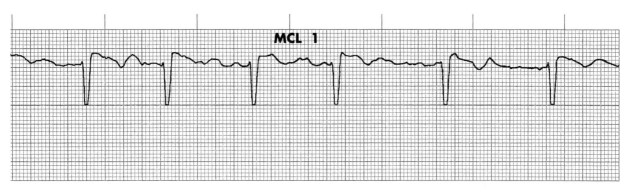

Regularity: _____ Heart rate: _____ PR interval: _____

P-waves: _____ QRS complex: _____

Interpretation: _____

#162

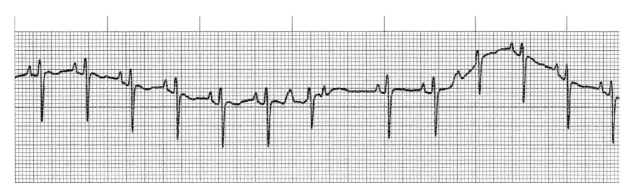

Regularity: _____ Heart rate: _____ PR interval: _____

P-waves: _____ QRS complex: _____

Interpretation: _____

#163

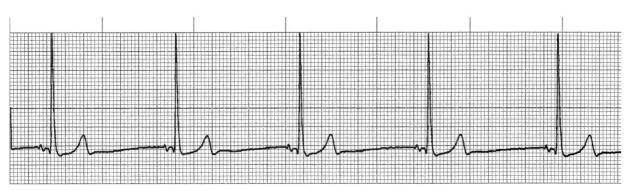

Regularity: _____ Heart rate: _____ PR interval: _____

P-waves: _____ QRS complex: _____

Interpretation: _____

#164

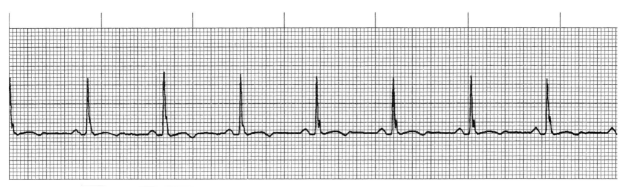

Regularity: _____ Heart rate: _____ PR interval: _____

P-waves: _____ QRS complex: _____

Interpretation: _____

#165

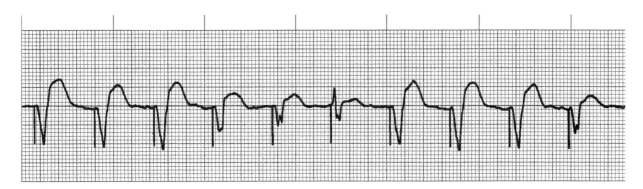

Regularity: _____ Heart rate: _____ PR interval: _____

P-waves: _____ QRS complex: _____

Interpretation: _____

#166

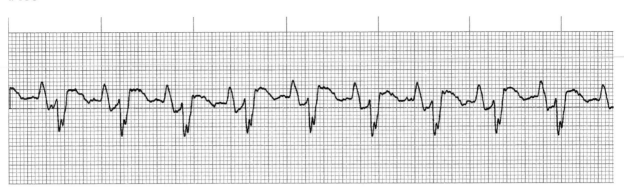

Regularity: _____ Heart rate: _____ PR interval: _____

P-waves: _____QRS complex: _____

Interpretation: _____

#167

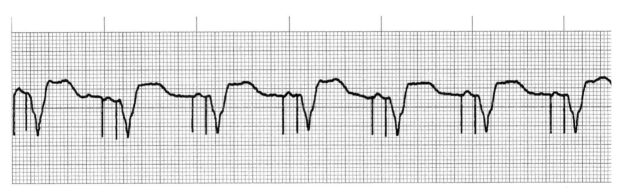

Regularity: _____ Heart rate: _____ PR interval: _____

P-waves: _____QRS complex: _____

Interpretation: _____

#168

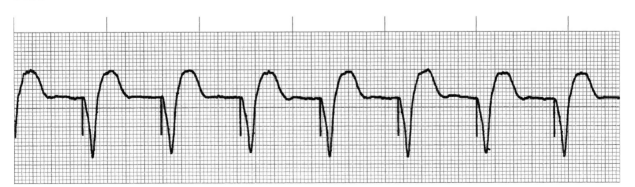

Regularity: _____ Heart rate: _____ PR interval: _____

P-waves: _____QRS complex: _____

Interpretation: _____

#169

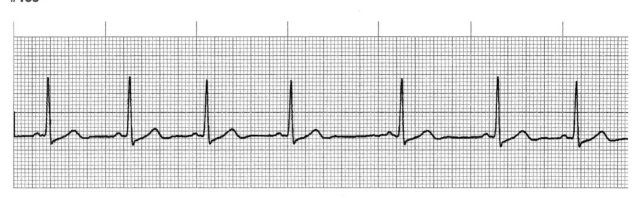

Regularity: _____ Heart rate: _____ PR interval: _____

P-waves: _____QRS complex: _____

Interpretation: _____

#170

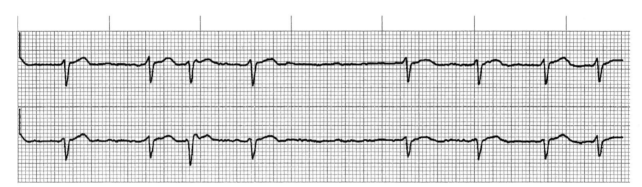

Regularity: _____ Heart rate: _____ PR interval: _____

P-waves: _____QRS complex: _____

Interpretation: _____

#171

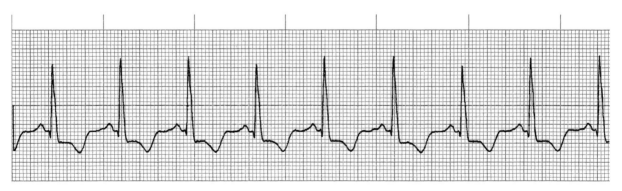

Regularity: _____ Heart rate: _____ PR interval: _____

P-waves: _____QRS complex: _____

Interpretation: _____

#172

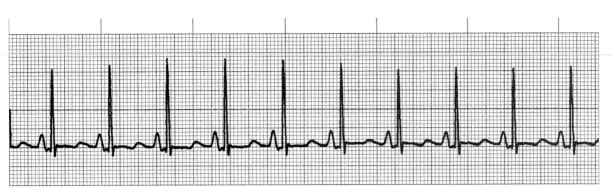

Regularity: _____ Heart rate: _____ PR interval: _____

P-waves: _____QRS complex: _____

Interpretation: _____

#173

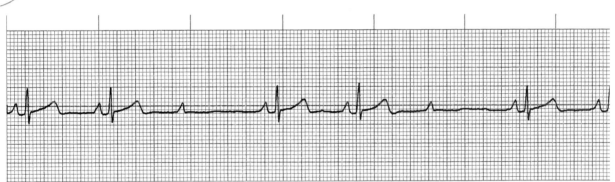

Regularity: _____ Heart rate: _____ PR interval: _____

P-waves: _____QRS complex: _____

Interpretation: _____

#174

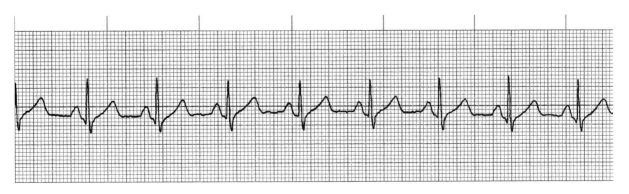

Regularity: _____ Heart rate: _____ PR interval: _____

P-waves: _____QRS complex: _____

Interpretation: _____

#175

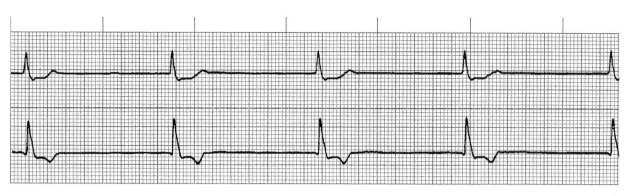

Regularity: _____ Heart rate: _____ PR interval: _____

P-waves: _____ QRS complex: _____

Interpretation: _____

#176

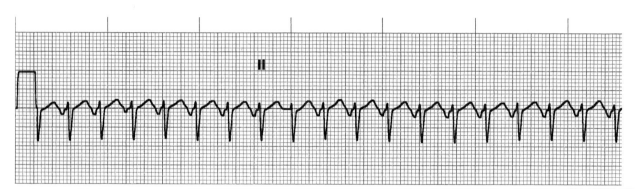

Regularity: _____ Heart rate: _____ PR interval: _____

P-waves: _____ QRS complex: _____

Interpretation: _____

#177

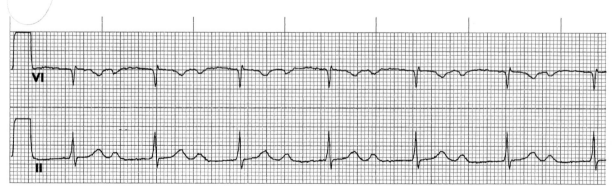

Regularity: _____ Heart rate: _____ PR interval: _____

P-waves: _____ QRS complex: _____

Interpretation: _____

#178

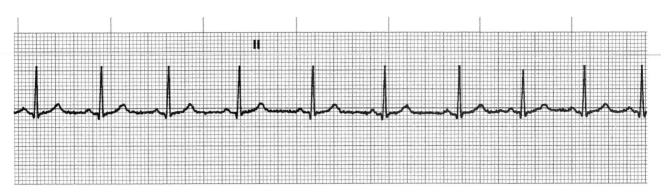

Regularity: _____ Heart rate: _____ PR interval: _____

P-waves: _____ QRS complex: _____

Interpretation: _____

#179

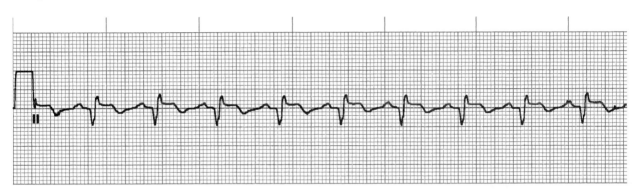

Regularity: _____ Heart rate: _____ PR interval: _____

P-waves: _____ QRS complex: _____

Interpretation: _____

#180

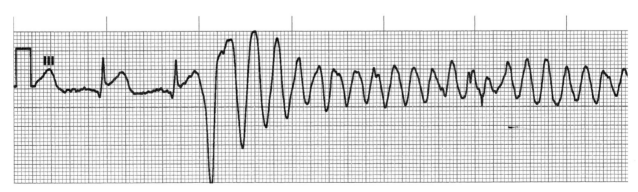

Regularity: _____ Heart rate: _____ PR interval: _____

P-waves: _____ QRS complex: _____

Interpretation: _____

#181

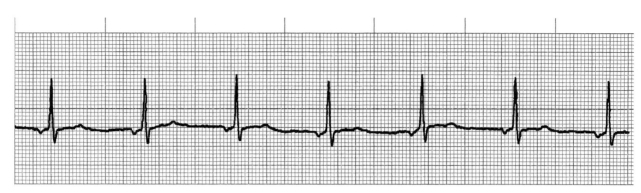

Regularity: _____ Heart rate: _____ PR interval: _____

P-waves: _____ QRS complex: _____

Interpretation: _____

#182

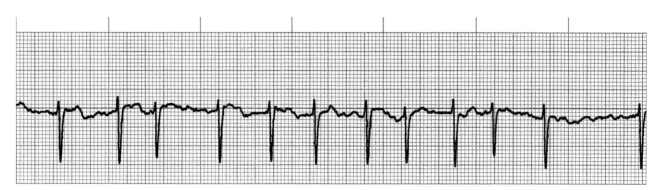

Regularity: _____ Heart rate: _____ PR interval: _____

P-waves: _____ QRS complex: _____

Interpretation: _____

#183

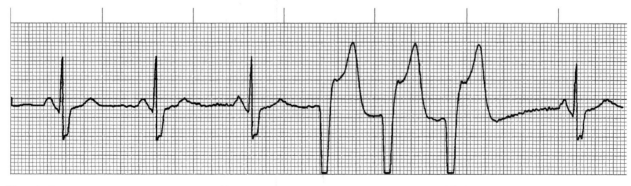

Regularity: _____ Heart rate: _____ PR interval: _____

P-waves: _____ QRS complex: _____

Interpretation: _____

#184

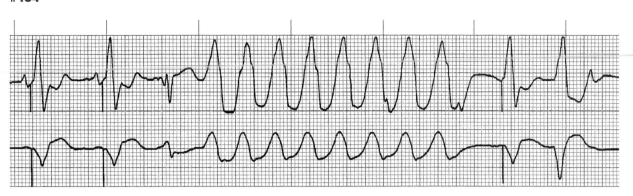

Regularity: _____ Heart rate: _____ PR interval: _____

P-waves: _____ QRS complex: _____

Interpretation: _____

#185

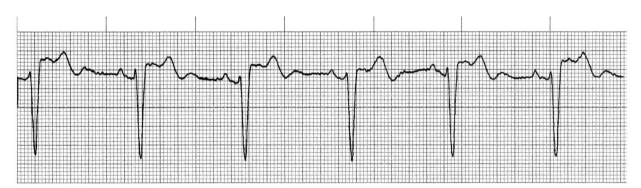

Regularity: _____ Heart rate: _____ PR interval: _____

P-waves: _____ QRS complex: _____

Interpretation: _____

#186

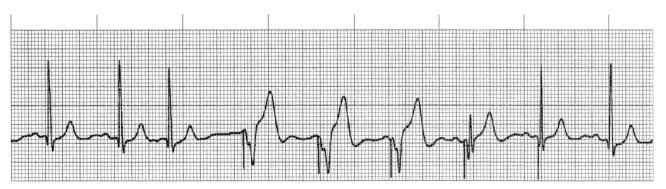

Regularity: _____ Heart rate: _____ PR interval: _____

P-waves: _____ QRS complex: _____

Interpretation: _____

#187

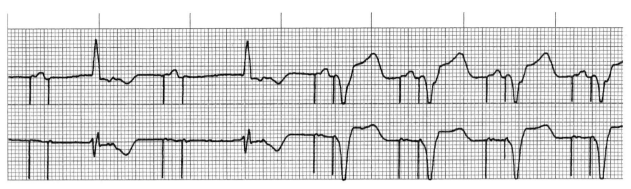

Regularity: _____ Heart rate: _____ PR interval: _____

P-waves: _____ QRS complex: _____

Interpretation: _____

#188

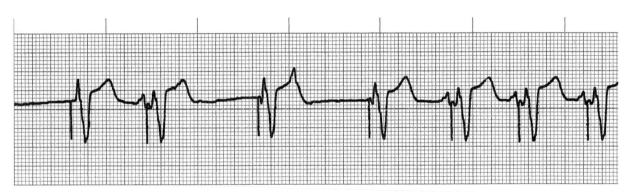

Regularity: _____ Heart rate: _____ PR interval: _____

P-waves: _____ QRS complex: _____

Interpretation: _____

#189

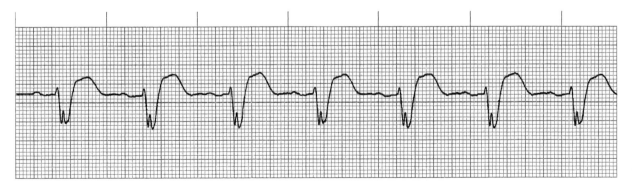

Regularity: _____ Heart rate: _____ PR interval: _____

P-waves: _____ QRS complex: _____

Interpretation: _____

#190

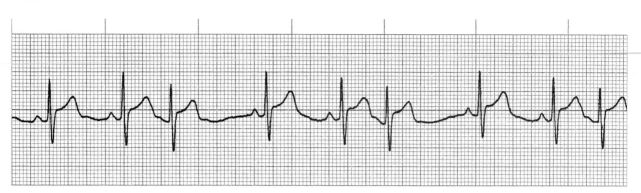

Regularity: _____ Heart rate: _____ PR interval: _____

P-waves: _____ QRS complex: _____

Interpretation: _____

#191

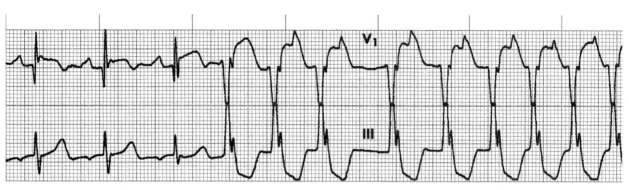

Regularity: _____ Heart rate: _____ PR interval: _____

P-waves: _____ QRS complex: _____

Interpretation: _____

#192

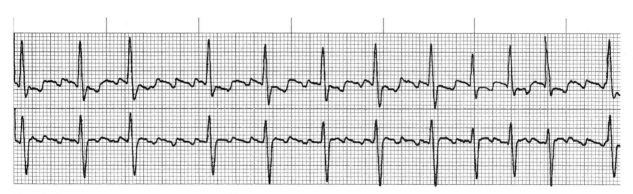

Regularity: _____ Heart rate: _____ PR interval: _____

P-waves: _____ QRS complex: _____

Interpretation: _____

#193

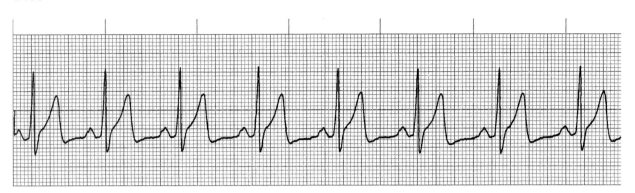

Regularity: _____ Heart rate: _____ PR interval: _____

P-waves: _____ QRS complex: _____

Interpretation: _____

#194

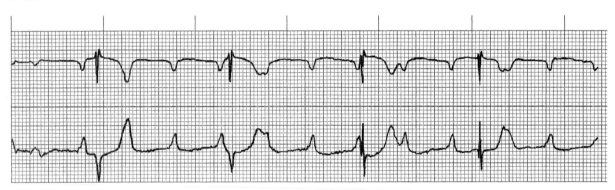

Regularity: _____ Heart rate: _____ PR interval: _____

P-waves: _____ QRS complex: _____

Interpretation: _____

#195

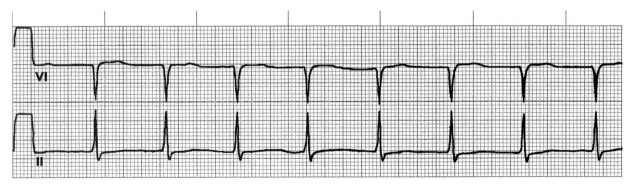

Regularity: _____ Heart rate: _____ PR interval: _____

P-waves: _____ QRS complex: _____

Interpretation: _____

#196

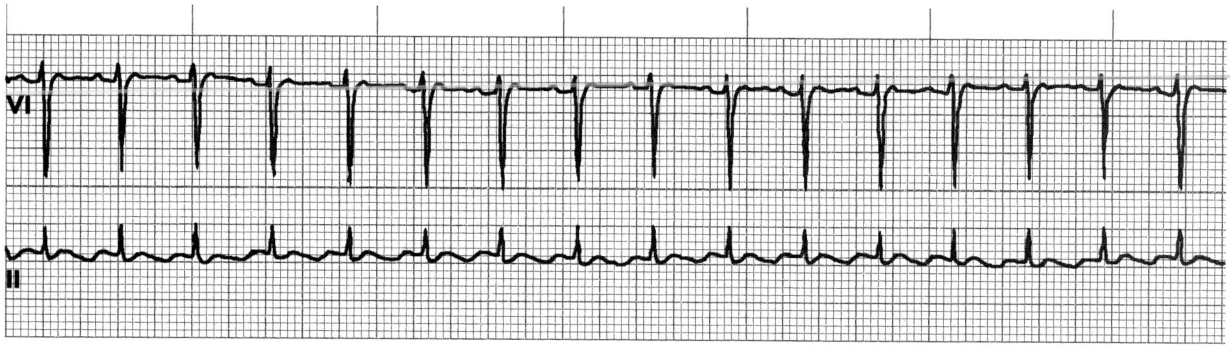

V1

II

Regularity: _____ Heart rate: _____ PR interval: _____

P-waves: _____ QRS complex: _____

Interpretation: _____

#197

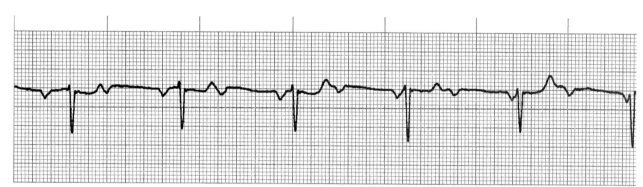

Regularity: _____ Heart rate: _____ PR interval: _____

P-waves: _____ QRS complex: _____

Interpretation: _____

#198

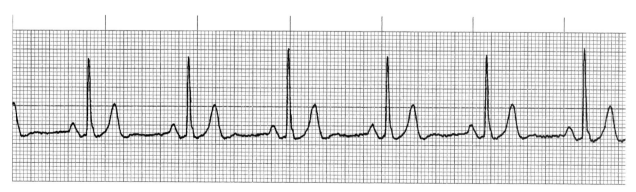

Regularity: _____ Heart rate: _____ PR interval: _____

P-waves: _____ QRS complex: _____

Interpretation: _____

Post-Test Questions

#199

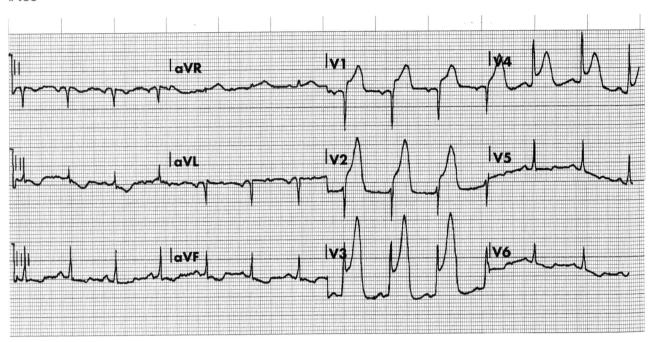

Regularity: _____ Heart rate: _____ PR interval: _____

P-waves: _____ QRS complex: _____

Interpretation: _____

#200

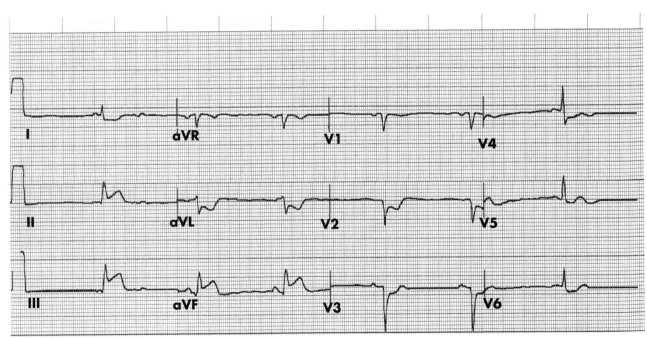

Regularity: _____ Heart rate: _____ PR interval: _____

P-waves: _____ QRS complex: _____

Interpretation: _____

Post-Test Answers

#1

Regularity: Regular except   Heart rate: 60 bpm (pacer rate: 90)

PR interval: 0.14 seconds

P-waves: Normal, all the same (pacemaker generated)

QRS complex: 0.12 seconds, all the same, pacemaker generated. The 3rd & 4th pacemaker P-waves have no QRS after them. Then there is a natural QRS (with no P-wave in front of it).

Interpretation: 100% AV sequential pacing with occasional ventricular noncapture and a junction escape beat (3rd QRS complex)

#2

Regularity: Irregular   Heart rate: atrial: 79 bpm, ventricular: 50 bpm

PR interval: Varies

P-waves: Normal, all the same, regular

QRS complex: 0.06 seconds, all the same, irregular

Interpretation: Sinus rhythm with 2nd degree AV block, type I

#3

Regularity: Irregular   Heart rate: 40 bpm

PR interval: 0.14 seconds

P-waves: Normal, all the same except the 3rd one which is inverted and has a short PR Interval

QRS complex: 0.08 seconds

Interpretation: Sinus bradycardia with sinus arrest or exit block (the junctional escape beat makes determination impossible) and junctional escape beat (3rd QRS complex)

#4

Regularity: Regular   Heart rate: 52 bpm

PR interval: Not measurable

P-waves: Inverted, occurring after QRS, deforming T-wave

QRS complex: 0.06 seconds, all the same, regular

Interpretation: Junctional rhythm

#5

Regularity: Regular   Heart rate: 103 bpm

PR interval: 0.12 seconds

P-waves: Normal, all the same

QRS complex: 0.12 seconds, all the same

Interpretation: Sinus tachycardia with bundle branch block

#6

Regularity: Regular   Heart rate: 107

PR interval: 0.16 seconds

P-waves: Normal, all the same

QRS complex: 0.14 seconds, all pacemaker generated

Interpretation: Sinus tachycardia with 100% ventricular pacing

Post-Test Answers

#7

Regularity: Irregular   Heart rate: Not measurable

PR interval: Not measurable

P-waves: None seen

QRS complex: Varies but all are wide

Interpretation: Atrial fibrillation with bundle branch block and PVCs with ventricular pacing without capture or sensing and R-on-T (near middle of strip) that causes ventricular fibrillation

#8

Regularity: Regular   Heart rate: 60 bpm

PR interval: Not measurable

P-waves: Normal, all the same (some buried in QRS complex or T-wave)

QRS complex: 0.18 seconds, all the same

Interpretation: Sinus rhythm with 3rd degree AV block and 100% ventricular pacing

#9

Regularity: Irregularly irregular   Heart rate: 80 bpm

PR interval: Not measurable

P-waves: None seen (wavy baseline)

QRS complex: 0.12 seconds

Interpretation: Atrial fibrillation with bundle branch block

#10

Regularity: Irregularly irregular   Heart rate: 60 bpm

PR interval: Not measurable

P-waves: None seen (wavy baseline)

QRS complex: Varies

Interpretation: Atrial fibrillation with 70% ventricular pacing and pseudofusion beat (5th beat)

#11

Regularity: Regular   Heart rate: 150 bpm

PR interval: Not clearly measurable because P-wave buried in preceding T-wave, but appears to be normal

P-waves: Peaked and buried in T-waves, regular, all the same

QRS complex: 0.06 seconds, all the same

Interpretation: Sinus tachycardia

#12

Regularity: Regular   Heart rate: 136 bpm

PR interval: 0.14 seconds

P-waves: Regular, all the same

QRS complex: 0.08 seconds, all the same

Interpretation: Sinus rhythm with inverted T-waves (abnormal)

#13

Regularity: Regular   Heart rate: 86 bpm

PR interval: 0.34 seconds

P-waves: All the same

QRS complex: 0.08 seconds

Interpretation: Sinus rhythm with 1st degree AV block

#14

Regularity: No complexes seen   Heart rate: 0 bpm

PR interval: Not measurable

P-waves: None seen

QRS complex: None seen

Interpretation: Asystole, 100% AV pacing with noncapture and nonsensing with chest compression artifact (confirmed in two leads) chest compression rate ~50 per minute, well below ANA recommendations

#15

Regularity: Irregularly irregular   Heart rate: Not measurable

PR interval: Not measurable

P-waves: None seen

QRS complex: None seen (wavy baseline), confirmed in two leads

Interpretation: Coarse ventricular fibrillation (confirm by checking pulse)

#16

Regularity: Regular   Heart rate: 143 bpm

PR interval: Not measurable

P-waves: P-wave obscured by somatic artifact

QRS complex: 0.08 seconds, all the same

Interpretation: Sinus rhythm with respiratory and somatic artifact, most likely respiratory due to loose lead (most prominent in bottom tracing)

#17

Regularity: Regular   Heart rate: 83 bpm

PR interval: 0.10 seconds

P-waves: Inverted (abnormal in this lead)

QRS complex: 0.10 seconds

Interpretation: Accelerated junctional rhythm

#18

Regularity: Regular except   Heart rate: 73 bpm

PR interval: 0.18 seconds

P-waves: Double-humped, all the same except the last beat

QRS complex: 0.08 seconds

Interpretation: Sinus rhythm with PAC (2nd to last beat) and prominent U-wave

#19

Regularity: Regular except   Heart rate: Atrial, 79 bpm; ventricular, 60 bpm

PR interval: 0.16 seconds

P-waves: Regular, all the same

QRS complex: 0.10 seconds, all the same, missing after 3rd and 6th P-waves

Interpretation: Sinus rhythm with 2nd degree AV block type II

#20

Regularity: Regular except   Heart rate: 77 bpm

PR interval: 0.16 seconds

P-waves: Notched, all the same except the premature beats

QRS complex: 0.06 seconds

Interpretation: Sinus rhythm with PAC (4th beat) and PJC (6th beat)

Post-Test Answers

#21
Regularity: Regular   Heart rate: 56 bpm
PR interval: Not measurable
P-waves: None seen
QRS complex: 0.06 seconds, all the same
Interpretation: Junctional rhythm

#22
Regularity: Regular except   Heart rate: 1st rhythm, atrial, 300 bpm; ventricular, 150 bpm;
PR interval: Not measurable   2nd rhythm, ventricular, 300 bpm
P-waves: All the same
QRS complex: 1st rhythm all the same, then varies in second rhythm
Interpretation: Atrial flutter (note the two consecutive F-waves visible after the first run on V-tach) with 2:1 AV block and
R-on-T PVCs generating self-terminating runs of ventricular tachycardia (these PVCs require treatment!)

#23
Regularity: Regular   Heart rate: 71 bpm
PR interval: 0.18 seconds
P-waves: All the same
QRS complex: 0.14 seconds, wide, all the same
Interpretation: Sinus rhythm with bundle branch block

#24
Regularity: Regular except   Heart rate: 90 bpm
PR interval: 0.18 seconds (best seen just after the PVCs)
P-waves: All the same
QRS complex: 0.10 seconds, all the same, except 2nd, 5th, and 8th beats
Interpretation: Sinus rhythm with unifocal trigeminal PVCs

#25
Regularity: Irregularly irregular   Heart rate: Not measurable
PR interval: Not measurable
P-waves: None seen
QRS complex: None seen (wavy baseline)
Interpretation: Coarse ventricular fibrillation (confirmed in two leads) and possible chest compression artifact best
seen in bottom lead.

#26
Regularity: Regular except   First: Heart rate: 63 bpm, second 136 bpm
PR interval: 0.14 seconds
P-waves: All the same
QRS complex: 0.14 seconds
Interpretation: Sinus rhythm with bundle branch block and four-beat run of unifocal ventricular tachycardia

#27
Regularity: Regular   Heart rate: 158 bpm
PR interval: Not measurable
P-waves: None seen
QRS complex: 0.14 seconds, all the same
Interpretation: Ventricular tachycardia (note retrograde P-waves at the end of some of the QRS complexes) with pacer
spikes and failure to capture (possibly nonsensing if ventricular pacemaker, but may not be if atrial pacemaker)

#28

Regularity: Regular   Heart rate: 71 bpm

PR interval: Difficult to determine

P-waves: Difficult to identify

QRS complex: 0.14 seconds

Interpretation: 100% ventricular pacing. Somatic artifact on the baseline with the gain level set too high (causing the flat-topping of the QRS complexes). Underlying rhythm is probably some type of sinus rhythm with AV dissociation, but because of the artifact, it is difficult to identify clearly.

#29

Regularity: None   Heart rate: None

PR interval: Not measurable

P-waves: None seen

QRS complex: None seen

Interpretation: Asystole (confirmed in two leads)

#30

Regularity: Irregularly irregular   Heart rate: 80 bpm

PR interval: 0.12 seconds

P-waves: All the same except 2nd beat

QRS complex: Varies

Interpretation: Sinus rhythm with atrial escape beat (2nd QRS complex), fusion beat (5th QRS complex), and accelerated idioventricular rhythm (last four QRS complexes)

#31

Regularity: Irregularly irregular   Heart rate: 180 bpm (1st rhythm varies, 2nd rhythm, 83 bpm)

PR interval: Not measurable

P-waves: None seen

QRS complex: Varies

Interpretation: Multifocal ventricular tachycardia (Torsades de pointes?) that self-terminates and is replaced by accelerated junctional rhythm

#32

Regularity: Regular   Heart rate: 107 bpm

PR interval: 0.08 seconds

P-waves: All the same

QRS complex: 0.16 seconds, all the same

Interpretation: Sinus tachycardia with 100% AV sequential pacing

#33

Regularity: Regular except   Heart rate: 50 bpm

PR interval: 0.16 seconds

P-waves: Normal, all the same except premature beats (2nd and 6th beats)

QRS complex: 0.08 seconds

Interpretation: Sinus bradycardia with PJCs

Post-Test Answers

#34

Regularity: Irregularly irregular   Heart rate: Atrial, 86 bpm; Ventricular, 30 bpm

PR interval: 0.20 seconds

P-waves: Regular, all the same

QRS complex: 0.12 seconds, wide, varying

Interpretation: Sinus rhythm with high-grade 2nd degree AV block (type II) with bundle branch block (switches
depending on which bundle branch is blocked) progressing to ventricular asystole

#35

Regularity: Regular   Heart rate: 71 bpm

PR interval: 0.26 seconds

P-waves: Regular, all the same

QRS complex: 0.08 seconds, all the same

Interpretation: Sinus rhythm with 1st degree AV block

#36

Regularity: Regular   Heart rate: 71 bpm

PR interval: Not measurable

P-waves: None seen

QRS complex: 0.16 seconds

Interpretation: 100% ventricular pacing

#37

Regularity: Regularly irregular   Heart rate: 70 bpm

PR interval: Varies

P-waves: Regular, notched, all the same

QRS complex: 0.06 seconds, all the same

Interpretation: Sinus rhythm with 2nd degree AV block type I (Wenckebach)

#38

Regularity: Regular except   Heart rate: 80 bpm

PR interval: 0.16 seconds

P-waves: Regular and all the same except one before 8th QRS complex

QRS complex: 0.08 seconds, all the same except the 3rd QRS complex

Interpretation: Sinus rhythm with PAC (7th beat) and PVC (3rd beat)

#39

Regularity: Regular except   Heart rate: 76 bpm

PR interval: 0.12 seconds

P-waves: Regular, all the same

QRS complex: Every other one is the same with 0.06 seconds, others are all different but wide and bizarre

Interpretation: Sinus rhythm with bigeminal, multifocal PVCs

#40

Regularity: Regular except   Heart rate: 60 bpm

PR interval: 0.26 seconds

P-waves: Regular, all the same except first one after the pause, which is inverted (there may be one at the very end of
the 3rd T-wave)

QRS complex: 0.10 seconds

Interpretation: Sinus rhythm with a 1st degree AV Block and pause (probably a blocked PAC after the 3rd QRS complex
note the "blip" at the end of the T-wave), followed by a junctional escape beat and returning to sinus rhythm again

#41

Regularity: Regular except   Heart rate: 70 bpm
PR interval: 0.22 seconds
P-waves: Regular, all the same
QRS complex: 0.10 seconds, all the same except 1st, 4th, and 7th
Interpretation: Sinus rhythm with 1st degree AV block and unifocal trigeminal PVCs

#42

Regularity: Regular except   Heart rate: Atrial, 67 bpm; ventricular, 50 bpm
PR interval: 0.20 seconds
P-waves: Regular, all the same
QRS complex: 0.08 seconds
Interpretation: Sinus rhythm (remember, the P-wave rate determines rhythm name) with 2nd degree AV block type II

#43

Regularity: Regular   Heart rate: 75 bpm
PR interval: 0.16 seconds
P-waves: Regular, all the same
QRS complex: 0.08 seconds, all the same
Interpretation: Sinus rhythm with inverted T-waves

#44

Regularity: Regular   Heart rate: 64 bpm
PR interval: Not measurable
P-waves: None seen
QRS complex: 0.10 seconds
Interpretation: Accelerated junctional rhythm (with elevated J-point, not true ST segment elevation)

#45

Regularity: Regular   Heart rate: 81 bpm
PR interval: 0.24 seconds
P-waves: Regular, notched (some obscured by baseline artifact)
QRS complex: 0.10 seconds, all the same
Interpretation: Sinus rhythm with possible inferior wall MI (note deep Q-wave that is more than one-third the QRS
    height in lead III and wider than one small box and slight ST-segment elevation)

#46

Regularity: Regular   Heart rate: 94 bpm
PR interval: Not measurable
P-waves: None seen, probably obscured by artifact
QRS complex: Appear normal, but can't measure due to artifact
Interpretation: Sinus rhythm (assumed from regularity) with significant baseline artifact. (In fact, this strip came from
    a patient on a chest percussion vest to loosen respiratory secretions. The sharp artifact is due to the repeated
    rhythmic motion of the vest. The patient was indeed in sinus rhythm, notice the interruptions to the regular artifact;
    these are the real QRS complexes.

Post-Test Answers

#47
Regularity: Regular except   Heart rate: 100 bpm
PR interval: 0.12 seconds
P-waves: Regular, all the same
QRS complex: 0.06 seconds, all the same except every 4th and 8th QRS complex
Interpretation: Sinus tachycardia with unifocal quadrigeminal PVCs

#48
Regularity: Regular   Heart rate: Atrial, 300 bpm; ventricular, 79 bpm
PR interval: Not measurable
P-waves: Multiple with each QRS complex, all the same
QRS complex: 0.06 seconds, all the same
Interpretation: Atrial flutter with 4:1 AV block

#49
Regularity: Regular   Heart rate: 86 bpm
PR interval: 0.42 seconds
P-waves: Peaked and taller than 2.5 mm, regular, all the same
QRS complex: 0.06 seconds, all the same
Interpretation: Sinus rhythm with 1st degree AV block

#50
Regularity: Regular   Heart rate: 65 bpm
PR interval: 0.14 seconds
P-waves: Regular, all the same
QRS complex: 0.06 seconds, all the same
Interpretation: Sinus rhythm with peaked T-waves (this dialysis patient had a potassium level of 7.2)

#51
Regularity: Regular   Heart rate: 70 bpm
PR interval: 0.16 seconds
P-waves: Regular, all the same
QRS complex: 0.06 seconds, all the same
Interpretation: Sinus rhythm with deeply inverted T-waves (suggests ischemia)

#52
Regularity: Regular except   Heart rate: 50 bpm
PR interval: 0.20 seconds
P-waves: Notched, regular, all the same except 4th beat
QRS complex: 0.08 seconds, all the same
Interpretation: Sinus bradycardia with PAC (4th beat)

#53
Regularity: Regular except   Heart rate: 70 bpm
PR interval: Not measurable
P-waves: None seen
QRS complex: 0.20 seconds, wide, all the same
Interpretation: 70% ventricular paced at 70 ppm, with unifocal trigeminal PVCs

#54

Regularity: Irregularly irregular   Heart rate: Atrial: 83 bpm, ventricular: 60 bpm
PR interval: Varies
P-waves: Regular, all the same
QRS complex: 0.08 seconds, all the same
Interpretation: Sinus rhythm with 2nd degree AV block type I (Wenckebach)

#55

Regularity: Regular   Heart rate: 88 bpm
PR interval: 0.16 seconds
P-waves: Regular, all the same
QRS complex: 0.10 seconds, all the same
Interpretation: Sinus rhythm with long QT interval (T-wave extends past halfway point to the next QRS complex QTc)

#56

Regularity: Regular   Heart rate: 115 bpm
PR interval: 0.22 seconds
P-waves: Regular, all the same
QRS complex: 0.08 seconds, all the same
Interpretation: Sinus tachycardia with 1st degree AV Block

#57

Regularity: Regular   Heart rate: Atrial, 88 bpm; ventricular, 44 bpm
PR interval: 0.24 seconds
P-waves: Regular, all the same, more than 1 per QRS complex
QRS complex: 0.08 seconds, all the same
Interpretation: Sinus rhythm with 2nd degree AV block (type II confirmed by a prior tracing) progressing to ventricular
   asystole

#58

Regularity: Irregularly irregular   Heart rate: 280 bpm
PR interval: Not measurable
P-waves: None seen
QRS complex: Varies
Interpretation: Multifocal ventricular tachycardia (Torsades de pointes)

#59

Regularity: Regular   Heart rate: 75 bpm
PR interval: 0.18 seconds
P-waves: Regular, all the same (accounting for baseline artifact), easiest to see at the beginning and end of the tracing
QRS complex: 0.06 seconds, all the same
Interpretation: Sinus rhythm with somatic artifact

#60

Regularity: Regular   Heart rate: 167 bpm
PR interval: 0.12 seconds
P-waves: Regular, all the same, inverted in lead II (abnormal)
QRS complex: 0.08 seconds, all the same
Interpretation: Atrial tachycardia (abnormal P-waves and heart rate over the 160-bpm threshold), but could be sinus
   tachycardia

Post-Test Answers

#61
Regularity: Slightly irregularly irregular   Heart rate: 80 bpm
PR interval: Varies
P-waves: Slightly irregular, more than three forms noted on tracing (1st, 2nd, 4th, 5th, and 6th)
QRS complex: 0.08 seconds, all the same
Interpretation: Wandering atrial pacemaker

#62
Regularity: Regular except   Heart rate: 100 bpm
PR interval: 0.16 seconds
P-waves: Regular, all the same except 4th and 5th beats
QRS complex: 0.06 seconds, all the same
Interpretation: Sinus tachycardia with PAC (4th beat) and atrial escape beat (5th beat)

#63
Regularity: Irregularly irregular   Heart rate: 140 bpm
PR interval: Not measurable
P-waves: None seen (wavy baseline)
QRS complex: 0.06 seconds, all the same
Interpretation: Atrial fibrillation with a rapid ventricular response (heart rate range, 100 to 167 bpm)

#64
Regularity: Irregularly irregular   Heart rate: 120 bpm
PR interval: Varies
P-waves: Irregular, more than three forms on tracing
QRS complex: 0.12 seconds, all the same
Interpretation: Multifocal atrial tachycardia with bundle branch block

#65
Regularity: Regular   Heart rate: 214 bpm
PR interval: Not measurable
P-waves: None seen (may be obscured due to high heart rate)
QRS complex: 0.08 seconds, all the same
Interpretation: SVT of unknown etiology. Rate precludes identifying P-wave presence or absence. (Obtain 12-lead ECG to help identify rhythm.)

#66
Regularity: Regular   Heart rate: 50 bpm
PR interval: 0.14 seconds
P-waves: Regular, biphasic (abnormal for this lead), all the same
QRS complex: 0.06 seconds, all the same
Interpretation: Ectopic atrial pacemaker

#67
Regularity: Regular   Heart rate: 70 bpm
PR interval: 0.10 seconds
P-waves: Regular, all the same, pacemaker generated
QRS complex: 0.12 seconds, all the same
Interpretation: 100% atrial pacing with bundle branch block

#68

Regularity: Regular   Heart rate: 70 bpm

PR interval: 0.16 seconds

P-waves: Regular, all the same

QRS complex: 0.14 seconds, all the same

Interpretation: Sinus rhythm with 100% ventricular pacing

#69

Regularity: Irregularly irregular   Heart rate: 90 bpm

PR interval: Not measurable

P-waves: None seen (wavy baseline)

QRS complex: 0.06 seconds, all the same

Interpretation: Atrial fibrillation (heart rate range, 63 to 115 bpm)

#70

Regularity: Regular except   Heart rate: Atrial, 91 bpm; ventricular, 70 bpm

PR interval: Varies

P-waves: Regular, all the same

QRS complex: 0.14 seconds, all the same except 5th and 9th beats

Interpretation: Sinus rhythm with 3rd degree AV block and accelerated idioventricular rhythm with occasional unifocal
   PVCs (5th and 9th beats)

#71

Regularity: Regularly irregular   Heart rate: 60 bpm

PR interval: 0.12 seconds

P-waves: Irregular, all the same

QRS complex: 0.08 seconds

Interpretation: Sinus arrhythmia

#72

Regularity: Irregularly irregular   Heart rate: 40 bpm

PR interval: Not measurable

P-waves: None seen

QRS complex: 0.10 seconds, all the same

Interpretation: Atrial fibrillation with slow ventricular response (heart rate range, 24 to 70 bpm)

#73

Regularity: None   Heart rate: None

PR interval: Not measurable

P-waves: None seen

QRS complex: None seen

Interpretation: Asystole confirmed in two leads; do pulse check

Post-Test Answers

#74

Regularity: Two different rhythms, first irregular, second appears regular

Heart rate: First, 160 bpm; second, 240 bpm

PR interval: Not measurable

P-waves: None seen

QRS complex: First rhythm, 0.08 seconds, all the same; second rhythm, 0.12 seconds, all the same

Interpretation: Atrial fibrillation with BBB and rapid ventricular response with a fusion beat (middle of strip 9th QRS complex) converting to unifocal ventricular tachycardia

#75

Regularity: Regular except   Heart rate: 80 bpm

PR interval: 0.12 seconds

P-waves: Regular, all the same except those after the 3rd and 6th QRS complexes

QRS complex: 0.12 seconds, all the same except 1st and 4th

Interpretation: Sinus rhythm with BBB and blocked PACs (after the 3rd and 6th QRS complexes) and ventricular escape beats (1st, 4th, and 7th beats)

#76

Regularity: Regular except   Heart rate: 46 bpm

PR interval: 0

P-waves: None

QRS complex: First four the same, wide

Interpretation: 100% ventricular pacing with noncapture and nonsensing (noted after the 2nd QRS complex) and ventricular escape rhythm

#77

Regularity: Regular   Heart rate: 79

PR interval: 0.18 seconds

P-waves: Small, but all the same

QRS complex: Wide, but all the same

Interpretation: 100% atrial pacing with bundle branch block

#78

Regularity: Regular   Heart rate: 83 bpm

PR interval: 0.10 seconds

P-waves: Normal, all the same

QRS complex: 0.14 seconds, wide, all the same

Interpretation: Sinus rhythm with 100% ventricular pacing

#79

Regularity: Regular except (the first three complexes are irregular)   Heart rate: 80 bpm

PR interval: 0.16 seconds

P-waves: Inverted (normal for this lead)

QRS complex: 0.06 seconds (except 1st and 3rd beats)

Interpretation: Sinus rhythm with ventricular pacing (with nonsensing 2nd paced QRS, and noncapture 3rd, 5th and 6th pacer spikes) 6th QRS is a fusion beat.

#80

Regularity: Regular except   Heart rate: Atrial, 83 bpm; ventricular, 60 bpm

PR interval: 0.14 seconds

P-waves: Regular, all the same

QRS complex: 0.08 seconds, all the same

Interpretation: Sinus rhythm with 2nd degree AV block type II

#81

Regularity: Slightly irregular   Heart rate: 70 bpm

PR interval: Varies

P-waves: Varies, some natural (2nd through 4th, 6th, etc) and some pacemaker generated (5th)

QRS complex: 0.16 seconds, wide, all pacemaker generated

Interpretation: Sinus rhythm with 100% ventricular sequential pacing and intermittent atrial pacing

#82

Regularity: Regular   Heart rate: 88 bpm

PR interval: Not measurable

P-waves: None seen

QRS complex: 0.06 seconds

Interpretation: Accelerated junctional rhythm

#83

Regularity: Regular except   Heart rate: 60 bpm

PR interval: 0.16 seconds (1st, 4th, and 7th beats 0.12)

P-waves: All the same except the premature beats (1st, 4th, and 7th)

QRS complex: 0.06 seconds, all the same

Interpretation: Sinus rhythm with trigeminal PACs (premature beats have inverted P-waves in lead II and normal PR
   interval)

#84

Regularity: Regular except   Heart rate: 80 bpm

PR interval: 0.24 seconds

P-waves: All the same

QRS complex: All the same (except 5th and 6th beats)

Interpretation: Sinus rhythm with 1st degree AV block and a unifocal ventricular couplet

#85

Regularity: Regular except   Heart rate: 90 bpm

PR interval: 0.14 seconds

P-waves: All the same

QRS complex: Alternate between two forms

Interpretation: Sinus rhythm with unifocal bigeminal PVCs

#86

Regularity: Irregularly irregular   Heart rate: Not measurable

PR interval: Not measurable

P-waves: None seen

QRS complex: None seen

Interpretation: Ventricular fibrillation (confirmed in second lead)

Post-Test Answers

#87

Regularity: Irregularly irregular   Heart rate: 200 bpm

PR interval: Not measurable

P-waves: None seen

QRS complex: Varies

Interpretation: Multifocal ventricular tachycardia

#88

Regularity: Regular   Heart rate: 100 bpm

PR interval: 0.22 seconds

P-waves: Regular, all the same

QRS complex: 0.08 seconds, all the same

Interpretation: Sinus tachycardia with 1st degree AV block

#89

Regularity: Regular   Heart rate: 60 bpm

PR interval: 0.28 seconds

P-waves: Small and nearly flat, but regular and all the same

QRS complex: 0.12 seconds, wide, all the same

Interpretation: Sinus rhythm with 1st degree AV block and bundle branch block

#90

Regularity: Regular   Heart rate: 52 bpm

PR interval: Not measurable

P-waves: None seen (? after QRS complexes in T-wave)

QRS complex: 0.10 seconds, all the same

Interpretation: Junctional rhythm

#91

Regularity: Regular except   Heart rate: 120 bpm

PR interval: 0.16 seconds

P-waves: Regular, all the same

QRS complex: 0.08 seconds, all the same except every third one is wide and bizarre

Interpretation: Sinus tachycardia with unifocal trigeminal PVCs (gain needs to be adjusted or lead changed because
the PVCs are "flat-topped")

#92

Regularity: None   Heart rate: None

PR interval: Not measurable

P-waves: None seen

QRS complex: None seen

Interpretation: Asystole, confirmed in two leads

#93

Regularity: Regular   Heart rate: Atrial, 115 bpm; ventricular, 41 bpm

PR interval: Varies

P-waves: Inverted (normal for this lead), all the same

QRS complex: 0.06 seconds, all the same

Interpretation: Sinus tachycardia with 3rd degree AV block (PR interval varies, see decision tree) and a junctional escape rhythm

#94

Regularity: Irregularly irregular   Heart rate: 100 bpm

PR interval: Not measurable

P-waves: None seen, possibly obscured by severe baseline artifact

QRS complex: 0.12 seconds, all the same (taking artifact into account)

Interpretation: Severe somatic artifact. Unable to determine rhythm, may be atrial fibrillation with bundle branch block, sinus tachycardia with bundle branch block and PACs, or multifocal atrial tachycardia with bundle branch block

#95

Regularity: Regular except   Heart rate: 60 bpm

PR interval: 0.10 seconds, only two measurable

P-waves: Only two seen, inverted (abnormal in this lead)

QRS complex: 0.06 seconds, all the same

Interpretation: Junctional rhythm with unifocal PJCs. (From a different junctional focus than the rhythm. The P-wave is inverted in lead II and the PR interval is less than normal.)

#96

Regularity: Irregularly irregular   Heart rate: Atrial, 273 bpm; ventricular, 90 bpm

PR interval: Not measurable

P-waves: Regular, multiple P-waves for each QRS complex (initial rhythm has two F-waves per QRS; second rhythm has four F-waves per QRS complex), all the same.

QRS complex: 0.08 seconds, all the same

Interpretation: Atrial flutter with 2:1 and 4:1 AV block changing back and forth

#97

Regularity: regular   Heart rate: 60 bpm

PR interval: 0.06 seconds

P-waves: Inverted (abnormal in this lead), regular, all the same

QRS complex: 0.08 seconds, all the same

Interpretation: Junctional rhythm

#98

Regularity: Regular   Heart rate: 63 bpm

PR interval: Not measurable

P-waves: Not seen, possibly because of artifact

QRS complex: 0.14 seconds, all the same (accounting for artifact)

Interpretation: Severe baseline artifact resulting in inappropriate pacemaker artifact recognition by monitoring equipment. Unable to determine rhythm, may or may not be paced rhythm, need artifact-free strip.

#99

Regularity: Regular   Heart rate: 111 bpm

PR interval: 0.16 seconds (the PQRST complex in the middle of the bottom tracing is the only one clearly measurable)

P-waves: Difficult to see due to artifact

QRS complex: 0.06 seconds, all the same

Interpretation: Sinus tachycardia with significant artifact (probably loose lead as the top strip indicates at least one patch is off).

Post-Test Answers

#100
Regularity: Regular   Heart rate: 70 bpm
PR interval: 0.18 seconds
P-waves: Regular, all the same
QRS complex: 0.10 seconds, all the same
Interpretation: Sinus rhythm

#101
Regularity: Irregularly irregular   Heart rate: Atrial, 250 bpm; ventricular, 90 bpm
PR interval: Not measurable
P-waves: F-waves, regular, all the same
QRS complex: 0.08 seconds, all the same
Interpretation: Atrial flutter with variable AV block. Heart rate range, 68 to 115 bpm

#102
Regularity: Irregularly irregular   Heart rate: 50 bpm
PR interval: 0.14 seconds
P-waves: Irregular, all the same except 4th beat
QRS complex: 0.08 seconds, all the same
Interpretation: Sinus arrhythmia with junctional escape beat (4th beat)

#103
Regularity: Irregular   Heart rate: atrial: 81 bpm, ventricular: 50 bpm
PR interval: Varies
P-waves: Normal, all the same, regular
QRS complex: 0.06 seconds, all the same, irregular
Interpretation: Sinus rhythm with 2nd degree AV block type I

#104
Regularity: Regular   Heart rate: Atrial, 79 bpm; ventricular, 50 bpm
PR interval: Varies
P-waves: Regular, all the same
QRS complex: 0.12 seconds, all the same
Interpretation: Sinus rhythm (based on atrial rate) with 3rd degree AV block and junctional vs ventricular escape rhythm

#105
Regularity: Regular   Heart rate: 136 bpm
PR interval: 0.14 seconds
P-waves: Regular, all the same
QRS complex: 0.06 seconds, all the same
Interpretation: Sinus tachycardia with significant artifact, probably loose lead and/or motion

#106
Regularity: Regular   Heart rate: 79 bpm
PR interval: 0.14 seconds
P-waves: Regular, all the same
QRS complex: 0.06 seconds, all the same
Interpretation: Sinus rhythm

#107

Regularity: Regular   Heart rate: 136 bpm

PR interval: 0.12 seconds

P-waves: Regular, all the same

QRS complex: 0.08 seconds, all the same

Interpretation: Sinus tachycardia

#108

Regularity: Regular   Heart rate: 44 bpm

PR interval: 0.18 seconds

P-waves: Regular, all the same

QRS complex: 0.06 seconds, all the same

Interpretation: Sinus bradycardia

#109

Regularity: Regular   Heart rate: 83 bpm

PR interval: 0.14 seconds

P-waves: Regular, slightly notched

QRS complex: 0.10 seconds, all the same

Interpretation: Sinus rhythm with deeply inverted T-wave. This patient had unstable angina, and the T-waves were indicative of ischemic changes.

#110

Regularity: Irregularly irregular   Heart rate: 80 bpm

PR interval: Varies (from 0.20 sec at the beginning, to 0.16 sec at the end)

P-waves: Changes from one form to another during tracing

QRS complex: 0.06 seconds

Interpretation: Sinus rhythm converting to ectopic atrial pacemaker. (This is not wandering atrial pacemaker. The reason there are multiple P-wave shapes is that the 3rd and 4th P-waves are fusion P-waves as both the atrial pacemaker and the sinus node depolarize the atria together.)

#111

Regularity: Regular except   Heart rate: 60 bpm

PR interval: 0.18 seconds

P-waves: Double-humped, regular, all the same

QRS complex: 0.08 seconds, all the same except every third

Interpretation: Sinus rhythm with unifocal trigeminal PVCs and 60-Hz interference artifact in bottom tracing (Note that the P-waves are not visible in the bottom tracing).

#112

Regularity: Regular   Heart rate: 94 bpm

PR interval: 0.16 seconds

P-waves: Regular, all the same

QRS complex: 0.06 seconds, all the same

Interpretation: Sinus rhythm with prominent U-wave. (This patient had a potassium level of 2.3.)

#113
Regularity: Both rhythms are regular   Heart rate: Initial rhythm, 130 bpm; second rhythm, 250 bpm
PR interval: 0.16 seconds
P-waves: First five are regular and all the same, 6th is early and different, no others are clearly visible
QRS complex: 0.06 seconds, all the same
Interpretation: Sinus tachycardia with PAC (6th beat) triggering a rapid SVT (possibly atrial flutter with 1:1 AV
    conduction, based on heart rate)

#114
Regularity: Regular except   Heart rate: 70 bpm
PR interval: 0.24 seconds
P-waves: Regular, all the same except for pause between 1st and 2nd beats
QRS complex: 0.06 seconds, all the same
Interpretation: Sinus rhythm with 1st degree AV block and blocked PAC (note the altered appearance of the 1st; there
    is a hidden P-wave there) and an atrial escape beat (2nd beat)

#115
Regularity: Regular except   Heart rate: 120 bpm
PR interval: 0.16 seconds
P-waves: Regular, all the same
QRS complex: 0.08 seconds, alternates forms
Interpretation: Sinus rhythm with bigeminal unifocal PVCs and fusion beats. P-waves are in the PVC QRS complexes
    and begin to reveal themselves toward the end of the tracing. When they do, the P-waves begin to depolarize some
    of the ventricles, altering the QRS complex form (the fusion beats).

#116
Regularity: Regular   Heart rate: 47 bpm
PR interval: Not measurable
P-waves: None seen
QRS complex: 0.06 seconds, all the same
Interpretation: Junctional rhythm

#117
Regularity: Regular except   Heart rate: 100 bpm
PR interval: 0.20 seconds
P-waves: Regular, all the same except 6th and 11th beats
QRS complex: 0.06 seconds, all the same
Interpretation: Tachycardia with PACs (6th and 11th beats)

#118
Regularity: Regular except   Heart rate: 77 bpm
PR interval: 0.14 seconds
P-waves: All the same except 7th and 8th beats
QRS complex: 0.08 seconds, all the same
Interpretation: Sinus rhythm with multifocal atrial couplet

#119

Regularity: Irregularly irregular   Heart rate: 80 bpm

PR interval: Varies

P-waves: Irregular, more than three forms on tracing (1st, 2nd, 7th, 8th)

QRS complex: 0.06 seconds, all the same

Interpretation: Wandering atrial pacemaker

#120

Regularity: regular   Heart rate: Atrial, 214 bpm; ventricular, 55 bpm

PR interval: Not measurable

P-waves: F-waves, regular, all the same

QRS complex: 0.18 seconds, wide, all the same

Interpretation: Either slow atrial flutter with a bundle branch block with a 4:1 AV block or atrial tachycardia with 4:1 conduction and a bundle branch block

#121

Regularity: Regular   Heart rate: 176 bpm

PR interval: 0.14 seconds

P-waves: Regular, upright (normal for this lead), all the same

QRS complex: 0.06 seconds, all the same

Interpretation: Atrial tachycardia (greater than 160 bpm threshold for sinus origin, but still could be sinus tachycardia)

#122

Regularity: Regular   Heart rate: 88 bpm

PR interval: 0.22 seconds (measured to the pacemaker spike)

P-waves: Regular, all the same

QRS complex: 0.12 seconds, all the same

Interpretation: Sinus rhythm with 1st degree AV block and 100% ventricular pacing

#123

Regularity: Regular except   Heart rate: 60 bpm

PR interval: 0.22 seconds

P-waves: Regular, all the same except P-wave after 5th QRS complex

QRS complex: 0.08 seconds, all the same

Interpretation: Sinus rhythm with 1st degree AV block and a blocked PAC (after 5th QRS complex, notice the altered T-wave)

#124

Regularity: Regular except   Heart rate: 90 bpm

PR interval: 0.20 seconds

P-waves: Regular, all the same except every third one

QRS complex: 0.08 seconds, all the same

Interpretation: Sinus rhythm with unifocal trigeminal PACs

#125

Regularity: Regular   Heart rate: Atrial, 23 bpm; ventricular, 37 bpm

PR interval: Varies

P-waves: Regular, all the same

QRS complex: 0.16 seconds, all the same

Interpretation: Sinus bradycardia with 3rd degree AV block and idioventricular escape rhythm (The AV node is not functioning. The last P-wave was far enough away from the QRS complex that it should have conducted.) The second P-wave appears to conduct but the QRS complex is unchanged indicating it started in the same place as the others.

Post-Test Answers

#126

Regularity: Irregularly irregular   Heart rate: 60 bpm

PR interval: Not measurable

P-waves: None seen (wavy baseline)

QRS complex: 0.06 seconds, all the same

Interpretation: Atrial fibrillation (heart rate range, 38 to 91 bpm)

#127

Regularity: Regular   Heart rate: Atrial, 250 bpm; ventricular, 60 bpm

PR interval: Not measurable

P-waves: F-waves, regular, all the same

QRS complex: 0.08 seconds, all the same

Interpretation: Atrial flutter with 4:1 AV block

#128

Regularity: Regular   Heart rate: 67 bpm

PR interval: 0.22 seconds

P-waves: Regular, all the same

QRS complex: 0.08 seconds, all the same

Interpretation: Sinus rhythm with 1st degree AV block with deeply inverted T-waves (suggesting ischemia of the right coronary artery, which could also explain the 1st degree AV block)

#129

Regularity: Regular   Heart rate: 158 bpm

PR interval: 0.12 seconds

P-waves: Regular, all the same

QRS complex: 0.08 seconds, all the same

Interpretation: Sinus tachycardia

#130

Regularity: Regularly irregular   Heart rate: 90 bpm

PR interval: 0.14 seconds

P-waves: Irregular, all the same

QRS complex: 0.08 seconds, all the same

Interpretation: Sinus arrhythmia (very small cyclical variation)

#131

Regularity: Regular   Heart rate: 115 bpm

PR interval: 0.14 seconds

P-waves: Regular, all the same, except unable to see last P-wave buried in, and distorting, the preceding T-wave

QRS complex: 0.08 seconds, all the same

Interpretation: Sinus tachycardia with PAC (Last beat on strip)

#132

Regularity: Regular   Heart rate: Atrial, 100 bpm; ventricular, 50 bpm

PR interval: 0.18 seconds

P-waves: Regular, all the same

QRS complex: 0.12 seconds

Interpretation: Sinus tachycardia with a BBB and 2nd degree AV block (unknown type, probably Type II due to wide QRS complex)

#133

Regularity: Regular   Heart rate: 150 bpm

PR interval: None seen

P-waves: None seen

QRS complex: 0.22 seconds, wide, all the same

Interpretation: Unifocal ventricular tachycardia

#134

Regularity: Regular   Heart rate: 55 bpm

PR interval: Varies

P-waves: Two kinds (pacemaker generated and sinus generated)

QRS complex: 0.08 seconds, all the same

Interpretation: Sinus rhythm and atrial pacing with 3rd degree AV block and junctional escape rhythm

#135

Regularity: Regularly irregular   Heart rate: 30 bpm

PR interval: Not measurable

P-waves: None seen

QRS complex: 0.26 seconds

Interpretation: Idioventricular rhythm (patient was pulseless and went asystole shortly after this strip was run)

#136

Regularity: Regular   Heart rate: 77 bpm

PR interval: 0.18 seconds

P-waves: Regular, all the same

QRS complex: 0.08 seconds, all the same

Interpretation: Sinus rhythm with 60-Hz interference

#137

Regularity: Regular   Heart rate: Atrial, 115; ventricular, 38 bpm

PR interval: Varies

P-waves: Regular, upright, all the same

QRS complex: 0.16 seconds

Interpretation: Sinus tachycardia with 3rd degree AV block and idioventricular escape rhythm

#138

Regularity: Regular   Heart rate: 64 bpm

PR interval: Not measurable

P-waves: None seen

QRS complex: 0.10 seconds, all the same (inverted normal in this lead)

Interpretation: Accelerated junctional rhythm

#139

Regularity: Regular   Heart rate: 83 bpm

PR interval: 0.30 seconds

P-waves: Regular, all the same

QRS complex: 0.08 seconds, all the same

Interpretation: Sinus rhythm with 1st degree AV block (notch at end of QRS complexes is NOT a buried P-wave because it does not march out regularly with the visible P-waves)

Post-Test Answers

#140
Regularity: Regular   Heart rate: 159 bpm
PR interval: Not measurable
P-waves: None seen
QRS complex: 0.14 seconds, wide, all the same
Interpretation: Ventricular tachycardia

#141
Regularity: Regular   Heart rate: 91 bpm
PR interval: Not measurable
P-waves: None seen
QRS complex: 0.08 seconds
Interpretation: Accelerated junctional rhythm

#142
Regularity: Regular except   Heart rate: 60 bpm
PR interval: None seen
P-waves: Small, barely perceptible
QRS complex: Wide, all the same except 5th beat
Interpretation: 100% AV sequential pacing with PVC (followed by a sinus beat with ventricular pacing)

#143
Regularity: Regular   Heart rate: 83
PR interval: 0.14 seconds
P-waves: Biphasic (normal for V_1), all the same
QRS complex: 0.14 seconds
Interpretation: Sinus rhythm with 100% ventricular pacing

#144
Regularity: Regular except   Heart rate: 90 bpm
PR interval: 0.18 seconds
P-waves: Regular, all the same except before 2nd, 6th, and 10th QRS complexes
QRS complex: 0.08 seconds, all the same (slight variation in 2nd, 6th, and 10th beats is due to premature beat)
Interpretation: Sinus rhythm with unifocal quadrigeminal PACs

#145
Regularity: Regular   Heart rate: Atrial, 88 bpm; ventricular, 33 bpm
PR interval: Varies
P-waves: Regular, all the same
QRS complex: 0.08 seconds, all the same
Interpretation: Sinus rhythm with 3rd degree AV block and junctional bradycardia escape rhythm

#146
Regularity: Regular   Heart rate: 83 bpm
PR interval: 0.14 seconds
P-waves: Regular, all the same
QRS complex: 0.12 seconds, all the same, pacemaker generated
Interpretation: Sinus rhythm with 100% ventricular pacing

#147
Regularity: Regular   Heart rate: 79 bpm
PR interval: 0.22 seconds
P-waves: Regular, all the same, pacemaker generated
QRS complex: 0.08 seconds, all the same
Interpretation: 100% atrial pacing with 1st degree AV block

#148
Regularity: Regularly irregular   Heart rate: Atrial, 231; ventricular, 80 bpm
PR interval: Not measurable
P-waves: F-waves, regular, all the same
QRS complex: 0.12 seconds, all the same
Interpretation: Atrial flutter with variable AV block (heart rate range, 75 to 107 bpm)

#149
Regularity: Irregularly irregular   Heart rate: 130 bpm
PR interval: Varies
P-waves: Irregular, more than three forms on tracing
QRS complex: 0.08 seconds, all the same
Interpretation: Multifocal atria tachycardia deteriorating into atrial fibrillation towards end of strip

#150
Regularity: Irregularly irregular   Heart rate: 130 bpm
PR interval: Not measurable
P-waves: None seen
QRS complex: 0.06 seconds, all the same
Interpretation: Atrial fibrillation with rapid ventricular response (heart rate range, 91 to 167 bpm)

#151
Regularity: Regular   Heart rate: 20 bpm
PR interval: Not measurable
P-waves: None seen
QRS complex: 0.20 seconds, all the same
Interpretation: Idioventricular rhythm

#152
Regularity: Regular except   Heart rate: 70 bpm
PR interval: 0.12 seconds
P-waves: Regular, all the same except after the 5th QRS complex, buried in T-wave
QRS complex: 0.08 seconds
Interpretation: Sinus rhythm with a blocked PAC (P-wave buried in T-wave after the 5th QRS complex)

#153
Regularity: Regular   Heart rate: 88 bpm
PR interval: 0.16 seconds
P-waves: Regular, all the same
QRS complex: 0.06 seconds, all the same
Interpretation: Sinus rhythm

Post-Test Answers

#154
Regularity: Regular   Heart rate: 100 bpm
PR interval: 0.16 seconds
P-waves: Inverted (due to pacemaker)
QRS complex: 0.16 seconds, wide, all the same
Interpretation: 100% AV sequential pacing

#155
Regularity: Regular   Heart rate: 53 bpm
PR interval: 0.14 seconds
P-waves: Regular, all the same
QRS complex: 0.10 seconds
Interpretation: Sinus bradycardia with inverted T-wave (abnormal in this lead)

#156
Regularity: Regular except   Heart rate: 88 bpm
PR interval: 0.16 seconds
P-waves: Regular, notched, all the same except 8th beat
QRS complex: 0.08 seconds, all the same
Interpretation: Sinus rhythm with PAC (8th beat)

#157
Regularity: Regular   Heart rate: 86 bpm
PR interval: 0.14 seconds
P-waves: Regular, all the same
QRS complex: 0.14 seconds, all the same
Interpretation: Sinus rhythm with bundle branch block

#158
Regularity: Regular except   Heart rate: 130 bpm
PR interval: 0.20 seconds
P-waves: Only one seen
QRS complex: 0.16 seconds, except for 8th beat
Interpretation: Ventricular tachycardia with pause and one sinus beat, followed by an R-on-T PVC and another run of
    ventricular tachycardia

#159
Regularity: Regular   Heart rate: 61 bpm
PR interval: 0.22 seconds
P-waves: Regular, all the same, pacemaker generated
QRS complex: 0.10 seconds, all the same
Interpretation: 100% atrial pacing

#160
Regularity: Irregularly irregular   Heart rate: 333 bpm; ventricular, 40 bpm
PR interval: Not measurable
P-waves: F-waves, regular, all the same (except some possible baseline distortion)
QRS complex: 0.08 seconds, all the same
Interpretation: Atrial flutter with variable AV block and slow ventricular response

#161

Regularity: Irregularly irregular   Heart rate: 60 bpm

PR interval: Not measurable

P-waves: None seen (wavy baseline)

QRS complex: 0.12 seconds, wide, all the same

Interpretation: Atrial fibrillation with bundle branch block (heart rate range, 50 to 68 bpm)

#162

Regularity: Regular except   Heart rate: 110 bpm

PR interval: 0.16 seconds

P-waves: Regular, all the same except before and after the 7th beat

QRS complex: 0.08 seconds, all the same

Interpretation: Sinus tachycardia with PACs (7th beat), blocked PAC (P-wave after the 7th beat), and significant respiratory artifact (peaks are about 5 seconds apart, corresponding to the patient's respiratory rate of 12 per minute).

#163

Regularity: Regular   Heart rate: 43 bpm

PR interval: 0.12 seconds

P-waves: Regular, biphasic, all the same

QRS complex: 0.08 seconds, all the same

Interpretation: Sinus bradycardia

#164

Regularity: Regular   Heart rate: 71 bpm

PR interval: 0.16 seconds

P-waves: Regular, all the same

QRS complex: 0.06 seconds, all the same

Interpretation: Sinus rhythm

#165

Regularity: Regular except   Heart rate: 94 bpm

PR interval: Not measurable

P-waves: None seen (wavy baseline)

QRS complex: Varies

Interpretation: Atrial fibrillation with 90% ventricular pacing and fusion beasts (4th, 5th, and 10th beats) and a pseudofusion beat (6th beat; note QRS complex is normal width, indicating it came from the bundle branches normally)

#166

Regularity: Regular   Heart rate: 88 bpm

PR interval: 0.18 seconds

P-waves: Regular, peaked, all the same

QRS complex: 0.14 seconds, all the same

Interpretation: Sinus rhythm with bundle branch block (and peaked P-waves)

#167

Regularity: Regular   Heart rate: 63 bpm

PR interval: 0.14 seconds

P-waves: All pacemaker generated, normal

QRS complex: 0.20, all the same

Interpretation: 100% AV sequential pacing

Post-Test Answers

#168
Regularity: Regular   Heart rate: 71 bpm
PR interval: Not measurable
P-waves: None seen
QRS complex: 0.16 seconds, all the same
Interpretation: 100% ventricular pacing

#169
Regularity: Irregularly irregular   Heart rate: 60 bpm
PR interval: 0.14 seconds
P-waves: All the same
QRS complex: 0.10 seconds, all the same
Interpretation: Sinus arrhythmia

#170
Regularity: Irregularly irregular   Heart rate: 80 bpm
PR interval: Not measurable
P-waves: None seen (wavy baseline)
QRS complex: 0.06 seconds, all the same
Interpretation: Atrial fibrillation (heart rate range, 39 to 150 bpm)

#171
Regularity: Regular   Heart rate: 79 bpm
PR interval: 0.16 seconds
P-waves: Regular, all the same
QRS complex: 0.10 seconds, all the same
Interpretation: Sinus rhythm with inverted T-waves

#172
Regularity: regular   Heart rate: 94 bpm
PR interval: 0.14 seconds
P-waves: Regular, all the same
QRS complex: 0.06 seconds, all the same
Interpretation: Sinus rhythm

#173
Regularity: Regular   Heart rate: Atrial, 65 bpm; ventricular, 50 bpm
PR interval: 0.16 seconds
P-waves: Regular, all the same
QRS complex: 0.06 seconds, all the same
Interpretation: Sinus rhythm with 2nd degree AV block type II

#174
Regularity: Regular   Heart rate: 75 bpm
PR interval: 0.16 seconds
P-waves: Regular, all the same
QRS complex: 0.08 seconds, all the same
Interpretation: Sinus rhythm

#175

Regularity: Regular   Heart rate: 38 bpm

PR interval: Not measurable

P-waves: None seen

QRS complex: 0.10 seconds

Interpretation: Junctional bradycardia

#176

Regularity: Regular   Heart rate: 159 bpm

PR interval: 0.08 seconds

P-waves: Regular, inverted (abnormal in this lead), all the same

QRS complex: 0.08 seconds

Interpretation: Junctional tachycardia

#177

Regularity: Regular   Heart rate: 65 bpm

PR interval: 0.52 seconds

P-waves: Regular, all the same

QRS complex: None seen

Interpretation: Sinus rhythm with 1st degree AV block

#178

Regularity: Regularly irregular   Heart rate: 79 bpm

PR interval: 0.16 seconds

P-waves: Regular, all the same

QRS complex: 0.08 seconds, all the same

Interpretation: Sinus arrhythmia

#179

Regularity: Regular   Heart rate: 91 bpm

PR interval: 0.16 seconds

P-waves: Regular, all the same

QRS complex: 0.10 seconds, all the same

Interpretation: Sinus rhythm with deep Q-wave and mild ST segment elevation, indicating probable evolving inferior wall MI

#180

Regularity: Regular, then irregularly irregular   Heart rate: 79 bpm

PR interval: 0.18 seconds

P-waves: Regular, then none seen

QRS complex: 0.08 seconds, then varies

Interpretation: Sinus rhythm with Q-wave and ST segment elevation indicating possible inferior wall MI and R-on-T PVC
   triggering ventricular tachycardia that quickly deteriorates to ventricular fibrillation

#181

Regularity: Regular   Heart rate: 59 bpm

PR interval: 0.10 seconds

P-waves: Inverted (abnormal in this lead)

QRS complex: 0.08 seconds

Interpretation: Junctional rhythm

#182
Regularity: Irregularly irregular   Heart rate: 110 bpm
PR interval: Not measurable
P-waves: None seen (wavy baseline)
QRS complex: 0.08 seconds, all the same
Interpretation: Atrial fibrillation with rapid ventricular response (acceptable increased heart rate due to the loss of
   atrial kick) (heart rate range, 60 to 142 bpm)

#183
Regularity: Regular except   Heart rate: 70 bpm
PR interval: 0.14 seconds
P-waves: All the same
QRS complex: 0.14 seconds, all the same except for 4th through 6th
Interpretation: Sinus rhythm with bundle branch block and a three-beat run of acclerated idioventricular rhythm
   (ventricular salvo)

#184
Regularity: Regular except   Heart rate: 1st rhythm, 79 bpm; 2nd rhythm, 167 bpm
PR interval: 0.10 seconds
P-waves: Regular, all the same
QRS complex: 0.20 seconds, wide, all the same
Interpretation: Sinus rhythm with an R-on-T PVC and eight-beat run of unifocal ventricular tachycardia (note P-waves in
   the T-waves during V-tach after 6th and 8th beats)

#185
Regularity: Regular   Heart rate: 51 bpm
PR interval: 0.16 seconds
P-waves: Regular, all the same
QRS complex: 0.14 seconds, all the same
Interpretation: Sinus bradycardia with bundle branch block and a U-wave (common with bradycardia rhythms)

#186
Regularity: Regular except   Heart rate: 75 bpm, then changes
PR interval: 0.18 seconds
P-waves: Regular, all the same, then changes
QRS complex: 0.08 seconds, all the same, then changes
Interpretation: Sinus rhythm with PAC (3rd beat) and three-beat ventricular pacing escape rhythm, followed by a fusion
   beat and pseudofusion beats and the resumption of the sinus rhythm.

#187
Regularity: Regular   Heart rate: 44 to 79 bpm
PR interval: 0.18 seconds (when present)
P-waves: All the same, all pacemaker generated (excepted inverted P-waves after 1st and 2nd QRS complex)
QRS complex: First two, natural and 0.08 seconds, rest all the same, pacemaker generated and 0.16 seconds
Interpretation: 100% atrial pacing with ventricular failure to capture and junctional escape rhythm. Then converts to
   100% AV sequential pacing with 100% capture. (In fact, this strip is from an external, transvenous pacemaker and
   the failure to capture was a result of the initial programming of the device.)

#188

Regularity: Irregularly irregular converting to regular   Heart rate: 60 bpm

PR interval: 0.12 seconds

P-waves: All the same except the ones buried in the 2nd and 3rd T-waves. (Note notches on 2nd T-wave and the large point on the 3rd T-wave)

QRS complex: 0.18 seconds wide, all the same

Interpretation: Sinus rhythm with blocked PACs and 100% ventricular pacing with occasional atrial triggering

#189

Regularity: Regular   Heart rate: 65 bpm

PR interval: 0.26 seconds

P-waves: Regular, all the same

QRS complex: 0.18 seconds, wide, all the same

Interpretation: Sinus rhythm with bundle branch block

#190

Regularity: Regular except   Heart rate: 80 bpm

PR interval: 0.14 seconds

P-waves: Regular, all the same except every third beat

QRS complex: 0.10 seconds, all the same

Interpretation: Sinus rhythm with unifocal trigeminal PACs

#191

Regularity: Regular, then irregularly irregular   Heart rate: 79 bpm, then 120 bpm

PR interval: 0.22 seconds

P-waves: Regular, all the same, then none seen

QRS complex: 0.10 seconds, first two the same, then changes

Interpretation: Sinus rhythm with 1st degree AV block and ST segment elevation, with fusion beat (3rd beat) and ventricular tachycardia

#192

Regularity: Irregularly irregular   Heart rate: 110 bpm

PR interval: Not measurable

P-waves: F-waves, regular, all the same

QRS complex: 0.08 seconds, all the same

Interpretation: Atrial flutter with variable AV block (heart rate range, 71 to 150 bpm)

#193

Regularity: Regular   Heart rate: 75 bpm

PR interval: 0.16 seconds

P-waves: Regular, all the same

QRS complex: 0.10 seconds, all the same

Interpretation: Sinus rhythm (elevated J-point)

#194

Regularity: regular   Heart rate: Atrial, 125 bpm; ventricular, 41 bpm

PR interval: Varies

P-waves: Regular, all the same

QRS complex: 0.06 seconds

Interpretation: Sinus tachycardia with 3rd degree AV block and junctional escape rhythm

#195
Regularity: Regular   Heart rate: 79 bpm
PR interval: Not measurable
P-waves: None seen
QRS complex: 0.08 seconds, all the same
Interpretation: Accelerated junctional rhythm

#196
Regularity: Regular   Heart rate: Atrial, 273; ventricular, 143
PR interval: Not measurable
P-waves: F-waves, regular, all the same
QRS complex: 0.08 seconds, all the same
Interpretation: Atrial flutter with 2:1 AV block (seen best in lead II tracing)

#197
Regularity: Regular   Heart rate: Atrial, 94 bpm; ventricular, 49 bpm
PR interval: Varies
P-waves: Regular, all the same
QRS complex: 0.08 seconds, all the same
Interpretation: Sinus rhythm with 3rd degree AV block and junctional escape rhythm

#198
Regularity: Regular   Heart rate: 56 bpm
PR interval: 0.18 seconds
P-waves: Regular, all the same
QRS complex: 0.08 seconds, all the same
Interpretation: Sinus bradycardia

#199
Regularity: Regular   Heart rate: 81 bpm
PR interval: 0.18 seconds
P-waves: Regular, all the same
QRS complex: 0.08 seconds
Interpretation: Sinus rhythm with hyperacute T-waves and ST segment elevation indicating acute MI in the anterior and
    septal leads (V1 through V4) with reciprocal changes (II, III, and aVF)

#200
Regularity: Regular   Heart rate: 38 bpm
PR interval: 0.16 seconds
P-waves: Regular, all the same
QRS complex: 0.10 seconds
Interpretation: Sinus bradycardia with ST segment elevation indicating acute MI in inferior leads, with reciprocal changes
    in leads I and aVL

Appendix 1
Heart Rate Tables

HR	Small	Large	HR	Small	Large
1500	1		94	16	
750	2		88	17	
500	3		83	18	
375	4		79	19	
300	5	1	75	20	4
250	6		71	21	
214	7		68	22	
188	8		65	23	
167	9		63	24	
150	10	2	60	25	5
136	11		58	26	
125	12		56	27	
115	13		54	28	
107	14		52	29	
100	15	3	50	30	6

HR	Small	Large	HR	Small	Large
48	31		33	46	
47	32		32	47	
45	33		31	48	
44	34		31	49	
43	35	7	30	50	10
42	36		29	51	
41	37		29	52	
39	38		28	53	
38	39		28	54	
38	40	8	27	55	11
37	41		27	56	
36	42		26	57	
35	43		26	58	
34	44		25	59	
33	45	9	25	60	12

HR	Small	Large	HR	Small	Large
48	31		33	46	
47	32		32	47	
45	33		31	48	
44	34		31	49	
43	35	7	30	50	10
42	36		29	51	
41	37		29	52	
39	38		28	53	
38	39	8	28	54	
38	40		27	55	11
37	41		27	56	
36	42		26	57	
35	43		26	58	
34	44		25	59	
33	45	9	25	60	12

HR	Small	Large	HR	Small	Large
1500	1		94	16	
750	2		88	17	
500	3		83	18	
375	4		79	19	
300	5	1	75	20	4
250	6		71	21	
214	7		68	22	
188	8		65	23	
167	9		63	24	
150	10	2	60	25	5
136	11		58	26	
125	12		56	27	
115	13		54	28	
107	14		52	29	
100	15	3	50	30	6

accelerated idioventricular rhythm (AIVR) An abnormal ectopic cardiac rhythm originating in the ventricular conducting system. This may occur intermittently after myocardial infarction and occurs at a rate of 40 to 99 beats per minute.

accelerated junctional rhythm An electrocardiographic rhythm arising in the atrioventricular junction. It appears on an electrocardiogram as a narrow QRS complex that lacks an upright P wave preceding it in lead II and occurs at a rate of 60 to 99 beats per minute.

accelerated An increase in the frequency of cardiac tissue depolarization from the intrinsic rate of that tissue.

action potential The change in electrical potential of nerve or muscle fiber when it is stimulated; depolarization followed by repolarization.

ACLS algorithm (advanced cardiac life support algorithm) A set of algorithms published by the American Heart Association for solving problems in patients with cardiac dysrhythmias most commonly present and life-threatening during cardiopulmonary resuscitation efforts.

agonal Related to death or dying. An ECG rhythm that is incompatible with life and usually is the final rhythm present before asystole.

alternating current A current that periodically flows in opposite directions; may be either sinusoidal or nonsinusoidal. The alternating current wave usually used therapeutically is the sinusoidal.

amiodarone An antiarrhythmic drug with a complex pharmacology that is effective in the treatment of both atrial and ventricular rhythm disturbances. Its side effects include pulmonary fibrosis and thyroid dysfunction.

angina pectoris An oppressive pain or pressure in the chest caused by inadequate blood flow and oxygenation to heart muscle. It is usually produced by atherosclerosis of the coronary arteries and in Western cultures is one of the most common emergent complaints bringing adult patients to medical attention. It typically occurs after (or during) events that increase the heart's need for oxygen, such as increased physical activity, a large meal, exposure to cold weather, or increased psychological stress.

> **stable** Angina that occurs with exercise or other stressor and is predictable; usually promptly relieved by rest or nitroglycerin.

> **unstable** Angina that has changed to a more frequent and more severe form. It can occur during rest and may be an indication of impending myocardial infarction. Unstable angina should be treated.

antidysrhythmic A drug or physical force that acts to control or prevent cardiac dysrhythmias.

aorta The main trunk of the arterial system of the body.

aortic valve The valve at the junction of the left ventricle and the ascending aorta; composed of three segments (semilunar cusps). The aortic valve prevents regurgitation.

arrhythmia Irregularity or loss of rhythm, especially of the heart.

arteriosclerosis A disease of the arterial vessels marked by thickening, hardening, and loss of elasticity in the arterial walls. Atherosclerosis is the single most important cause of disease and death in Western societies.

artifact 1. Anything artificially produced. **2.** In electronics, the appearance of a spurious signal not consistent with results expected from the signal being studied. For example, an electrocardiogram may contain artifacts produced by a defective machine, electrical interference, patient movement, or loose electrodes.

> **60-cycle interference** Artifact produced by improperly grounded electrical equipment in close proximity to the ECG monitoring equipment manifested by thicker-than-normal baseline with approximately 12 mini P-waves per large box.

> **baseline sway** Artifact in ECGs that results in the tracing migrating above the baseline and below the baseline in a repeating manner, usually related to respirations.

> **chest compression** Artifact generated from the muscle movement or muscle stimulation related to chest compressions during resuscitation efforts.

> **large-muscle** Artifact in ECGs generated by electrical signals to large muscle groups, such as the pectoralis major muscles of the chest.

> **loose lead** Artifact generated by loose leads causing intermittent contact of the electrode gel with the patient's skin.

> **pacemaker** Artifact generated by the pacemaker depolarizing when generating a signal.

> **somatic** Artifact generated from the patient's body. It may be related to small muscle tremors, seizures, or other patient movement.

asystole Literally means, "without contraction". Cardiac standstill; absence of electrical activity and contractions of the heart evidenced on the surface electrocardiogram as a flat (isoelectric) line during cardiac arrest. In most instances, asystole is an electrocardiographic confirmation that a patient has died.

atherosclerosis The most common form of arteriosclerosis, marked by cholesterol-lipid-calcium deposits in the walls of arteries.

atrial fibrillation The most common cardiac dysrhythmia, affecting as many as 10% of people age 70 and over. It is marked by rapid, irregular electrical activity in the atria, resulting in ineffective ejection of blood into the ventricles. Blood that eddies in the atria may occasionally form clots that may embolize (especially to the brain, but also to other organs). As a result, AF is an important risk factor for stroke. It may also contribute to other diseases and conditions, including congestive heart failure, dyspnea on exertion, and syncope.

atrial flutter A cardiac dysrhythmia marked by rapid (from 250 to 350 beats per minute) regular atrial depolarizations and usually a regular ventricular response (whose rate may vary depending on the conduction of electrical impulses from the atria through the atrioventricular node). On the electrocardiogram, the fluttering of the atria is best seen in leads II, III, and aVF as "saw-tooth" deflections between the

Glossary

QRS complexes. Atrial flutter may convert to sinus rhythm with low-voltage direct current (DC) cardioversion or atrial pacing and may deteriorate to atrial fibrillation without conversion.

atrial kick The term used to indicate the amount (usually a percentage) of blood ejected from the atria during atrial contraction. In contrast to the amount of blood passively transferred from the atria, before contraction. This amount may be as much as 30% of the ventricular volume.

atrial tachycardia A rapid regular heart rate arising from an irritable focus in the atria, with a rate of more than 100 beats per minute (bpm) but less than 220 bpm.

atrioventricular (AV) node Specialized cardiac muscle fibers in the lower interatrial septum that receive impulses from the sinoatrial node and atrium and transmit them to the bundle of *His.* This tissue is capable of generating spontaneous signals itself.

atrium (and atria) A chamber or cavity communicating with another structure. One of two of the upper chambers of the heart whose role is to fill the ventricles as efficiently as possible. Atria is the plural form.

atropine A medication used to increase heart rate in patients in whom the SA or AV node is properly functioning. A vagolytic medication that decreases the influence of the vagus nerve in slowing the heart.

augmented leads ECG limb leads that are unipolar, requiring some kind of augmentation in amplitude to appear a reasonable size on the ECG tracing.

automaticity The unique property of cardiac muscle tissue to contract without nervous stimulation.

AV block A condition in which the depolarization impulse is delayed or blocked at the atrioventricular (A-V) node or a more distal site. There are various degrees of AV block that indicate the amount of dysfunction present in the AV node.

  1st degree Delayed conduction through or from the atrioventricular node, marked on the electrocardiogram by a prolonged PR interval. Usually no treatment is necessary.

  2nd degree type I (Mobitz I) A form of atrioventricular block in which only some atrial impulses are conducted to the ventricles. In this form, the PR intervals become progressively longer until a QRS complex is dropped. Because of the dropped beats, the QRS complexes appear to be clustered (a phenomenon called *grouped beating*) on the electrocardiogram.

  2nd degree type II (Mobitz II) A form of atrioventricular block in which only some atrial impulses are conducted to the ventricles. In Mobitz II, PR intervals have a constant length but QRS complexes are dropped periodically, usually every second, third, or fourth beat.

  3rd degree A form of atrioventricular block in which no atrial impulses are conducted to the ventricles. The result is that the atria and the ventricles conduct and contract independently. This results in a loss of atrial kick and a decrease in cardiac output. Frequently referred to by the incorrect name of *complete heart block.*

  classic 2nd degree Synonym for 2nd degree AV block, type II or Mobitz II.

  complete heart block A technically incorrect name for a condition in which there is a complete dissociation between atrial and ventricular systoles. Ventricles may beat from their own pacemakers at a rate of 30 to 40 beats per minute while atria beat independently.

  high-grade 2nd degree Second-degree AV block type II with multiple consecutive nonconducted P-waves.

  pathologic An AV block that does not occur in normal AV node tissue. The heart rate is such that the AV node should be able to conduct all atrial impulses, but due to some disease process, the AV node blocks one or more of the signals.

  physiologic A normal expected function of the involved tissue. An AV block that occurs in normal AV node tissue to protect the ventricles from excessive atrial rates present in some rhythms such as atrial fibrillation or atrial flutter.

  ratio The relationship in degree or number between two things. Particular ratios are listed under the first word.

  wenckebach A form of incomplete heart block in which, as detected by electrocardiography, there is progressive lengthening of the P-R interval until there is no ventricular response; and then the cycle of increasing P-R intervals begins again. Synonymous with Mobitz I and second-degree AV block type I.

AV block, pathologic AV block that occurs due to a disease process or dysfunction of the AV nodal tissue, despite reasonable heart rate, where the AV node should normally conduct.

AV block, physiologic AV block that is caused by the normal rate-limiting features of the AV node, such as found in atrial flutter or rapid atrial fibrillation.

AV node See *atrioventricular node.*

baseline The ECG line that occurs between the end of the T-wave of one beat and before the P-wave of the next beat. This represents the electrical level of the body while the heart is not conducting any signals. Also known as isoelectric line.

beta blockers Beta-adrenergic blocking agent. Medications in this group are known to decrease heart rate, cardiac contractility, and blood pressure.

bigeminal Double; paired. Occurring in a group such as a normal beat and an abnormal beat occurring in a repeating pattern.

biphasic Consisting of two phases. A waveform that goes above and below the baseline.

bipolar Pertaining to the use of two poles in electrocardiography.

blockage Referring to an occlusion, particularly in a blood vessel or in the conduction of an electrical signal.

bradycardia A slow heartbeat marked by a pulse rate below the intrinsic rate of the specific tissue of origin. This is 60 beats per minute in sinus and atrial rhythms, 40 beats per minute in junctional rhythms, and 20 beats per minute in ventricular tissue in an adult.

British Pacing Group (BPG) A group assigned the task of monitoring pacemaker coding for the British.

bundle branch block (BBB) Defect in the heart's electrical conduction system in which there is failure of conduction down one of the main branches of the bundle of *His*. On the surface electrocardiogram, the QRS complex is >0.12 seconds and its shape is altered.

> **left** Defect in the conduction system of the heart in which electrical conduction down the left bundle branch is delayed. On the 12-lead EKG, it gives the QRS complex a widened QS complex in lead V_1.

> **right** Defect in the conductive system of the heart in which electrical conduction down the right bundle branch is delayed. On the 12-lead EKG, it gives the widened QRS complex an RSR appearance in leads V_1.

bundle of *His* The atrioventricular (AV) bundle, a group of modified muscle fibers, the Purkinje fibers, forming a part of the impulse-conducting system of the heart. It arises in the AV node and continues in the interventricular septum as a single bundle, the crus commune, which divides into two trunks that pass respectively to the right and left ventricles, fine branches passing to all parts of the ventricles. It conducts impulses from the atria to the ventricles, which initiate ventricular depolarization and hopefully ventricular contraction.

CABG (coronary artery bypass graft) Surgical establishment of a shunt that permits blood to travel from the aorta or internal mammary artery to a branch of the coronary artery at a point past an obstruction. It is used in treating coronary artery occlusive disease.

calcium channel blockers Any of a group of drugs that slow the influx of calcium ions into smooth muscle cells, resulting in decreased arterial resistance and oxygen demand. These drugs are used to treat angina, hypertension, vascular spasm, intracranial bleeding, congestive heart failure, and supraventricular tachycardia. Because hypotension occurs as both an intended and occasionally an unwelcome effect, blood pressure must be monitored especially closely during the initial treatment period. These drugs also slow the rate of depolarization of the SA node and AV node due to their dependence on calcium ion movement for depolarization.

calcium A silver-white metallic element; atomic number 20, atomic weight 40.08. An important electrolyte in electrical signal conduction and muscle contraction in the human body.

calipers A hinged instrument for measuring thickness or diameter.

cardiac output The amount of blood discharged from the left or right ventricle per minute. Cardiac output is determined by multiplying the stroke volume by the heart rate. Normal cardiac output range is 5 to 8 liters per minute

cardioversion The restoration of normal sinus rhythm by chemical or electrical means. When performed medicinally, the procedure relies on the oral or intravenous administration of antiarrhythmic drugs. Electrical cardioversion relies instead on the delivery of synchronized shock of direct electrical current across the chest wall. It is used to terminate arrhythmias such as atrial fibrillation, atrial flutter, supraventricular tachycardia, and well-tolerated ventricular tachycardia. Unlike defibrillation, which is an unsynchronized shock applied during dire emergencies, electrical cardioversion is timed to avoid the T wave of cardiac repolarization to avoid triggering malignant arrhythmias. A patient will almost always require sedation and analgesia before the procedure.

cardioversion, synchronized Synonym for cardioversion above.

catecholamine One of many biologically active amines, including metanephrine, dopamine, epinephrine, and norepinephrine, derived from the amino acid tyrosine. They have a marked effect on the nervous and cardiovascular systems, metabolic rate, temperature, and smooth muscle. They increase heart rate, cardiac contractility, blood pressure, and irritability of cardiac tissue.

channels 1. A conduit, groove, or passageway through which various materials may flow. **2.** In cell biology, a passageway in the cell membrane through which materials may pass.

chaotic atrial pacemaker Synonym for ectopic atrial pacemaker.

cholesterol A chemical widely distributed in animal tissues and occurring in egg yolks, various oils, fats, myelin in brain, spinal cord and axons, liver, kidneys, and adrenal glands. An important metabolic molecule. necessary for normal body function but in the wrong location can accumulate over time and cause blockage of the coronary arteries, resulting in angina or myocardial infarction.

> **HDL** Plasma lipids bound to albumin, consisting of lipoproteins. They contain more protein than either very-low-density lipoproteins or low-density lipoproteins. High-density lipoprotein cholesterol is the so-called good cholesterol; therefore, a high level is desirable.

> **LDL** Plasma lipids that carry most of the cholesterol in plasma. Bound to albumin, LDLs are a proven cause of atherosclerosis; lowering LDLs with a low-fat diet or with drugs helps to prevent and treat coronary artery disease. The so-called bad cholesterol.

compensation Making up for a defect, as cardiac circulation compensates to meet demands regardless of valvular defect.

complete cardiac standstill Cessation of contractions of the heart.

complex An atrial or ventricular signal as it appears on an electrocardiograph tracing.

concave ST elevation ST-segment elevations that branch off from the QRS complex at a concave angle analogous to a smile shape.

conduction system The path an electrical signal follows as it is transmitted to adjacent portions of a tissue or cell, so that the signal is transmitted to remote points. Conduction occurs not only in the fibers of the nervous system but may also occur in muscle fibers.

congenital long-QT syndrome A congenital anomaly that results in a person having an abnormally long-QT interval on his or her ECG. This condition puts the person at increased risk of sudden cardiac death.

convex ST elevation ST-segment elevation where the ST segment leaves the QRS complex at a convex angle analogous to a frown shape.

coronary artery One of a pair of arteries that supply blood to the myocardium of the heart. They arise within the right and left aortic sinuses at the base of the aorta. Decreased flow of blood through these arteries induces attacks of angina pectoris, while blockage at any point along these arteries results in a heart attack.

couplet A pair of consecutive ECG complexes that originate in the same portion of the heart (atria, AV node, or ventricles).

decompensation Failure of the heart to maintain adequate circulation, or failure of other organs to work properly during stress or illness.

defibrillation 1. Termination of ventricular fibrillation (vfib) with electrical countershock(s). This is the single most important intervention a rescuer can take in patients who have suffered cardiac arrest due to vfib or pulseless ventricular tachycardia. **2.** A term formerly used to signify termination of atrial fibrillation. The contemporary terms for this are *conversion* or *cardioversion*.

Glossary

deflection Movement of the ECG tracing above (positive deflection) or below (negative deflection) the isoelectric line.

depolarization A reversal of charges at a cell membrane; an electrical change in an excitable cell in which the inside of the cell becomes positive (less negative) in relation to the outside. This is the opposite of polarization and is caused by a rapid inflow of sodium ions.

diastole The period of cardiac muscle relaxation, alternating in the cardiac cycle with systole or contraction. During diastole, the cardiac muscle fibers lengthen and the chambers fill with blood.

dobutamine A synthetic beta-agonist whose primary effect is to increase cardiac contractility, with little effect on systemic vascular resistance. It produces less tachycardia than dopamine and has no effect on renal blood flow. It is of use in congestive heart failure and cardiogenic shock.

dopamine A catecholamine synthesized by the adrenal gland; it is used to treat cardiogenic and septic shock. Its effects on receptors in the kidneys, blood vessels, and heart vary with the dose of the drug that is given. Lower doses (up to 10.0 μg/kg per min) increase the force of heart muscle contraction, improve cardiac output, and increase heart rate. Higher doses (greater than 10.0 μg/kg per min) elevate blood pressure by causing vasoconstriction and may cause excessive increase in heart rate, especially in patients who are dehydrated.

dual chamber Relating to or affecting separate chambers as in dual-chamber pacemaker.

dysrhythmia Abnormal, disordered, or disturbed rhythm.

ectopic atrial pacemaker An endogenous cardiac pacemaker that originates in the atrial tissue and controls the heart's rhythm for several consecutive beats or longer.

electrocardiograph A device for recording changes in the electrical energy produced by the action of heart muscles.

electrode 1. An electrical terminal or lead. 2. A conductive medium. 3. In electrotherapy, an instrument with a point or surface from which to discharge current to a patient's body.

electromechanical dissociation Outdated synonym for pulseless electrical activity.

electronic pacemaker 1. Anything that influences the rate and rhythm of occurrence of some activity or process. 2. In cardiology, a specialized cell or group of cells that automatically generates impulses that spread to other regions of the heart. The normal cardiac pacemaker is the sinoatrial node, a group of cells in the right atrium near the entrance of the superior vena cava. 3. A generally accepted term for artificial cardiac pacemaker.

electrophysiology study (EPS) A procedure used to determine the cause of life-threatening cardiac arrhythmias and the effect of treatments to prevent them. EPS is used typically after an episode of sudden death caused by ventricular tachycardia or ventricular fibrillation or in patients at high risk of death from these arrhythmias. Electrodes are placed within the heart and used to stimulate rhythm disturbances; the response of the heart can be studied after administration of antiarrhythmic drug therapy or under other controlled conditions.

epinephrine $C_9H_{13}NO_3$; a catecholamine produced by the adrenal gland, secreted when the sympathetic nervous system is stimulated. In the physiological response to stress, it is responsible for maintaining blood pressure and cardiac output, keeping airways open wide, and raising blood sugar levels. All of these functions are useful to frightened, traumatized, injured, or sick humans and animals. The therapeutic uses of epinephrine are diverse. As one of the key agents used in advanced cardiac life support, it is helpful in treating asystole, ventricular arrhythmias, and other forms of cardiac arrest. It counteracts the effects of systemic allergic reactions and is an effective bronchodilator. It helps control local hemorrhage by constricting blood vessels; because of this action, it prolongs the effects of local anesthesia.

escape beat A heartbeat that occurs after a prolonged pause or failure of the sinus node to stimulate the heart to contract.

external pacemaker An electronic pacemaker where at least part of the device is external to the patient's body.

failure to capture A pacemaker malfunction where there is a pacemaker spike that is not followed by cardiac tissue depolarization.

failure to fire (failure to pace) A pacemaker malfunction where there is an extended period of time without a natural or artificial paced beat. If this occurs frequently or during a particularly slow natural rhythm, it can be fatal.

failure to sense A pacemaker problem where the patient's natural rhythm is not sensed. This can result in R-on-T phenomenon and ventricular fibrillation.

fascicle (left anterior and left posterior) Little bundle. A fasciculus, a branch off of a larger bundle.

fibrillate Refers to the mechanical state of the heart where there is no coordinated contraction but instead a quivering of the specific chambers of the heart.

fibrillatory waves (f-waves) A fibrillatory wave seen as the wavy base line on the electrocardiogram tracing of atrial fibrillation or ventricular fibrillation. These waves are caused by multiple ectopic foci in the atria, or ventricles respectively.

fluid bolus A large amount of fluid given over a short period of time to correct cardiovascular problems such as low blood pressure or pulseless electrical activity.

flutter wave (F-wave) Flutter waves in atrial flutter, detectable on the electrocardiogram at 250 to 350 per minute.

focus (foci) 1. The starting point of a disease process. 2. A point where the electrical depolarization of the heart originates.

fusion beat A beat that occurs when two different foci begin to depolarize the ventricles simultaneously, resulting in a QRS complex that has characteristics of beats that originate in the two disparate locations.

gain In electronics, the term used to describe the amplification factor for a given circuit or device.

gatekeeper Tissue that determines how quickly signals in the heart's electrical system may be propagated. The end result is that the gatekeeper has a significant impact on heart rate.

heart attack Myocardial infarction.

idio- Prefix indicating individual, distinct, or unknown.

idiojunctional A junctional rhythm with a heart rate between 40 and 60 bpm that corresponds to the intrinsic heart rate for the AV node.

idioventricular rhythm (IVR) A cardiac rhythm that arises from pacemakers in ventricular muscle and has a heart rate in the range of 20 to 40 bpm.

infarction Death of tissue that results from deprivation of its blood supply.

inferior vena cava The principal vein draining blood from the lower portion of the body. It is formed by junction of the two common iliac veins and terminates in the right atrium of the heart.

inhibit, inhibition, inhibited A normal function of artificial pacemakers where the pacemaker is caused to not fire when a natural beat is sensed.

injury Blunt or penetrating trauma or damage to a part of the body. In the heart, a amalgam of changes that are present on the ECG that suggest tissue that is most at risk of death.

internodal A pathway that connects the two separate nodes in the cardiac conduction system—the AV node and the SA node.

interval 1. A space or time between two objects, periods or complexes.

intra-atrial Within one or both atria of the heart.

intraventricular conduction defect (IVCD) A delay in the conduction of the cardiac electrical signal as it travels through the ventricles. The QRS duration will be greater than 0.10 seconds.

irregular Not regular.

irregularly irregular Refers to a rhythm where the QRS complexes are not evenly spaced and there is no identifiable pattern to their occurrence.

ischemia A temporary deficiency of blood flow to an organ or tissue. The deficiency may be caused by diminished blood flow either through a regional artery or throughout the circulation.

isoelectric line Synonym for baseline. The flat line of the ECG from one T-wave to the following P-wave where there is no electrical signal generated from the heart's electrical conduction system.

J-point On the electrocardiogram, the juncture between the end of the QRS complex and the beginning of the T wave; that is, between the representations of ventricular depolarization and repolarization.

junctional bradycardia A heart rhythm originating in the AV node with a heart rate slower than 40 bpm.

junctional rhythm An electrocardiographic rhythm arising in the atrioventricular junction. It appears on an electrocardiogram as a narrow QRS complex that lacks an upright P wave preceding it. The heart rate must be between 40 and 60 bpm.

junctional tachycardia A heart rhythm originating in the AV node with a heart rate faster than 100 bpm.

large-box method A method for estimating heart rate in regular rhythms where the number of large boxes between consecutive QRS complexes are determined and divided into 300 (the number of large boxes in 1 minute).

lead 1. Insulated wires connecting a monitoring device to a patient. **2.** A conductor attached to an electrocardiograph. The three limb leads are lead I, right arm to left arm; lead II, right arm to left leg; lead III, left arm to left leg. These are also known as standard leads, bipolar limb leads, or indirect leads.

left anterior descending (LAD) coronary artery One branch of the left main coronary artery.

left anterior fascicle The portion of the left bundle branch that is responsible for sending the signal to the anterior portion of the left ventricle.

left circumflex (LCx) coronary artery The second branch of the left main coronary artery.

left main coronary artery (LMCA) The coronary artery that branches from the left side of the aorta to deliver blood to the left circumflex and left anterior descending arteries.

left posterior fascicle The portion of the left bundle branch that is responsible for sending the signal to the posterior portion of the left ventricle.

lidocaine A local anesthetic drug. Trade name is Xylocaine. Used in treating symptomatic ventricular dysrhythmias.

limb leads Any lead, unipolar or bipolar, in which a limb is the location of the positive electrode.

magnesium A white mineral element found in soft tissue, muscles, bones, and to some extent in the body fluids. Concentration of magnesium in the serum is between 1.5 and 2.5 mmol/L. Magnesium deficiency is frequently associated with a dangerous form of multifocal ventricular tachycardia known as Torsades de pointes.

MATCH×5ED An acronym used to remember the most common differential diagnoses associated with asystole and pulseless electrical activity.

millivolts One thousandth of a volt.

mitral valve The valve that closes the orifice between the left atrium and the left ventricle during ventricular systole.

modified chest leads ECG leads that approximate the precordial leads in systems that do not offer true 12-lead capability.

morphology The science of structure and form of ECG waveforms without regard to function.

multifocal ventricular tachycardia A dangerous heart rhythm that originates in multiple locations in the ventricles. The QRS complexes will vary in shape and or size, indicating that each starts at different foci.

multifocal atrial tachycardia A cardiac arrhythmia that sometimes is confused with atrial fibrillation because the heart rate is greater than 100 beats per minute and the ventricular response is irregular. However, in MAT, p waves are clearly visible on the electrocardiogram, and they have at least three distinct shapes. MAT is seen most often in patients with poorly compensated chronic obstructive lung disease. It may resolve with management of the underlying respiratory problem, or decrease in demands placed on the heart.

multifocal Concerning or arising from many locations or foci.

Glossary

myocardial infarction The loss of living heart muscle as a result of coronary artery occlusion. MI usually occurs when an atheromatous plaque in a coronary artery ruptures and the resulting clot obstructs the injured blood vessel. Perfusion of the muscular tissue that lies downstream from the blocked artery is lost. If blood flow is not restored within a few hours, the heart muscle dies.

myocardium The middle layer of the walls of the heart, composed of cardiac muscle.

myopotential Electrical potential associated with muscle cells.

narrow complex A QRS complex whose duration falls in the normal range of 0.04 to 0.10 seconds.

narrow complex tachycardia Tachycardia in which the duration of the QRS complex is less than 0.12 seconds. Most narrow complex tachycardias originate from a pacemaker above the ventricles and are therefore supraventricular tachycardias.

NBG generic code A code used to describe pacemaker basic functions. Developed by NASPE (North American Society for Pacing and Electrophysiology) and the BPEG (British Pacing and Electrophysiology Group), each giving a letter to the generic code's name.

necrosis The death of cells, tissues, or organs.

nodal tissue A portion of the AV node area.

North American Society of Pacing and Electrophysiology (NASPE) The group responsible for pacing nomenclature in the United States.

NSTEMI (Non–ST-segment elevation myocardial infarction) A myocardial infarction that does not demonstrate ST-segment elevation during the acute phase and does not demonstrate Q-waves in the post-MI phase.

occlusion A blockage of the blood flow through a coronary artery or one of its branches.

overdrive suppression A method of controlling excessive heart rate by electronically pacing the heart at a faster rate than the natural rhythm and, once the pacemaker controls the heart rate and rhythm, slowing the heart rate to more reasonable levels.

oversense A pacemaker complication where the pacemaker senses inappropriate electrical activity as a natural beat. Most commonly occurs when the T-wave is sensed as a QRS complex, resulting in an abnormally long delay in pacemaker depolarization.

oxygen 1. A medicinal gas used in the management of anemia, bleeding, ischemia, shock, pulmonary edema, pneumonia, respiratory distress, ventilatory failure, obstructive lung diseases, pulmonary embolism, myocardial infarction, mountain sickness, smoke inhalation, carbon monoxide or cyanide poisoning, gangrene, and other illnesses where its presence in the body is temporarily or chronically insufficient. **2.** Symbol: O. A nonmetallic element occurring freely in the atmosphere (approximately 21% at sea level) as a colorless, odorless, tasteless gas; atomic weight, 15.9994; atomic number, 8. It is a constituent of animal, vegetable, and mineral substances and is essential to respiration for most living organisms. At sea level, it represents 10% to 16% of venous blood and 17% to 21% of arterial blood.

PAC premature atrial complex.

pace To control the heart rate and rhythm with a pacemaker, natural or artificial.

pacemaker cells Cells that are capable of depolarizing spontaneously and controlling the heart rate and rhythm without external stimulation.

pacemaker 1. Anything that influences the rate and rhythm of occurrence of some activity or process. **2.** In cardiology, a specialized cell or group of cells that automatically generates impulses that spread to other regions of the heart. The normal cardiac pacemaker is the sinoatrial node, a group of cells in the right atrium near the entrance of the superior vena cava. **3.** A generally accepted term for artificial cardiac pacemaker.

asynchronous (competitive) pacing Cardiac pacing that is set at a rate that is independent of the heart's own pacemakers. This type of pacemaker will discharge at set intervals without regard to the patient's rhythm or need for the pacemaker's assistance. This also puts the patient at risk of R-on-T phenomenon and ventricular fibrillation and is rarely used today.

capture The normal response of the heart to an electrical impulse from the cardiac conduction system or an artificial pacemaker.

dual chamber A pacemaker that is also known as an atrioventricular sequential pacemaker because it stimulates both atria and ventricles sequentially.

electronic An artificial pacemaker.

epicardial Electrical pacing of the heart by conductive leads inserted surgically, usually during bypass graft or valvular operations. The leads are used in the postoperative period for the management of heart blocks or dysrhythmias and are removed as the patient stabilizes.

external A pacemaker that is not completely enclosed in the patient's body.

internal A cardiac pacemaker placed within the body.

leads Insulated wires connecting a pacemaker device to a patient. It may allow detection of natural beats as well as allowing delivery of a depolarization signal to the heart.

mode A pacemaker setting that tells the pacemaker when and how often to fire.

permanent A pacemaker that is permanently implanted within the patient.

preferred The part of the heart's electrical conduction system that is the normal pacemaker—the SA node.

sensitivity A pacemaker setting that tells the pacemaker how much energy must be sensed from the patient before a natural beat is presumed.

single chamber A pacemaker that only controls one heart chamber.

spike A vertical deflection on the ECG tracing indicating that a pacemaker discharged.

stimulus The signal sent to the heart by the pacemaker.

synchronous (demand) pacing A pacemaker mode where the pacemaker is capable of sensing the patient's natural rhythm and can alter its own function so as not to compete with it.

transcutaneous An artificial cardiac pacemaker that is located outside the body. The electrodes for delivering the stimulus are located on the chest wall, and deliver the energy through the skin.

transesophageal A pacemaker whose electrode sits in the esophagus and stimulates the heart from behind by sending the depolarization signal through the relatively thin esophageal tissue.

transthoracic A cardiac pacemaker connected to electrodes passed through the chest wall, usually used only in emergency situations, on a temporary basis.

transvenous A pacemaker whose leads are passed to the heart through a vein such as the subclavian or femoral veins.

trigger A pacemaker setting that will allow the pacemaker to fire in response to a natural electrical signal. Useful to maintain atrial kick. To initiate or start with suddenness.

wires Pacemaker electrode.

pacing Setting the rate or pace of an event, especially the heartbeat.

pacing interval The number of milliseconds the pacemaker is programmed to wait from the last depolarization (natural or artificial) before depolarizing again.

PCTA (percutaneous transluminal coronary angioplasty) A method of treating localized coronary artery narrowing. A special double-lumen catheter is designed so that a cylindrical balloon surrounds a portion of it. After the catheter is inserted transcutaneously in the artery, inflation of the balloon with pressure between 9 and 15 atmospheres (approximately 135 to 225 psi) dilates the narrowed vessel. This technique may be used on narrowed arteries other than the coronaries.

pericarditis Inflammation of the pericardium, marked by chest pain, fever, and an audible friction rub.

PJC Premature junctional complex.

polarization The electrical state that exists at the cell membrane of an excitable cell at rest; the inside is negatively charged in relation to the outside. The difference is created by the distribution of ions within the cell and in the extracellular fluid.

potassium A mineral element that serves as both the principal cation in intracellular fluid and an important electrolyte in extracellular fluid. Along with other electrolytes (e.g., sodium, magnesium, calcium, chloride), potassium participates in many functions, including cell membrane homeostasis, nerve impulse conduction, and muscle contraction. Significantly excessive or inadequate levels are associated with potentially life-threatening cardiac conduction disturbances.

precordial Pertinent to the precordium or epigastrium. Refers to leads that wrap around the chest from the right sternal border to the left midaxillary line in the typical 12-lead ECG placement.

premature atrial complex (PAC) The depolarization of the cardiac ventricle prior to the normal time, caused by an electrical impulse to the ventricle arising from a site in the atrial tissue. The PAC may be a single event or occur several times in a minute or in pairs or groups. Three or more PACs in a row constitute a separate atrial rhythm.

premature beat A heartbeat that arises from a site other than the sinus node and occurs early in the cardiac cycle before the expected beat.

premature junctional complex The depolarization of the cardiac ventricle before the normal time caused by an electrical impulse to the ventricle arising from a site in the AV nodal tissue. The PJC may be a single event or occur several times in a minute or in pairs or groups. Three or more PJCs in a row constitute a separate junctional rhythm.

premature ventricular complex (PVC) The depolarization of the cardiac ventricle before the normal time caused by an electrical impulse to the ventricle arising from a site in the ventricular tissue. The PVC may be a single event or occur several times in a minute or in pairs or groups. Three or more PVCs in a row constitute a separate ventricular rhythm.

PR interval In the electrocardiogram, the period between the onset of the P wave and the beginning of the QRS complex.

procainamide hydrochloride An antiarrhythmic drug used to treat atrial and ventricular cardiac rhythm disturbances; its adverse effects may include proarrhythmia and lupus-like syndromes, among others.

PR segment The line on an electrocardiogram that begins with the end of the P wave and ends with the beginning of the QRS. It represents the depolarization of the AV node, and the bundle branches.

pseudo-fusion beats A QRS complex that appears normal in all respects but has a ventricular pacemaker spike just before or at the very beginning of the QRS complex, suggesting a fusion beat.

pseudo-pseudo-fusion beats An uncommon finding, present only with dual-chamber pacemakers, where the atrial pacemaker spike appears just before, or at the beginning of, the QRS complex, suggesting a fusion or pseudo-fusion beat.

pulmonary arteries The artery that takes blood from the right ventricle to the lungs. They are the only arteries to contain deoxygenated blood.

pulmonary veins One of the four veins that takes blood from the lungs to the left atrium. They are the only veins in the body to contain oxygenated blood.

pulmonic valve The valve at the junction of the right ventricle and pulmonary artery. It is composed of three semilunar cusps and prevents regurgitation of blood from the pulmonary artery to the right ventricle.

pulseless electrical activity (PEA) A form of cardiac arrest in which the continuation of organized electrical activity in the heart is not accompanied by a palpable pulse or effective circulation of blood. Replaces the outdated and occasionally incorrect term electro-mechanical dissociation (EMD).

Purkinje fibers A cardiac muscle cell beneath the endocardium of the ventricles of the heart. These extend from the bundle branches to the ventricular myocardium and form the last part of the cardiac conduction system.

Glossary

PVC Premature ventricular complex.

P-wave A wave of an electrocardiogram caused by the depolarization of the atria, whose electrical changes in turn cause atrial contraction.

quadrigeminal Fourfold; having four symmetrical parts. Refers to a rhythm with beats occurring in groups of four, such as three normal beats followed by one abnormal beat.

QRS complex The pattern traced on the surface electrocardiogram by depolarization of the ventricles. The complex normally consists of a small initial downward deflection (Q wave), a large upward deflection (R wave), and a second downward deflection (S wave). The normal duration of the complex is 0.06 to 0.10 seconds. Longer QRS complexes are seen in premature ventricular beats, bundle branch blocks, pacemaker rhythms, and ventricular arrhythmias.

QRS interval In the electrocardiogram, the interval that denotes depolarization of the ventricles between the beginning of the Q wave and the end of the S wave. The normal interval is less than or equal to 0.10 seconds.

QT interval The representation on the electrocardiogram of ventricular depolarization and repolarization, beginning with the QRS complex and ending with the T wave.

QTc interval (corrected QT interval) In electrocardiography, the duration of the QT interval adjusted for the patient's heart rate. Prolonged QTcs are associated with an increased risk of ventricular dysrhythmia and sudden death. It is calculated by dividing the measured QT interval by the square root of length (in time) of the previous R-to-R interval.

Q-wave A downward or negative wave of an electrocardiogram following the P wave. It is usually not prominent and may be absent without significance. New Q waves are frequently present on the electrocardiogram after patients suffer myocardial infarction. The Q-wave must be the first negative deflection of the QRS complex. If any positive deflection occurs first, then negative deflections are referred to as S-waves.

  significant A Q-wave that is at least one small box wide or at least 25% or more the height of the entire QRS complex. They strongly suggest prior myocardial damage from a myocardial infarction.

R-to-R interval The amount of time between two consecutive QRS complexes. Usually measured from the peak of one R-wave to the following R-wave.

R-on-T phenomenon A dangerous occurrence where a new ventricular depolarization begins before the ventricles are completely repolarized. It may be precipitated by a PVC or a pacemaker discharge that occurs during the last half of the T-wave. May initiate a sudden onset of ventricular fibrillation.

reciprocal changes ST-segment depression and T-wave inversion in ECG leads that point to areas of the heart that are not being damaged in an acute myocardial infarction. Their presence is strongly supportive of acute myocardial infarction.

refractory **1.** Resistant to ordinary treatment. **2.** Resistant to stimulation; used of muscle or nerve.

refractory period

  absolute The brief period during depolarization of a neuron or muscle fiber when the cell does not respond to any stimulus, no matter how strong. Usually associated with the QRS complex and the first half of the T-wave.

  relative The brief period during repolarization of a neuron or muscle fiber when excitability is depressed. If stimulated, the cell may respond, but a stronger-than-usual stimulus is required. Usually associated with the second half of the T-wave.

regular except A rhythm that, with the exception of a clearly identified portion or portions, would be regular and occur at regular intervals.

regular **1.** Conforming to a rule or custom. **2.** Methodical, steady in course, as a pulse. **3.** Occuring at set intervals.

regularly irregular A rhythm, while not regular, does appear to have a regular recurring pattern. An example is sinus arrhythmia.

repolarization Restoration of the polarized state at a cell membrane after depolarization in muscle or nerve fibers.

retrograde impulse transmission A signal that follows the reverse path of normal signals. A signal that travels from the ventricles to the atria via the AV node.

right coronary artery (RCA) The coronary artery that arises from the right base of the aorta.

R-wave A wave of an electrocardiogram that corresponds to depolarization of ventricular muscle. Any deflection of the QRS complex above the isoelectric line.

salvo An older term group of three, consecutive premature ventricular complexes.

segment A part or section of an ECG tracing. Particularly that area that falls between two waves or complexes.

sense The ability of an artificial pacemaker to detect an electrically conducted signal produced by the heart, such as a P wave or QRS complex.

sinus arrest Condition in which the sinus node of the heart does not initiate impulses for heartbeat. If this condition persists, or recurs at frequent intervals it usually requires implantation of a permanent cardiac pacemaker.

sinus arrhythmia Cardiac irregularity marked by variation in the interval between sinus beats and evident on the electrocardiogram as alternately long and short intervals between P waves. Sinus arrhythmia may occur with respiration (evidenced as an increased heart rate during inspiration and a decreased heart rate on expiration) or may result from the use of digitalis glycosides. In older patients, presence of sinus arrhythmia is common and is statistically linked with an increased risk of sudden death.

sinus bradycardia A slow sinus rhythm with a heart rate below 60 beats per minute in an adult or 70 beats per minute in a child.

sinus exit block A rhythm where the sinus node continues to discharge at its normal rate but one or more signals get trapped in the sinus node and do not cause atrial depolarization or a P-wave on the ECG.

sinus tachycardia A rapid heart rate (over 100 beats per minute) originating in the sinoatrial node of the heart. It may be caused by fever, exercise, dehydration, bleeding, stimulant drugs (e.g., epinephrine, aminophyline), thyrotoxicosis, or many other diseases or conditions.

sinoatrial node (or sinus node, or SA node) A specialized group of cardiac muscle cells in the wall of the right atrium at the entrance of the superior vena cava. These cells depolarize spontaneously and rhythmically to initiate normal heartbeats.

six-second method A method of estimating heart rate. The number of ECG complexes in 6 seconds is calculated, and the result is multiplied by 10.

small-box method The most precise method for determining heart rate by counting the number or small boxes between consecutive ECG complexes and dividing the result into 1500 (the number of small boxes in 1 minute).

sodium The most abundant cation in extracellular fluids. It is the main contributor to osmotic pressure and hydration, participates in many specialized pumps and receptors on cell membranes, and plays a fundamental part in the electrical activities of the body (e.g., nerve impulse transmission and muscular contraction).

stent Any material or device used to hold tissue in place, to maintain open blood vessels, or to provide a support for a graft or anastomosis while healing is taking place.

drug-eluting A stent that is impregnated with a medication to decrease the risk of reocclusion of the repaired coronary artery.

sternum The narrow, flat bone in the median line of the thorax in front. It consists of three portions: the manubrium, the body or gladiolus, and the ensiform or xiphoid process.

stroke volume The amount of blood ejected by the left ventricle at each heartbeat. The amount varies with age, sex, and exercise but averages 60 to 100 mL.

ST segment The line on an electrocardiogram that begins with the end of the QRS complex and ends at the beginning of the T wave. The level of the ST segment is normally equal to that of the PR interval and the TP interval. ST segment elevation is found in patients with acute myocardial infarction and other conditions. ST segment depression is an indicator of coronary ischemia, or may suggest acute myocardial infarction in another area of the heart.

depression An ECG finding where the ST segment is lower than the isoelectric line. May be associated with cardiac ischemia, digoxin administration, or ventricular conduction disturbances.

elevation An ECG finding where the ST segment is higher than the isoelectric line. May be associated with cardiac injury, pericarditis, or ventricular conduction disturbances.

STEMI (ST segment elevation myocardial infarction) A myocardial infarction that is associated with ST segment elevation during the acute phase and with a Q-wave in the recovery phase.

superior vena cava The principal vein draining blood from the upper portion of the body. It is formed by the junction of the right and left brachiocephalic veins and empties into the right atrium of the heart.

supraventricular tachycardia (SVT) A rapid, regular tachycardia in which the pacemaker is found in the sinus node, the atria, or the atrioventricular junction, i.e., above the ventricles.

S-wave A wave of an electrocardiogram that corresponds to depolarization of ventricular muscle. Any negative deflection of the QRS complex after the occurrence of the R-wave on the ECG.

systole Contraction of the chambers of the heart. The myocardial fibers shorten, making the chamber smaller and forcing blood out. In the cardiac cycle, atrial systole precedes ventricular systole, which pumps blood into the aorta and pulmonary artery.

tachycardia An abnormally rapid heart rate, greater than 100 beats per minute in adults.

tachydysrhythmia A dysrhythmia associated with an elevated heart rate above 100 bpm.

thrombolytic Pertinent to or causing the breaking up of a blood clot.

toll booth A device associated with entry to a highway that can limit the number and/or speed of cars attempting to gain entry to the highway.

Torsade de pointes A rapid, unstable form of multifocal ventricular tachycardia in which the QRS complexes appear to twist, or shift, electrical orientation around the isoelectric line of the electrocardiogram. It often occurs as a life-threatening effect of a medication (e.g., quinidine, amiodarone, or a tricyclic antidepressant) that prolongs the Q-T interval but may also complicate congenital long–Q-T syndromes. Intravenous magnesium sulfate may be used to treat this arrhythmia.

transvenous pacemaker A pacemaker whose leads are delivered to the cardiac tissue through a vein.

tricuspid valve The valve that closes the orifice between the right cardiac atrium and right ventricle during ventricular systole.

trigeminal Found in a grouping of three as when two normal beats are followed by an abnormal beat in a repeated grouping.

triplet A combination of three of a kind. In ECG tracing, three beats from the same area of the heart that occur consecutively, such as PACs, PJCs, or PVCs.

T-wave The portion of the electrical activity of the heart that reflects repolarization of the ventricles.

hyperacute Extremely or excessively acute: tall and peaked or pointed. Usually found in the early stages of an acute myocardial infarction.

inverted T-waves that are deflected in the opposite direction of the preceding QRS complex. Usually indicative of cardiac ischemia or ventricular conduction disturbances.

undersense (nonsensing) A pacemaker malfunction where the patient's natural rhythm is not sensed correctly by the pacemaker. This can result in R-on-T phenomenon and ventricular fibrillation.

unifocal Applied to the origin of cardiac complexes; indicates that all the complexes originated in one location or focus.

unipolar A rhythm or beat that originates from a single foci or location; an ECG lead that relies on one actual patch and one imaginary patch.

unsynchronized shock Synonym for defibrillation.

Glossary

U-wave In the electrocardiogram, a low-amplitude deflection that follows the T wave. It is exaggerated in hypokalemia bradycardia and with digitalis use and negative in ventricular hypertrophy.

valsalva maneuver An attempt to forcibly exhale with the glottis, nose, and mouth closed. This maneuver causes increased intrathoracic pressure, slowing of the pulse, decreased return of blood to the heart, and increased venous pressure. If the eustachian tubes are not obstructed, the pressure on the tympanic membranes also will be increased. When this maneuver is done with just the glottis closed, only intrathoracic pressure will increase. This maneuver may be helpful in converting supraventricular tachycardias to normal sinus rhythm or in clearing ears that have become blocked during a descent from a high altitude.

vector Any force or influence that is a quantity completely specified by magnitude, direction, and sense, which can be represented by a straight line of appropriate length and arrow indicating direction.

ventricle **1.** A small cavity. **2.** Either of two lower chambers of the heart that, when filled with blood, contract to propel it into the arteries. The right ventricle forces blood into the pulmonary artery and then into the lungs; the left pumps blood into the aorta to the rest of the body.

ventricular bradycardia A heart rhythm that originates in the ventricles and has a heart rat of less than 20 bpm.

ventricular fibrillation A frequently treatable but lethal dysrhythmia present in nearly half of all cases of cardiac arrest. It is marked on the electrocardiogram by rapid, chaotic nonrepetitive waveforms and clinically by the absence of effective circulation of blood (pulselessness). Rapid defibrillation (applying unsynchronized electrical shocks to the heart) is the key to treatment. Basic measures, such as opening the airway and providing rescue breaths and chest compressions, should be undertaken until the defibrillator is available.

> **coarse** A form of ventricular fibrillation with wide undulations from the baseline. Usually associated with less time in ventricular fibrillation, and may resemble multifocal ventricular tachycardia in certain leads.

> **fine** A form of ventricular fibrillation with slight undulations from the baseline. Usually associated with a longer time in ventricular fibrillation, and may resemble asystole in certain leads.

ventricular flutter Ventricular depolarizations of the heart at 250 to 350 beats per minute, creating a high-amplitude, saw-tooth, or sinusoidal pattern on the surface electrocardiogram. The rhythm is lethal unless immediate life support and resuscitation are provided.

ventricular response The rate at which the ventricles respond to atrial depolarization. Particularly used in atrial fibrillation and preceded by the terms *slow, normal* (controlled), or *rapid.*

ventricular standstill Cessation of ventricular contractions.

ventricular tachycardia Three or more consecutive ventricular ectopic complexes (duration greater than 120 ms) occurring at a rate of 100 to 250 beats per minute. Although nonsustained VT may occasionally be well-tolerated, it often arises in hearts that have suffered ischemic damage or cardiomyopathic degeneration and may be a cause of sudden death. Nonsustained VT lasts less than 30 seconds. Sustained VT lasts more than 30 seconds and is much more likely to produce loss of consciousness or other life-threatening symptoms.

> **slow** A term commonly applied to ventricular tachycardia with a heart rate slower than 150 bpm. It may be better tolerated than fast ventricular tachycardia.

> **fast** A term commonly applied to ventricular tachycardia with a heart rate faster than 150 bpm. It is usually poorly tolerated due to the decreased ventricular filling time.

verapamil A calcium channel blocker, administered orally or intravenously to manage hypertension, angina pectoris, Prinzmetal's angina, and supraventricular arrhythmias. It is sometimes given to prevent migraine headaches. Its therapeutic classes are antianginal, antiarrhythmic, antihypertensive, and vascular headache suppressant. It should not be given to a patient in V-tach.

wandering atrial pacemaker A cardiac arrhythmia in which the site of origin of the pacemaker stimulus shifts from one site to another, usually from the atrioventricular node to some other part of the atrium. This results in three or more different P-wave shapes and a slightly irregular rhythm.

wave An oscillation seen in the recording of an electrocardiogram.

wide-complex tachycardia An arrhythmia with a sustained rate of more than 100 beats per minute in which the surface electrocardiogram reveals QRS complexes lasting at least 120 msec. WCT is usually caused by ventricular tachycardia, although it may occasionally result from a supraventricular tachycardia whose conduction through the ventricles produces an abnormally wide QRS complex.

widow maker A colloquial term associated with complete occlusion of the proximal left anterior descending artery or the left main coronary artery. Name due to the fact that such an occlusion is commonly associated with sudden death.

Suggested Readings

ACLS textbook, American Heart Association

Antman, EM, Anbe, DT, Armstrong, PW, et al. ACC/AHA guidelines for the management of patients with ST-elevation myocardial infarction—executive summary: a report of the American College of Cardiology/American Heart Association Task Force on Practice Guidelines (Writing Committee to Revise the 1999 Guidelines for the Management of Patients With Acute Myocardial Infarction). Circulation 2004, 110:588.

Bernstein, AD, Daubert, JC, Fletcher, RD, et al. The revised NASPE/BPEG generic code for antibradycardia, adaptive-rate, and multisite pacing. North American Society of Pacing and Electrophysiology/British Pacing and Electrophysiology Group. Pacing Clin Electrophysiol 2002, 25:260.

http://www.blaufuss.org/SVT/index.html, last accessed November 22, 2005.

Braat, SH, Brugada, P, De Zwaan, C, et al. Value of electrocardiogram in diagnosing right ventricular involvement in patients with an acute inferior wall myocardial infarction. Br Heart J 1983, 49:368.

Buxton, AE, Marchlinski, FE, Doherty, JU, et al. Hazards of intravenous verapamil for sustained ventricular tachycardia. Am J Cardiol 1987, 59:1107.

Casas, RE, Marriott, HJL, Glancy, DL. Value of leads V7-V9 in diagnosing posterior wall acute myocardial infarction and other causes of tall R waves in V1-V2. Am J Cardiol 1997, 80:508.

http://www.emedicine.com/ekgotwindexbytitle.html, last accessed November 22, 2005.

Goldberger, AL. Myocardial Infarction: Electrocardiographic Differential Diagnosis, 4th ed., Mosby Year Book, St Louis 1991.

Goldstein, J. Pathophysiology and management of right heart ischemia. J Am Coll Cardiol 2002, 40:841.

Gupta, AK, Thakur, RK. Wide QRS complex tachycardias. Med Clin North Am 2001, 85:245.

http://heart.healthcentersonline.com/arrhythmia/?WT.srch=1, last accessed November 22, 2005.

Josephson, ME. Clinical Cardiac Electrophysiology: Techniques and Interpretations. 2nd ed., Lea Febiger, Philadelphia, 1993.

Kastor, JA. Multifocal atrial tachycardia. N Engl J Med 1990, 322:1713.

Kinch, JW, Ryan, TJ. Right ventricular infarction. N Engl J Med 1994, 330:1211.

Knight, BP, Pelosi, F, Michaud, GF, et al. Physician interpretation of electrocardiographic artifact that mimics ventricular tachycardia. Am J Med 2001, 110:335.

Lamas, GA, Ellenbogen, KA. Evidence base for pacemaker mode selection: from physiology to randomized trials. Circulation 2004, 109:443.

Levine, JH, Michael, JR, Guarnieri, T. Multifocal atrial tachycardia: A toxic effect of theophylline. Lancet 1985, 1:12.

http://www.mdchoice.com/ekg/ekg.asp, last accessed November 22, 2005.

http://medlib.med.utah.edu/kw/ecg/tests/, last accessed November 22, 2005.

Mirvis, DM, Goldberger, AL. Electrocardiography. In: Heart Disease: A Textbook of Cardiovascular Medicine, 7th ed., Braunwald, E, Zipes, DP, Libby, P, (Eds), W.B. Saunders Company, Philadelphia 2004.

Ornato, JP. Chest pain emergency centers: improving acute myocardial infarction care. Clin Cardiol 1999, 22:IV3.

Peuch, P, Groileau, R, Guimond, C. Incidence of different types of A-V block and their localization by His bundle recordings. In: The Conduction System of the Heart, Wellens, HJJ, Lie, KI, Janse, MJ (Eds), Stenfert, Leiden, 1976, p. 467.

Pope, JH, Ruthazer, R, Beshansky, JR, et al. Clinical features of emergency department patients presenting with symptoms suggestive of acute cardiac ischemia: a multicenter study. J Thromb Thrombolysis 1998, 6:63.

Robalino, BD, Whitlow, PL, Underwood, DA, Salcedo, EE. Electrocardiographic manifestations of right ventricular infarction. Am Heart J, 1989, 118:138.

http://www.skillstat.com/ECG_Sim_demo.html, last accessed November 22, 2005.

http://sprojects.mmi.mcgill.ca/heart/egcyhome.html, last accessed November 22, 2005.

Wang, K, Asinger, RW, Marriott, HJ. ST-segment elevation in conditions other than acute myocardial infarction. N Engl J Med 2003, 349:2128.

Answer Key

Chapter 1

1. The heart has **four** chambers.

2. The two upper chambers are called **atria**.

3. The two lower chambers are called **ventricles**.

4. A change in **pressure** is the primary reason that valves open and close.

5. You can increase the cardiac output by increasing **heart rate** or **stroke volume**.

6. The heart receives its blood supply from the **coronary arteries** that start at the base of the **aorta**.

7. The large, flat bone in front of the heart is the **sternum**.

8. The **mitral (bicuspid)** valve separates the left atrium from the left ventricle, and the **tricuspid** valve separates the right atrium from the right ventricle.

9. Starling's Law states that increased **pressure or stretch** results in increased strength of **contraction** up to a point.

10. When the right ventricle is contracting, the **pulmonic** valve is open and the **tricuspid** valve is closed.

11. Label the parts of the heart in the picture below:

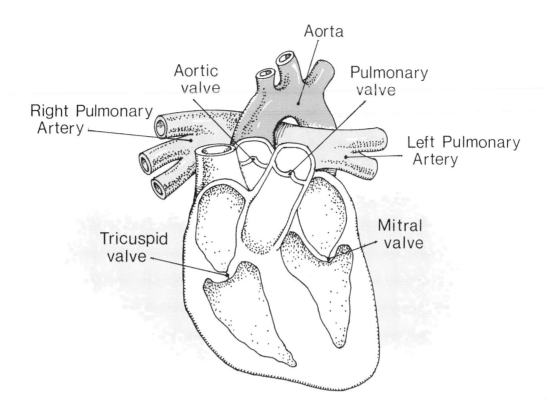

Aorta

Aortic valve

Pulmonary valve

Right Pulmonary Artery

Left Pulmonary Artery

Tricuspid valve

Mitral valve

Chapter 2

1. The **cell membrane** controls the depolarization of the cardiac cell.

2. The **sinus node** is a group of cells that is the heart's preferred pacemaker.

3. **Calcium** is the positive ion responsible for actually causing the muscle cell to contract.

4. The cell membrane has a normal resting charge of about **−90 mV**.

5. **Inter**atrial pathways transmit the signal from the sinus node to the AV node.

6. **Intra**-atrial pathways transmit the signal from the sinus node to the left atrium.

7. The **AV node** normally holds on to the signal for a brief period of time before sending it on.

Chapter 3

1. One small box equals **0.04** seconds horizontally and **0.1** mV vertically.

2. One large box equals **5** small boxes.

3. One large box represents **0.20** seconds horizontally.

4. There are **1500** small boxes and **300** large boxes in 1 minute.

5. There are **25** small boxes and **5** large boxes in 1 second.

6. Why can't the small-box method of calculating heart rate give you an accurate heart rate for an irregular rhythm? **The number of small boxes between different pairs of QRS complexes would be too different.**

7. Which method of calculating heart rate is the most accurate for a regular rhythm? **The small-box method is the most accurate for regular rhythms.**

8. Why are there extra markings for time on the ECG strip? **To quickly identify important intervals such as 1, 3, or 6 seconds for rate estimation.**

9. What additional information should always be on a rhythm strip? **The patient's name, date, time, lead, and any signs or symptoms that precede or coincide with a rhythm strip change.**

10. Circle the lead designation and the computer's calculated heart rate and fill in the appropriate information for the following 10 strips:

    A. Is the rhythm regular or irregular?

    B. Use the 6-second method to determine the heart rate.

    C. Use the large-box method to determine the heart rate.

    D. Use the small-box method to determine the heart rate.

3–1

1st Regular/2nd Irregular	**50 bpm**	**1st 75 bpm/N/A**	**1st 79 bpm/N/A**
Regular/Irregular	Six-second rate	Large-box rate	Small-box rate

3–2

Regular	**70 bpm**	**75 bpm**	**71 bpm**
Regular/Irregular	Six-second rate	Large-box rate	Small-box rate

3–3

Irregular	**80 bpm**	**N/A**	**N/A**
Regular/Irregular	Six-second rate	Large-box rate	Small-box rate

3–4

Regular	**50 bpm**	**50 bpm**	**54 bpm**
Regular/Irregular	Six-second rate	Large-box rate	Small-box rate

3–5

Regular	**160 bpm**	**150 bpm**	**158 bpm**
Regular/Irregular	Six-second rate	Large-box rate	Small-box rate

3–6

Irregular	**80 bpm**	**N/A**	**N/A**
Regular/Irregular	Six-second rate	Large-box rate	Small-box rate

3–7

Irregular	**60 bpm**	**N/A**	**N/A**
Regular/Irregular	Six-second rate	Large-box rate	Small-box rate

3–8

Irregular	**130 bpm**	**N/A**	**N/A**
Regular/Irregular	Six-second rate	Large-box rate	Small-box rate

3–9

Regular	**150 bpm**	**150 bpm**	**150 bpm**
Regular/Irregular	Six-second rate	Large-box rate	Small-box rate

3–10

Irregular	**170 bpm**	**N/A**	**N/A**
Regular/Irregular	Six-second rate	Large-box rate	Small-box rate

Chapter 4

1. A vector can be represented by an **arrow**.

2. The ECG tracing represents the **average** of all of the electrical vectors in the heart.

3. Name four impediments that can interfere with the electrical signal: **Oil, sweat, dry skin, bone, hair, lotions, irritated skin.**

4. Silver chloride (AgCL) is used as an electrical **conductor** in many ECG patches.

5. Which leads are limb leads? **Limb leads are I, II, III, aVF, aVR, and aVL.** Which leads are precordial leads? **Precordial leads are V$_1$, V$_2$, V$_3$, V$_4$, V$_5$, and V$_6$.**

6. Which leads are unipolar? **Unipolar leads are aVR, aVL, aVF, V$_1$, V$_2$, V$_3$, V$_4$, V$_5$, and V$_6$.** Which are bipolar? **Bipolar leads are I, II, and III.**

7. Bipolar leads use two **actual** electrodes. Unipolar leads use one **actual** lead and one **imaginary** electrode, which is an average of the remaining electrodes.

8. Match the electrode with its proper location:

   A. White   a. 4th intercostal space left sternal border

   B. Black   b. 5th intercostal space midaxillary line

   C. Red   c. Right arm (shoulder area)

   D. Green   d. Left arm (shoulder area)

   E. V$_1$ (MCL$_1$)   e. 5th intercostal space midclavicular line

   F. V$_2$ (MCL$_2$)   f. 4th intercostal space right sternal border

   G. V$_3$ (MCL$_3$)   g. 5th intercostal space anterior axillary line

   H. V$_4$ (MCL$_4$)   h. Left leg (left midclavicular line on abdomen)

   I. V$_5$ (MCL$_5$)   i. Right leg (right midclavicular line on abdomen)

   J. V$_6$ (MCL$_6$)   j. Midway between V$_2$ and V$_4$

   Answers: (A, c) (B, d) (C, h) (D, i) (E, f) (F, a) (G, j) (H, e) (I, g) (J, b)

Chapter 5

1. Label all of the parts of the ECG tracing in the following 10 strips:

   5–1

   P-wave: **F–0.12 seconds**   PR interval: **A–0.14 seconds**   QRS complex: **C–0.10 seconds**

   T-wave: **B–0.16 seconds**   QT interval: **E–0.36 seconds**

   ST segment: **D–0.12 seconds**   TP segment: **H–0.54 seconds**

   5–2

   P-wave: **F–0.12 seconds**   PR interval: **C–0.16 seconds**   QRS complex: **H–0.14 seconds**

   T-wave: **G–0.20 seconds**   QT interval: **A–0.42 seconds**   ST segment: **B–0.12 seconds**

   TP segment: **D–0.24 seconds**

   5–3

   P-wave: **E–0.10 seconds**   PR interval: **B–0.16 seconds**   QRS complex: **G–0.10 seconds**

   T-wave: **D–0.16 seconds**   QT interval: **A–0.40 seconds**

   ST segment: **H–0.12 seconds**   TP segment: **C–0.42 seconds**

5–4

P-wave: **D–0.10 seconds**   PR interval: **E–0.14 seconds**   QRS complex: **A–0.08 seconds**

T-wave: **G–0.18 seconds**   QT interval: **F–0.42 seconds**   ST segment: **C–0.12 seconds**

TP segment: **B–0.24 seconds**

5–5

P-wave: **E–0.10 seconds**   PR interval: **A–0.20 seconds**   QRS complex: **C–0.08 seconds**

T-wave: **D–0.20 seconds**   QT interval: **H–0.44 seconds**   ST segment: **B–0.10 seconds**

TP segment: **F–0.08 seconds**

5–6

P-wave: **E–0.12 seconds**   PR interval: **D–0.18 seconds**   QRS complex: **H–0.08 seconds**

T-wave: **F–0.16 seconds**   QT interval: **G–0.38 seconds**   ST segment: **C–0.10 seconds**

TP segment: **B–0.26 seconds**

5–7

P-wave: **H–0.10 seconds**   PR interval: **G–0.14 seconds**   QRS complex: **A–0.10 seconds**

T-wave: **E–0.16 seconds**   QT interval: **F–0.34 seconds**   ST segment: **C–0.08 seconds**

TP segment: **B–0.32 seconds**

5–8

P-wave: **G–0.12 seconds**   PR interval: **A–0.18 seconds**   QRS complex: **D–0.08 seconds**

T-wave: **B–0.28 seconds**   QT interval: **C–0.56 seconds**   ST segment: **H–0.14 seconds**

TP segment: **E–0.52 seconds**

5–9

P-wave: **E–0.10 seconds**   PR interval: **F–0.16 seconds**   QRS complex: **A–0.08 seconds**

T-wave: **H–0.24 seconds**   QT interval: **D–0.48 seconds**   ST segment: **C–0.16 seconds**

TP segment: **B–0.14 seconds**

5–10

P-wave: **C–0.12 seconds**   PR interval: **A–0.16 seconds**   QRS complex: **G–0.10 seconds**

T-wave: **D–0.20 seconds**   QT interval: **B–0.40 seconds**   ST segment: **F–0.12 seconds**

TP segment: **H–0.42 seconds**

2. The PR interval begins at the **beginning** of the P-wave and ends at the **beginning** of the QRS complex.

3. A segment connects two **waves**.

4. An interval includes at least one **wave** and/or one **segment**.

5. A complex is defined as a group of **waves**.

6. A wave begins when the ECG tracings leaves the **baseline**, or **isoelectric line**, with a rounded curve or straight line.

Chapter 6

1. If the PR interval is too short, what effect does that have on the cardiac output?
Cardiac output is decreased because the atria do not have enough time to contract and empty before the ventricles begin contracting.

2. The PR interval is made up of the **P-wave** and the PR **segment**.

3. When does the P-wave occur in relation to the QRS complex? **The P-wave may occur before, during, or after the QRS complex.**

4. A rhythm can have one, no, or many **P-waves** for each QRS complex.

5. All PR intervals must be carefully examined because PR intervals can **vary** throughout a tracing.

6. In the following 10 rhythm strips, identify all of the P-waves and measure the PR interval if that is appropriate:

6-1

PR interval: **0.26 seconds**

6-2

PR interval: **0.20 seconds**

6-3

PR interval: **0.22 seconds**

6-4

PR interval: **0.16 seconds**

6-5

PR interval: **0.40 seconds**

6-6

PR interval: **0.24 seconds**

6-7

PR interval: **0.28 seconds**

6-8

PR interval: **0.16 seconds**

6-9

PR interval: **0.14 seconds**

6-10

PR interval: **0.28 seconds**

Chapter 7

1. The QRS complex represents the signal traveling through the **terminal Purkinje fibers**, and depolarizing the ventricles.

2. There are **two** main bundle branches.

3. The **left anterior** bundle branch, or **fascicle**, sends the signal to the front, or anterior portion, of the left ventricle.

4. The **left posterior** bundle branch, or **fascicle**, sends the signal to the back, or **posterior portion**, of the left ventricle.

5. The normal length of the QRS complex is between **0.06** and **0.10** seconds.

6. Most QRS complexes consist of **straight lines**, unlike the P-wave and T-wave.

7. The J-point is the point where the QRS complex begins to **bend or curve**.

8. The J-point marks the **end** of the QRS complex.

9. Measure the QRS complex width in the following 10 strips:

    7–9

    QRS width: **0.08 seconds**

    7–10

    QRS width: **0.16 seconds**

    7–11

    QRS width: **0.12 seconds**

    7–12

    QRS width: **0.06 seconds**

    7–13

    QRS width: **0.08 seconds**

    7–14

    QRS width: **0.14 seconds**

    7–15

    QRS width: **0.08 seconds**

    7–16

    QRS width: **0.06 seconds**

    7–17

    QRS width: **0.16 seconds**

    7–18

    QRS width: **0.14 seconds**

Chapter 8

1. An ECG tracing originating in the sinus node with a heart rate of 52 bpm would be described as **sinus bradycardia**.

2. An ECG tracing originating in the sinus node with a heart rate of 89 bpm, with two consecutive premature ventricular contractions, would be described as **sinus rhythm** with a **ventricular couplet**.

3. Accelerated junctional rhythm could have a heart rate from **60** to **100** bpm.

4. Any rhythm with a heart rate above 100 bpm is considered a **tachycardia**.

5. A rhythm that has a heart rate of 56 bpm, originates in the junctional tissue, and has two beats followed by a premature ventricular complex (PVC) in a repeating cycle would be called **junctional rhythm** with **trigeminal PVCs**.

6. Junctional tachycardia originates in the **AV node** and has a heart rate of at least **100** bpm.

7. When a rhythm has premature atrial contractions (PACs) that come from different locations, the PACs are considered **multifocal**.

Chapter 9

1. In a regular rhythm, the distance between consecutive QRS complexes varies by less than **3** small boxes.

2. In an irregularly irregular rhythm, there is no **pattern** to the occurrence of the QRS complexes.

3. In a **regular except** rhythm, one or more complexes disturb an otherwise regular rhythm.

4. Identifying P-wave morphology can help determine where the rhythm **originates**.

5. PR interval measurements can be a fixed number, **variable** or **not measurable**.

6. Answer the questions in the five areas for the following five strips:

9–1

Regularity: **Regularly irregular**   Heart rate: **60 bpm**

P-waves: **All the same, more than 1 per QRS**   PR interval: **Variable**

QRS complex: **0.06 seconds**

9–2

Regularity: **Regular**   Heart rate: **63 bpm**

P-waves: **Regular, all the same**   PR interval: **0.18 seconds**

QRS complex: **0.06 seconds**

9–3

Regularity: **Regular**   Heart rate: **71 bpm**

P-waves: **None**   PR interval: **Not measurable**

QRS complex: **0.10 seconds**

9–4

Regularity: **Irregularly irregular**   Heart rate: **60 bpm**

P-waves: **All the same, more than 1 per QRS**   PR interval: **Variable**

QRS complex: **0.10 seconds**

9–5

Regularity: **Regular except**   Heart rate: **80 bpm**

P-waves: **All the same except the third and eighth beats**   PR interval: **0.20 seconds**

QRS complex: **0.12 seconds**

Chapter 10

1. The sinus node has an intrinsic rate of **60–99 bpm**.

2. If the heart rate is less than 60 bpm but otherwise meets the criteria for sinus rhythm, it is called sinus **bradycardia**.

3. Sinus tachycardia meets all of the criteria for sinus rhythm except the heart rate, which is between **100 and 160 bpm**.

4. Name six causes of sinus tachycardia:

   (Answer: Any six of the conditions listed in Table 10–3.)

5. Fill in the regularity of the following sinus node–generated rhythms:

Sinus rhythm	**Regular**
Sinus bradycardia	**Regular**
Sinus tachycardia	**Regular**
Sinus arrhythmia	**Regularly irregular**
Sinus exit block	**Regular except**
Sinus arrest	**Regular except**

6. What is the potential effect of atropine on the heart rate? **Atropine increases the heart rate.**

7. In sinus **exit block**, the P-wave after the pause occurs at the usual interval because the sinus node is not reset.

8. The PR interval for sinus rhythms is between **0.12** and **0.20** seconds.

9. Sinus tachycardia usually occurs **gradually**, whereas other tachyarrhythmias usually occur **suddenly**.

10. Fill in the information for the following forty rhythm strips, all of which originate in the sinus node:

    10–1

    Regularity: **Regular**   Heart rate: **80**   PR interval: **0.16 seconds**

    P-waves: **Normal, all the same**   QRS complex: **0.08 seconds**

    Interpretation: **Sinus rhythm**

    10–2

    Regularity: **Regular**   Heart rate: **77**   PR interval: **0.16 seconds**

    P-waves: **Normal, all the same**   QRS complex: **0.06 seconds**

    Interpretation: **Sinus rhythm**

    10–3

    Regularity: **Regular**   Heart rate: **71**   PR interval: **0.18 seconds**

    P-waves: **Normal, all the same**   QRS complex: **0.08 seconds**

    Interpretation: **Sinus rhythm with inverted T-wave**

    10–4

    Regularity: **Regular**   Heart rate: **63**   PR interval: **0.16 seconds**

    P-waves: **Normal, all the same**   QRS complex: **0.10 seconds**

    Interpretation: **Sinus rhythm with inverted T-wave and Q-wave**

    10–5

    Regularity: **Regular**   Heart rate: **103**   PR interval: **0.16 seconds**

    P-waves: **Normal, all the same**   QRS complex: **0.06 seconds**

    Interpretation: **Sinus tachycardia**

10–6

Regularity: **Regularly irregular**   Heart rate: **80**   PR interval: **0.12 seconds**

P-waves: **Normal, all the same**   QRS complex: **0.08 seconds**

Interpretation: **Sinus arrhythmia**

10–7

Regularity: **Regular**   Heart rate: **56**   PR interval: **0.16 seconds**

P-waves: **Normal, all the same**   QRS complex: **0.08 seconds**

Interpretation: **Sinus bradycardia**

10–8

Regularity: **Regular**   Heart rate: **77**   PR interval: **0.12 seconds**

P-waves: **Normal, all the same**   QRS complex: **0.08 seconds**

Interpretation: **Sinus rhythm**

10–9

Regularity: **Regular**   Heart rate: **107**   PR interval: **0.16 seconds**

P-waves: **Normal, all the same**   QRS complex: **0.10 seconds**

Interpretation: **Sinus tachycardia**

10–10

Regularity: **Regular**   Heart rate: **167**

PR interval: **>0.12 seconds (P-wave partly buried in T-wave; difficult to measure)**

P-waves: **Normal, all the same**   QRS complex: **0.08 seconds**

Interpretation: **Sinus tachycardia** (may have rate up to 180 bpm)

10–11

Regularity: **Regular**   Heart rate: **107**   PR interval: **0.14 seconds**

P-waves: **Normal, all the same**   QRS complex: **0.06 seconds**

Interpretation: **Sinus tachycardia**

10–12

Regularity: **Regular**   Heart rate: **83**   PR interval: **0.16 seconds**

P-waves: **Normal, all the same**   QRS complex: **0.08 seconds**

Interpretation: **Sinus rhythm**

10–13

Regularity: **Regular**   Heart rate: **85**   PR interval: **0.16 seconds**

P-waves: **Normal, all the same**   QRS complex: **0.10 seconds**

Interpretation: **Sinus rhythm**

10–14

Regularity: **Regular**   Heart rate: **53**   PR interval: **0.16 seconds**

P-waves: **Normal, all the same**   QRS complex: **0.08 seconds**

Interpretation: **Sinus bradycardia**

10–15

Regularity: **Regular**   Heart rate: **103**   PR interval: **0.14 seconds**

P-waves: **Normal, all the same**   QRS complex: **0.08 seconds**

Interpretation: **Sinus tachycardia**

10–16

Regularity: **Regular**   Heart rate: **83**   PR interval: **0.12 seconds**

P-waves: **Normal, all the same**   QRS complex: **0.08 seconds**

Interpretation: **Sinus rhythm**

10–17

Regularity: **Regular**   Heart rate: **107**   PR interval: **0.16 seconds**

P-waves: **Normal, all the same**   QRS complex: **0.08 seconds**

Interpretation: **Sinus rhythm**

10–18

Regularity: **Regularly irregular**   Heart rate: **60**   PR interval: **0.16 seconds**

P-waves: **Normal, all the same**   QRS complex: **0.08 seconds**

Interpretation: **Sinus arrhythmia**

10–19

Regularity: **Regular**   Heart rate: **81**   PR interval: **0.14 seconds**

P-waves: **Normal, all the same**   QRS complex: **0.08 seconds**

Interpretation: **Sinus rhythm with inverted T-waves**

10–20

Regularity: **Regular**   Heart rate: **42**   PR interval: **0.16 seconds**

P-waves: **Normal, all the same**   QRS complex: **0.06 seconds**

Interpretation: **Sinus bradycardia**

10–21

Regularity: **Regular**   Heart rate: **130**   PR interval: **0.12 seconds**

P-waves: **Normal, all the same**   QRS complex: **0.10 seconds**

Interpretation: **Sinus tachycardia**

10–22

Regularity: **Regular**   Heart rate: **50**   PR interval: **0.20 seconds**

P-waves: **Normal, all the same**   QRS complex: **0.06 seconds**

Interpretation: **Sinus bradycardia**

10–23

Regularity: **Regular**   Heart rate: **125**   PR interval: **0.14 seconds**

P-waves: **Normal, all the same**   QRS complex: **0.08 seconds**

Interpretation: **Sinus tachycardia**

10–24

Regularity: **Regular except**   Heart rate: **96**   PR interval: **0.14 seconds**

P-waves: **Normal, all the same**   QRS complex: **0.08 seconds**

Interpretation: **Sinus rhythm with sinus exit block**

10–25

Regularity: **Regular**   Heart rate: **143**   PR interval: **0.12 seconds**

P-waves: **Normal, all the same**   QRS complex: **0.04 seconds**

Interpretation: **Sinus tachycardia**

10–26

Regularity: **Regular except**   Heart rate: **60**   PR interval: **0.16 seconds**

P-waves: **Normal, all the same**   QRS complex: **0.08 seconds**

Interpretation: **Sinus rhythm with sinus arrest**

10–27

Regularity: **Regular**   Heart rate: **39**   PR interval: **0.14 seconds**

P-waves: **Normal, all the same**   QRS complex: **0.06 seconds**

Interpretation: **Sinus bradycardia**

10–28

Regularity: **Regular**   Heart rate: **79**   PR interval: **0.16 seconds**

P-waves: **Normal, all the same**   QRS complex: **0.08 seconds**

Interpretation: **Sinus rhythm**

10–29

Regularity: **Regular**   Heart rate: **63**   PR interval: **0.14 seconds**

P-waves: **Normal, all the same**   QRS complex: **0.06 seconds**

Interpretation: **Sinus rhythm**

10–30

Regularity: **Regular**   Heart rate: **104**   PR interval: **0.18 seconds**

P-waves: **Normal, all the same**   QRS complex: **0.08 seconds**

Interpretation: **Sinus tachycardia**

10–31

Regularity: **Regular**   Heart rate: **88**   PR interval: **0.18 seconds**

P-waves: **Normal, all the same**   QRS complex: **0.10 seconds**

Interpretation: **Sinus rhythm**

10–32

Regularity: **Regular**   Heart rate: **104**   PR interval: **0.12 seconds**

P-waves: **Normal, all the same**   QRS complex: **0.08 seconds**

Interpretation: **Sinus tachycardia**

10–33

Regularity: **Regular**   Heart rate: **50**   PR interval: **0.16 seconds**

P-waves: **Normal, all the same**   QRS complex: **0.08 seconds**

Interpretation: **Sinus bradycardia**

10–34

Regularity: **Regular**   Heart rate: **62**   PR interval: **0.18 seconds**

P-waves: **Normal, all the same**   QRS complex: **0.06 seconds**

Interpretation: **Sinus rhythm**

10–35

Regularity: **Regular**   Heart rate: **142**   PR interval: **0.16 seconds**

P-waves: **Normal, all the same**   QRS complex: **0.06 seconds**

Interpretation: **Sinus tachycardia**

10–36

Regularity: **Regular**   Heart rate: **112**   PR interval: **0.16 seconds**

P-waves: **Normal, all the same**   QRS complex: **0.06 seconds**

Interpretation: **Sinus tachycardia**

10–37

Regularity: **Regular**   Heart rate: **50**   PR interval: **0.18 seconds**

P-waves: **Normal, all the same**   QRS complex: **0.08 seconds**

Interpretation: **Sinus bradycardia with prominent U-wave**

10–38

Regularity: **Regularly irregular**   Heart rate: **60**   PR interval: **0.14 seconds**

P-waves: **Normal, all the same**   QRS complex: **0.08 seconds**

Interpretation: **Sinus bradycardia with sinus arrhythmia**

10–39

Regularity: **Regular**   Heart rate: **63**   PR interval: **0.16 seconds**

P-waves: **Normal, all the same**   QRS complex: **0.10 seconds**

Interpretation: **Sinus rhythm**

10–40

Regularity: **Regular**   Heart rate: **77**   PR interval: **0.14 seconds**

P-waves: **Normal, all the same**   QRS complex: **0.06 seconds**

Interpretation: **Sinus rhythm**

Chapter 11

1. **Atrial fibrillation** has a wavy baseline and an irregularly irregular R-to-R pattern.

2. Atrial rhythms differ from sinus rhythms in the shape of the **P-wave.**

3. In atrial flutter, an irritable atrial focus can discharge from **250** to **350** times per minute.

4. To compute the AV block in atrial flutter, divide the **atrial** rate by the **ventricular** rate.

5. **Ectopic atrial pacemaker** occurs when a single irritable atrial focus discharges faster than the sinus node.

6. **Calcium channel blockers, beta blockers,** and digoxin are used to control the heart rate in atrial fibrillation.

7. Quinidine and amiodarone are used to convert **atrial fibrillation** to **sinus rhythm.**

8. **Wandering atrial pacemaker** has at least three differently shaped **P-waves**.

9. **Digoxin** toxicity, especially with coexistent **hypokalemia**, can cause atrial tachycardia.

10. Identify the atrial rhythm in the following 40 strips:

    11–1

    Regularity: **Regular**   Heart rate: **Atrial, ~250; ventricular, ~63**

    PR interval: **Not measurable**   P-waves: **F-waves**   QRS complex: **0.08 seconds**

    Interpretation: **Atrial flutter with a 4:1 AV block (250/63 = ~4)**

    11–2

    Regularity: **Irregularly irregular**   Heart rate: **Average, 90; minimum, 56; maximum, 111**

    PR interval: **Not measurable**   P-waves: **F-waves**   QRS complex: **0.10 seconds**

    Interpretation: **A-fib**

    11–3

    Regularity: **Irregular**   Heart rate: **90**   PR interval: **Variable**

    P-waves: **Abnormal, all different**   QRS complex: **0.08 seconds**

    Interpretation: **Wandering atrial pacemaker**

    11–4

    Regularity: **Regular except**   Heart rate: **125**   PR interval: **0.14 seconds**

    P-waves: **Normal, all the same, except before 5th and 12th beats**   QRS complex: **0.06 seconds**

    Interpretation: **Sinus tachycardia with PACs**

    11–5

    Regularity: **Irregularly irregular**   Heart rate: **Average, 90; minimum, 38; maximum, 143**

    PR interval: **Not measurable**   P-waves: **F-waves, all the same**   QRS complex: **0.08 seconds**
    except last two which are ventricular escape beats due to the slow rate

    Interpretation: **Atrial flutter with variable AV block and ventricular escape beats**

    11–6

    Regularity: **Irregularly irregular**   Heart rate: **Average, 110; minimum, 81; maximum, 136**

    PR interval: **Not measurable**   P-waves: **Wavy baseline**   QRS complex: **0.06 seconds**

    Interpretation: **A-fib with rapid ventricular response (RVR)**

11–7

Regularity: **Irregularly irregular**   Heart rate: **120**   PR interval: **Variable**

P-waves: **Abnormal, more than three different shapes**   QRS complex: **0.10 seconds**

Interpretation: **Multifocal atrial tachycardia**

11–8

Regularity: **First rhythm regular except, second rhythm regular**

Heart rate: **First rhythm, 140; second rhythm, 240**

PR interval: **First rhythm, 0.14 seconds; second rhythm, not measurable**

P-waves: **First rhythm normal, all the same except the last beat; second rhythm indiscernible**

QRS complex: **0.06 seconds**

Interpretation: **Rhythm starts out as sinus rhythm and then a PAC occurs (8th beat), triggering a run of atrial tachycardia.**

11–9

Regularity: **Regular**   Heart rate: **First half, 79; second half, 83**   PR interval: **0.16 seconds**

P-waves: **Normal, all the same until focus changes halfway through rhythm, producing a new shape**

QRS complex: **0.08 seconds**

Interpretation: **Ectopic atrial pacemaker converting to sinus rhythm when sinus node discharge rate surpasses atrial focus discharge rate. (This could technically be called wandering atrial pacemaker because there are three different shapes of P-waves; however, the last three P-waves are identical, suggesting the new P-waves will continue as the focus for a new rhythm.**

11–10

Regularity: **Regular except**   Heart rate: **70**

PR interval: **0.12 seconds in sinus beats, 0.10 seconds in atrial beats**

P-waves: **Normal, all the same, except P-wave after the pause (also note deformed T-wave just before the pause)**

QRS complex: **0.08 seconds**

Interpretation: **Sinus rhythm with blocked PACs and atrial escape beats. Deformed T-waves after the 2nd, 5th, QRS complexes each contain a blocked PAC. Then comes a pause, and the next P-wave is shaped differently than in the sinus beats. These are atrial P-waves and also atrial escape beats because they occur later than expected, not earlier.**

11–11

Regularity: **Irregular**   Heart rate: **Atrial, ~250; ventricular, ~70**   PR interval: **Not measurable**

P-waves: **F-waves**   QRS complex: **0.08 seconds**

Interpretation: **Atrial flutter with variable AV block (3:1 and 4:1)**

11–12

Regularity: **Irregularly irregular**   Heart rate: **Average: 170, minimum: 142, maximum: 214**
PR interval: **Not measurable**

P-waves: **None visible, wavy baseline**   QRS complex: **0.10 seconds**

Interpretation: **A-fib with RVR**

11–13

Regularity: **Regular**   Heart rate: **180**   PR interval: **Difficult to measure**

P-waves: **Appear all the same**   QRS complex: **0.06 seconds**

Interpretation: **Atrial tachycardia (due to heart rate convention but may be sinus tachycardia)**

11–14

Regularity: **Irregular**   Heart rate: **80**   PR interval: **Variable**

P-waves: **Abnormal, many different shapes**   QRS complex: **0.10 seconds**

Interpretation: **Wandering atrial pacemaker**

11–15

Regularity: **Irregularly irregular**   Heart rate: **Atrial, 214; ventricular, 70**   PR interval: **Not measurable**

P-waves: **F-waves**   QRS complex: **0.10 seconds**

Interpretation: **Atrial tachycardia (because of atrial rate) with variable block (not atrial flutter because of slow atrial rate)**

11–16

Regularity: **Slightly irregular**   Heart rate: **80**   PR interval: **Variable**

P-waves: **Abnormal, many different shapes**   QRS complex: **0.08 seconds**

Interpretation: **Wandering atrial pacemaker**

11–17

Regularity: **Regular**   Heart rate: **188**   PR interval: **0.10 seconds**

P-waves: **Normal, all the same**   QRS complex: **0.06 seconds**

Interpretation: **Atrial tachycardia**

11–18

Regularity: **Regular**   Heart rate: **94**   PR interval: **0.14 seconds**

P-waves: **Normal, all the same**   QRS complex: **0.06 seconds**

Interpretation: **Ectopic atrial pacemaker (This strip is from a patient that had large P-waves in sinus rhythm. This strip demonstrates how EAP can be mistakes for SR with knowing the patient.)**

11–19

Regularity: **Regular**   Heart rate: **Atrial, 273; ventricular, 72**   PR interval: **Not measurable**

P-waves: **F-waves**   QRS complex: **0.06 seconds**

Interpretation: **Atrial flutter with 4:1 AV block**

11–20

Regularity: **Irregularly irregular**   Heart rate: **120**   PR interval: **Variable**

P-waves: **Abnormal, many different shapes**   QRS complex: **0.08 seconds**

Interpretation: **Multifocal atrial tachycardia**

11–21

Regularity: **Irregularly irregular**   Heart rate: **Average, 60; minimum, 42; maximum, 65**

PR interval: **Not measurable**

P-waves: **None identifiable, wavy baseline**

QRS complex: **0.06 seconds**   Interpretation: **A-fib**

11–22

Regularity: **First rhythm regular, second rhythm regular except**   Heart rate: **~100**

PR interval: **First rhythm, 0.12 seconds; second rhythm, 0.16 seconds**

P-waves: **First rhythm all the same; conversion rhythm changing slightly as pacemaker site starts to move and ending with a premature beat; second rhythm all the same**

QRS complex: **0.06 seconds**

Interpretation: **Ectopic atrial pacemaker converting to sinus rhythm with PAC (9th beat with P-wave buried and deforming the preceding T-wave.)**

11–23

Regularity: **Regular**   Heart rate: **Atrial, 333; ventricular, 83**   PR interval: **Not measurable**

P-waves: **F-waves**   QRS complex: **0.08 seconds**

Interpretation: **Atrial flutter with 4:1 AV block**

11–24

Regularity: **Irregularly irregular**   Heart rate: **Average: 100, minimum: 68, maximum: 167**
PR interval: **Not measurable**

P-waves: **None visible, wavy baseline**   QRS complex: **0.08 seconds**

Interpretation: **A-fib**

11–25

Regularity: **Irregularly irregular**   Heart rate: **Atrial, 333; ventricular, 140**

PR interval: **Not measurable**   P-waves: **F-waves**   QRS complex: **0.08 seconds**

Interpretation: **Atrial flutter with RVR and variable AV block**

11–26

Regularity: **Irregularly irregular**   Heart rate: **Average, 70; minimum, 26; maximum, 136**

PR interval: **Not measurable**   P-waves: **None seen, wavy baseline**

QRS complex: **0.06 seconds**   Interpretation: **A-fib with 2.28 second pause**

11–27

Regularity: **Regular except**   Heart rate: **52**   PR interval: **0.16 seconds**

P-waves: **Every third wave different, otherwise all the same**   QRS complex: **0.06 seconds**

Interpretation: **Sinus bradycardia with trigeminal PACs**

11–28

Regularity: **Irregularly irregular**   Heart rate: **Average: 100, minimum: 81, maximum: 121**
PR interval: **Not measurable**

P-waves: **None seen, wavy baseline**   QRS complex: **0.06 seconds**

Interpretation: **A-fib**

11–29

Regularity: **Irregularly irregular**   Heart rate: **140**   PR interval: **N/A**

P-waves: **wavy baseline**   QRS complex: **0.10 seconds**

Interpretation: **A-fib with RVR**

11–30

Regularity: **Irregularly irregular**   Heart rate: **Atrial, 300; ventricular, 150**

PR interval: **Not measurable**   P-waves: **F-waves**   QRS complex: **0.06 seconds**

Interpretation: **Atrial flutter with variable AV block (start as 2:1, then short period of 4:1)**

11–31

Regularity: **Irregularly irregular**   Heart rate: **Average, 180; minimum, 136; maximum, 214**

PR interval: **Not measurable**   P-waves: **None seen, wavy baseline**

QRS complex: **0.10 seconds**   Interpretation: **A-fib with RVR followed by burst of SVT**

11–32

Regularity: **Regular**   Heart rate: **100 slowing to 83**   PR interval: **0.16 seconds**

P-waves: **All the same, change to another focus, at the end**   QRS complex: **0.08 seconds**

Interpretation: **Sinus rhythm with ectopic atrial beat not early or late.**

11–33

Regularity: **Regular**   Heart rate: **Atrial, 333; ventricular, 167**   PR interval: **Not measurable**

P-waves: **F-waves**   QRS complex: **0.06 seconds**

Interpretation: **Atrial flutter with 2:1 AV block**

11–34

Regularity: **Irregularly irregular**   Heart rate: **130**   PR interval: **Variable**

P-waves: **More than three different shapes**   QRS complex: **0.10 seconds**

Interpretation: **Multifocal atrial tachycardia**

11–35

Regularity: **Regular**   Heart rate: **Atrial, 333; ventricular, 86**   PR interval: **Not measurable**

P-waves: **F-waves**   QRS complex: **0.06 seconds**   Interpretation: **Atrial flutter with 4:1 AV block**

11–36

Regularity: **Irregularly irregular**   Heart rate: **130**   PR interval: **Not measurable**

P-waves: **F-waves**   QRS complex: **0.08 seconds**

Interpretation: **Atrial flutter with variable AV block (begin as 2:1, slows to become variable and the F-waves become clear)**

11–37

Regularity: **Regular**   Heart rate: **Average, 140; minimum, 115; maximum, 167**

PR interval: **Not measurable**   P-waves: **f-waves**   QRS complex: **0.06 seconds**

Interpretation: **A-fib with RVR**

11–38

Regularity: **Irregularly irregular**   Heart rate: **100**   PR interval: **Variable**

P-waves: **More than three different shapes**   QRS complex: **0.08 seconds**

Interpretation: **Wandering atrial pacemaker or multifocal atrial tachycardia (depends on how you view the heart rate the rest of the time.)**

11–39

Regularity: **Regular except**   Heart rate: **94**   PR interval: **0.14 seconds**

P-waves: **Normal, all the same except every third beat**   QRS complex: **0.06 seconds**

Interpretation: **Sinus rhythm with multifocal trigeminal PACs**

11–40

Regularity: **Regularly irregular**   Heart rate: **100**   PR interval: **0.16 seconds**

P-waves: **Normal, all the same in an alternating pattern**   QRS complex: **0.08 seconds**

Interpretation: **Sinus rhythm with bigeminal PACs**

Chapter 12

1. The main difference among sinus rhythms, atrial rhythms, and junctional rhythms is found in the **P-wave**.

2. The main similarity among sinus rhythms, atrial rhythms, and junctional rhythms is found in the **QRS complex**.

3. The PR interval in junctional rhythms, if measurable, should be less than **0.12 seconds**.

4. An important distinction between atrial fibrillation and junctional rhythm is whether or not the rhythm is **regular**.

5. **Supraventricular tachycardia** is the generic term for all rhythms faster than **100 bpm** and originating in the sinus node, atrial tissue, or AV node.

6. To compensate for the loss of atrial kick, **accelerated junctional rhythm** is the preferred junctional rhythm in most cases.

7. The P-wave in lead II is always **inverted** in junctional rhythms.

8. **Multifocal** PJCs have P-waves that look the same but appear in different locations relative to the QRS complex.

9. The intrinsic rate for junctional tissue is **40** to **60** bpm.

10. Identify the junctional rhythm in the following thirty strips:

12–1

Regularity: **Regular except**   Heart rate: **97**   PR interval: **0.10 seconds**

P-waves: **All the same**   QRS complex: **0.10 seconds**

Interpretation: **Accelerated Junctional Rhythm**

12–2

Regularity: **Regular**   Heart rate: **34**   PR interval: **Not measurable**

P-waves: **Inverted P-wave just after QRS in lead II.**   QRS complex: **0.08 seconds**

Interpretation: **Junctional bradycardia**

12–3

Regularity: **Regular except**   Heart rate: **97**   PR interval: **0.10 seconds**

P-waves: **All the same except after beat 9 (blocked PAC) and before beat 10 (junctional escape beat)**

QRS complex: **0.10 seconds**

Interpretation: **Sinus rhythm with blocked PAC and junctional escape beat**

12–4

Regularity: **Regular**   Heart rate: **68**   PR interval: **0.08 seconds**

P-waves: **All the same (upright in V_1)**   QRS complex: **0.08 seconds**

Interpretation: **Accelerated junctional rhythm**

12–5

Regularity: **Regular**   Heart rate: **90**   PR interval: **Not measurable**

P-waves: **None visible**   QRS complex: **0.08 seconds**

Interpretation: **Accelerated junctional rhythm**

12–6

Regularity: **Regular except**   Heart rate: **88**   PR interval: **0.20 seconds**

P-waves: **All the same when visible**   QRS complex: **0.08 seconds**

Interpretation: **Sinus rhythm with PJCs (beats 1, 3, 9, and 10)**

12–7

Regularity: **Regular**   Heart rate: **136**   PR interval: **0.10 seconds**

P-waves: **All the same, inverted in lead II**   QRS complex: **0.06 seconds**

Interpretation: **Junctional tachycardia**

12–8

Regularity: **Regular**   Heart rate: **43**   PR interval: **Not measurable**

P-waves: **None visible except before 5th QRS**   QRS complex: **0.08 seconds**

Interpretation: **Junctional rhythm with a PAC.**

12–9

Regularity: **Regular**   Heart rate: **58**   PR interval: **Not measurable**

P-waves: **None visible**

QRS complex: **0.06 seconds**

Interpretation: **Junctional rhythm**

12–10

Regularity: **Regular**   Heart rate: **38**   PR interval: **Not measurable**

P-waves: **None visible**   QRS complex: **0.06 seconds**

Interpretation: **Junctional bradycardia**

12–11

Regularity: **Regular, irregular, then regular again**

Heart rate: **Variable; average, 130; minimum, 88; maximum, 214**   PR interval: **Variable**

P-waves: **All the same in the first two, difficult to identify in the middle, then all the same but different from initial P-waves**

QRS complex: **0.08 seconds**

Interpretation: **Sinus tachycardia with PJC (beat 3) triggering run of SVT (beats 4–10), then ectopic atrial pacemaker**

12–12

Regularity: **Regular**   Heart rate: **36**   PR interval: **Not measurable**

P-waves: **None visible**   QRS complex: **0.06 seconds**

Interpretation: **Junctional bradycardia**

12–13

Regularity: **Regular**   Heart rate: **67**   PR interval: **Variable**

P-waves: **Visible before beats 1, 2, 8, and 9. P-waves distort the beginning of the QRS in beats 3, 4, and 7.**

QRS complex: **0.08 seconds**

Interpretation: **Sinus rhythm converting to accelerated junctional rhythm and back to sinus rhythm**

12–14

Regularity: **Regular**   Heart rate: **71**   PR interval: **0.08 seconds**

P-waves: **All the same**   QRS complex: **0.06 seconds**

Interpretation: **Accelerated junctional rhythm**

12–15

Regularity: **Regular**   Heart rate: **94**   PR interval: **0.12 seconds**

P-waves: **All the same**   QRS complex: **0.06**

Interpretation: **Accelerated junctional rhythm**

12-16

Regularity: **Regular**   Heart rate: **52**   PR interval: **Not measurable**

P-waves: **(Three possible seen but not related to QRS: more about this in future chapters.) None visible**   QRS complex: **0.08 seconds**

Interpretation: **Junctional rhythm**

12-17

Regularity: **Regular**   Heart rate: **68**   PR interval: **0.10 seconds**

P-waves: **All the same**   QRS complex: **0.10 seconds**

Interpretation: **Accelerated junctional rhythm**

12-18

Regularity: **Regular**   Heart rate: **94**   PR interval: **Not measurable**

P-waves: **Inverted at the end of the QRS**   QRS complex: **0.08 seconds**

Interpretation: **Accelerated junctional rhythm**

12-19

Regularity: **Regular**   Heart rate: **~20**   PR interval: **Not measurable**

P-waves: **None visible**   QRS complex: **0.10 seconds**

Interpretation: **Junctional bradycardia**

12-20

Regularity: **Regular except**   Heart rate: **94**   PR interval:**0.18 seconds**

P-waves: **All the same except the one after beat 5, which deforms the T-wave.**

QRS complex: **0.08 seconds**

Interpretation: **Sinus rhythm with blocked PAC and junctional escape beat**

12-21

Regularity: **Regular**   Heart rate: **97**   PR interval: **0.18 seconds then 0.10 seconds**

P-waves: **Variable throughout strip—initially upright, then inverted**   QRS complex: **0.08 seconds**

Interpretation: **Sinus rhythm converting to accelerated junctional rhythm**

12-22

Regularity: **Irregular**   Heart rate: **90**   PR interval: **0.18 seconds**

P-waves: **All the same except before beat 7 (junctional escape beat) and before beats 5 and 9**
QRS complex: **0.06 seconds**

Interpretation: **Sinus rhythm with PACs (beats 5 and 9) and junctional escape beat (beat 7)**

12-23

Regularity: **Regular**   Heart rate: **94**   PR interval: **Variable**

P-waves: **Clearly visible just before QRS**

QRS complex: **0.10 seconds**

Interpretation: **Accelerated junctional rhythm at a rate slightly higher than the sinus rate**

12-24

Regularity: **Regular** Heart rate: **58** PR interval: **Variable**

P-waves: **Clearly visible before beats 1 and 2, clearly seen in T-wave after beats 5 and 6**

QRS complex: **0.06 seconds**

Interpretation: **Sinus rhythm converting to accelerated junctional rhythm at a rate slightly higher than the sinus rate**

12-25

Regularity: **Regular** Heart rate: **40** PR interval: **Not measurable**

P-waves: **None visible** QRS complex: **0.06 seconds**

Interpretation: **Junctional rhythm**

12-26

Regularity: **Regular except** Heart rate: **83** PR interval: **0.18 seconds**

P-waves: **All the same except after beat 4. P-wave also distorts QRS of beat 5 (junctional escape beat).**

QRS complex: **0.08 seconds**

Interpretation: **Sinus rhythm with blocked PAC and junctional escape beat**

12-27

Regularity: **Regular** Heart rate: **60** PR interval: **Not measurable**

P-waves: **None seen** QRS complex: **0.06 seconds**

Interpretation: **Junctional rhythm with trigeminal PJCs**

12-28

Regularity: **Regular** Heart rate: **31** PR interval: **Not measurable**

P-waves: **Possibly inverted at the end of the QRS** QRS complex: **0.10 seconds**

Interpretation: **Junctional bradycardia**

12-29

Regularity: **Regular** Heart rate: **75** PR interval: **0.08 seconds**

P-waves: **All the same** QRS complex: **0.06 seconds**

Interpretation: **Accelerated junctional rhythm**

12-30

Regularity: **Regular except** Heart rate: **75** PR interval: **0.18 seconds**

P-waves: **All the same except before 4th QRS** QRS complex: **0.08 seconds**

Interpretation: **Sinus rhythm with PJC**

Chapter 13

1. Increased **irritability** of the ventricular cells is one cause of ventricular rhythms.

2. Unless verified in at least one other lead, **ventricular fibrillation** can be mistaken for asystole, leading to improper treatment.

3. The QRS duration is **greater than or equal to 0.12 seconds** in ventricular rhythms.

4. Key characteristics of ventricular beats are **wide** and **bizarre** QRS complexes with the **T-wave** in the direction opposite to most of the QRS complex.

5. The **idio-** prefix indicates that the ventricles are depolarizing on their own, not being triggered by another pacemaker site.

6. List at least four causes of asystole. **[Any four causes listed in the MATCH(×5)ED table.]**

7. The intrinsic rate for ventricular tissue is **20** to **40** bpm.

8. Why is slow ventricular tachycardia sometimes treated differently from fast V-tach? **The cardiac output in slow ventricular tachycardia is frequently sufficient to perfuse the body.**

9. Ventricular fibrillation can be described as **coarse** or **fine**.

10. In addition to decreasing atrial kick, fast V-tach decreases cardiac output by reducing **ventricular filling time**.

11. Ventricular fibrillation is a dangerous rhythm because no effective **ventricular contractions** are occurring, and therefore there is no cardiac output.

12. When V-tach has a pulse, **synchronized** cardioversion is used, but when it doesn't have a pulse, **defibrillation** is used.

13. Identify the rhythm for the following 30 ECG strips:

13–1

Regularity: **None**   Heart rate: **0**   PR interval: **None**

P-waves: **None**   QRS complex: **None**

Interpretation: **Asystole (the rounded undulations accur at a rate of approximately 100 per minute and are caused by chest compressions at the AHA recommended rate.**

13–2

Regularity: **Irregular**   Heart rate: **Variable**   PR interval: **None**

P-waves: **None visible**   QRS complex: **Variable**

Interpretation: **Multifocal v-tach deteriorating to V-fib**

13–3

Regularity: **Regular except**   Heart rate: **~80 counting PVCs**   PR interval: **0.16 seconds**

P-waves: **Normal, all the same**   QRS complex: **0.10 seconds when following P-wave, 0.14 seconds otherwise**

Interpretation: **Sinus rhythm with unifocal PVCs and a unifocal couplet**

13–4

Regularity: **Regular**   Heart rate: **150**   PR interval: **None**

P-waves: **None seen**   QRS complex: **0.14 seconds**   Interpretation: **V-tach**

13–5

Regularity: **Both rhythms regular**   Heart rate: **First rhythm, 83; second rhythm, 188**

PR interval: **First rhythm, 0.18 seconds; second rhythm, none**

P-waves: **First rhythm normal, all the same; second rhythm, none seen**

QRS complex: **First rhythm, 0.10 seconds; second rhythm, 0.16 seconds**

Interpretation: **Sinus rhythm converting to V-tach**

13–6

Regularity: **Regular except 3rd and 7th beats are early**   Heart rate: **~60**   PR interval: **0.20 seconds**

P-waves: **Normal, all the same**   QRS complex: **0.10 seconds; early QRSs, 0.14 seconds**

Interpretation: **Sinus rhythm with PVCs**

13–7

Regularity: **Regular except 4th and 6th QRSs**   Heart rate: **60**   PR interval: **0.20 seconds**

P-waves: **All the same**   QRS complex: **0.10 seconds; early QRSs 0.16 seconds**

Interpretation: **Sinus rhythm with unifocal PVCs**

13–8

Regularity: **Slightly Irregular**   Heart rate: **~100**   PR interval: **Variable**

P-waves: **More than three on the strip**

QRS complex: **0.06 seconds with P-waves, 0.12 seconds without**

Interpretation: **WAP with 4-beat run of V-tach**

13–9

Regularity: **Regular**   Heart rate: **167**   PR interval: **None**   P-waves: **None seen**

QRS complex: **Difficult to measure because of sinusoidal QRSs, but definitely wide**

Interpretation: **Ventricular tachycardia**

13–10

Regularity: **Irregular**   Heart rate: **Atrial ~30, ventricular 0**   PR interval: **None**

P-waves: **Normal, all the same**   QRS complex: **None**

Interpretation: **Sinus bradycardia with sinus arrhythmia and ventricular asystole**

13–11

Regularity: **Regular**   Heart rate: **50**   PR interval: **None**

P-waves: **None**   QRS complex: **0.18 seconds**

Interpretation: **Accelerated idioventricular rhythm**

13–12

Regularity: **Regular**   Heart rate: **167**   PR interval: **None**

P-waves: **None seen**   QRS complex: **0.14 seconds**

Interpretation: **V-tach**

13–13

Regularity: **Both rhythms regular**   Heart rate: **First: 42, second: 150**   PR interval: **0.16 seconds**

P-waves: **Normal, all the same**

QRS complex: **0.06 seconds with P-waves, 0.12 seconds without P-waves**

Interpretation: **Sinus bradycardia converting to V-tach. The P-wave just before the V-tach has not had time to conduct.**

13–14

Regularity: **Regular**   Heart rate: **52**   PR interval: **None**

P-waves: **None seen**   QRS complex: **0.20 seconds**

Interpretation: **Accelerated idioventricular rhythm**

13–15

Regularity: **Regular**   Heart rate: **33**   PR interval: **None**

P-waves: **None seen**   QRS complex: **0.22 seconds**

Interpretation: **Idioventricular rhythm**

13–16

Regularity: **Irregularly irregular**   Heart rate: **140**   PR interval: **Not measurable**

P-waves: **None**   QRS complex: **0.06 seconds**

Interpretation: **A-fib with rapid ventricular response and 5-beat run of multifocal V-tach after the 6th QRS**

13–17

Regularity: **Irregular**   Heart rate: **0**   PR interval: **None**   P-waves: **None seen**

QRS complex: **None**   Interpretation: **Coarse V-fib**

13–18

Regularity: **None**   Heart rate: **0**   PR interval: **None**   P-waves: **None seen**

QRS complex: **None**   Interpretation: **Complete asystole**

13–19

Regularity: **Irregular**   Heart rate: **0**   PR interval: **None**   P-waves: **None seen**

QRS complex: **None seen**   Interpretation: **Coarse V-fib**

13–20

Regularity: **Both rhythms regular**   Heart rate: **First, 136; second, 267**   PR interval: **Variable**

P-waves: **Hard to see**   QRS complex: **First, 0.06 seconds; second, 0.12 seconds**

Interpretation: **SVT (can't tell what kind because of difficulty seeing P-waves, but probably A-flutter with 2:1 AVB) converting to V-tach due to PVC**

13–21

Regularity: **Regular**   Heart rate: **~300**   PR interval: **None**   P-waves: **None seen**

QRS complex: **0.12 seconds**   Interpretation: **V-tach**

13–22

Regularity: **None**   Heart rate: **0**   PR interval: **None**   P-waves: **None seen**

QRS complex: **None**   Interpretation: **Complete asystole**

13–23

Regularity: **Irregular**   Heart rate: **0**   PR interval: **None**   P-waves: **None seen**

QRS complex: **None**   Interpretation: **V-fib**

13–24

Regularity: **Regular except 4th and 5th beat**   Heart rate: **83**   PR interval: **0.24 seconds**

P-waves: **Normal, all the same**   QRS complex: **0.08 seconds with P-wave**

Interpretation: **Sinus rhythm (with 1st-degree AV block) with multi focus ventricular couplet**

13–25

Regularity: **Irregular**   Heart rate: **0**   PR interval: **None**   P-waves: **None seen**

QRS complex: **None**   Interpretation: **Coarse V-fib converting to asystole**

13–26

Regularity: **Irregularly irregular**   Heart rate: **Not measurable**   PR interval: **Not measurable**

P-waves: **None**   QRS complex: **Not measurable**   Interpretation: **Fine V-fib**

13–27

Regularity: **Regular**   Heart rate: **Ventricular, 125 in first half, then 0**   PR interval: **None**

P-waves: **None seen**   QRS complex: **0.12 seconds**

Interpretation: **V-tach converting to complete asystole**

13–28

Regularity: **Regular except**   Heart rate: **~50**   PR interval: **None**

P-waves: **None seen before QRSs. After PVCs there are inverted P-waves visible**   QRS complex:
Small complexes, 0.08 seconds; tall complexes, 0.16 seconds

Interpretation: **Junctional rhythm with bigeminal PVCs**

13–29

Regularity: **Regular except beats 2, 4, and 7**   Heart rate: **75**

PR interval: **0.14 seconds**   P-waves: **Normal, all the same**

QRS complex: **0.08 seconds with P-waves, 0.14 seconds without P-waves**

Interpretation: **Sinus rhythm with unifocal PVCs**

13–30

Regularity: **Regular except 3rd and 4th QRSs**   Heart rate: **73**   PR interval: **Not measurable**

P-waves: **F-waves**   QRS complex: **0.06 seconds**

Interpretation: **A-Flutter with 4:1 AV block and ventricular couplet (probably unifocal but slightly
different because of flutter waves), the third beat is an escape beat due to the longer than normal pause before it. The fourth beat is a PVC.**

13–31

Regularity: **Regular except**   Heart rate: **60**

PR interval: **0.16**   P-waves: **All the same except absent before 2nd and 5th beats**

QRS complex: **0.10 seconds: 2nd and 5th 0.14**

Interpretation: **Sinus rhythm with unifocal PVCs**

13–32

Regularity: **Irregular**   Heart rate: **Atrial, ~300; ventricular, 130**   PR interval: **Not measurable**

P-waves: **F-waves**   QRS complex: **Normal complexes, 0.06 seconds; side complexes, 0.12 seconds**

Interpretation: **Atrial flutter with variable AV block and premature ventricular couplet**

13–33

Regularity: **Regular except**   Heart rate: **97**

PR interval: **0.16 seconds**   P-waves: **Normal, all the same**

QRS complex: **0.08 seconds with P-waves, 0.16 seconds without P-waves**

Interpretation: **Sinus rhythm with unifocal PVCs**

13–34

Regularity: **Regular except**   Heart rate: **88**   PR interval: **0.20 seconds**

P-waves: **Normal, all the same**   QRS complex: **0.08 seconds**

Interpretation: **Sinus rhythm with blocked PACs (after 7th and 10th QRSs), converting to bigeminal, unifocal PVCs**

13–35

Regularity: **Regular**   Heart rate: **300**   PR interval: **None**

P-waves: **None seen**   QRS complex: **Difficult to measure, but wide**

Interpretation: **V-tach**

13–36

Regularity: **Regular except**   Heart rate: **115**

PR interval: **0.15 seconds**   P-waves: **Normal, all the same**

QRS complex: **0.10 seconds with P-waves, 0.12 seconds without P-waves**

Interpretation: **Sinus tachycardia with bigeminal unifocal PVCs**

13–37

Regularity: **Irregularly irregular**   Heart rate: **~110**   PR interval: **None**

P-waves: **None seen**   QRS complex: **0.06 to 0.16 seconds**

Interpretation: **A- fib with RVR and a 3-beat run of unifocal V-tach (ventricular salvo)**

13–38

Regularity: **Regular except 3rd, 8th, 9th, and 10th QRSs**   Heart rate: **107**

PR interval: **0.14 seconds**   P-waves: **Normal, all the same**   QRS complex: **0.08 seconds**

Interpretation: **Sinus rhythm with PVC (3rd QRS) and 3-beat run of unifocal V-tach or ventricular salvo (8th, 9th, and 10th QRSs)**

13–39

Regularity: **Irregular**   Heart rate: **~80**

PR interval: **0.14 seconds**   P-waves: **Normal, all the same**

QRS complex: **0.10 seconds with P-waves, 0.14 seconds without P-waves**

13–40

Regularity: **Regular except**   Heart rate: **65**   PR interval: **0.16 seconds**

P-waves: **Normal, all the same**

QRS complex: **0.08 seconds with P-waves, 0.16 seconds without P-waves**

Interpretation: **Sinus rhythm with 1 PVC**

Chapter 14

1. The AV node normally holds on to signals from the atria for approximately **0.10** seconds before send-ing them to the ventricles.

2. **First-** degree and second-degree type **II** are the types of AV block in which the PR interval does not change.

3. The two types of AV block that most frequently have regular ventricular rhythms are **first degree** and **third degree**.

4. Lidocaine, and other medications that reduce ventricular irritability, should be avoided in patients exhibiting **third-degree** AV block.

5. **First-degree AV block** is not really a true block but simply an abnormally long delay of the signal in the AV node.

6. The criteria for second-degree type I AV block include **regular** P-waves, **lengthening** PR intervals, and **more** P-waves than QRS complexes.

7. Which part of the ECG tracing do AV blocks affect? **The PR interval.**

8. Identify the rhythm and type of AV block present in the following 20 ECG strips:

14–1

Regularity: **Regular**   Heart rate: **97**   PR interval: **0.24 seconds**

P-waves: **Regular, all the same**   QRS complex: **0.08 seconds**

Interpretation: **Sinus rhythm with 1st-degree AV block**

14–2

Regularity: **Regular**   Heart rate: **73**   PR interval: **0.24 seconds**

P-waves: **Regular, all the same**   QRS complex: **0.08 seconds**

Interpretation: **Sinus rhythm with 1st-degree AV block**

14–3

Regularity: **Regularly irregular**   Heart rate: **Atrial, 79; ventricular, ~60**

PR interval: **Not measurable**   P-waves: **Regular, all the same**   QRS complex: **0.06 seconds**

Interpretation: **Sinus rhythm with 2nd-degree AV block (Wenckebach or Mobitz I)**

14–4

Regularity: **Regular**   Heart rate: **Atrial, 111; ventricular, 115**

PR interval: **Variable (shortens slightly throughout the strip)**

P-waves: **Regular, all the same**   QRS complex: **0.06 seconds**

Interpretation: **Sinus tachycardia with 3rd-degree AV block. Although subtle, the slight difference in PR intervals, as well as atrial and ventricular heart rates, clinches the interpretation.**

14–5

Regularity: **Regular**   Heart rate: **50**   PR interval: **0.26 seconds**

P-waves: **Regular, all the same**   QRS complex: **0.06 seconds**

Interpretation: **Sinus bradycardia with 1st-degree AV block**

14–6

Regularity: **Regularly irregular**   Heart rate: **Atrial, 91; ventricular, 70**

PR interval: **0.06 seconds**   P-waves: **Regular, all the same**   QRS complex: **0.06 seconds**

Interpretation: **Sinus rhythm with 2nd-degree AV block (Wenckebach or Mobitz I)**

14–7

Regularity: **Irregular**   Heart rate: **70**   PR interval: **0.18 seconds**

P-waves: **Regular, more than 1 per QRS**   QRS complex: **0.08 seconds**

Interpretation: **Sinus rhythm with 2nd-degree AV block (Classic or Mobitz II)**

14–8

Regularity: **Regular**   Heart rate: **121**   PR interval: **0.22 seconds**

P-waves: **Regular, all the same**   QRS complex: **0.08 seconds**

Interpretation: **Sinus tachycardia with 1st-degree AV block**

14–9

Regularity: **Irregular**   Heart rate: **Atrial, 77; ventricular, ~60**   PR interval: **Variable**

P-waves: **Regular, all the same**   QRS complex: **0.06 seconds**

Interpretation: **Sinus rhythm with 2nd-degree AV block (Wenckebach or Mobitz I)**

14–10

Regularity: **Regular**   Heart rate: **Atrial, 120; ventricular, 52**   PR interval: **Variable**

P-waves: **Regular, all the same**   QRS complex: **0.08 seconds**

Interpretation: **Sinus tachycardia with 3rd-degree AV block and junctional escape rhythm. The sinus node is discharging faster to try to increase cardiac output, but with this type of block it fails.**

14–11

Regularity: **Regular**   Heart rate: **Atrial, 79; ventricular, 49**   PR interval: **Variable**

P-waves: **Regular, all the same**   QRS complex: **0.12 seconds**

Interpretation: **Sinus rhythm with probable ventricular escape rhythm**

14–12

Regularity: **Regular**   Heart rate: **63**   PR interval: **0.32 seconds**

P-waves: **Regular, all the same**   QRS complex: **0.10 seconds**

Interpretation: **Sinus rhythm with 1st-degree AV block**

14–13

Regularity: **Regular**   Heart rate: **Atrial, 75; ventricular, 59**   PR interval: **Variable**

P-waves: **Regular, all the same**   QRS complex: **0.10 seconds**

Interpretation: **Sinus rhythm with 3rd-degree AV block and junctional escape rhythm**

14–14

Regularity: **Irregular**   Heart rate: **90**   PR interval: **0.14 seconds**

P-waves: **Regular, all the same**   QRS complex: **0.08 seconds**

Interpretation: **Sinus tachycardia with 2nd-degree AV block (Classic or Mobitz II)**

14–15

Regularity: **Irregular**   Heart rate: **Atrial, 111; ventricular, 40**   PR interval: **0.18 seconds**

P-waves: **Regular, all the same**   QRS complex: **0.06 seconds**

Interpretation: **Sinus tachycardia with high-grade (advanced 2-degree) AV block**

14–16

Regularity: **Regular**   Heart rate: **88**   PR interval: **0.34 seconds**

P-waves: **Regular, all the same**   QRS complex: **0.06 seconds**

Interpretation: **Sinus rhythm with 1st-degree AV block**

14–17

Regularity: **P-waves and QRSs both regular at different rates**   Heart rate: **Atrial, 100; ventricular, 67**

PR interval: **Variable**   P-waves: **Regular, all the same**   QRS complex: **0.08 seconds**

Interpretation: **Sinus tachycardia with 3rd-degree AV block and accelerated junctional escape rhythm**

14–18

Regularity: **Regularly irregular**   Heart rate: **Atrial, 94; ventricular, ~80**   PR interval: **Variable**

P-waves: **Regular, all the same except inverted P-wave after 4th QRS deforming the T-wave**
QRS complex: **0.06 seconds**

Interpretation: **Sinus rhythm with 2nd-degree AV block and junctional escape beat (beat 4). The long delay after the blocked P-wave produces a junctional beat.**

14–19

Regularity: **Regular**   Heart rate: **47**   PR interval: **0.40 seconds**

P-waves: **Regular, all the same**   QRS complex: **0.10 seconds**

Interpretation: **Sinus bradycardia with 1st-degree AV block**

14–20

Regularity: **Irregular**   Heart rate: **Atrial, 75; ventricular, ~50**   PR interval: **Variable**

P-waves: **Regular, all the same**   QRS complex: **0.06 seconds**

Interpretation: **Sinus rhythm with 2nd-degree AV block (Wenckebach or Mobitz I) with two junctional escape beats (3rd and 4th beats). Although there is a P-wave before the third QRS, the PR interval is too short to allow conduction. The next P-wave reaches the AV node, which is still refractory because of the junctional beat and doesn't conduct.**

Chapter 15

1. What is a bundle branch block? **A disturbance in the conduction from the atria to the ventricles that delays depolarization of the ventricles, lengthening the QRS interval.**

2. List three ECG features that point to ventricular tachycardia. **QRS complex ≥0.16 seconds; P-waves that are not associated with QRSs; rabbit ears in V$_1$, with the second peak taller than the first positive precordial ventricular concordance, QRS changes shape from known BBB.**

3. List three ECG features that point to supraventricular tachycardia with a bundle branch block. **QRS complex ≤0.14 seconds; P-waves that are associated with QRSs; rabbit ears in V$_1$, with the second peak taller than the first QRS shape unchanged from slower rate, decreased heart rate with valsalva maneuver.**

4. What drug should never be given to a patient with ventricular tachycardia and why not? **Verapamil, because it may cause or worsen a severe hypotension that is difficult to correct.**

5. How do you treat a patient with a wide-complex tachycardia when you can't differentiate between SVT with a BBB and V-tach? **Treat for V-tach first. If treatment is unsuccessful, try treating as SVT. If treatment is still unsuccessful, revert to ventricular tachycardia therapy.**

6. In the following five strips, identify the rhythm as V-tach or SVT with a BBB. Note the feature or features that support your choice.

   15–1

   V-tach. The QRS is greater than 0.16 seconds, no P-waves are visible, and the rhythm is regular.

   15–2

   SVT with a BBB. P-Waves are visible in front of each QRS and appear related. The rhythm is regular except for the 6th beat, which is a PAC with a BBB.

   15–3

   SVT with a BBB (actually sinus tachycardia with a BBB). Small P-waves appear before every QRS. The QRS is 0.12 seconds.

   15–4

   V-tach. The P-wave just before the wide-complex tachycardia is too close to the QRS to have caused it. Because we know the AV node works, the wide QRS must come from a different location, namely the ventricles.

   15–5

   V-tach. The second and fourth complexes are PVCs. The waveform of the wide-complex tachycardia following the second PVC is nearly identical in shape and size to the PVCs, suggesting that they started at the same spot and followed the same path. Therefore, the rhythm is ventricular.

7. Identify the rhythm in the following 10 strips:

   15–6

   Regularity: **Regular**   Heart rate: **86**   PR interval: **0.18 seconds**

   P-waves: **Regular, all the same**   QRS complex: **0.12 seconds**

   Interpretation: **Sinus rhythm with BBB**

15–7

Regularity: **Regular**   Heart rate: **75**   PR interval: **0.16 seconds**

P-waves: **Regular, all the same**   QRS complex: **0.14 seconds**

Interpretation: **Sinus rhythm with BBB**

15–8

Regularity: **Irregularly irregular**   Heart rate: **Maximum, 75; minimum, 43; average, 50**

PR interval: **Not measurable**   P-waves: **None seen**   QRS complex: **0.12 seconds**

Interpretation: **A-fib with BBB (wavy baseline, no P-waves, and irregularly irregular)**

15–9

Regularity: **Regular except**   Heart rate: **86**   PR interval: **0.14 seconds**

P-waves: **Regular, all the same**   QRS complex: **0.12 seconds**

Interpretation: **Sinus rhythm with BBB and PVC (3rd QRS). Notice that the shape of the 3rd QRS is much different than all the others**

15–10

Regularity: **Regular**   Heart rate: **115**   PR interval: **0.14 seconds**

P-waves: **Regular, all the same**   QRS complex: **0.12 seconds**

Interpretation: **Sinus tachycardia with BBB**

15–11

Regularity: **Regular except**   Heart rate: **68**   PR interval: **0.20 seconds**

P-waves: **Regular, all the same except 2nd and 6th which are different shapes and early**
QRS complex: **0.20 seconds**

Interpretation: **Sinus rhythm with BBB and multifocal PACs (beats 2 and 6)**

15–12

Regularity: **Regular**   Heart rate: **58**   PR interval: **0.20 seconds**

P-waves: **Regular, all the same**   QRS complex: **0.16 seconds**

Interpretation: **Sinus bradycardia with BBB**

15–13

Regularity: **Regular**   Heart rate: **94**   PR interval: **0.20 seconds**

P-waves: **Regular, all the same**   QRS complex: **0.16 seconds**

Interpretation: **Sinus rhythm with BBB**

15–14

Regularity: **Regular**   Heart rate: **86**   PR interval: **0.16 seconds**

P-waves: **Regular, all the same**   QRS complex: **0.14 seconds**

Interpretation: **Sinus rhythm with BBB**

15–15

Regularity: **Regular**   Heart rate: **58**   PR interval: **0.18 seconds**

P-waves: **Regular, all the same**   QRS complex: **0.14 seconds**

Interpretation: **Sinus bradycardia with BBB**

Chapter 16

1. Why are transcutaneous pacemakers used only as a stopgap measure? **They use more energy, are less reliable than other types, and may cause significant discomfort.**

2. The pacemaker's electrical discharge should show up on the ECG strip as a small **spike.**

3. Describe how a VVI pacemaker functions. **It paces only the ventricles, senses natural ventricular activity, and is inhibited from firing if it senses a ventricular beat.**

4. What condition precludes the use of an AAI pacemaker? **AV node dysfunction.** Why? **The pacemaker senses and paces only the atria. If the AV node does not transmit the signal to the ventricles, heart rate and cardiac output may be seriously compromised.**

5. Why are asynchronous pacemakers less popular than they used to be? **They don't sense natural activity and compete with the patient's own heart rhythm, with potentially serious consequences.**

6. Why is pacemaker inhibition an important feature? **If the pacemaker can sense a natural beat, it should be inhibited to prevent competition with the patient's intrinsic rhythm.**

7. Why is triggering an important pacemaker feature? **It helps to maximize cardiac output by maintaining proper coordination between atrial and ventricular contraction.**

8. How do you calculate the percentage of heartbeats generated by the pacemaker? **Count the number of paced beats in a given period (e.g., 6 seconds) and divide by the total number of beats in the same six seconds.**

9. Where is the ventricular lead located in most permanent pacemakers? **In the lower portion of the right ventricle.**

10. Match the pacemaker malfunctions with their identifying features:

    A. Failure to Fire   a. Paced beats consistently occurring late

    B. Failure to capture   b. A long interval with no natural or paced beats.

    C. Undersensing   c. Pacemaker spikes occurring when expected with no PQRST following

    D. Oversensing   d. Pacemaker spikes occurring too close to the previous beat.

    Answers: *(A, b) (B, c) (C, d) (D, a)*

11. Identify the rhythms in following 25 strips involving pacemakers and identify any malfunctions:

    16–1

    Base rhythm: **Junctional (beats 3-5)**   Type of pacing: **Dual chamber (beats 1 and 2)**

    Paced rate: **70**   Percentage of pacing: **50% (2 of 4 beats)**

    Malfunctions? **Failure to fire. The pacemaker should have fired before the 3rd QRS but didn't.**

    Interpretation: **Junctional rhythm with 50% AV sequential pacing and failure to fire**

    16–2

    Base rhythm: **Paced**   Type of pacing: **Atrial only**

    Percentage of pacing: **100% (all P-waves are pacemaker generated)**   Malfunctions? **None**

    Interpretation: **100% atrial pacing**

16–3

Base rhythm: **Sinus rhythm**   Type of pacing: **Ventricular only**

Percentage of pacing: **100% (all QRS complexes are pacemaker generated)**   Malfunctions? **None**

Interpretation: **Sinus rhythm with 100% ventricular pacing**

16–4

Base rhythm: **Probably A-fib (wavy baseline)**   Type of pacing: **Ventricular**

Percentage of pacing: **100%**   Malfunctions? **None**

Interpretation: **A-fib with 100% ventricular pacing**

16–5

Base rhythm: **A-fib**   Type of pacing: **Ventricular**   Percentage of pacing: **22% (occasional)**

Malfunctions? **None**

Interpretation: **A-fib with RVR and occasional ventricular pacing**

16–6

Base rhythm: **Atrial flutter (P-wave rate 250) with 3rd-degree AVB (no flutter waves conduct during the pause)**

Type of pacing: **Probably ventricular (atrial pacing not usually used with A-fib, A-flutter, or 3rd-degree AVB)**

Percentage of pacing: **No successful pacing is observed.**

Malfunctions? **Failure to fire–the pacemaker should have taken over the rhythm after the 3rd QRS but didn't. Failure to sense–the pacemaker fired on the T-wave just before the pause but didn't capture.**

16–7

Base rhythm: **Sinus rhythm with BBB**   Type of pacing: **Ventricular**   Percentage of pacing: **25%**

Malfunctions? **None**

Interpretation: **Sinus rhythm with BBB and 25% ventricular pacing. Alternatively, sinus rhythm with BBB converting to 100% ventricular pacing (if the paced rhythm continues).**

16–8

Base rhythm: **Unknown**   Type of pacing: **Atrial**   Percentage of pacing: **71%**

Malfunctions? **None**   Interpretation: **Atrial pacing with PAC (3rd QRS)**

16–9

Base rhythm: **Asystole (possibly fine V-fib)**   Type of pacing: **Dual**   Percentage of pacing: **100%**

Malfunctions? **Failure to capture. There are no P-waves or QRSs after any pacemaker spike.**

Interpretation: **Asystole with 100% AV sequential pacing and failure to capture**

16–10

Base rhythm: **Paced with 3-beat run of V-tach**   Type of pacing: **Ventricular**

Percentage of pacing: **100%**   Malfunctions? **Failure to sense**

Interpretation: **100% ventricular pacing with a 3-beat run of V-tach and failure to sense**

16–11

Base rhythm: **Sinus rhythm**   Type of pacing: **Ventricular**   Percentage of pacing: **50%**

Pacer rate: **60; notice P-wave at start of 3rd QRS as sinus discharge rate increases and takes over.**

Malfunctions? **None**

Interpretation: **Sinus rhythm with 50% ventricular pacing. Notice the points of the buried P-wave just before the 3rd paced beat. The sinus node increased its rate and eventually discharged faster than the pacemaker's programmed rate. The fastest pacemaker wins.**

16–12

Base rhythm: **Sinus or Atrial tachycardia**   Type of pacing: **Ventricular**   Percentage of pacing: **100%**

Malfunctions? **None, but pacemaker should be reprogrammed to ignore the P-waves; VVI might be a better mode.**

Interpretation: **Atrial tachycardia with 100% ventricular pacing. The P-waves are difficult to see in this strip. The P-waves triggered the pacemaker to discharge at such a fast rate.**

16–13

Base rhythm: **Asystole**   Type of pacing: **Dual**   Percentage of pacing: **100%**

Malfunctions? **Failure to fire (after beat 3)**

Interpretation: **100% AV sequential pacing with failure to fire, resulting in a 2.24-second pause**

16–14

Base rhythm: **Ventricular (unknown rate)**   Type of pacing: **Ventricular**   Percentage of pacing: **60%**

Malfunctions? **Failure to sense. The last beat has a spike in the T-wave, and the previous beat is an R-on-T paced beat. Because the beat falls so close to the previous QRS, the pacemaker is not expected to capture it.**

Interpretation: **Idioventricular rhythm and ventricular pacing with failure to sense.**

16–15

Base rhythm: **Sinus rhythm**   Type of pacing: **Ventricular**   Percentage of pacing: **100%**

Malfunctions? **None**

Interpretation: **Sinus rhythm with 100% VVI pacing (ventricular pacing is independent of the P-waves)**

PS 16–16

Base rhythm: **Sinus rhythm**   Type of pacing: **Ventricular**

Percentage of pacing: **100%**   Malfunctions? **None**

Interpretation: **100% Sinus rhythm with ventricular pacing**

PS 16–17

Base rhythm: **A-fib/A-flutter**   Type of pacing: **Ventricular**

Percentage of pacing: **100%**   Malfunctions? **None**

Interpretation: **100% ventricular pacing (VVI mode due to large number of f-waves)**

PS 16–18

Base rhythm: **Unknown**   Type of pacing: **Atrial**   Percentage of pacing: **100%**   Malfunctions? **None**

Interpretation: **100% atrial pacing (with normal AV node connection)**

PS 16–19

Base rhythm: **Sinus rhythm**   Type of pacing: **Ventricular**

Percentage of pacing: **100%**   Malfunctions? **None**

Interpretation: **100% ventricular pacing (may be VAT or DDD)**

PS 16–20

Base rhythm: **Sinus bradycardia**   Type of pacing: **Ventricular**

Percentage of pacing: **50%**   Malfunctions? **None**

Interpretation: **Sinus bradycardia with bigeminal ventricular pacing**

PS 16–21

Base rhythm: **Unknown**   Type of pacing: **Atrial**   Percentage of pacing: **100%**

Malfunctions? **None (6th pacemaker spike probably does produce a P-wave, obscured by the PVC)**

Interpretation: **100% atrial pacing with 1 PVC**

PS 16–22

Base rhythm: **Unknown**   Type of pacing: **Dual**   Percentage of pacing: **100%**

Malfunctions? **None**

Interpretation: **100% AV pacing**

PS 16-23

Base rhythm: **Sinus rhythm with ventricular standstill**   Type of pacing: **Ventricular**

Percentage of pacing: **100% (all QRSs are caused by pacemaker spikes)**

Malfunctions? **Failure to capture, then failure to fire (first 4 QRSs are paced; next 2 pacemaker spikes fail to capture, then failure to fire.)**

Interpretation: **Sinus rhythm with 100% ventricular pacing with failure to capture progressing to failure to fire**

PS 16–24

Base rhythm: **Unknown**   Type of pacing: **Atrial**   Percentage of pacing: **100%**

Malfunctions? **None. The pacemaker spike in the PVC is not a malfunction. The atrial lead fired because it didn't sense a P-wave.**

Interpretation: **100% Atrial pacing with 1 PVC**

PS 16–25

Base rhythm: **Asystole**   Type of pacing: **Dual**   Percentage of pacing: **100%**

Malfunctions? **Failure to fire. The set rate is 70, measured by the 2nd half of the strip. Therefore there should be more paced beats in the 1st half of the strip.**

Interpretation: **100% AV pacing with failure to fire**

Chapter 17

1. Baseline sway caused by breathing may be corrected by **moving** some ECG patches.

2. During resuscitation it's important to periodically **stop** chest compressions because the artifact they generate may interfere with rhythm identification.

3. **Sixty-cycle (or 60-Hz) interference** can be caused by any electrical device that leaks current.

4. In which rhythms can pulseless electrical activity occur? **Any ECG-recorded rhythm may have electrical activity but not generate a pulse.**

5. List at least three possible causes of PEA. **Tension pneumothorax, pericardial tamponade, significant blood loss, pulmonary embolism, myocardial infarction, electrolyte disturbance.**

6. Artifact can occur because the ECG patches transmit **all** electrical signals that reach them; not just those from the heart's electrical system.

7. Some rhythm strips do not have artifact because the monitoring equipment has built-in **algorithms** to filter the electrical signals received from the ECG Patches.

8. It's impossible to obtain a patient's **pulse** from the ECG monitor.

9. Identify which of the following 20 strips have artifact and the probable cause for the artifacts:

17–1

Underlying rhythm: **Probably sinus rhythm with PAC**   Artifact: **Toothbrush tachycardia**

Cause of artifact: **Possibly motion of muscles under the patch or intermittent contact with the patch**

17–2

Underlying rhythm: **Indeterminable; probably asystole**

Artifact: **Motion**   Cause of artifact: **Chest compressions**

17–3

Underlying rhythm: **Sinus rhythm**   Artifact: **Patient motion or loose lead**

Cause of artifact: **Large muscle movements, possibly with a loose or dry patch**

17–4

Underlying rhythm: **Probably sinus rhythm (P-waves before first 2 small QRSs, heart rate in 90s). Artifact makes it look like V-fib or asystole.**

Artifact: **Loose or detached patch**

Cause of artifact: **Loosening of lead required for the bottom tracing; this strongly affects the top tracing.**

17–5

Underlying rhythm: <u>**Sinus tachycardia**</u>   Artifact: <u>**Baseline sway**</u>

Cause of artifact: <u>**Probably respirations, with excessive rate about 38 per minute**</u>

17–6

Underlying rhythm: <u>**Known sinus rhythm; artifact makes it look like atrial flutter.**</u>

Artifact: <u>**Patient motion**</u>   Cause of artifact: <u>**Parkinson-like tremors**</u>

17–7

Underlying rhythm: <u>**Sinus tachycardia**</u>   Artifact: <u>**Baseline sway**</u>

Cause of artifact: <u>**Respirations with rate approximately 15 per minute**</u>

17–8

Underlying rhythm: <u>**Probably sinus tachycardia**</u>

Artifact: <u>**60-cycle interference (not all 60 cycles are visible)**</u>

Cause of artifact: <u>**Electrical appliance**</u>

17–9

Underlying rhythm: <u>**Sinus tachycardia with BBB**</u>   Artifact: <u>**Motion or lead contact**</u>

Cause of artifact: <u>**Patient motion, or possibly interference with proper lead contact, such as from dried gel, lotion, oil, or hair**</u>

17–10

Underlying rhythm: <u>**Sinus tachycardia**</u>   Artifact: <u>**Baseline sway**</u>

Cause of artifact: <u>**Respirations with rate approximately 12 per minute**</u>

17–11

Underlying rhythm: <u>**Atrial fibrillation with a PVC**</u>

Artifact: <u>**60-cycle interference noted in bottom tracing only**</u>

Cause of artifact: <u>**Electrical appliance**</u>

17–12

Underlying rhythm: <u>**Sinus rhythm with BBB**</u>   Artifact: <u>**Loose lead, patient motion, or both**</u>

Cause of artifact: <u>**Loose lead or patch with dried gel**</u>

17–13

Underlying rhythm: <u>**Sinus rhythm**</u>   Artifact: <u>**Toothbrush tachycardia**</u>

Cause of artifact: <u>**Patient motion or tremor that causes intermittent lead disruption**</u>

17–14

Underlying rhythm: <u>**Unknown**</u>   Artifact: <u>**Motion**</u>

Cause of artifact: <u>**Significant patient motion**</u>

17–15

Underlying rhythm: **Unknown, but patient was having PEA.**

Artifact: **Motion**   Cause of artifact: **Chest compressions**

17–16

Underlying rhythm: **Asystole with a single QRS**   Artifact: **Motion**

Cause of artifact: **Chest compressions**

17–17

Underlying rhythm: **Sinus rhythm**   Artifact: **Motion**

Cause of artifact: **Significant patient motion**

17–18

Underlying rhythm: **Sinus rhythm with probable blocked PAC after the 3rd QRS, junctional escape beat (4th QRS), and PAC (last beat)**

Artifact: **Motion**

Cause of artifact: **Patient tapping on MCL$_1$ patch. Lower tracing shows less effect and therefore the rhythm is easier to identify.**

17–19

Underlying rhythm: **Sinus rhythm with premature supraventricular beats**

Artifact: **Toothbrush tachycardia**   Cause of artifact: **Patient motion**

17–20

Underlying rhythm: _____ **Sinus rhythm with bundle branch block** _____.

Artifact: _____ **Sharp pointed waveforms at the end of the strip** _____

Cause of artifact: _____ **Motion artifact is the actual cause in this strip** _____

Chapter 18

1. The T-wave should end before the **halfway** point between two consecutive QRS complexes.

2. The normal values for QT intervals vary according to **heart rate**.

3. During the **absolute refractory period**, no stimulus, no matter how large, can initiate another QRS complex.

4. The **relative** refractory period begins approximately at the **middle** of the T-wave and ends at the end of the T-wave.

5. In **fusion beats,** which are benign, QRS complexes are formed by two different locations initiating ventricular depolarization at the same time.

6. **R on T phenomenon** may cause ventricular fibrillation because a new stimulus tries to depolarize the ventricles before they are fully ready.

7. Identify the pacemaker timing anomalies in the following eight strips:

18–1

Beat 4 is a pseudo–pseudo-fusion beat. The first spike is the atrial spike, which can't affect the natural QRS it's embedded in. Beat 5 demonstrates ventricular failure to capture. Beat 6 shows a combination of the natural QRS (seen in beat 4) and the pacemaker-generated QRS (beats 1–3) resulting from a true fusion beat.

18–2

This tracing comes from a single-chamber ventricular pacemaker that can be triggered by atrial activity. Beat 2 demonstrates R on T phenomenon; the pacemaker spike falls during the down-sloping portion of the T-wave. Beat 3 is a pseudo-fusion beat; the spike falls at the end of the QRS, well before the vulnerable period at the end of the T-wave.

18–3

On this tracing, beat 2 raises two issues. The first spike is atrial and therefore is a pseudo–pseudo-fusion beat because it can't affect the QRS it's embedded in. The second spike occurs at the peak of the T-wave and represents an R on T phenomenon. Because it doesn't capture, there is no QRS.

18–4

Beat 4 is a fusion beat. The QRS is a hybrid between the paced and natural QRSs. It is smaller than the natural QRSs that follow it because the pacemaker QRSs are negative and drag the height of the fusion beat down.

18–5

Beat 3 is a pseudo-fusion beat. The rhythm is ventricular, but not because of the pacemaker. All of the QRSs are identical, whether or not they are immediately preceded by a pacemaker spike. Therefore they all originated from the same site, which may be the patient's natural pacemaker site.

18–6

The first two QRSs are fully pacemaker generated. The 3rd, although it appears identical in the lower tracing, is clearly a fusion beat when viewed in the upper tracing. The next beat is a pseudo-fusion beat—it's identical in both leads to the next beat, which is natural. Beat 8 is again a fusion beat.

18–7

The 6th and 12th QRSs are fusion beats.

18–8

Beat 6 is a pseudo–pseudo-fusion beat. The atrial pacemaker spike couldn't have caused the premature QRS.

Chapter 19

1. ST segment **depression** can be a sign of ischemia in a cardiac patient.

2. ST segment **elevation** can be a sign of cardiac cell injury.

3. Early repolarization is a benign cause of **ST segment elevation.**

4. The AV node receives its blood supply from the **right coronary artery, in most patients.**

5. Blockage of the left anterior descending artery is associated with which type of myocardial infarction? **Anterior wall.**

6. If a patient is having an acute inferior wall MI, which additional ECG lead should you check? Why? **Lead V4R, which helps identify right ventricular MIs.**

7. Identify the features associated with MIs in the following five strips:

19–1

Diagnosis: **Significant ST segment elevation in leads II, II, and aVF, indicating an inferior wall MI in progress.**

19–2

Diagnosis: **Significant ST segment elevation in leads V_1 through V_5, indicating an anterior wall MI in progress.**

19–3

Diagnosis: **Significant ST segment elevation in leads I and aVL, indicating a lateral wall MI in progress.**

19–4

Diagnosis: **Significant ST segment elevation in leads II, III, and aVF, indicating an inferior wall MI in progress. Also, the Q-waves in leads V_1 through V_4 indicate that the patient has previously had both an anterior wall MI and a septal wall MI.**

19–5

Diagnosis: **Early repolarization. There is diffuse, slight ST segment elevation (only 1–2 small boxes) in leads II, III, aVF, and V_3 through V_6. Also, the ST segment has a "smiley face" configuration (concave elevation), most evident in lead II.**

Index

Index

Index